WAR PSYCHIATRY

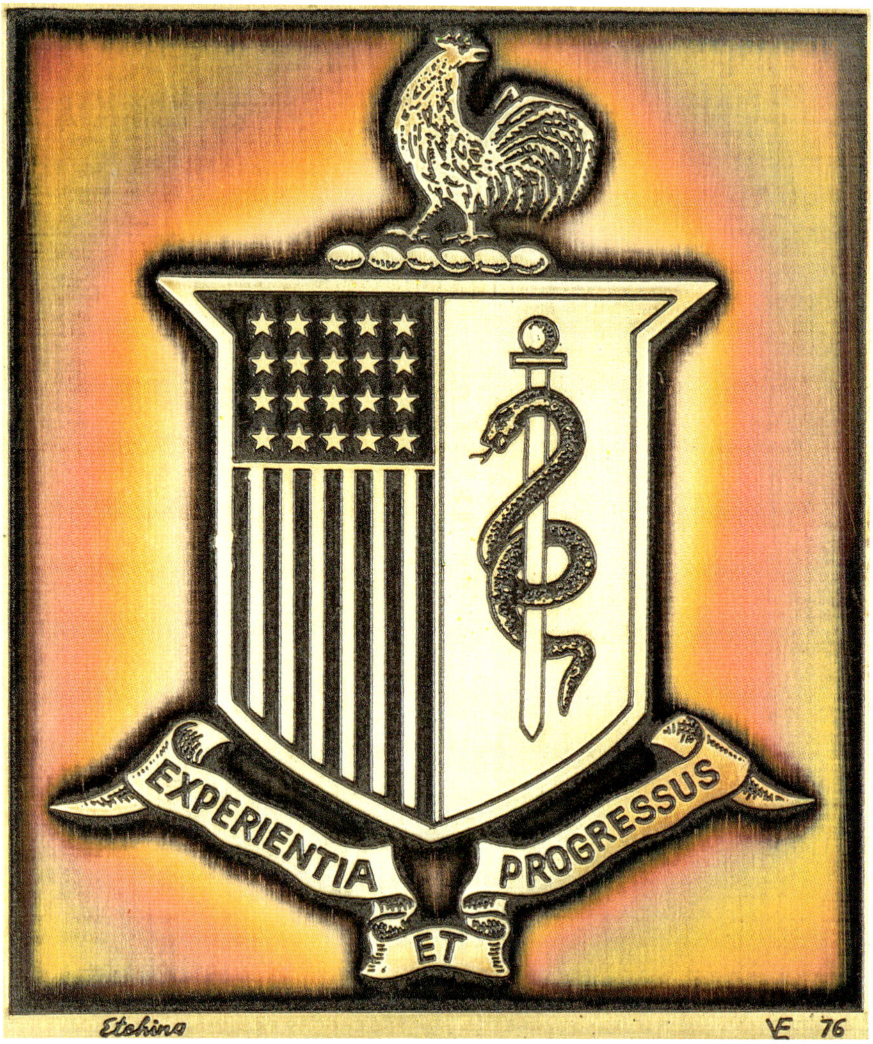

The Coat of Arms
1818
Medical Department of the Army

A 1976 etching by Vassil Ekimov of an original color print that appeared in *The Military Surgeon*, Vol XLI, No 2, 1917

The first line of medical defense in wartime is the combat medic. Although in ancient times medics carried the caduceus into battle to signify the neutral, humanitarian nature of their tasks, they have never been immune to the perils of war. They have made the highest sacrifices to save the lives of others, and their dedication to the wounded soldier is the foundation of military medical care.

Textbook of Military Medicine

Published by

Office of The Surgeon General
United States of America

Editor in Chief
Brigadier General Russ Zajtchuk, MC, U.S. Army
Director, Borden Institute
Commander
U.S. Army Medical Research and Materiel Command
Professor of Surgery
F. Edward Hébert School of Medicine
Uniformed Services University of the Health Sciences

Officer in Charge and Managing Editor
Colonel Ronald F. Bellamy, MC, U.S. Army
Borden Institute
Associate Professor of Military Medicine,
Associate Professor of Surgery,
F. Edward Hébert School of Medicine
Uniformed Services University of the Health Sciences

Managing Editor 1987–1993
Donald P. Jenkins, Ph.D.

The TMM Series

Part I. *Warfare, Weaponry, and the Casualty*

Medical Consequences of Nuclear Warfare (1989)

Conventional Warfare: Ballistic, Blast, and Burn Injuries (1991)

Military Psychiatry: Preparing in Peace for War (1994)

War Psychiatry (1995)

Medical Aspects of Chemical and Biological Warfare

Military Medical Ethics

Part II. *Principles of Medical Command and Support*

Medicine and War

Medicine in Low-Intensity Conflict

Part III. *Disease and the Environment*

Occupational Health: The Soldier and the Industrial Base (1993)

Military Dermatology (1994)

Military Preventive Medicine: Mobilization and Deployment

Environmental Hazards and Military Operations

Part IV. *Surgical Combat Casualty Care*

Anesthesia and Perioperative Care of the Combat Casualty (1995)

Combat Injuries to the Head, Face, and Neck

Combat Injuries to the Trunk

Combat Injuries to the Extremities and Spine

Rehabilitation of the Injured Soldier

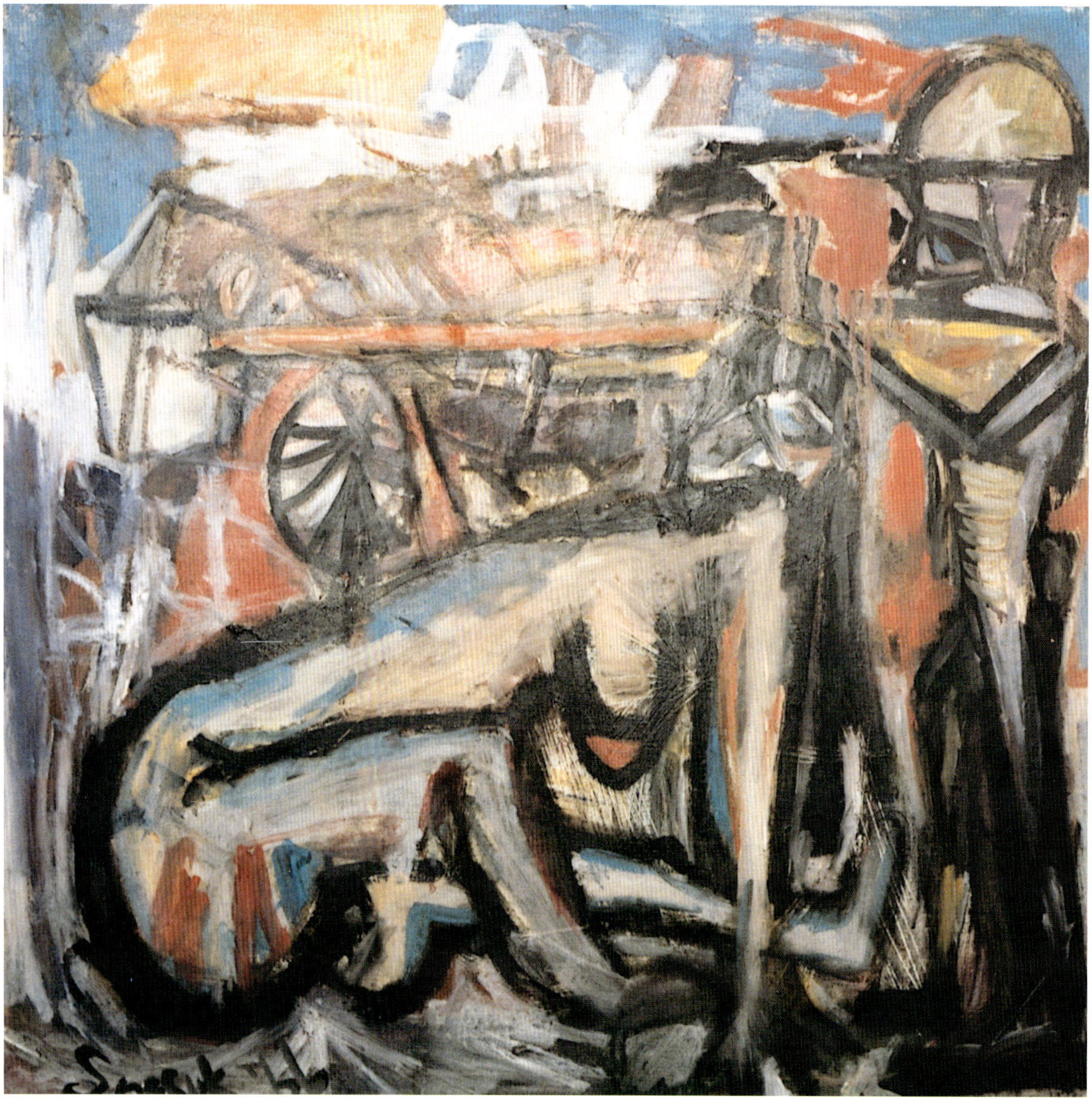

Soo Suk Kim	*War*	1966

Soo Suk Kim, a 22-year-old art student, painted *War* in 1966 as a gift to his brother-in-law, Captain Franklin D. Jones, who was serving as a division psychiatrist in Vietnam. Soo Kim had experienced war first-hand as a 6-year-old refugee during the North Korean occupation of Seoul, hiding from a communist edict calling for the execution of his prominent family. The painting depicts his childhood recollection of the horrors and chaos of war.

WAR PSYCHIATRY

Specialty Editors

FRANKLIN D. JONES, M.D., F.A.P.A.
LINETTE R. SPARACINO, M.A.
VICTORIA L. WILCOX, Ph.D.
JOSEPH M. ROTHBERG, Ph.D.
JAMES W. STOKES, M.D.

Office of The Surgeon General
United States Army
Falls Church, Virginia

United States Army Medical Department Center and School
Fort Sam Houston, Texas

Walter Reed Army Institute of Research
Washington, D.C.

Uniformed Services University of the Health Sciences
Bethesda, Maryland

1995

Lorraine B. Davis
Senior Editor

This volume was prepared for military medical educational use. The focus of the information is to foster discussion that may form the basis of doctrine and policy. The volume does not constitute official policy of the United States Department of Defense.

Dosage Selection:

The authors and publisher have made every effort to ensure the accuracy of dosages cited herein. However, it is the responsibility of every practitioner to consult appropriate information sources to ascertain correct dosages for each clinical situation, especially for new or unfamiliar drugs and procedures. The authors, editors, publisher, and the Department of Defense cannot be held responsible for any errors found in this book.

Use of Trade or Brand Names:

Use of trade or brand names in this publication is for illustrative purposes only and does not imply endorsement by the Department of Defense.

Neutral Language:

Unless this publication states otherwise, masculine nouns and pronouns do not refer exclusively to men

---

Published by the Office of The Surgeon General at TMM Publications
Borden Institute
Walter Reed Army Medical Center
Washington, DC 20307-5001

Library of Congress Cataloging–in–Publication Data

War psychiatry / specialty editors, Franklin D. Jones . . . [et al.].
p. cm. — (Textbook of military medicine. Part I, Warfare, weaponry, and the casualty)
Includes bibliographical references and index.
1. War Neurosis. 2. Military psychiatry—United States.
I. Jones, Franklin D., 1935- . II. Series.
[DNLM: 1. Combat Disorders. 2. War. 3. Military Psychiatry. WH 390 T355 pt 1 1989 v.4]
RC971.T48 1989
[RC550]
616.9'8023 s—dc20
[616.85'212]
DNLM/DLC
for Library of Congress 95-18334
CIP

PRINTED IN THE UNITED STATES OF AMERICA

04, 03, 02, 01, 00, 99, 98, 97, 96, 5 4 3 2 1

Contents

Frontispiece Plates

Foreword

This volume of the *Textbook of Military Medicine* addresses the delivery of mental health services during wartime. The foreseeable future of the U.S. military includes the potential for involvement in a variety of conflicts, ranging from peace-keeping missions to massive deployments of personnel and materiel and possible nuclear, biological, and chemical threats as was seen in the Persian Gulf War. The medical role in wartime is critical to success of the mission. For the mental health disciplines, this role encompasses identification and elimination of unfit personnel, improvement of marginal personnel to standards of acceptability, prevention of psychiatric casualties, and their treatment when prevention fails. All of these efforts must be guided by past experience and sound principles of human behavior.

The identification and elimination of unfit personnel must be prudently managed. During World War II, medical personnel mistakenly believed that soldiers who had exhibited any prior symptoms of anxiety would be prone to breakdown. However, review of casualty breakdown in World War II revealed that breakdown was largely related to unit and battle conditions rather than predisposition.

Prevention of psychiatric casualties must address the factors known to be important in soldier efficiency and breakdown. These can be grouped into biological, interpersonal, and intrapsychic factors. Of these, interpersonal factors may be the most critical. Soldiers living and working together in conditions of shared danger and hardship will foster unit cohesion, which is known to reduce the risk of psychiatric breakdown. Thus, producing cohesive combat forces has become a mainstay of psychiatric prevention.

The soldier brings with him many, sometimes conflicting, intrapsychic beliefs and attitudes, including a strong sense of invulnerability. These contribute to his psychological defense against the rigors of the battlefield. It is the loss of such defenses that produces breakdown on an individual basis. The treatment of the combat psychiatric casualty near the front with replenishment of physiological deficits and expectation of return to one's unit shores up these failing defenses.

I strongly recommend that all commanders and medical officers read this book and heed its central theme: the stresses of combat are significant, but with appropriate and timely prophylaxis and treatment, the majority of these soldiers can be returned to their units as functional members of their group.

Lieutenant General Alcide M. LaNoue
The Surgeon General
U.S. Army

July 1995
Washington, D.C.

Preface

The stresses of the military environment are diverse and significant—the potential for deployment and combat, long and arduous training missions, and separations from families. A companion volume, *Military Psychiatry: Preparing in Peace for War*, addresses these issues in a peacetime military. As stressful as garrison life can be, it pales when compared to the stresses of combat. These stresses are greatest during actual combat, but begin with notification of a deployment, and often continue after the fighting is over as the participants deal with the aftermath of the battlefield, which may include post-traumatic stress disorder, especially if they have been prisoners of war or experienced mutilating injuries. This volume discusses the evolution of the concept of combat stress reaction, the delivery of mental health care on the various battlefields our soldiers are likely to experience, and the psychological consequences of having endured the intensity and lethality of modern combat.

The concept of the stress casualty has changed considerably from times past when the symptoms of stress breakdown were thought to be evidence of cowardice and thus were punished rather than treated. As our understanding of the dynamics of the stress casualty and the battlefield environment have increased, we have discovered that the most important lesson learned from previous wars is the need for timely and appropriate handling of stress casualties. Psychiatric casualties should be seen as close to the battlefield as possible (proximity) and as quickly as possible (immediacy), and should be provided with rest and nutrition. They should be told that their symptoms are normal in combat and that they will recover (expectancy). These are the principles of proximity, immediacy, and expectancy, known by the PIE acronym. Psychiatric casualties treated under these principles are more likely to recover than those for whom treatment is delayed or occurs far from the battlefield. These principles can also be utilized in debriefing groups exposed to unusual stress whether in combat or in disasters (critical incident debriefing). This early intervention often prevents later development of chronic post-traumatic stress disorders.

While the principles of combat psychiatry are relatively universal, their application may vary in the different military services, depending on the mission. Thus, service-specific scenarios and issues are presented in separate chapters on combat psychiatry in the U.S. Army, the U.S. Air Force, and the U.S. Navy. An important area addressed in this volume is the need for uniform psychiatric procedures in joint operations, which will likely be more common in the future.

The prevention and treatment of combat stress reaction is not simply the domain of the mental health provider. Commanders must also play an active role by maintaining contact with soldiers when they are temporary casualties and welcoming them back to the unit after they have rested and recovered. This increases the likelihood of continued long-term functioning and enhances unit cohesion. It is also the honorable thing to do for those individuals who have temporarily been overcome by the horrors of battle, but are now ready to rejoin their unit to continue the fight.

Brigadier General Russ Zajtchuk
Medical Corps, U.S. Army

July 1995
Washington, D.C.

The current medical system to support the U.S. Army at war is a continuum from the forward line of troops through the continental United States; it serves as a primary source of trained replacements during the early stages of a major conflict. The system is designed to optimize the return to duty of the maximum number of trained combat soldiers at the lowest possible level. Far-forward stabilization helps to maintain the physiology of injured soldiers who are unlikely to return to duty and allows for their rapid evacuation from the battlefield without needless sacrifice of life or function.

Medical Force 2000 (MF2K)
PATIENT FLOW IN A THEATER OF OPERATIONS

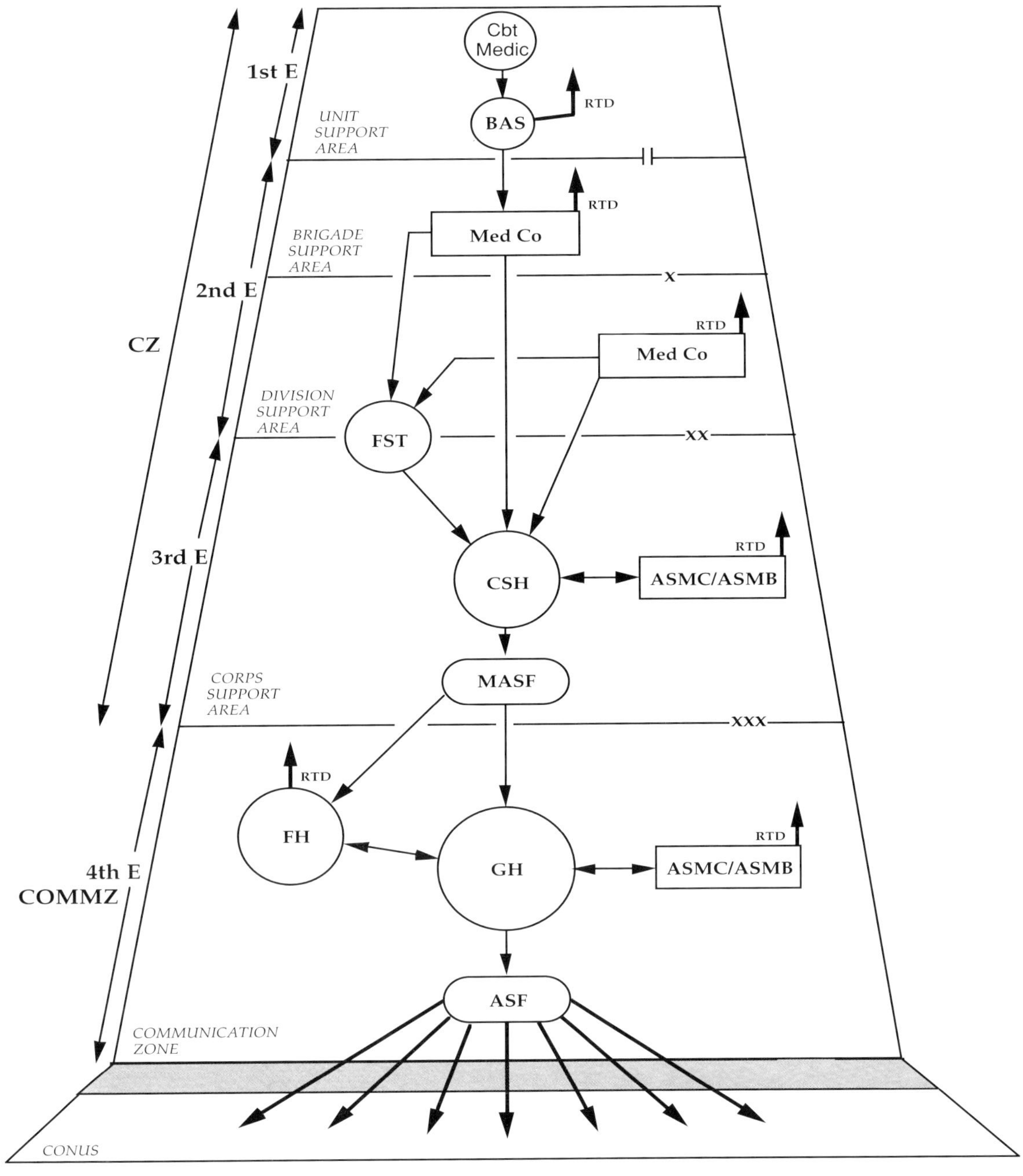

ASF:	Aeromedical Staging Facility, USAF	E:	Echelon
ASMB:	Area Support Medical Battalion	FH:	Field Hospital
ASMC:	Area Support Medical Company	FST:	Forward Surgical Team
BAS:	Battalion Aid Station	GH:	General Hospital
Cbt Medic:	Combat Medic	MASF:	Mobile Aeromedical Staging Facility, USAF
CSH:	Combat Support Hospital	Med Co:	Medical Company
COMMZ:	Communication Zone	RTD:	Return to Duty
CZ:	Combat Zone		

Chapter 1

PSYCHIATRIC LESSONS OF WAR

FRANKLIN D. JONES, M.D., F.A.P.A.*

*Colonel (ret), Medical Corps, U.S. Army; Clinical Professor, Uniformed Services University of the Health Sciences, Bethesda, Maryland; Past President and Secretary and current Honorary President of the Military Section, World Psychiatric Association; formerly Psychiatry and Neurology Consultant, Office of The Surgeon General, U.S. Army

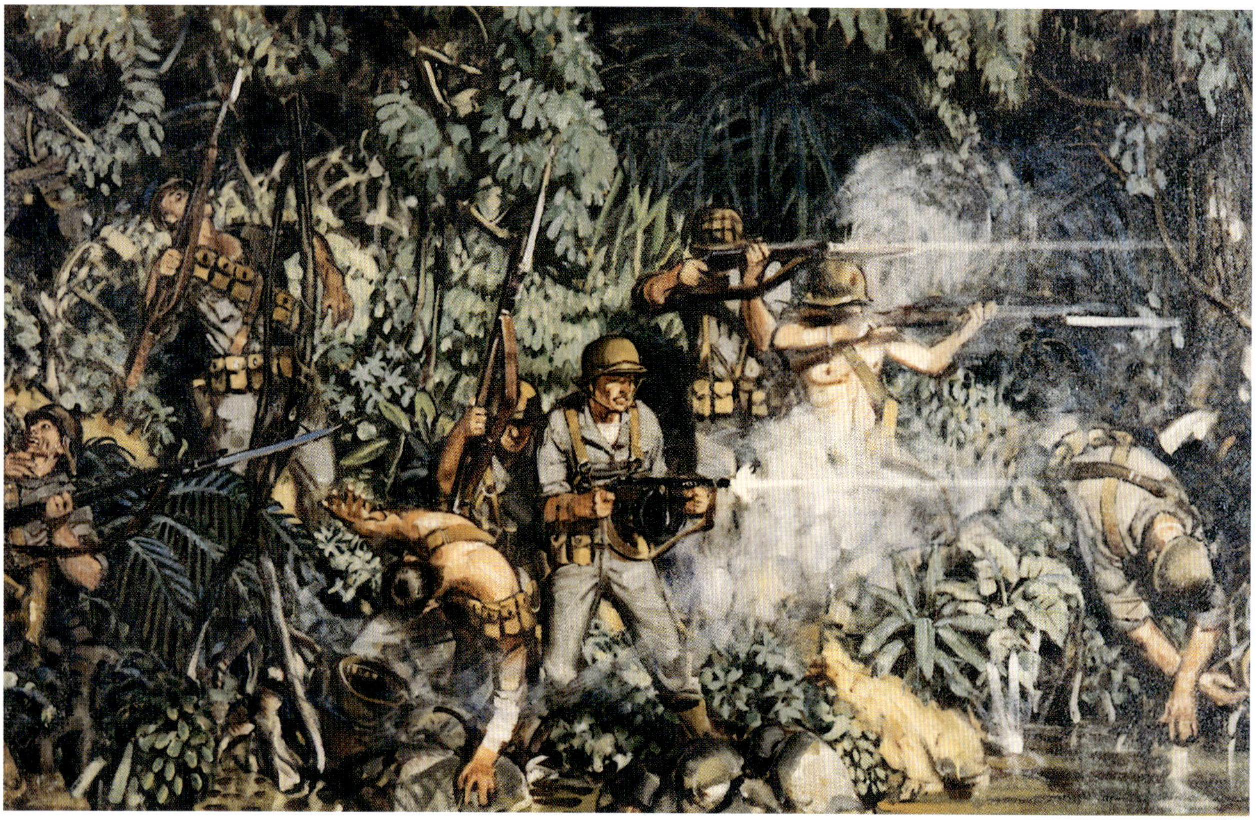

Richard W. Baldwin *Fighting at Guadalcanal* 1943

This painting by Richard W. Baldwin, who was a sergeant in the U.S. Army Air Forces, depicts World War II jungle fighting in the South Pacific at Guadalcanal, which was characterized by environmental deprivation, disease, and isolation. The psychiatric lessons of World War I had to be relearned and expanded during World War II to include physical stressors.

Art: Courtesy of US Center of Military History, Washington, DC.

INTRODUCTION

War, with its lesser elaborations such as competitive sports, has been an enduring aspect of human existence. Survival for the prehuman individual and the species was largely dependent on the evolution of physical attributes until fairly late in human development. The ability of prehumans and humans to organize into groups resulted in the supplanting of biological evolution with social evolution. Social evolution was so powerful an agency that while modern humans are less well developed physically than their human and prehuman ancestors, they are nevertheless more capable of survival. Social evolution has necessarily been accompanied by psychological evolution such that the two cannot be separated. In modern wars, beyond a minimal level of physical fitness and technical learning of how to fight, the soldier's most important training is in social-psychological reaction patterns, particularly the handling of fear and aggression and the bonding with a group for accomplishing the military mission.

While wars differ along many dimensions ranging from ideology to technology, the human element remains the same. After millions of years of evolutionary molding, the human organism is reasonably well equipped physically to fight the solitary or group combat that our Stone-Age ancestors endured. This physical development alone, however, would never have allowed humans to achieve dominion over the natural world. This dominion resulted from the development of implements of combat and a social structure that facilitated cooperation in battle. Part of this social structure included the ability of protomen to band together on hunting expeditions as well as their ability to discover and then propagate the knowledge of how to make and use weapons. It is a striking observation that men through all periods of recorded history have fought ultimately as small groups consisting of from 2 to 20 or 30 persons.[1]

The same cultural evolution of groups that maximized warrior skills in the past, however, has increasingly prepared homo sapiens for peace rather than war. Individual psychology, reflecting family and cultural influences, often hinders rather than facilitates successful adaptation to combat. This can be seen, for example, in religious prohibitions against violence, which when internalized by any of a variety of processes, may even overcome near-instinctive behaviors for self-preservation.[2(p512)]

Erikson[3] gave a classic example of the interaction of the biological, interpersonal, and intrapsychic factors in the breakdown and later elaborations of symptoms in a World War II combat veteran.

Case Study: A Combat Crisis in a Marine.

The patient, a young teacher in his thirties, primarily suffered from severe headaches. History at a veterans' clinic revealed that he was with a group of medical corpsmen who lay in pitch darkness on a South Pacific beachhead, pinned down by enemy fire, with little supporting fire from U.S. Navy ships. The group experienced mounting anger and fear; however, the patient seemed unaffected by the group anxiety. The patient did not drink, smoke, or even swear, and had chosen to be a medical corpsman because he could not bring himself to carry a gun.

During the night, he had only isolated memories of a dreamlike quality: the corpsmen were ordered to unload ammunition; the medical officer became angry, swearing abusively; someone thrust a submachine gun into the corpsman's hands. By morning he was a patient sedated in the improvised hospital, with severe intestinal fever. At nightfall, the enemy attacked by air. The patient was immobilized and unable to care for the sick and wounded. He felt fear, and next day he was evacuated. At the rear area hospital he was initially calmer, but became upset and crawled under his sheets when the first meal was served. The metallic clanging of the mess kits sounded like salvos of incoming shots. He was plagued by severe headaches and when not suffering from them remained apprehensive, jumpy, easily startled. Although the fever which could have justified the initial headache was cured, his other symptoms persisted and he was evacuated home as a "war neurosis."

Erikson found that the patient's family had been in economic and moral decline. At age 14, the patient had left home after his mother, in a drunken rage, threatened him with a gun. He had secured the secret help of his principal, a fatherly man who protected and guided him, asking in exchange that he never drink, swear, indulge himself sexually, or touch a gun.

Erikson was able to separate out the biosociopsychological vulnerabilities that produced the breakdown. In the biological area were exhaustion and sleeplessness coupled with subliminal infection and fever. In the sociological area were the lowering of group morale and growth of group panic, immobilization under enemy fire, the inducement to give up in the hospital bed, and finally immediate evacuation creating a conflict between the desire to escape and the call to duty to care for his mates. In the psychological area were the loss of support for an idealized father substitute when the medical officer swore, and conflict over his identity as a noncombatant when a submachine gun was pressed on him, for "the gun had become the symbol of his family's downfall and represented all ... which he had chosen not to do."[3(p44)] The subsequent headaches represented "the unconscious wish to continue to suffer in order to overcompensate psychologically for the weakness of having let others down; for many of these escapists were more loyal than they knew. Our conscientious man, too, felt 'shot through the head' by excruciating pain whenever he seemed definitely better."[3(p44)]

Comment: This case illustrates not only the tripartite elements of combat breakdown but also the sequelae of improper treatment (evacuation) of such breakdown, in this case a chronic traumatic neurosis, which would currently be called post-traumatic stress disorder (PTSD). This chapter will, through historical analysis, show the importance of these elements in understanding combat breakdown and the importance of appropriate interventions.

Withstanding the Stress of Combat

The three groups of factors—*biological* (inherent propensities and physical attributes), *interpersonal* (cultural, social), and *intrapsychic* (individual psychological)—can affect positively or negatively the soldier's ability to withstand the stresses of combat. Such stresses are multidimensional: injury; disease; physical and psychological fatigue; and fears of death, maiming, showing cowardice, and releasing aggressive and destructive tendencies. Recognition of these factors was slow to develop. Prior to the 20th century, most soldiers who broke down in combat were considered to be cowards or weaklings, an attitude that persists to this day in some settings. The result of this attitude was usually unfortunate for the soldier and the unit. The term "decimate," for example, originally referred to the policy of killing every tenth soldier in a unit that had shown lack of fighting will in combat. When breakdown was recognized as medically legitimate before the 20th century, it was considered to be of organic causation, and terms such as "nostalgia" and "exhausted heart" were sometimes used. The recognition of biological/interpersonal/intrapsychic factors and their successful manipulation to prevent breakdown in combat or disasters and to facilitate recovery is the special province of military psychiatry.[4]

Exhibit 1-1 illustrates a number of stressors found to be important in combat breakdown, also called combat stress reaction (CSR). This listing obviously is not all-inclusive, because the human mind is infinitely adaptive in the service of physical and psychological survival. In addition, some stressors may overlap, they may interact to exacerbate each other, and specific factors will be of greater or lesser significance in a given individual and in a particular situation. The history of psychiatry in warfare is a study of the recognition of stressors that lead to psychiatric breakdown and the development of pre-

EXHIBIT 1-1

COMBAT STRESS FACTORS

Biological Factors
- Fatigue
- Dehydration and hunger
- Sleep and sensory deprivation
- Adverse environments (heat, cold)
- Disrupted circadian rhythms
- Infectious, inflammatory, and metabolic disorders

Situational Factors
- Military situation (static situations have more casualties, and attacking and retreating maneuvers have fewer casualties)
- Indirect fire (artillery, bombs)
- Unexpected weapons
- Surprise attack

Intrapsychic Factors
- Fear of death, maiming
- Fear of showing cowardice
- Belief or nonbelief in the cause
- Belief war is being won or lost
- Breakdown of Ur (narcissistic) defenses:
  - Loss of feeling of invulnerability
  - Loss of belief that others care (social security)
  - Loss of faith in a celestial order

Interpersonal Factors
- Disruption of unit cohesion
- Impaired leadership
- Loss of a "buddy"

Adapted with permission from Jones FD, Crocq L, Adelaja O, et al. Psychiatric casualties in modern warfare: Evolution of treatment. In: Pichot P, Berner P, Wolf R, Thau K, eds. *Psychiatry: The State of the Art*. Vol. 6. New York: Plenum; 1985: 461.

TABLE 1-1

PSYCHIATRIC LESSONS OF WAR

War	Lessons Learned/Relearned	Lessons Available But Not Learned
Before 20th century	Homesickness (nostalgia) is a form of stress casualty	Nostalgia is nonorganic "Soldier's heart" is a masked casualty
Russo-Japanese War	There are multiple types of nonorganic casualties	Contagious stress symptoms may be evacuation syndromes
World War I	Combat stress reaction can be nonorganic Forward treatment conserves the fighting strength Nonpsychiatric labeling reduces stress casualties Contagious stress symptoms may be an evacuation syndrome	Trench foot and frostbite may be voluntary casualties
World War II	Forward treatment minimizes casualties Screening is not useful Personality is not important for presentation of symptoms Stress reaction depends on combat intensity Fatigue contributes to stress reaction Morale (cohesion) prevents breakdown Cumulative stress is a factor in breakdown	Family concerns may contribute to stress reactions
Korean Conflict	Rotation policy reduces casualties End-of-tour indiscipline is a short-timer syndrome Frostbite may be a voluntary casualty	Alcohol and drug abuse and venereal disease are nostalgic casualties
Vietnam Conflict	Alcohol and drug abuse, venereal disease, and antisocial acts are nostalgic casualties Malaria may be a voluntary casualty	Conscientious objectors, peace marchers, medically certified as unfit to be drafted are masked casualties Stress casualties may be delayed (PTSD)
Yom Kippur War: 1973	Forward treatment conserves the fighting strength Concurrent stress is a factor in combat stress Mass casualties generate stress casualties Personality is important for prognosis of combat reaction Dehydration may be a voluntary casualty	Normal battle reactions may be overdiagnosed Stress casualties may be delayed (PTSD)
Lebanon War: 1982	Preassessment of unit factors can reduce breakdown	Stress casualties may be delayed (PTSD)
Falklands War: 1982	Poor sleep discipline contributes to stress casualties	
Grenada Invasion: 1983	Poor water discipline contributes to stress casualties	
Panama Invasion: 1989	Combat units can effectively include women	
Persian Gulf War: 1991	Critical incident debriefing prevents casualties	Predeployment family support minimizes concurrent stress

PTSD: post-traumatic stress disorder
Adapted with permission from Jones FD, Crocq L, Adelaja O, et al. Psychiatric casualties in modern warfare: Evolution of treatment. In: Pichot P, Berner P, Wolf R, Thau K, eds. *Psychiatry: The State of the Art*. Vol. 6. New York: Plenum; 1985: 462, with subsequent updates.

ventive and treatment measures to alleviate their effects. It is most appropriate and logical to discuss stressors and treatment chronologically as they have been discovered in the contexts of various wars.

The historical approach has practical value. An understanding of how military medicine dealt with combat stress breakdown in the past can enable mental health professionals to avoid mistakes made earlier and to devise new ways to deal with modern stress. Lessons both learned and not learned but available are outlined in Table 1-1. One example of a lesson not learned in the Russo-Japanese War is that providing a medical label for stress symptoms results in the development of such symptoms by other soldiers as an honorable way out of combat.[5]

PRE-20TH CENTURY CONCEPTIONS OF PSYCHIATRIC CASUALTIES

While combat stress breakdown and some of its causative factors were described in the epic accounts of early cultural mythology, not until the late 17th century were some of them given a particularly medical cognizance in the form of the diagnosis, *nostalgia*. Initially called "the Swiss disease" because of its prevalence among young Swiss uprooted from their villages and placed in mercenary armies, it was soon recognized as a more universal ailment. By the mid-18th century it was firmly established in the medical terminology with excellent clinical descriptions, as was discussed by Leopold Auenbrugger in his *Inventum Novum* of 1761:

> When young men who are still growing are forced to enter military service and thus lose all hope of returning safe and sound to their beloved homeland, they become sad, taciturn, listless, solitary, musing, full of sighs and moans. Finally, they cease to pay attention and become indifferent to everything which the maintenance of life requires of them.
>
> This disease is called nostalgia. Neither medicaments, nor arguments, nor promises nor threats of punishment are able to produce any improvement. While all thought is directed toward ungratified desires, the body wastes away, with a dull sound (*sonitus obscuras*) on one side of the chest. [Some cases of nostalgia were undoubtedly linked with tuberculosis and other chest diseases. Such diseases were noted in the author's descriptions of autopsy reports.—Au.]
>
> Some years ago this disease was rather common but now occurs very rarely since the wise arrangement was instituted of limiting the period of military service to a definite number of years. As a result the young men retain the hope of leaving military service after this period has elapsed, and of being able to return to their homes and enjoy their civic rights.[6(pp344–345)]

French physicians of the Napoleonic Era recognized numerous factors important in producing or preventing nostalgia; many of the same factors influence combat breakdown in the modern era. These physicians assessed the importance of conditions ranging from cultural (rural vs urban conscripts), and social (boredom vs rigorous activity and organized vs disorganized camp conditions), to environmental (clement vs inclement weather), and battle (victorious armies suffering few cases of nostalgia vs those experiencing reverses having many cases). Exhibit 1-2 discusses factors currently thought to promote or prevent nostalgic casualties.

Baron Larrey, Napoleon's Chief Surgeon, prescribed a course of treatment that, while ostensibly biologically oriented, reveals a keen awareness of social factors and is surprisingly close to modern handling of combat psychiatric casualties, both preventively and curatively:

> [T]o prevent this sort of cerebral affection in soldiers who have lately joined their corps, it is necessary not to suffer those individuals who are predisposed to it more repose than is necessary to recruit their strength, exhausted during the day; to vary their occupations, and to turn their labours and recreations to their own advantage, as well as to that of society. Thus, after the accustomed military exercises, it is desirable that they should be subjected to regular hours, gymnastic amusements, and some mode of useful instruction. It is in this manner, especially, that mutual instruction, established among the troops of the line, is beneficial to the soldier and the state. Warlike music, during their repasts, or at their hours of recreation, will contribute much to elevate the spirits of the soldier, and to keep away those gloomy reflections which have been traced above.[6(p348)]

One could hardly ask for a better prescription to ensure physical bodily integrity and thus to produce a conviction of health, to give a sense of mastery of weapons and, as Larrey points out, especially to effect an integration into the unit through "mutual instruction, established among the troops of the line."[6(p348)] This regimen prevents evacuation home (the treatment approach of earlier physicians) and minimizes any secondary gain from illness.

EXHIBIT 1-2

FACTORS AND CHARACTERISTICS OF NOSTALGIC CASES

Aggravating Conditions	Ameliorating Conditions
Initial separation from home	Prior separations handled successfully
Dependent personality traits	Independent personality traits
Family stress	Absence of family stress
Breakup of dyadic love relationship ("Dear John" letter)	Intact or absent dyadic love relationship
"Culture shock"	Dislocation to similar milieu
Boredom	Rigorous discipline
Disorganized camp conditions	Organized camp conditions
Inclement weather	Clement weather
Static warfare or reverses in combat	Victorious battles
Anticipated defeat or prolonged warfare	Anticipated victory or brief war
War unpopular at home	War supported by home society (popular war)
Poor communication with command	Open, candid, two-way communication with command
Denigrating treatment by superiors	Respectful treatment by superiors
No sense of participation in the mission	Subordinates feel they own the mission
Superiors indifferent to subordinates' welfare	Subordinates believe superiors are committed to their welfare
Commanders lie to subordinates	Commanders tell subordinates the truth
Fragmented social relations among soldiers	Soldiers depend on and trust each other

Characteristics of Nostalgic Cases

Constricted affect	Chronic post-traumatic stress disorders
Social estrangement	Delayed post-traumatic stress disorders
Disciplinary problems	Mistrust of command
Explosive aggression	Alienation from military goals and values
Substance abuse	Alienation from state institutions
Sexual problems	

Adapted with permission from Jones FD. Psychiatric lessons of low-intensity wars. *Ann Med Milit Fenn* [Finland]. 1985;60:131.

In parallel with their European colleagues, American physicians considered nostalgia to be a disorder associated with the military. No significant data are available concerning psychiatric casualties prior to the American Civil War, except that problems of alcoholism and desertion were not uncommon. Physicians during those times dealt almost entirely with surgical and infectious cases, leaving morale and discipline problems for commanders to handle.[7(p4)]

The Civil War, however, saw the first appearance of recognized nostalgic casualties in significant numbers. Approximately three cases of nostalgia per 1,000 troops per year were reported among Union soldiers, mainly among teenage conscripts.[8] Apparently lacking any knowledge of Larrey's published insights, Civil War physicians urged screening as the primary method of preventing nostalgia. Surgeon General William A. Hammond in 1862 recommended that the minimum age of recruits be fixed at 20 years to screen out those prone to this condition; despite this effort, the rate did not change appreciably.[8] It was recognized, however, that group cohesion was important in preventing nostalgia and that the battle experience could forge these cohesive bonds.[9] Writing in a textbook of psychiatry 20 years after the Civil War, Hammond[10] recommended an army activity program similar to that of

Larrey. He wrote: "The best means of preventing nostalgia is to provide occupation both for the mind and the body ... soldiers placed in hospitals near their homes are always more liable to nostalgia than those who are inmates of hospitals situated in the midst of or in the vicinity of the army to which they belong."[10(p34)] Hammond referred to Bauden's account of the Crimean War in which similar principles were applied. He further stated that "in some cases it may be necessary for the military surgeon to send the nostalgic soldier to his home in order to save his life. This, however, should be done with all possible precautions to prevent his comrades becoming acquainted with the fact."[10(p35)]

From 1861 to 1865 the Union Army officially recognized 2,600 cases of "insanity" and 5,200 cases of "nostalgia" requiring hospitalization at the Government Hospital of the Insane (now St. Elizabeths) in Washington, D.C.[7] Probably still in the realm of psychiatric casualties, in this same conflict there were 200,000 Union deserters and 160,000 cases of "constipation," the latter reminiscent of the "precombat syndrome."[11]

Other psychiatric entities of the Civil War included malingering, which usually took the form of exaggerated trivial conditions or neurological symptoms, and the irritable and exhausted heart of DaCosta.[8] This latter condition was not recognized as a psychiatric entity and may well have included rheumatic and other heart disease. However, most cases diagnosed as exhausted heart were probably functional, secondary to anxiety. They may have resembled the neurocirculatory asthenia of World War I.[7(p3)]

In addition to innovations in treatment of surgical wounds and application of similar procedures pioneered by Florence Nightingale in the Crimean War a decade earlier, the major medical accomplishment during the Civil War was the establishment of the specialty of neurology by such pioneers as S. Weir Mitchell, W.W. Keen, G.R. Morehouse, and William A. Hammond.[8] The development of neurology laid the foundations for differentiating combat disorders with organic causes from those with psychological causes.

Following the Civil War, alcoholism, venereal diseases, and disciplinary infractions continued to be present in soldiers fighting the Indian Wars, the Spanish-American War, and the Philippine Insurrection, but these psychiatric problems in U.S. forces were not so labeled until World War I. Recognition of these and other aberrant behaviors as psychiatric problems first occurred during the Russo-Japanese War.[12]

20TH CENTURY COMBAT PSYCHIATRY

In the decade immediately preceding the outbreak of World War I, Russian physicians during the Russo-Japanese War (1904–1906) reportedly first utilized psychiatric specialists in the treatment of combat stress casualties both at the front and upon return to home territory.[12] This war also provided the first good description of war neurosis. Emphasis was placed on treatment of "insane" soldiers (an unfortunate term suggesting incurability), and no distinction was made between psychotic and neurotic soldiers. Although some psychiatric casualties were returned to combat, evacuation home, usually accompanied by psychiatric personnel, was the standard treatment. As this evacuation policy became known among the troops, the number of psychiatric patients increased 6- to 10-fold at some collecting points.[12] Nevertheless, such psychiatric casualties were not recognized as a significant source of personnel lost in battle until World War I.

Development of Principles

"Shell shock" was the popular label given to most World War I (1914–1918) neuropsychiatric casualties.[2(p311)] Jones, Belenky, and Marlowe[13(pp1-2)] have discussed the impact of labeling in producing adverse outcomes in such casualties:

> The interaction between label and belief and behavior was particularly striking in the consequences of the use of the term shell shock in World War I .... As a metaphor for the new shape of battle that characterized that war, it was particularly appropriate. In no previous conflict had men, pinned into place by the stasis of trench warfare, been subjected to artillery exchanges of such regularity, intensity and magnitude. The tactics of the day ensured that artillery shells and other explosive devices would be the primary cause of death, wounding, and stress. In a professional world in which most psychiatry was articulated to a neurological base, shell shock was initially seen as a species of actual shock to the central nervous system—a "commotional" syndrome that was the result of the effects of a blast pressure wave that was coupled to the body of the victim. Although the German, Oppenheim, had hypothesized a "molecular derangement" of brain cells as the pathologic agency,[14] a number of observations discredited this theory. Soldiers nowhere near an explosion devel-

oped "shell shock." German prisoners of war exposed to shelling or bombing did not develop "shell shock" while their allied captors did. Soldiers exposed, or thinking themselves exposed, to toxic gases developed "shell shock." Finally, Farrar,[15] after observing scores of Canadian soldiers with severe head injuries from shrapnel and gunshot wounds, noted that symptoms of psychosis or traumatic neurosis practically never occurred. He concluded " ... trench neuroses occur usually in unwounded soldiers."[15(p16)]

In spite of the fact that British and French psychiatrists rapidly came to understand that the great majority of "shell-shocked" soldiers were the victims of transient stress-induced psychological disorders, the label and the beliefs and behaviors associated with it continued to exercise a major influence on the battlefield. While the clinicians dispensed with "shell-shock," the troops did not. It became part of the self-diagnostic and self-labeling nomenclature of the soldier.[13(pp1-2)]

British and French forces during World War I discovered the importance of proximity or forward treatment. The British had been evacuating neuropsychiatric casualties back to England and finding them most refractory to treatment. By 1917, when Salmon (Figure 1-1) made his famous report on "shell shock" among British and French soldiers, one seventh of all discharges for disability from the British Army had been due to mental conditions; of 200,000 soldiers on the pension list of England, one fifth suffered from war neurosis.[2] However, within a few months of the onset of hostilities, British and French physicians had noted that patients with war neuroses improved more rapidly when treated in permanent hospitals near the front than at the base, better in casualty clearing stations than even at the advanced base hospitals, and better still when encouragement, rest, persuasion, and suggestion could be given in a combat organization itself. The importance of immediate treatment quickly became obvious when vicissitudes of combat prevented early treatment of war neuroses even in forward settings. Those who were left to their own devices due to a large influx of casualties were found more refractory to treatment and more likely to need further rearward evacuation.[2(p508)]

As an emissary of the U.S. Army Surgeon General, Thomas Salmon in 1917 observed and synthesized the British and French experience into a comprehensive program for the prevention and treatment of shell shock cases, which were renamed "war neuroses." Salmon's program, which involved placing psychiatrists in the divisions with forward hospitals to support them, was the first rational system of echelon psychiatry in U.S. military forces. American Expeditionary Forces (AEF) physicians fine-tuned this design based on their own experiences.[16(p313)] When fully conceptualized by Artiss,[17] three principles—proximity, immediacy, and expectancy—became the cornerstones of combat psychiatric casualty treatment. They referred to treating the combat psychiatric casualty in a safe place as close to the battle scene as possible (*proximity*), as soon as possible (*immediacy*), with simple treatment such as rest, food, and perhaps a warm shower (*simplicity*), and most importantly an explicit statement that he is not ill and will soon be rejoining his comrades (*expectancy*). Proximity and immediacy are important because the soldier's time away from his unit weakens his bonds with it and allows time for consolidation of his rationalization of his symptoms. The patient's rationalization may take many forms but basically consists of a single line of logic: "If I am not sick, then I am a coward who has abandoned his buddies. I cannot accept being a coward, therefore I am sick." The psychiatrist offers an alternative hypothesis: "You are neither sick nor a coward. You are just tired and will recover when rested."

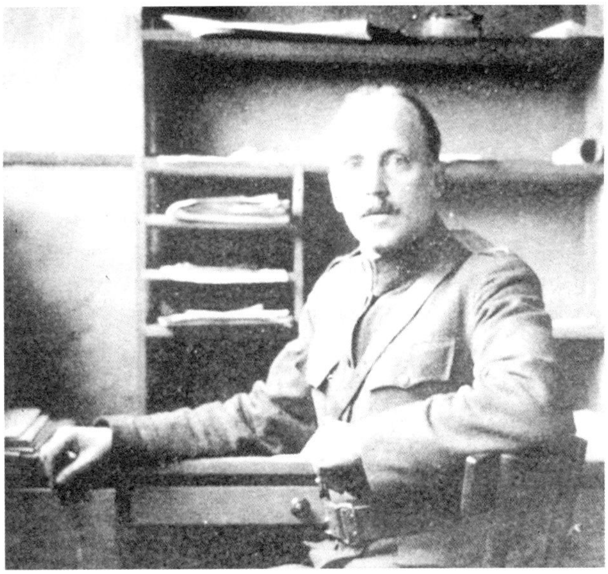

Fig. 1-1. Thomas Salmon inaugurated the principles of forward treatment of combat psychiatry casualties and was the Neuropsychiatry Consultant to the American Expeditionary Forces in World War I. He subsequently held many distinguished positions, including Presidency of the American Psychiatric Association, and is remembered for championing the mental health movement started by Clifford Beers.

Expectancy is the central principle from which the others derive. A soldier who is treated near his unit in space (proximity) and shortly after leaving it (immediacy) can expect to return to it. Distance in space or time decreases this expectancy. Similarly, the principle of simplicity derives from the concept of expectancy. The application of involved treatments such as narcosynthesis or electroshock treatment may only strengthen the soldier's rationalization that he is ill physically or mentally. The occasional use of these more elaborate procedures in refractory cases actually reinforces the preeminent role of expectation; they convey the message: "Yes, you had a mild ailment; however, we have applied a powerful cure, and you are well."

The role of expectancy can be seen in the labeling of these psychiatric casualties. Soldiers in World War I who were called "shell-shocked" indeed acted as though they had sustained a shock to the central nervous system. As recounted by Bailey, Williams, and Komora, "There were descriptions of cases with staring eyes, violent tremors, a look of terror, and blue, cold extremities. Some were deaf and some were dumb; others were blind or paralyzed."[18(p2)] When it was realized that concussion was not the etiologic agent, the term "war neurosis" was used. This was hardly an improvement because even the lay public was aware that Freud had used William Cullen's 1777 nonspecific term, "neurosis," to describe chronic and sometimes severe mental illnesses. The soldier could readily grasp this medical diagnosis as proof of illness. This problem was remedied when medical personnel were instructed to tag such casualties as "N.Y.D. (nervous)" for "not yet diagnosed (nervous)." The term "N.Y.D. (nervous)" gave soldiers nothing definite to cling to and no suggestion had been made to help them in formulating their disorder into something that was generally recognized as incapacitating and requiring hospital treatment, thus honorably releasing them from combat duty. This left them open to the suggestion that they were only tired and a little nervous and with a short rest would be fit for duty. Eventually, many of these cases began to be referred to simply as "exhaustion," then, with the rediscovery of the principles during World War II, as "combat exhaustion." Finally, during World War II, the term "combat fatigue" came to be preferred in that it conveyed more exactly the expectation desired.[19(p993)]

Another finding of World War I was the "contagiousness" of medical disorders that allow honorable escape from combat. This occurs particularly in situations of ambiguity when such escape behavior can become an "evacuation syndrome," as described by Belenky and Jones:

> An evacuation syndrome develops in combat or in field training exercises when through accident or ignorance an evacuation route, usually through medical channels, opens to the rear for soldiers displaying a certain constellation of symptoms and signs.... In the First World War, lethal gases were used in combat. In one battle, an incident occurred in which soldiers from a certain division came to their medical aid stations in large numbers complaining of being gassed. This division had taken heavy casualties, but now was involved in a desultory holding action, with no particular aim or object. The soldiers in the division had been expecting to be relieved following the previous heavy fighting and when they had not been, morale had declined precipitously. During the current action, there was some gas shelling, but not of sufficient intensity to produce any serious casualties. Nevertheless, soldiers usually in groups of comrades were coming to their battalion aid stations complaining of cardiorespiratory symptoms. The medical personnel seeing these men evacuated them to the rear. An initial trickle of soldiers turned into a flood, and very soon this inappropriate evacuation of men—for symptoms only—turned into a significant source of manpower loss. Once the line commanders became aware of the magnitude of the ongoing loss they intervened and sought consultation from the division psychiatrist. The psychiatrist reorganized the system of evacuation by treating the soldiers coming to the aid station with a complaint of gas exposure and cardiorespiratory symptoms as psychiatric casualties. He gave them a brief rest, a warm drink, and a change of clothes, and rapidly returned them to their unit. The flow of men with cardiorespiratory complaints slowed and finally stopped. Overall the incident lasted over a week before it was finally terminated.[20(pp140–141)] [Similarly, during the Vietnam conflict, Jones reported an "epidemic" of sleepwalking, which is described in Chapter 2, Traditional Warfare Combat Stress Casualties.—Au.]

Following World War I, the principles of forward treatment were gradually lost to the U.S. military. The psychoanalytic notion that the origin of psychiatric disorders could be traced to childhood trauma prevailed. A natural consequence of this theory was that evidence of such trauma could be detected, and such potential casualties screened out. The Spanish Civil War revealed an interesting admixture of this faith in screening along with a pragmatic application of forward treatment of combat stress casualties.

Application of Principles

The Spanish Civil War (1936–1939) was a struggle between a monarchist-military faction supported with money, equipment, and volunteers by Germany and Italy and a republican-socialist faction supported by France, the United States, and the Soviet Union. Much of the combat psychiatry learned in this war was not available until after World War II because those who learned the proper handling of psychiatric casualties were on the losing side and were scattered. Mira, the psychiatrist who set up the mental health program for the Spanish Republican Army, gave the Thomas W. Salmon Memorial Lecture in 1942 and later expanded it into a book. His work was not published until late in World War II, by which time U.S. forces had relearned the lessons of World War I. Mira made two main contributions to the literature of combat psychiatry: (1) the revalidation of forward treatment for psychiatric casualties, and (2) the value of psychiatric screening. The latter point will be addressed first.

Mira[21] described a written psychiatric questionnaire to be filled out by potential recruits for the Spanish Republican Army. The 17 questions, when skillfully interpreted, allowed the physician to assess motivation, intelligence, and, it was believed, the probability that men were "likely to suffer from war neurosis." After demographic questions, the following were then asked: "Do you ever faint?" "Do you suffer from dizziness?" "How often do you have sexual relations?" "How often would you like to have a 7-day leave if it were possible? Where and how would you spend the time?"[21(p68)]

According to Mira,

> Broadly speaking, the cases of mental and neurotic disorders occurring subsequently in the group of approximately twenty thousand troops selected in this way were three times less frequent than among those not given any such examination. This suggests that considerable value would be derived from the adoption of this or similar methods of selection and group testing at the recruiting centers.[21(p69)]

Although Mira attributed the very low rate of psychiatric casualties to screening, it seems more likely, based on U.S. experience in World War II and Vietnam, that the policy of forward treatment, including "forward evacuation," was far more critical than screening in accounting for the low figures. The forward treatment program reported by Mira seems to have worked well.

Late in the war (July 1938), Mira organized the various psychiatric services that had developed during the war into a coordinated program of 5 centers with 32 psychiatrists.[21(p73)] Not all of the rear area military psychiatric casualties were evacuated to the central psychiatric clinic (in the civilian zone) but some were sent toward the forward emergency psychiatric center of the corresponding battle sector. In Mira's words, "They were surprised that instead of going backward they were moved ahead when they complained of mental disorder! The purpose was to avoid the encouragement of malingering or the exaggeration of nervous symptoms as a means of escape from the hardships of military life."[21(p74)] Psychiatric casualties in the front lines were "not to be put to bed but treated boldly by suggestive measures and directly transferred ... where much gymnastic and kinetic exercise was the basis of their readjustment."[21(p75)] The average percentage of recovery of psychiatric casualties from the front centers was reported to be 93.6%, and the total percentage of men temporarily discharged because of war neurosis was not greater than 1.5%.[21(p73)] Subsequent experience with similar procedures suggests that the high recovery and low discharge rates were primarily attributable to forward evacuations. The Israelis in the 1982 Lebanon War also successfully utilized "forward evacuation" and a stringent physical fitness program for psychiatric casualties.[22]

Unfortunately, the forward treatment methods used in the Spanish Civil War were unknown by U.S. physicians at the inception of World War II and had to be painfully relearned. Furthermore, American recruiters shared Mira's view of the efficacy of psychiatric screening, resulting in the rejection of hundreds of thousands of potentially effective soldiers during World War II. World War II studies suggest that beyond minimal screening to eliminate severe mental disorders such as schizophrenia or brain deficits, mass screening is inefficient.[23]

Rediscovery and Extensive Application of Principles

The United States became involved in World War II in 1941, 2 years after its outbreak in Europe. At the outset, American medical personnel were unprepared to carry out the program of forward psychiatry that had been devised by World War I psychiatrists. No psychiatrists were assigned to combat divisions and no provisions for special psychiatric treatment units at the field army level or communications zone had been made.[24] American planners under the guidance of Harry Stack Sullivan had believed that potential psychiatric casualties could be screened out prior to induction.[7(p21)]

To minimize these casualties, physicians at the outset of hostilities did not select draft registrants who had any significant history of psychiatric disturbance, especially those with anxiety symptoms. Furthermore, soldiers showing symptoms after induction were expeditiously discharged. In effect, production of psychiatric symptoms as an honorable way of avoiding induction produced a massive loss of manpower reminiscent of an evacuation syndrome.

Although about 1,600,000 registrants were classified as unfit for induction during World War II because of mental disease or educational deficiency (a disqualification rate about 7.6 times as high as in World War I), separation rates for psychiatric disorders in World War II were 2.4 times as high as in World War I.[24] Not only was screening ineffective in preventing breakdown, but also the liberal separation policy for those presenting with neurotic symptoms threatened the war effort. For instance, in September 1943 more soldiers were being eliminated from the U.S. Army than accessed; most of those separated were for psychoneurosis (35.6/1,000/y).[24(p740)]

Studies attempting to find predisposition to psychiatric breakdown in combat have revealed more similarities between psychiatric casualties and their fellow soldiers than differences. For example, in a comparison of the combat records of 100 men who suffered psychiatric breakdowns requiring evacuation to a U.S. Army hospital in the United States and an equivalent group of 100 surgical casualties, Pratt[25] found no significant difference in numbers of awards for bravery. Glass remarked, "Out of these experiences came an awareness that social and situational determinants of behavior were more important than the assets and liabilities of individuals involved in coping with wartime stress and strain;..."[19(p1024)] The reliance on screening to prevent psychiatric casualties was recognized as a failure when large numbers of these casualties occurred during fighting in North Africa. Because no provision for treatment had been made, they were shipped to distant centers from which they never returned to combat.

World War I-style forward treatment was relearned during two battles of the Tunisian Campaign in March and April 1943.[26] Captain Frederick Hanson (Figure 1-2), a U.S. Army psychiatrist from Canada who may have been familiar with the Salmon Lectures, avoided evacuation and returned more than 70% of 494 neuropsychiatric patients to combat after 48 hours of treatment, which basically consisted of resting the soldier and indicating to him that he would soon rejoin his unit.[26(p9)] On April 26, 1943, in response to the recommendations of his surgeon, Colonel Long, and psychiatrists, Captain Hanson and Major Tureen, General Omar Bradley issued a directive that established a holding period of 7 days for psychiatric patients and further prescribed the term "exhaustion" as the initial diagnosis for all combat psychiatric cases.[26(pp9–10)] The word exhaustion was chosen because it conveyed the least implication of mental disturbance and came closest to describing how the patients really felt. The World War I principles had been rediscovered![26(p10)]

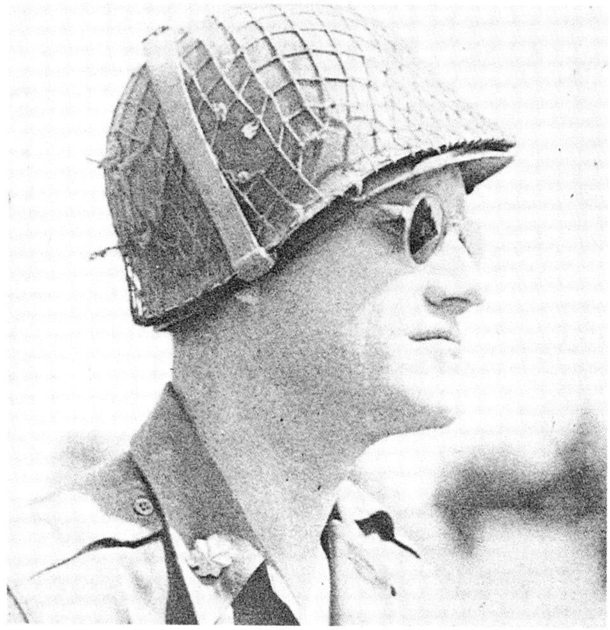

Fig. 1-2. Frederick Hanson, an American who volunteered for duty with the Canadian military before entry of the United States into World War II, was later assigned to the U.S. Army as a consultant to General Omar Bradley's forces. He rediscovered the principles of forward treatment in the North Africa campaign.

Discovery of Mediating Principles

In addition to rediscovering the principles of treatment applied so effectively in World War I, and the ineffectiveness of large-scale screening, World War II psychiatrists learned about the epidemiology of combat stress casualties (direct relationship to intensity of combat, modified by physical and morale factors) and the importance of unit cohesion both in preventing breakdown and in enhancing combat effectiveness. During the war, prospective

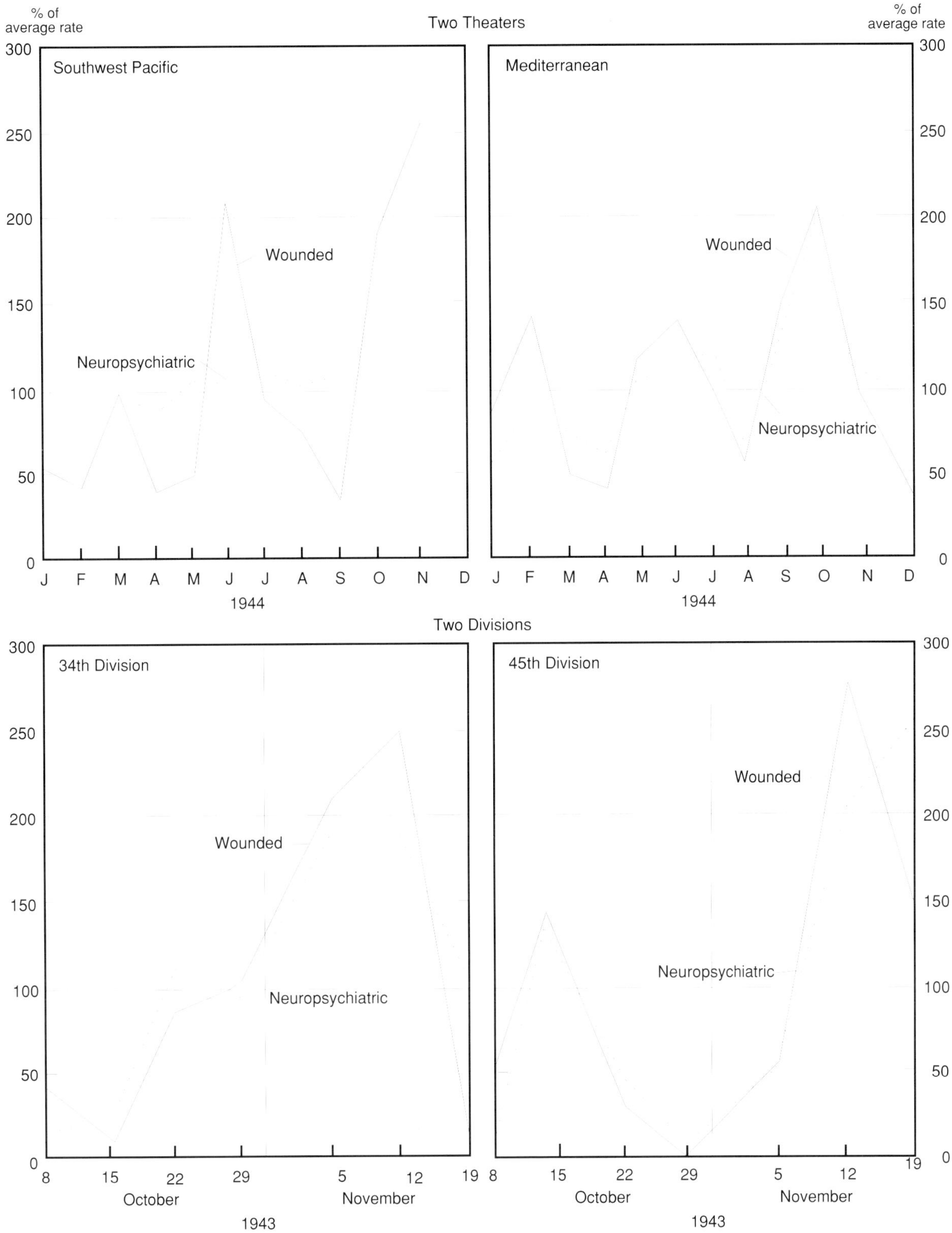

Fig. 1-3. Relation between rates for neuropsychiatric and wounded admissions in World War II. These figures illustrate the dependent relationship of combat stress casualties to combat intensity, as measured by rates of wounded in action. The absence of such a relationship in the Southwest Pacific Theater may represent a phenomenon of sporadic combat or may represent a data collection problem. Reprinted with permission from Beebe GW, De Bakey ME. *Battle Casualties: Incidence, Mortality, and Logistic Considerations*. Springfield, Ill: Charles C Thomas; 1952: 28.

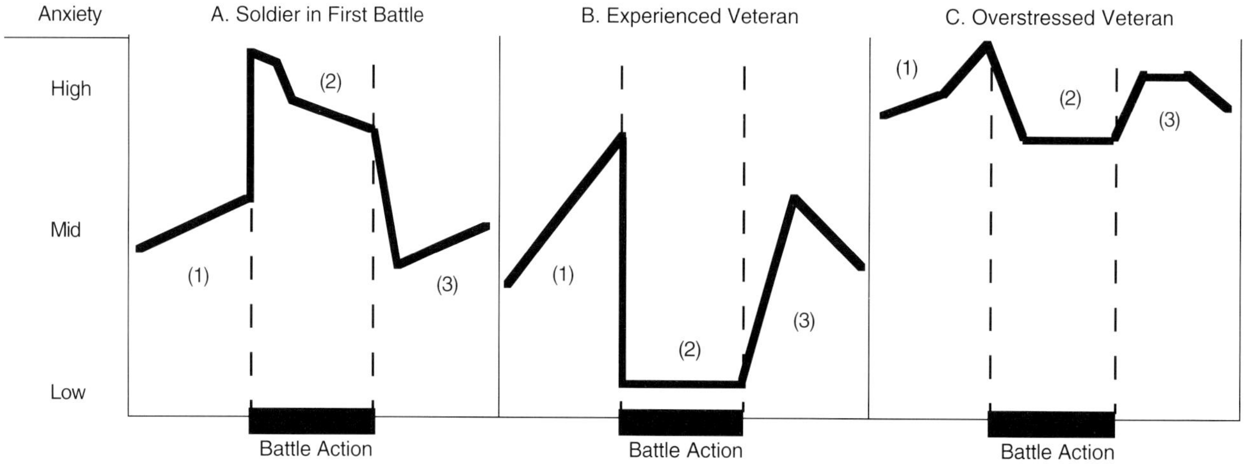

Fig. 1-4. Anxiety, fear, and arousal at different stages in combat tour. A soldier new to battle is more likely to break down than an experienced soldier; however, a soldier exposed to combat for a long period of time is also likely to be a stress casualty. Reprinted from US Department of the Army. *Leaders' Manual for Combat Stress Control.* Washington DC: DA; 1994. Field Manual 22-51: 2-10.

studies conducted by Stouffer and colleagues[27] conclusively showed that units with good morale and leadership had fewer combat stress casualties than those without these attributes when variables such as combat intensity were comparable.

The dependent relationship of combat stress casualties to combat intensity, as measured by rates of wounded in action, can be seen in Figure 1-3 taken from Beebe and De Bakey.[28(p28)] The absence of such a relationship in the Southwest Pacific Theater was explained by Beebe and De Bakey as a collection problem; however, this may be a phenomenon of sporadic combat. In such warfare, neuropsychiatric casualties take the form of venereal disease, alcohol and drug abuse, and disciplinary problems. This phenomenon, which has been detailed by Jones[29] for subsequent wars, will be discussed later.

Another finding during World War II was the chronology of breakdown in combat. It had long been recognized that inexperienced troops were more likely to become stress casualties. Green troops have usually accounted for over three fourths of stress casualties; however, with increasing exposure to combat after 1 or 2 combat months, an increasing rate of casualty generation also occurs. Figure 1-4 addresses battle stress relative to combat experience. Sobel[30] described the anxious, depressed soldier who broke down after having lived through months of seeing friends killed, as "the old sergeant syndrome." Today, it would probably be called chronic post-traumatic stress disorder. Swank and Marchand[31] discussed the relationship of combat exposure and combat effectiveness. The author has devised a graph showing the relationship of psychiatric morbidity to experiences in battle and nonbattle settings (Figure 1-5). Thus, the theory of ultimate vulnerability was promulgated and usually expressed as "everyone has his breaking point." Hanson and Ranson[32] found that while a soldier

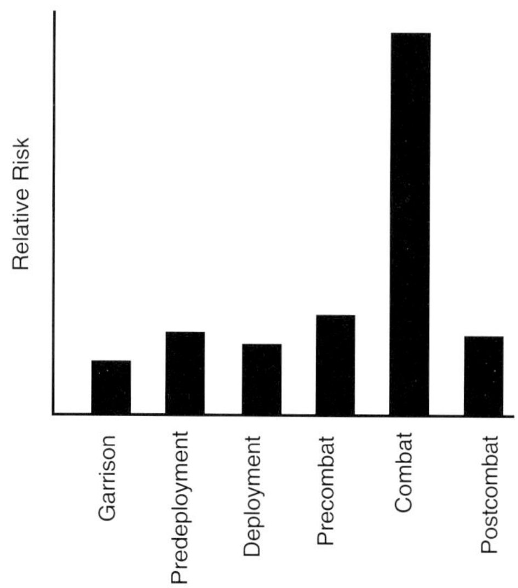

Fig. 1-5. Relationship of psychiatric morbidity to experiences in battle and nonbattle settings. This figure illustrates the risk of psychiatric breakdown in troops ranging from garrison settings through combat and postcombat situations. As is apparent, troops are at greatest risk during combat; however, increased risk of breakdown precedes and follows combat.

who broke down after his unit experienced 4 to 5½ months of combat exposure could be returned to full combat duty in 70% to 89% of cases, those exposed over 1 year returned in only 32% to 36% of cases.

Beebe and Appel[33] analyzed the World War II combat attrition of a cohort of 1,000 soldiers from the European Theater of Operations (ETO). They found that the breaking point of the average rifleman in the Mediterranean Theater of Operations (MTO) was 88 days of company combat, that is, days in which the company sustained at least one casualty. A company combat day averaged 7.8 calendar days in the MTO and 3.6 calendar days in the ETO. They found that due to varying causes of attrition in both theaters, including death, wounding, and transfers, by company combat day 50, nine of 10 "original" soldiers had departed. In their projections, Beebe and Appel found that if only psychiatric casualties occurred, there would be a 90% depletion by company combat day 210; however, due to other causes of attrition (transfer, death, wounding, illness), the unit would be virtually depleted by company combat day 80 or 90, approximately the breaking point of the median man.[33(p92)]

Noy[34] reviewed the work of Beebe and Appel and found that soldiers who departed as psychiatric casualties had actually stayed longer in combat duties than medical and disciplinary cases and that their breakdowns were more related to exposure to battle trauma than were medical and disciplinary cases.

From studies of cumulative stress such as these as well as observations of the efficacy of a "point system" (so many points of credit toward rotation from combat per unit of time in combat or so many combat missions of aircrews) used during World War II, the value of periodic rest from combat and of rotation came to be understood.[19(p1002)]

The final and perhaps most important lesson of World War II was the importance of group cohesion not only in preventing breakdown,[19] but also in producing effectiveness in combat. This latter point is demonstrated by Marshall's[35] account of soldiers parachuted into Normandy. The imprecision of this operation resulted in some units being composed of soldiers who were strangers to each other and others with varying numbers who had trained together. Uniformly, those units of strangers were completely ineffective. In *Men Against Fire*, Marshall[36] had also observed that only a small percentage (about 15%) of soldiers actually fired their rifles at the enemy during World War II but that in group firing activities, among members of crew-served weapons teams such as machine guns, the percentage was much higher.

This element of group cohesion has already been alluded to in terms of morale and leadership. Marshall again probably made the point best in reviewing his experiences in World War I, World War II, Korea, and various Arab-Israeli wars:

> When fire sweeps the field, be it in Sinai, Pork Chop Hill or along the Normandy coast, nothing keeps a man from running except a sense of honor, of bound obligation to people right around him, of fear of failure in their sight which might eternally disgrace him.[37(p304)]

Cohesion is so important in both prevention and treatment of psychiatric casualties that Matthew D. Parrish, an eminent psychiatrist who served in combat aircrews during World War II and as U.S. Army Neuropsychiatry Consultant in Vietnam, has suggested it as another principle of forward treatment.[38] Parrish observed that combat fatigue patients who had regular visits from their units in which they were welcomed to return, were far more likely to do so. He suggested that this preventive and curative principle be termed "membership."

In the words of Parrish,

> [T]he principles of *proximity, immediacy, simplicity, expectancy* ... seem to imply that the medics are trying to get the individual so strong within his own separate self that he will be an effective soldier. Thus we would have a newly pre-combat person with a strong character and therefore could be predicted to perform well. There is no ... mention of the principle [of] ... the maintenance of his bonded membership in his particular crew, squad or team (at least no larger than company). This bonding maintained, he never faces combat alone. In Vietnam, when possible, the entire such primary group would visit the casualty, keep him alive to the life of the group and show him the other members' need for him. Often an "ambassador" would visit and leave a sign on the casualty's bed announcing that he was a proud member of his unit. (This sort of thing was effective for some medical and surgical casualties too, who could easily have developed the evacuation syndrome.)
> What did we call this 5th principle? All I can think of is *membership*. Of course, like everything else in psychiatry, it is ultimately a command responsibility—yet its effectiveness is in the hands of team leaders and the troops themselves....[38]

In summary, World War II taught combat psychiatrists that psychiatric casualties are an inevitable consequence of life-threatening hostilities, that they cannot be efficiently screened out ahead of time, that their numbers depend on individual, unit, and combat environmental factors, and that appropriate interventions can return the majority to combat duty.

Validation and Limitations of Principles

Just as in the initial battles of World War II, provisions had not been made for psychiatric casualties in the early months of the Korean conflict (1950–1953). As a result they were evacuated from the combat zone. Due largely to the efforts of Colonel Albert J. Glass (Figure 1-6), a veteran of World War II, who was assigned as Theater Neuropsychiatry Consultant, the U.S. combat psychiatric treatment program was soon in effect and generally functioning well.[39] Since only 5 years had elapsed, the lessons of World War II were still well known and the principles learned during that war were applied appropriately. Combat stress casualties were treated forward, usually by battalion surgeons and sometimes by an experienced aidman or even the soldiers' "buddies," and returned to duty. Psychiatric casualties accounted for only about 5% of medical out-of-country evacuations, and some of these (treated in Japan) were returned to the combat zone.[39] To prevent psychiatric casualties, a rotation system was in effect (9 months in combat or 13 months in support units).[39] In addition, attempts were made to rest individuals ("R and R" or rest and recreation) and, if tactically possible, whole units. Marshall[40] warned of the dangers to unit cohesion of rotating individuals, but this lesson was not to be learned until the Vietnam conflict.

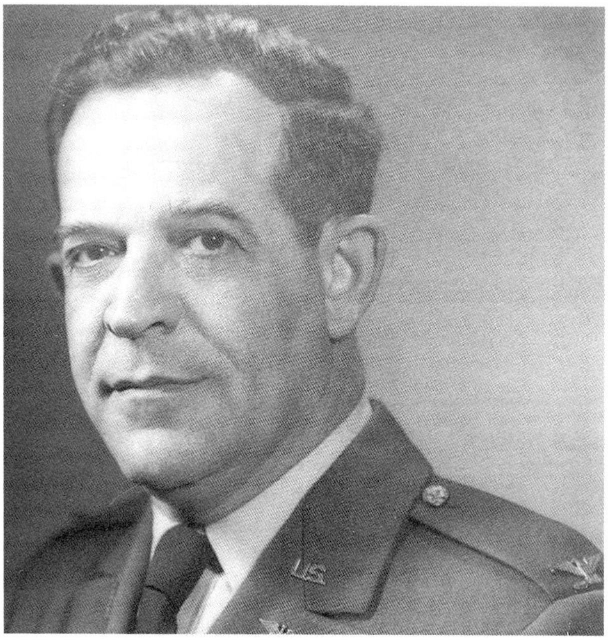

Fig. 1-6. Albert Julius Glass taught and popularized the principles of forward treatment throughout his life. He was a division psychiatrist in World War II, where his experiences shaped his views of appropriate care of stress casualties. In the Korean conflict, as Theater Neuropsychiatry Consultant, he instituted policies that maximized the effectiveness of treatment of psychiatric casualties. Subsequently, he applied these principles to the garrison military as Psychiatry and Neurology Consultant to the U.S. Army Surgeon General, resulting in closure of five of the six U.S. Army prisons. After his retirement from the military, he edited *Neuropsychiatry in World War II*, the two-volume official history of neuropsychiatry in the Zone of the Interior (Vol 1) and the Overseas Theaters (Vol 2).

These procedures appear to have been quite effective with two possible exceptions. One was the development of frostbite as an evacuation syndrome. This condition, which was the first psychiatric condition described in the British literature during World War I,[41] was almost completely preventable, yet accounted for significant numbers of "ineffectives."

The other problem was an unrecognized portent of the psychiatric problems of rear-area support troops. As the war progressed, U.S. support troops increased in number until they greatly outnumbered combat troops. These support troops were seldom in life-endangering situations. Their psychological stresses were related more to separation from home and friends, social and sometimes physical deprivations, and boredom. Paradoxically, support troops who may have avoided the stress of combat, according to a combat veteran and military historian, were deprived of the enhancement of self-esteem provided by such exposure.[42] To an extent the situation resembled that of the nostalgic soldiers of prior centuries. In these circumstances the soldier sought relief in alcohol abuse (and, in coastal areas, in drug abuse)[43] and sexual stimulation. These often resulted in disciplinary infractions. Except for attempts to prevent venereal diseases, these problems were scarcely noticed at the time, a lesson not learned.

The Korean conflict revealed that the appropriate use of the principles of combat psychiatry could result in the return to battle of up to 90% of combat psychiatric casualties; however, there was a failure to recognize the types of casualties that can occur among rear-echelon soldiers.[11] These "garrison casualties" later became the predominant psychiatric

TABLE 1-2

SELECTED CAUSES OF ADMISSION TO HOSPITAL AND QUARTERS AMONG ACTIVE DUTY U.S. ARMY PERSONNEL IN VIETNAM, 1965–1970

	Rate Expressed as Number of Admissions (per 1,000 Average Strength)					
Cause	**1965**	**1966**	**1967**	**1968**	**1969**	**1970**
Wounded in Action	61.6	74.8	84.1	120.4	87.6	52.9
Neuropsychiatric Conditions	11.7	12.3	10.5	13.3	15.8	25.1
Viral Hepatitis	5.7	4.0	7.0	8.6	6.4	7.2
Venereal Disease (includes CRO*)	277.4	281.5	240.5	195.8	199.5	222.9
Venereal Disease (excludes CRO*)	3.6	3.8	2.6	2.2	1.0	1.4

*CRO: Carded for record only, ie, not hospitalized
Adapted from Neel S. *Vietnam Studies: Medical Support of the US Army in Vietnam, 1965–1970.* Washington, DC: US Department of the Army; 1973: 36.

casualties of the Vietnam conflict.[11] Vietnam and the Arab-Israeli wars revealed limitations to the traditional principles of combat psychiatry.

America's longest conflict, Vietnam (1961–1975), can best be viewed from a psychiatric perspective as encompassing three phases: (1) an advisory period with few combatants and almost no psychiatric casualties; (2) a build-up period with large numbers of combatants but few psychiatric casualties; and (3) a withdrawal period in which relatively large numbers of psychiatric casualties took forms other than traditional combat fatigue symptomatology.

During the initial phases of the build-up in Vietnam, the psychiatric program was fully in place, with abundant mental health resources and psychiatrists fairly conversant with the principles of combat psychiatry. Combat stress casualties, however, failed to materialize. Throughout the entire conflict, even with a liberal definition of combat fatigue, less than 5% (and nearer to 2%) of casualties were placed in this category.[11]

The Vietnam conflict produced a number of paradoxes in terms of the traditional understanding of psychiatric casualties. Most spectacular was the low rate of identified psychiatric casualties generally and, in particular, the relative absence of the transient anxiety states currently termed combat fatigue or combat reaction. Table 1-2, taken from statistics compiled by Neel,[44] reveals that the Vietnam conflict was unusual in that the psychiatric casualty rate did not vary directly with the wounded-in-action rate. Despite the decline of the wounded-in-action rate by more than half in 1970 compared with the high in 1968, the neuropsychiatric casualty rate in 1970 was almost double the 1968 rate. In other words, wounded-in-action and neuropsychiatric casualty rates showed an inverse relationship that was unique to the Vietnam conflict until the 1982 Lebanon War.

This was contrary to prior experience and expectations. For example, Datel,[45] in reviewing neuropsychiatric rates since 1915, showed that in the U.S. Army the rates had previously peaked coincidentally with combat intensity (1918, 1943, and 1951) but in the Vietnam conflict they peaked after the war was over (1973), as seen in Figure 1-7.

In one study of combat psychiatric casualties in Vietnam[46] during the first 6 months of 1966, less than 5% of cases were labeled "combat exhaustion." Most cases presented with behavioral or somatic complaints.

This initially (1965–1967) low incidence of neuropsychiatric cases in Vietnam was posited by Jones[47] to reflect the low incidence of combat fatigue in Vietnam compared to other wars. This low incidence of combat fatigue was in turn attributed to the 12-month rotation policy, the absence of heavy and prolonged artillery barrages, and the use of seasoned and motivated troops. Because the rate of psychiatric cases did not increase with increased utilization of drafted troops in 1966 as compared to 1965, the latter consideration seems less important. Other explanations of the low incidence of psychiatric cases included thorough training of troops,

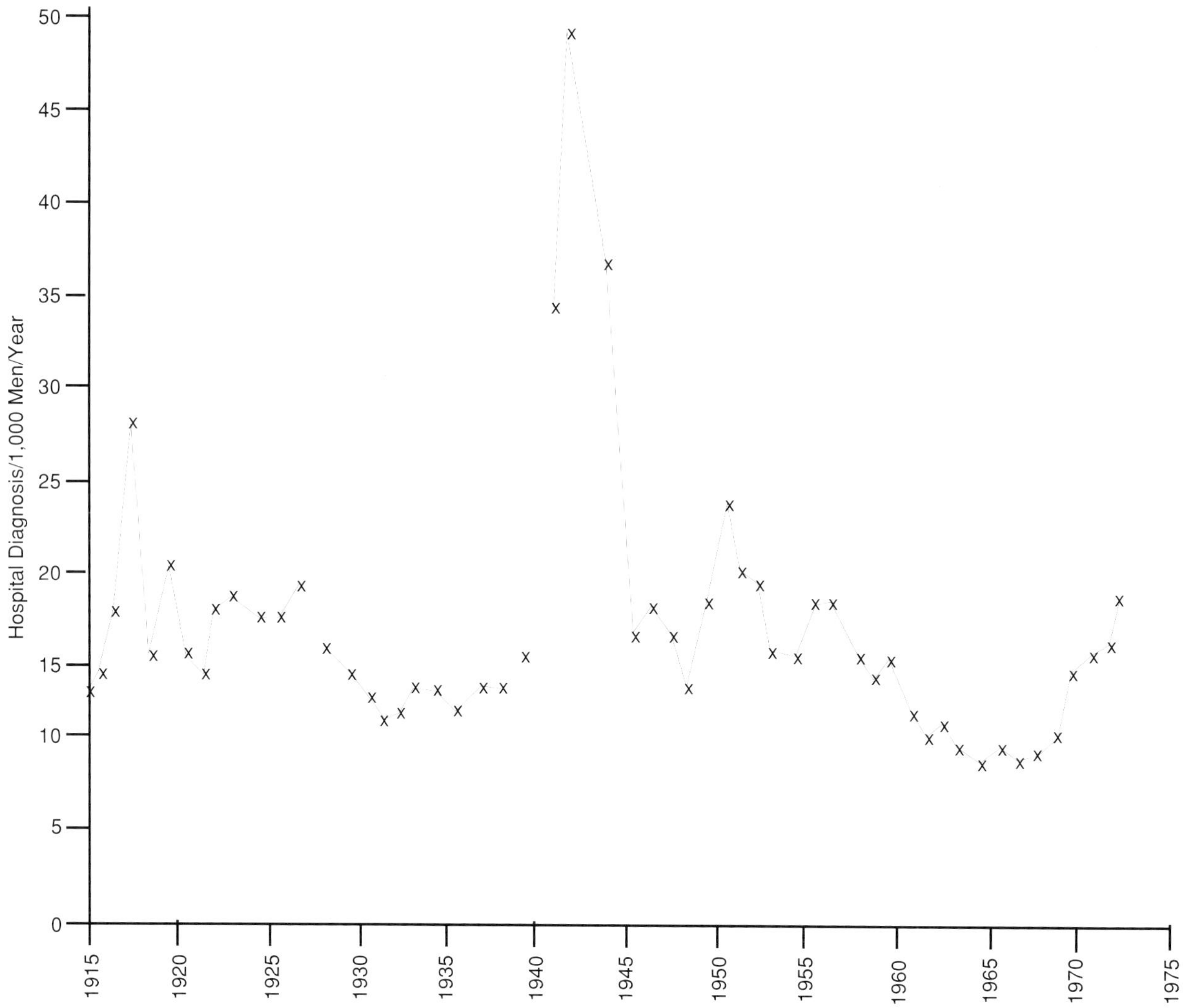

Fig. 1-7. Incidence of neuropsychiatric disorders, U.S. Army worldwide, active duty, 1915–1975. The incidence of neuropsychiatric disorders peaks during and immediately after major wars. Reprinted from Datel WE. *A Summary of Source Data in Military Psychiatric Epidemiology*. Alexandria, Va: Defense Technical Information Center (ADA 021265); 1976.

troops' confidence in their weapons and means of mobility, helicopter evacuation of wounded, early treatment of psychiatric casualties in an atmosphere of strong expectation of rapid return to duty, and a type of combat that consisted largely of brief skirmishes followed by rests in a secure base camp. Fatigue and anxiety did not have a chance to build up.[11]

Huffman[48] suggested that a factor in the low incidence of psychiatric cases was the effectiveness of stateside psychiatric screening of troops being sent to Vietnam. This possibly affected in a sporadic way the initial deployment of troops because some company level commanders did attempt to eliminate "oddballs" from their units in anticipation of future noneffectiveness; however, no organized screening program beyond basic combat and advanced individual training was in effect.

In an interesting sociological and psychodynamic analysis of 1,200 U.S. Marine Corps and U.S. Navy personnel serving in the Vietnam combat zone, Renner[49] suggested that the true picture was not one of diminished psychiatric casualties but rather of hidden casualties manifested in various character and behavior disorders. These character and behavior disorders were "hidden" in the sense that they did not present with classical fatigue or anxiety symptoms but rather with substance abuse and disciplinary infractions. Renner developed evidence supporting an explanation of character and behavior disorders based on a general alienation of the soldier from the goals of the military unit. He contrasted support units with combat units, noting that the former faced less external danger, allowing greater expression of the basic alienation that he regarded as present among virtually all U.S. troops in Vietnam. He attributed this alienation to the lack of group cohesiveness largely resulting from the policy of rotating individuals and disillusionment with the war after 12 months. The result was that the prime motivative behaviors became personal survival, revenge for the deaths of friends, and enjoyment of unleashing aggression. These in turn produced not only disordered behavior reflected in increased character and behavior disorder rates but also feelings of guilt and depression. Alienation from the unit and the U.S. Army led to the formation of regressive alternative groups based on race, alcohol or drug consumption, delinquent and hedonistic behavior, and countercultural life styles.

A second paradox in the Vietnam conflict was the development of greatly increased rates of psychosis in U.S. Army troops[11] (Figure 1-8). Datel[45] showed that this was a worldwide phenomenon of all active duty personnel, but especially of U.S. Army troops (see Figure 1-7). Like the total neuropsychiatric incidence rate previously mentioned, the psychosis rate also peaked after active combat. Previous experience had shown only minor increases in the psychosis rate during wartime. In both combat and noncombat situations the psychosis rate had remained stable at approximately two or three per 1,000 troops per year.[7]

Hayes[50] suggested two hypotheses to explain the increase in psychoses. One was the increased precipitation of schizophrenia and other psychotic reactions in predisposed persons by their use of psychoactive drugs. The other was the tendency of recently trained psychiatrists to classify borderline syndromes as latent schizophrenia, while more experienced psychiatrists would have chosen a different nosological category (presumably character and behavior disorders).

Jones and Johnson[11] suggested that the doubling of the psychosis rate in the U.S. Army Vietnam (USARV) troops in 1969 was due not to drug precipitation of schizophrenia or styles of diagnosis per se but rather due to the influence of drugs in confusing the diagnosis. Holloway[51] showed that large scale abuse of drugs other than marijuana and alcohol began about 1968. Approximately 5% of departing soldiers were excreting detectable heroin products in the summer of 1971; however, this fell to about 3% when the screening became publicized. Soldiers frequently took potent hallucinogens as well as marijuana and heroin. Jones and Johnson[11] showed that out-of-country evacuations were essentially reserved for psychotics until the beginning of 1971 (Figure 1-9) but with the advent of emphasis on drug abuse identification and rehabilitation, often by detoxification and evacuation to stateside rehabilitation programs, an alternative diagnosis was available. Finding a new diagnostic category for soldiers who just did not belong in a combat zone, namely, drug dependence, the evacuating psychiatrists stopped using the schizophrenia label. This is reflected in the decline in psychosis back to approximately two per 1,000 troops per year.[11] Also, fluctuation began to increase due to the smaller samples.

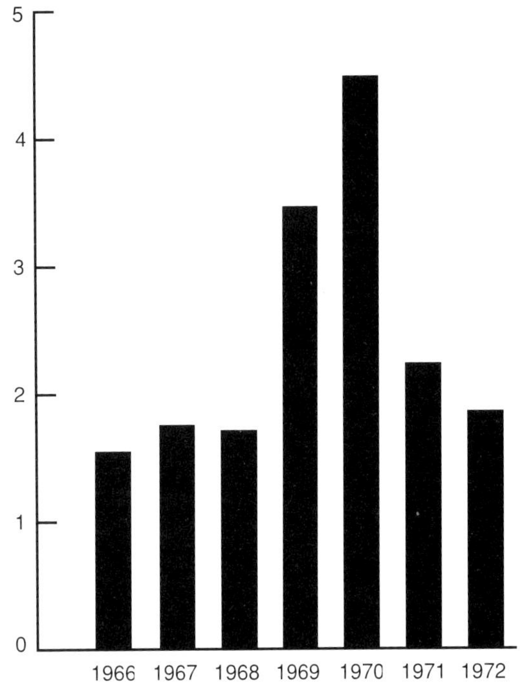

Fig. 1-8. Annual psychosis rates, U.S. Army Vietnam, per 1,000 strength, 1966–1972. In all kinds of military settings, combat and noncombat, the rate of psychosis in troops averaged about 2 per 1,000 per year until the war in Vietnam. The paradox, that is the doubling of the normal psychosis rate of military troops in Vietnam in 1969 and 1970, was thought by the author to be due to the influence of illegal drugs in confusing the diagnosis. This rate declined when drug abuse treatment facilities became available in 1971. Adapted with permission from Jones FD, Johnson AW. Medical and psychiatric treatment policy and practice in Vietnam. *J Soc Issues.* 1975;31(4):63.

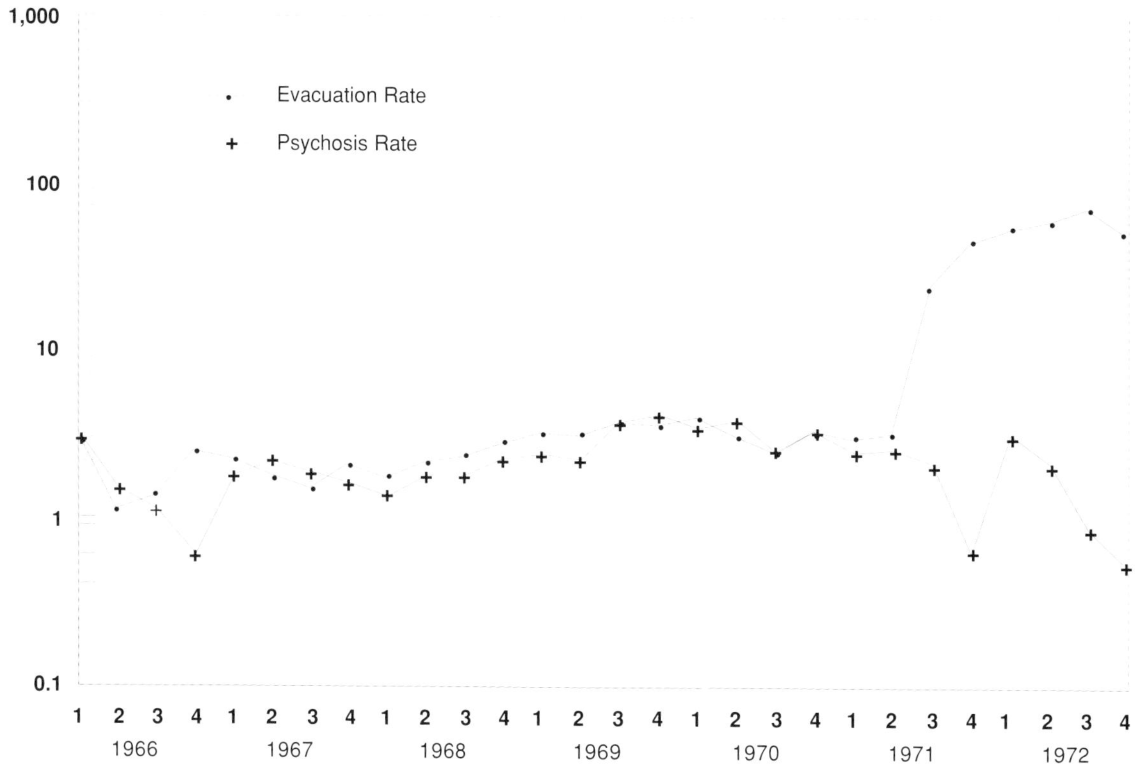

Fig. 1-9. Quarterly psychosis and out-of-country psychiatric evacuation rates, U.S. Army Vietnam, per 1,000 strength, 1966–1972. This figure illustrates that out-of-country evacuations were predominantly reserved for psychotics until the beginning of 1971. With the advent of emphasis on drug abuse identification and rehabilitation, often by detoxification and evacuation to stateside drug programs, an alternative diagnosis was available. The result was a decline of the psychosis rate to its expected level of about 2 per 1,000 troops per year, but an exponential increase in out-of-country evacuations, primarily drug-abusing patients, to a level exceeding 100 per 1,000 troops per year. Adapted with permission from Jones FD, Johnson AW. Medical and psychiatric treatment policy and practice in Vietnam. *J Soc Issues*. 1975;31(4):62.

In other overseas areas the U.S. Army policy of not evacuating persons with character and behavior problems, including drug dependence, still held; therefore, the psychiatrist seeing a patient who did not belong overseas might label him with a psychosis, especially if the patient described perceptual distortions and unusual experiences. Such a psychiatrist might be applying a broad categorization of schizophrenia as Hayes suggests. Because U.S. Air Force and U.S. Navy psychiatrists have generally had more latitude in being permitted to evacuate patients with character and behavior problems than have U.S. Army psychiatrists, one would expect their rates of psychosis to be lower, and, in fact, they were. This may explain the discrepancy between Datel's worldwide psychosis rate with diagnoses by U.S. Navy, U.S. Air Force, and U.S. Army psychiatrists and Jones and Johnson's Vietnam psychosis rate with diagnoses by U.S. Army psychiatrists only.

Vietnam revealed the limits of World War II-type psychiatric treatment policy in a low-intensity, prolonged, unpopular conflict. Such conflicts, if they cannot be avoided, must be approached with primary prevention as the focus. Career soldiers with strong unit cohesion will not endanger themselves, their fellows, or their careers by abusing alcohol or drugs. When casualties do occur, the Larrey treatment for nostalgia, mentioned earlier, can be used as a model.[6]

Since World War II (as, indeed, long before World War II), the Middle East has experienced essentially continual conflict of every conceivable nature. Exhibit 1-3 illustrates the variety of these conflicts, ranging from state-sponsored terrorism, in which countries fight indirectly and often by proxy, through low-intensity and guerrilla warfare to high-intensity and even chemical warfare. The significance of terrorist activities should not be minimized. In 1983, a single terrorist suicide attack killed 241 U.S. Marines on a peace-keeping mission

EXHIBIT 1-3

POST-WORLD WAR II MIDDLE-EAST CONFLICTS

1948: Israel fought the Arab League in a civil war which became Israel's war of independence

1956: Egypt fought the tripartite powers (France, Great Britain, and Israel) when they attempted to prevent Egypt from asserting sovereignty over the Suez Canal; ie, repulsion of former colonial powers

1962: Egypt fought against the Royalists in the Yemen Civil War, somewhat similar to the U.S. involvement in Vietnam, a guerrilla war

1967: Israel launched a preemptive surprise attack on Egypt and her allies, a conventional medium-intensity war but of brief duration

1968–1970: Arab-Israeli War of Attrition, a war with a static front and primarily indirect fire, thus having some similarity to World War I

1973: Egypt launched a surprise attack on the Israelis in what became an example of high-intensity, high-technology, continuous combat

1982: Israel bombed a nuclear reactor in Iraq, thus even a "nuclear" war (but radioactive material had not yet been acquired by Iraq)

1982: Israel attacked Palestine Liberation Organization forces in Lebanon, a state within a state. This was a war fought in an area of high-density civilian population, with besieged cities reminiscent of the latter phases of World War II

1980-1988: Iraq-Iran War, primarily a conventional war but with the use of chemical agents

1989–1990: Intifada in Israeli-occupied Palestinian territories. Urban guerrilla war carried out largely by adolescents repressed by Israeli army

1991: Persian Gulf War; U.S.-led coalition war against Iraq was primarily an uncontested aerial attack for 5 weeks followed by a 4-day ground assault using conventional weapons

1991: Iraqi war between the established government and Shiite and Kurdish minorities

Adapted from Jones FD. Lessons of the Middle Eastern Wars. Originally presented at Grand Rounds, Psychiatry Department, Walter Reed Army Medical Center; March 15, 1984 with subsequent updates; Washington, DC.

in Beirut, producing nearly as many deaths as the Spanish-American War.[52,53]

The periodic wars between Israel and its Arab neighbors have served as a human factors laboratory as well as a testing ground for technological developments in weapons systems (see Exhibit 1-3). In 1967, Egyptian ground troops, surprised by Israel with its air superiority, had a feeling of helplessness that resulted in large numbers of psychiatric casualties. Having been surprised by Israel in the 1967 Six Day War, the Arabs had learned the effectiveness of surprise so well that Israel was almost defeated before it could organize its defenses against the sudden 1973 Arab attack. From the perspective of psychiatric breakdown, the 1973 Yom Kippur War is most instructive. For the first time Israel suffered significant combat stress casualties, initially reported as 10% of total casualties, but later estimated to be from 30% to 50%.[54] The 10% rate was artificially low because casualties treated at forward medical facilities and returned to duty were not counted; only those disabled longer than 4 days and sent to rear hospitals were counted. In addition, soldiers who were psychiatrically disabled but also had light wounds were not counted as psychiatric casualties but as wounded in action. Finally, psychiatric casualties occurring after 26 October 1973 (2 days after the cease-fire) were not counted.

The Egyptians also reported high psychiatric casualties, but most occurred later when the tide of battle began to favor Israel. El Sudany El Rayes[55] reported that in some units "the surgical and psychiatric casualties were equal." The Egyptians treated psychiatric casualties according to then-Soviet doctrine, which called for forward treatment similar to that advocated by the U.S. Army. They were unable to apply this doctrine, however, because there was no safe forward area. As a result, casualties were sent to distant facilities where they became chronically disabled. The author saw some of these patients on a consultant visit to Maadhi

Military Hospital, Cairo in 1984. Their symptoms were of severe PTSD.

Unexpectedly, the rate of the 1973 Israeli combat stress casualties was highest among support personnel who, although sometimes exposed to hostile fire, were probably responding primarily to the trauma of seeing their dead and mutilated comrades. Israeli support troops additionally felt comparatively helpless during this threat to national survival. According to a former Deputy Surgeon General of the Israeli Defence Forces,[56] many support personnel took up weapons and fought alongside combat troops. These Israeli combat support soldiers have traditionally been considered to have less aptitude for the military; those with higher intelligence and leadership ability are allocated to combat units.

Factors contributing to psychiatric casualties in all units in the 1973 war were surprise, fear of national destruction, lack of expectation or preparation for psychiatric casualties, and the hasty constitution of reserve units by personnel who had not trained together (impaired cohesion).[22]

However, the primary generator of initial stress casualties may be the unparalleled intensity of sustained combat with numerous mutilated victims. This is suggested by results in the June 1982 Lebanon War, which again saw a relatively high (23%) stress casualty rate.[57] Because the factors of combat other than intensity (surprise, lack of cohesion, and national vulnerability) were absent, intensity alone may be a predominant factor in producing combat stress casualties. It must be noted that the majority of acute combat stress casualties occurred during 2 weeks early in June when fighting was intense though not as intense as that during the first week of the 1973 war. The role of expectancy may have contributed to the relatively high rates of psychiatric casualties in Lebanon, where frequent visits of field psychologists to units may have produced an expectancy that psychiatric casualties would occur. This may have led to overdiagnosis of soldiers with normal battle reaction symptoms as casualties and may have conveyed the impression that becoming a psychiatric casualty was acceptable.[57]

As in the 1973 Yom Kippur War, during the 1982 Lebanon War, some psychiatric casualties were evacuated to civilian treatment facilities far rearwards, bypassing the forward treatment teams. Very few of these soldiers returned to combat. In contrast, about half of the stress casualties were treated in forward facilities, and almost all of these soldiers returned to their combat units.[22]

After the Lebanon War, large numbers of delayed or chronic post-traumatic stress disorders appeared, perhaps similar to the experience after Vietnam. Both were wars in which many civilian bystanders became casualties. Belenky[57] has reported that after the initial casualties related to the active combat in June 1982 (25%, with most occurring during the 2 weeks of active combat), there was a continuing influx of psychiatric patients among the participants. Ultimately the majority of cases developed subsequent to combat.

The Arab-Israeli conflicts have continued to validate the significance of factors preventing or promoting breakdown in combat, and they have validated the efficacy of forward treatment.[58] These conflicts have also revealed the weaknesses of this treatment approach in high-intensity, high-technology, mobile, and sustained combat in which there may be no relatively safe forward area at which rest and recuperation can occur. Treatment is further jeopardized by inadequate capability to return the casualty to his unit because of the high mobility and wide dispersion of combat units in actions. These conflicts have not yielded treatment approaches that can prevent chronic and delayed post-traumatic stress disorders.

As in so many prolonged wars, the 1980 Soviet military assistance to the unpopular leaders of its client state, Afghanistan (1980–1989), led not to a quick return to ante-bellum stability but rather to a prolonged conflict with no foreseeable resolution. The Soviet lack of military success against determined guerrilla forces, despite sophisticated weaponry including chemical agents,[59] has been likened to the U.S. experience in Vietnam. In fact, Soviet combat casualties have been reported at about 70,000, of which approximately 13,000 were killed.[60]

Afghan partisans viewed the presence of over 110,000 Soviet soldiers as just another invasion by their ancient Russian enemies, thus their morale in protecting their homeland remained high. Soviet soldiers, fighting on foreign soil against elusive enemies remarkably similar to the friends whom they came to help, reportedly experienced problems with alcoholism, drug abuse, and disciplinary infractions.[61] Similarly, returning soldiers have suffered from PTSD.[62]

An adverse morale factor for combatants on both sides of a conflict consists of observing the displacement of friendly or enemy civilians, usually women, children, and the elderly, from their homes. This was seen in the dislocation of large numbers of Vietnamese civilians by the strategic hamlet policy to neutralize the guerrilla support bases. Similarly, the Afghan War resulted in the generation of hundreds of thousands of refugees, most of whom fled to Pakistan.[63] Thus, Afghanistan is an object lesson in the problems met by industrialized nations in fighting low-intensity, unpopular foreign wars against indigenous guerrilla forces. Except with strictest government censorship (not available in a democratic country), refugee flight engenders antiwar sentiments, lack of public support for the war, and ultimately poor soldier morale.

In the midst of the turmoil that characterized the Iranian revolution in 1980, forces from neighboring Iraq seized control of disputed border territories, thereby initiating a conflict that raged about 8 years (1980–1988). An unusual mixture of high- and low-technology fighting, the Iraq-Iran War resembled World War I in the use of chemical agents and the relatively static front. Casualty patterns initially were similar to those in World War I. Early reports of Iranian psychiatric casualties indicated that many of them suffered from "explosion blow," which resembled the "shell shock" of World War I. Initially attributed to concussion, these cases were later viewed by Iranian psychiatrists as having psychogenic causes and requiring treatment similar to that given combat fatigue cases of more recent wars.[64] An additional similarity of this war to World War I was the report of the Iraqi use of chemical agents.[65] This may have been particularly terrifying to Islamic soldiers who believed that for death in battle in a holy war to lead them to the Islamic paradise, the combat must involve the shedding of blood. Anecdotal reports indicate that this morale problem was alleviated by Islamic holy men who informed the soldiers that the chemicals altered the blood to render it useless in a way analogous to its being shed. Post-traumatic stress disorders occurred primarily among displaced civilians.[66]

Although low-intensity, guerrilla-type conflicts have recently occurred or are occurring in numerous parts of the world (Ulster, Cambodia, Angola, Sri Lanka, Nicaragua, El Salvador, Peru, Colombia, West Irian, and the Philippines, to name a few), there are no data to suggest that psychiatric casualties have been a significant variable even though many of these conflicts might be characterized as psychological warfare. Some psychiatric lessons and casualty figures are presented below from the Falkland Islands War in 1982, the U.S. invasion of Grenada in 1983, the U.S. invasion of Panama in 1989, and the Persian Gulf War in 1991.

The Falkland Islands War lasted only 73 days, 45 of which involved significant combat.[67–69] This conflict involved high-technology weaponry in the midst of harsh environmental conditions and primitive hand-to-hand combat. Apparently intending only a limited police action to publicize their territorial claims, Argentine forces occupied the major part of the Falkland Islands. While this action quelled political unrest at home, it was so popular that public opinion did not allow the Argentine forces to withdraw expeditiously. The result was a short, bitterly fought land, sea, and air war with Britain.

Most of the British soldiers had ample opportunity to prepare and acclimate in the leisurely 2-week transatlantic cruise from England. British troops were also able to practice amphibious assault landings on St. George's Island, which was still under British control.[70] Airplane pilots, however, often flew directly to the combat zone. Benzodiazepine hypnotics were successfully used to regulate sleep and prevent fatigue in pilots.[67]

Major casualties on both sides occurred from naval fighting. Of the over 1,700 Argentine forces killed and wounded, 368 seamen (of the 1,000 aboard) were killed when a British nuclear submarine sank an Argentine cruiser.[68] Most of the approximately 1,000 British casualties (250 dead, 750 wounded[69]) occurred during the destruction of five ships by air-launched bombs and missiles.[71]

Psychiatric casualties among combatants on both sides were surprisingly low. This may have been due to the fact that becoming a psychiatric casualty did not result in evacuation. In British forces psychiatric casualties were reported as less than 2% of total casualties; however, 20% of the land forces casualties were from immersion foot.[67] The latter probably resulted more from the terrain and weather than from psychogenic causes. Collazo[72] reported that psychiatric casualties were also quite low in Argentine forces, representing about 4% to 5% of total combat casualties (wounded in action [WIA] and killed in action [KIA]). These figures are probably equivalent to the British figures if the British figures were to exclude medical casualties (immersion foot, infections, etc.) and include WIA and KIA only. In one Argentine unit exposed to heavy naval and air bombardment for 45 days, however, psychiatric casualties represented 14% of total casualties.[72] One surprise among Argentine psychiatric casualties was that the percentage of officers afflicted was higher than that of enlisted men. This may simply reflect the greater likelihood of enlisted to be wounded compared with officers. Significant numbers of post-traumatic stress disorder cases were reported among British forces after the war.[73]

The Falkland Islands War reveals again that while psychiatric casualties are rare in elite forces (British), they do occur. Furthermore, the absence of an evacuation route for psychiatric casualties (Argentine forces) contributes to low rates of such casualties. When becoming a psychiatric casualty does not offer an evacuation from combat, there is little reinforcement for becoming a casualty. In future wars, the possible use of drugs to regulate sleep and improve performance in combatants who have been rapidly deployed across multiple time zones is suggested by the British use of temazepam (Restoril) and triazolam (Halcion) for some of their airplane pilots.

In late October 1983, American forces invaded the small Caribbean island country of Grenada, whose leadership had been assassinated by a Communist splinter group. Operation Urgent Fury was undertaken to insure the safety of about 1,000 Americans, including 700 medical students, and to restore order as requested by Grenada's neighboring island countries.[74] Most of the 19 Americans killed in Grenada died from accidents, although U.S. forces did meet stiff resistance from 600 well-armed and professionally trained Cuban soldiers.[74] Because elite forces (Rangers, SEALS [SEa Air Land commandos], and airborne units) made the assault, few psychiatric casualties were expected, and few occurred (three so designated in 3,000 invading troops with 19 KIA and 73 WIA).[52]

Dehydration and heat exhaustion casualties accounted for most of the preventable casualties. Fullerton[74] debriefed most of the commanders after combat had ended. He reported that one battalion suffered 29 heat casualties in a single day but another battalion suffered only two heat casualties on the same day, while both engaged in virtually identical tasks. The commander of the latter battalion had emphasized water discipline.

Some of the wounded soldiers suffered delayed post-traumatic stress disorders.[74,75] Mateczun and Holmes-Johnson[52] had an interesting opportunity to compare the psychological adjustment of U.S. Marines wounded in the Grenada invasion with those wounded in the Beirut massacre when casualties from both incidents arrived almost simultaneously at Bethesda Naval Hospital in Maryland. About 25 U.S. Marines, more from Beirut than Grenada, were treated in a psychiatric consultation-liaison model with "group therapy" as the primary intervention. The group therapy was modeled after Marshall's[76] group debriefing technique; however, the Beirut casualties had less to recount because they were sleeping when the bomb exploded. Their memories centered on feelings of helplessness and fear of dying before rescuers could reach them. Survivor guilt was high among Beirut casualties but almost absent among Grenada casualties. Both groups had post-traumatic stress symptoms (nightmares, intrusive thoughts, anxiety), but Grenada casualties had high morale and a strong desire to return to the combat unit. In contrast, the Beirut casualties wanted to go home. These differences in symptoms are attributable to the different forms of combat. In Beirut, the U.S. Marines had no clear enemies or mission, and some viewed themselves as vulnerable targets, whereas U.S. forces in Grenada had a clear mission with a known enemy and had numerical and logistical superiority.

Belenky[75] interviewed a dozen men wounded in Grenada who had been evacuated to Walter Reed Army Medical Center in Washington, D.C. The main lessons reported from Belenky's observations included the need to emphasize self/buddy aid, communication, and water discipline. He also noted that clear evacuation channels for the wounded were necessary.

In December 1989, U.S. combined forces invaded Panama in Operation Just Cause to oust the military dictator Manuel Noriega and his loyal soldiers. The experience was similar to that of Grenada. One difference was the presence of women in military police units who engaged in combat. With few exceptions they acquitted themselves well.

Stokes,[77] in his capacity as the Combat Stress Action Officer for the U.S. Army Medical Department Center and School, reviewed mental health issues in Operation Just Cause. He reports that no unit mental health personnel or formal stress holding capability was deployed to Panama in conjunction with the operation due to the priority given to combatants and weaponry. During the combat phase of the operation, which lasted only a few days, some soldiers evidencing symptoms of combat stress reaction were given nonstressful duties in their units without being evacuated. Stokes reports only one case in which medical personnel (U.S. Air Force nurses at Howard Air Force Base in Panama) successfully held and returned to duty a "classic" battle fatigue casualty. This occurred on the third or fourth night of Operation Just Cause (after the surgical mass casualty was over).[77]

Many soldiers with potentially "return to duty" medical conditions, including Rangers and Airborne, were evacuated to military hospitals in San Antonio, Texas through the mobile aeromedical staging facility (MASF) at Howard Air Force Base over the first several days. These cases included minor orthopedic injuries (most parachute-assault related), heat exhaustion, and other conditions such as headache in a soldier whose helmet had been struck by a bullet (but not penetrated) while he was shielding his dead buddy who had been killed by a sniper. These evacuations were because Howard Air Force Base had only surgical teams, very limited x-ray and laboratory capability, no holding personnel, and many surgical casualties.[77]

Many of these elite soldiers were mortified that they had been evacuated to San Antonio for what to them were "dishonorable" or "shameful" injuries. One broke down crying on being told that his ankle was only sprained. One officer was going to refuse the Purple Heart he was to receive on television, on grounds that he didn't deserve it (although the combat assault in which he had injured himself was from 250 feet altitude, on a moonless night, under fire, with full combat load, onto a concrete runway). He was finally persuaded by the chief ward nurse to take it without making a scene. Some soldiers left behind the decorations they had been given when they were evacuated further to home base. Informal follow-up has indicated that some of these elite soldiers suffered post-traumatic stress symptoms and sought treatment covertly at a Department of Veterans Affairs center or left the service.[77]

Two soldiers were sent to a nearby U.S. military hospital several days after they had presented with stress-type symptoms. The hospital was not staffed, configured, or geographically located to function as a combat stress recovery unit or restoration center. These two soldiers were evaluated in the busy admissions area and admitted on the psychiatric ward. After several more days, both were administratively/medically evacuated to the continental United States via Brooke Army Medical Center in Texas with psychiatric labels. Stokes interviewed both at Brooke Army Medical Center, and considered both evacuations to have been inappropriate, although one became inevitable once the soldier was admitted to the psychiatric ward and reacted by behaving like the adolescent psychiatric patient she was expected to be.

After soldiers returned to their home bases, there were several instances in which units consulted with mental health professionals to deal with lingering issues pertaining to experiences in Panama. For instance, Fort Bragg and the XVIII Corps called in an outside consultant in post-Vietnam PTSD to give training, because of symptoms among a unit that had performed mortuary duties for Panamanian civilian casualties. The division and U.S. Army Medical Department mental health staff treated cases of post-traumatic stress disorder, especially from small units which had had especially horrible experiences such as the death of a pregnant woman at a roadblock. Stokes also noted that a military police company at Fort Drum requested and received stress debriefing from the division social work officer about 1 month after homecoming.[77]

The Department of Military Psychiatry of the Walter Reed Army Institute of Research, as part of their ongoing research relating unit cohesion and combat readiness, sent debriefing teams to the 7th Infantry Division (Light), the 5th Infantry Division (Mountain), and the 82d Airborne Division, all units that had been part of Operation Just Cause. The teams found numerous examples of unresolved combat memories which could become post-traumatic stress disorder months after returning from Panama.[77]

Anecdotal evidence suggests that a Ranger battalion's attrition rate from the U.S. Army was high after return from Panama. Attrition was also high in the months following Urgent Fury (Grenada), according to a physician assistant who jumped in with one of the Ranger battalions. The physician assistant told Stokes that he had talked with many of his Ranger comrades during their preretirement medical outprocessing. A common explanation for retiring was, "My wife wants me to; she worried about me in Grenada." Only with careful questioning would it become clear that the wife had accepted the danger in Grenada, but was worried that her husband had come home changed, with symptoms of PTSD. She felt that if he left the military, he would get back to being the man she had married. Finally, some of the Rangers shared with the physician assistant their traumatic memories, often involving survivor guilt.

Stokes reported a number of lessons learned in Panama,[77] which have subsequently been incorporated into U.S. Army doctrine.[78,79] Very short, victorious campaigns such as Operation Urgent Fury in Grenada and Operation Just Cause in Panama are just long enough for soldiers (especially the highly-trained elite units) to experience the "Stage of Alarm"[80] and suboptimal combat performance.[31] The combat is not long enough to achieve the "Stage of Resistance"[80] and the enhanced combat skills of the experienced veteran. The soldiers, including the leaders, often return with their confidence in themselves and their comrades shaken, but are hesitant to share such thoughts with anyone (even their peers) for fear of being thought weaklings. This observation supports the need for routine after-action debriefing within the units themselves.

Stokes[77] suggested that even a very austere holding capability could enable keeping stress casualties and highly motivated minor disease/nonbattle injury (DNBI) cases in theater for return to duty. Many of the elite soldiers with minor injuries in Operation Just Cause would have volunteered to sleep on the ground, in an airfield hanger or keep watch in a foxhole, M16 in hand, with their ankle wrapped and ibuprofen (or nothing) for the pain. If, after 1 to 2 days, they were not able to return to their units' headquarters for limited duty and required further x-rays or treatment, they could have been evacuated without shame. This would decrease post-traumatic stress disorder, guilt over failure, and attrition of good soldiers from the U.S. Army.

Doctrine[79] now states that division mental health sections (and the new combat stress control units) should be deployed in brief contingency operations such as Operation Just Cause. Even if they don't arrive until after combat is over (due to limited space on aircraft), they can debrief units in theater, soon after action, at the scene of the action. This is far more effective than waiting until after the units come home and return from family leave with problems already locked in. The mental health personnel also gain the knowledge, experience, and credibility with the units that will enable them to be much more helpful to soldiers who are experiencing difficulty over the following months.

Stokes[77] also reviewed deployment of mental health resources during the Persian Gulf War which involved the largest deployment of U.S. forces in the 20 years since the withdrawal of U.S. forces from Vietnam. The Persian Gulf War rivaled the Vietnam conflict in total forces in a combat zone at a given time. It was reported that during the Persian Gulf War the 540,000-member U.S. forces had 148 killed in action and 467 wounded.[81] Of these, 35 were killed and 78 wounded in fratricidal incidents. Iraq's military is estimated to have lost between 30,000 and 100,000 killed and 100,000 to 300,000 wounded. There were an estimated 60,000 to 70,000 Iraqi prisoners of war by war's end.[82]

During the peacetime interim between the Vietnam conflict and the Persian Gulf War, division mental health sections had been preoccupied with clinic mental health and U.S. Army Medical Department PROFIS (Professional Officer Filler System) duties. Thus they lacked field experience and cohesion with their divisions. Fortunately, the prolonged mobilization phase (Operation Desert Shield) of the Persian Gulf War allowed most to correct this before combat started.

Most division mental health sections found it advisable to send one of the mental health officers (social worker, psychologist, or psychiatrist) forward to augment the behavioral science specialist (91G NCO) which doctrine said should be with every brigade. In the Persian Gulf War, the brigades were the principal fighting element. The division's main support medical companies were often left far to the rear.

Ideally the function of these officer/NCO combat stress control teams was like that of the original World War I division psychiatrists: to educate, triage, and *prevent* the evacuation of any stress cases who could be managed in their own organizations. The ability to hold for treatment at that forward echelon is minimal, which is why expert triage to prevent overevacuation is so crucial. Like the World War I psychiatrists, the mental health personnel's place in the Persian Gulf War during combat was at the main triage point (now the medical company in the brigade support area, and sometimes forward at the ambulance exchange points).[83,84] These teams also provided preventive debriefings and consultation to command following traumatic incidents.

Stokes[77] provided several examples of the appropriate treatment of combat stress casualties during the Persian Gulf War. For instance, the Tiger Brigade was attached to a U.S. Marine Division for the frontal assault on Iraqi defenses around Kuwait City. Four stress casualties were evacuated to the U.S. Marine's Surgical Support Company, which had been augmented by the U.S. Navy with a Combat Stress Center. Three of the four soldiers were returned to duty to their units shortly after the brief campaign was over. The remaining case, who had more severe psychopathology, was evacuated.

The U.S. Navy's creative improvisation in support of the U.S. Marines is another example. In mid-January, the U.S. Navy psychiatrist aboard the USNS *Comfort* began a move in concert with the Specialty Advisor for Psychiatry and the Medical Officer of the U.S. Marine Corps to move neuropsychiatric resources forward of the hospital ships and fleet hospitals.[85] Four combat stress centers, each with a psychiatrist and a psychologist (or two psychologists, under the supervision of the nearby combat stress center which had a psychiatrist), were established at each of the four surgical support companies. These were assisted by a mix of psychiatrically-trained or on-the-job-trained corpsmen and nurses. The combat stress centers had a 40-cot holding capability. Fortunately, the battle did not require weeks of fighting in chemically-contaminated trenches, which could have generated mass stress casualties to fill those cots.

The regimental surgeon of one U.S. Army armored cavalry regiment requested and received a combat stress control team from the corps, which consisted of two psychiatrists, a social worker, and an enlisted technician.[86] The team accompanied the medical troop into Iraq, went forward to interact with the line troops, and conducted debriefings following traumatic incidents. They also advised the command regarding pre- and post-homecoming activities.

Three medical (psychiatric) detachments (OM teams) were activated and deployed to the Persian Gulf War. The one active component detachment, the 528th, became XVIII Corps' combat stress control asset. It did not reach Saudi Arabia until late October, but immediately set up a brief restoration program collocated with a combat support hospital and sent mobile teams to provide consultation/education at the battalion aid stations and dispensaries. This produced a marked decrease in the evacuation of "psychiatric" cases, and also of cases with stress-related somatic complaints who were being evacuated with other tentative diagnoses. Most of the cases held for treatment and returned to duty by this detachment were from the corps-level combat support/combat service support units. This may have been in part because the division personnel were geographically more distant, and had their own division mental health sections to prevent unnecessary evacuation or referral. The combat support/combat service support personnel in corps were also often reservists who had been called up unexpectedly, with unresolved homefront problems.

The combat support/combat service support personnel were also working the hardest during the buildup phase of the Persian Gulf War. Some worked extremely long hours under difficult and dangerous environmental conditions. When the 528th psychiatric detachment deployed forward in late December and divided into teams to provide backup support to each division in 18th Corps (in accordance with evolving doctrine[79]) the evacuation of "psychiatric casualties" began to rise again.[77]

Two Reserve OM teams were activated and deployed in December 1990. The 531st from Baltimore, Maryland became the combat stress control asset for 7th Corps, and divided into teams to provide backup support for each division. The 467th from Madison, Wisconsin was initially assigned to provide echelon above corps support at Riyadh, Saudi Arabia. As the ground campaign approached, it continued that mission while splitting off three teams. One team established a combat stress control restoration/reconditioning center collocated with a hospital at King Khalid Military City. The other two teams reinforced the 528th and 531st psychiatric detachments which were supporting the two corps. The stress control teams were integrated into the medical task forces which deployed forward behind the ground offensive. Along with surgical and preventive medicine teams, some of them reached the Euphrates River. Hospital psychiatry was not neglected by the forward deployment of these teams. The neuropsychiatry sections of two evacuation hospitals combined to form a stress recovery unit which followed the principles of combat psychiatry. Between 16 February 1991 and 9 March 1991, it admitted 22 cases and returned 21 to duty after an average stay of 4 days.[87]

Stokes[77] observed that total stress casualties in the Persian Gulf War from 16 January 1991 (the start date of the air war against Iraq) through early March 1991 would include all those held in division clearing stations for over 24 hours, in the OM team facilities collocated with hospitals, and in the hospitals themselves. These have not been tabulated and may never be fully counted. However, it requires only 94 cases from all the services held for treatment in the theater between 16 January 1991 and mid-March 1991 to constitute the "standard" one to five ratio for the 467 wounded in action. The distinction between "combat stress" and "noncombat stress" casualties becomes unclear when the Scud missile threat was greater in the rear than near the front, and driving a truck long distances on the Tapline Road was at least as likely to result in death as driving a tank against Iraqi armor and infantry.[77]

Nostalgic casualties were few because the host country (Saudi Arabia), in keeping with Muslim tradition, did not allow importation of alcoholic beverages or prostitution. Accidents reportedly were one third the rate of other U.S. forces due to absence of alcohol. However, casualties secondary to substance abuse did occur when soldiers attempted to make homemade alcohol and died from methanol ingestion. Clear grain alcohol was available at stores along the Tapline Road, disguised as bottles of drinking water, for those who knew how to ask and were willing to pay.[77] Only a few drug-related incidents occurred, including that of a U.S. Air Force pharmacist who used and distributed drugs illegally.

Some of the lessons learned from the Persian Gulf War appear to have been of a negative nature. On the evening of 21 February 1991, a Scud missile holding a ton of explosives struck the 14th Quartermaster's barracks at Dhahran, Saudi Arabia, killing or mortally wounding 13 members of the 69-member unit, including the first woman soldier killed in Persian Gulf combat. The missile wounded 37 others. The doctrinal requirement to send the combat stress control teams forward to support the combat arms had left the corps area with little combat stress control support for such a large area. Consequently, when the Scud missile caused mass casualties in Dhahran, there was no mobile combat stress control team available to provide immediate command consultation and debriefing. A critical incident debriefing did not occur. There was also ambivalence by unit officers and troops' suspicion of military mental health officers. Even worse, days later the survivors were shipped far from the front to a European-based hospital for evaluation and eventual evacuation to the United States.[88] One official U.S. Army Medical Department lesson learned from the Persian Gulf War was to support the fielding of the new TO&E (Table of Organization and Equipment) combat stress control units and their doctrine. At one of the lessons-learned conferences, the senior U.S. Army Medical Department leaders in the Persian Gulf War declared combat stress control "one of the success stories" of the operation, but added that there were not enough combat stress control units to be everywhere they were needed. It was also recommended that each divisional brigade, separate brigade, and armored cavalry regiment should have a predesignated (if not organic) officer/NCO combat stress control team.[77]

The Persian Gulf deployment left 17,000 children of single parents or two-soldier couples temporarily without any parents during the war. How significant this will be in the subsequent development of these children is unknown.[89] Schneider and Martin discuss these issues in greater detail.[90]

The United States has continued involvement in mercy and peacekeeping roles in Somalia (Operation Restore Hope), Macedonia (to contain the civil war in Bosnia), and Haiti. These relatively small and brief operations may be the main role of the military in the future as the responsibilities of the U.S. military are expanded to add peacekeeping and humanitarian missions to those of fighting wars and deterring aggression.[91] However, these operations will not necessarily be without combat stress casualties. At least one Ranger who was in the battle of the Olympic Hotel in Mogadishu, Somalia (October 1994) was dropped from the Rangers (although not from the U.S. Army) as a result of misconduct that was clearly related to undiagnosed post-traumatic stress disorder.[77] The cause of his survivor guilt was identified (and quickly dispelled) during a group debriefing one year later.

SUMMARY AND CONCLUSION

This history of warfare reveals certain recurring themes concerning soldiers who persevere in combat versus those who break down in combat. Both groups are often quite similar as individuals (and may even be the same individuals); however, their social situations are markedly different. The social situations consist of a matrix of factors that determine whether the soldier excels or breaks down.

Thus, in adapting to combat, as in all survival-relevant activities, humans respond holistically. Their physical, intrapsychic, and social states form this matrix of factors, which influences their responses to environmental danger. In combat, deep urgings for individual survival often conflict with socially conditioned expectations, requirements, and desires for "soldierly conduct," which have been embodied in ideals such as patriotism, discipline, loyalty to comrades, and identification with the leader.

To prevent combat breakdown, the presence of mission-oriented small group cohesion is essential. Cohesion is fostered by good leadership and by having soldiers train, live, and experience stress together. Further preventive measures include adequate rest, sleep, and nutrition so that chronic or acute fatigue does not develop. Rest from battle should ideally occur through small group rotation so that group support is continuous. Commanders should be open and honest with their subordinates to build trust and vertical cohesion, and to enhance the soldier's understanding of the importance of his contribution to the unit mission and the national interest. The soldier must believe that his entire society supports him in his privations and sacrifices.

Factors that foster psychiatric breakdown are the negatives of the preventive factors: poor leadership, cohesion and training; inadequate social support; and the buildup of fatigue. Factors that emphasize perceptions of individual or collective vulnerability increase the probability of psychiatric breakdown. This accounts for the strong relationship between intensity of combat (as measured by wounded and killed in action) and numbers of stress casualties. It also accounts for the observation that the death of a comrade was the most common precipitant of breakdown during World War II. A feeling of helplessness in controlling one's fate also exacerbates stress and weakens resistance. This is seen in the increased stress casualties that occur in circumstances of indirect fire such as artillery or bombing barrages, or gas attacks compared with the direct fire situation (even though the wounded and killed rate may be the same or higher than under indirect fire).

After a soldier has become a psychiatric casualty, it is important to restore as many positive factors as possible: rest, sleep, and nutrition. Bonds to the unit are kept intact with expectation of return to the unit, hence the importance of treating as far forward and as quickly as possible. Treatment must be kept simple to emphasize the normality of the soldier's experience rather than give an imputation of mental illness. In garrison or rear-echelon settings, prevention is even more important because the disorders that occur (alcohol and drug abuse, character disorders, and sexual problems) are even more difficult to treat than combat stress disorders. In rear-echelon settings, attention should be paid to discipline, morale-enhancing activities, and recognition of the critical role played by support troops. Communication between support troops and those they support should be encouraged. Temporary assignment to combat units should be available. Infractions should be dealt with through forward rather than rearward evacuation to minimize secondary gain from misbehavior.

Prevention of combat stress casualties is primarily a command responsibility but the medical person, through consultation with command and avoidance of medical "evacuation syndromes," plays a critical role in this endeavor.

REFERENCES

1. Marlowe DH. Personal Communication, 1985.

2. Salmon TW. The care and treatment of mental diseases and war neurosis ("shell shock") in the British Army. In: Bailey P, Williams FE, Komora PA, Salmon TW, Fenton N, eds. *Neuropsychiatry*. Vol 10. In: *The Medical Department of the United States Army in the World War*. Washington, DC: Office of The Surgeon General, US Army; 1929: Appendix; 497–523.

3. Erikson EH. *Childhood and Society*. New York: WW Norton; 1950: 43–44.

4. Jones FD. Combat stress: Tripartite model. *Int Rev Army Navy Air Force Med Serv*. 1982;55:247–254.

5. Jones FD, Crocq L, Adelaja O, et al. Psychiatric casualties in modern warfare: Evolution of treatment. In: Pichot P, Berner P, Wolf R, Thau K, eds. *Psychiatry: The State of the Art*. Vol 6. New York: Plenum; 1985: 459–464.

6. Rosen G. Nostalgia: A "forgotten" psychological disorder. *Psychol Med*. 1975;5:340–354.

7. Glass AJ. Army psychiatry before World War II. In: Glass AJ, Bernucci RJ, eds. In: *Zone of Interior*. Vol 1. In: *Neuropsychiatry in World War II*. Washington, DC: Office of The Surgeon General, US Army; 1966: 3–23.

8. Deutsch A. Military psychiatry: The Civil War, 1861–1865. In: Hall JK, Zilboorg G, Bunker HA, eds. *One Hundred Years of American Psychiatry: 1844–1944*. New York: Columbia University Press; 1944: 367–384.

9. Calhoun JT. Nostalgia as a disease of field service. *Buff Med Surg Rep*. 1864;11:130–132.

10. Hammond WA. *A Treatise on Insanity in its Medical Relations*. New York: Appleton; 1883.

11. Jones FD, Johnson AW. Medical and psychiatric treatment policy and practice in Vietnam. *J Soc Issues*. 1975;31(4):49–65.

12. Richards RL. Mental and nervous disorders in the Russo-Japanese War. *Milit Surg* [now *Milit Med*]. 1910;26(2): 177–193.

13. Jones FD, Belenky GL, Marlowe DH. Shell shock and battle fatigue: The importance of a name. Presented at the World Psychiatric Association-American Psychiatric Association Regional Meeting entitled Critical Issues in Psychiatry for the 80s; October 30–November 3, 1981; New York.

14. Laughlin HP. *The Neuroses.* Washington, DC: Butterworths; 1967: 838–839.

15. Farrar CB. War and neurosis. *Am J Insanity* [now *Am J Psychiatry*]. 1917;73(12):112–116.

16. Salmon TW, Fenton N, eds. In the American Expeditionary Forces [Section 2]. *Neuropsychiatry.* Vol. 10. In: *The Medical Department of the United States Army in the World War.* Washington, DC: Office of The Surgeon General, US Army; 1929.

17. Artiss KL. Human behavior under stress: From combat to social psychiatry. *Milit Med.* 1963;128(10):1011–1015.

18. Bailey P, Williams FE, Komora PO, eds. Introduction [Section I]. In: *Neuropsychiatry.* Vol 10. In: *The Medical Department of the United States Army in the World War.* Washington, DC: Office of The Surgeon General, US Army; 1929: 1–22.

19. Glass AJ. Lessons learned. In: Glass AJ, ed. *Overseas Theaters.* Vol 2. In: *Neuropsychiatry in World War II.* Washington, DC: Office of The Surgeon General, US Army; 1973: 989–1027.

20. Belenky GL, Jones FD. The evacuation syndrome in military exercises: A model of the psychiatric casualties of combat. In: Mangelsdorff AD, Furukawa PT, eds. *Proceedings, User's Workshop on Combat Stress.* US Army Academy of Health Sciences, Fort Sam Houston, Tex. Defense Technical Information Center, Cameron Station, Alexandria, Va, Document #ADA152464; 1981: 140–142.

21. Mira E. *Psychiatry in War.* New York: WW Norton; 1943: 68–75.

22. Belenky GL, Tyner CF, Sodetz FJ. *Israeli Battle Shock Casualties: 1973 and 1982.* Report WRAIR NP-83-4. Washington, DC: Walter Reed Army Institute of Research; Defense Technical Information Center Document ADA133359; 1983.

23. Arthur RJ. Success is predictable. *Milit Med.* 1971;136(6):539–545.

24. Glass AJ. Lessons learned. In: Glass AJ, Bernucci R, eds. *Zone of Interior.* Vol 1. In: *Neuropsychiatry in World War II.* Washington, DC: Office of The Surgeon General, US Army; 1966: 735–759.

25. Pratt D. Combat record of psychoneurotic patients. *Bull US Army Med Dept.* 1947;7:809–811.

26. Drayer CS, Glass AJ. Introduction. In: Glass AJ, ed. *Overseas Theaters.* Vol 2. In: *Neuropsychiatry in World War II.* Washington, DC: Office of The Surgeon General, US Army; 1973: 1–23.

27. Stouffer SA, DeVinney LC, Star SA, Williams RM. *The American Soldier.* Vol 2. Princeton, NJ: Princeton University Press; 1949.

28. Beebe GW, De Bakey ME. *Battle Casualties: Incidence, Mortality, and Logistic Considerations.* Springfield, Ill: Charles C Thomas; 1952: 28.

29. Jones FD. Psychiatric lessons of low-intensity wars. *Ann Med Milit Fenn* [Finland]. 1985;60:128–134.

30. Sobel R. Anxiety-depressive reactions after prolonged combat experience: The "old sergeant syndrome." Supplement on Combat Psychiatry. *Bull US Army Med Dept.* 1949;9:137–146.

31. Swank RL, Marchand F. Combat neuroses: Development of combat exhaustion. *Arch Neurol Psychiatry* [superseded in part by *Arch Neurol* and *Arch Gen Psychiatry*]. 1946;55:236–247.

32. Hanson FR, Ranson SW. Statistical studies. Supplement on Combat Psychiatry. *Bull US Army Med Dept.* 1949;9:191–204.

33. Beebe GW, Appel JW. Psychological breakdown in relation to stress and other factors. In: *Variation in Psychological Tolerance to Ground Combat in World War II, Final Report*. Washington, DC: National Academy of Sciences; 1958: 88–131.

34. Noy S. Battle intensity and length of stay on the battlefield as determinants of the type of evacuation. *Milit Med*. 1987;152(12):601–607.

35. Marshall SLA. *Night Drop: The American Airborne Invasion of Normandy*. Boston, Mass: Little, Brown; 1962: 15–21.

36. Marshall SLA. *Men Against Fire*. New York: William Morrow; 1950: 54–58.

37. Marshall SLA. Combat leadership. In: *Preventive and Social Psychiatry*. Washington, DC: GPO; 1957: 303–307.

38. Parrish MD. Written Communication, 1991.

39. Glass AJ. Psychiatry in the Korean Campaign (Installment 1). *US Armed Forces Med J*. 1953;4:1387–1401.

40. Marshall SLA. *Pork Chop Hill*. New York: William Morrow; 1958: xii, xv.

41. Fearnsides EG, Culpin M. Frost-Bite. *Br Med J*. January 1915;1:84.

42. Kirkland F. Personal Communication, 1991.

43. Glass AJ. Personal Communication, 1982.

44. Neel S. *Vietnam Studies: Medical Support of the US Army in Vietnam, 1965–1970*. Washington, DC: Department of the Army; 1973: 36.

45. Datel WE. *A Summary of Source Data in Military Psychiatric Epidemiology*. Defense Technical Information Center, Cameron Station, Alexandria, Va, Document ADA021265; 1976.

46. Bowman J. *Recent Experiences of Combat Psychiatry in Vietnam*. Washington, DC: Division of Neuropsychiatry, Walter Reed Army Institute of Research; 1967. Typescript.

47. Jones FD. Experiences of division psychiatrist in Vietnam. *Milit Med*. 1967;132(12):1003–1008.

48. Huffman RE. Which soldiers break down: A survey of 610 psychiatric patients in Vietnam. *Bull Menninger Clin*. 1970;34(6):343–351.

49. Renner JA. The changing patterns of psychiatric problems in Vietnam. *Compr Psychiatry*. 1973;14(2):169–180.

50. Hayes FW. Military aeromedical evacuation and psychiatric patients during the Vietnam war. *Am J Psychiatry*. 1969;126:658–666.

51. Holloway HC. Epidemiology of heroin dependency among soldiers in Vietnam. *Milit Med*. 1974;139:108–113.

52. Mateczun J, Holmes-Johnson E. The psychiatric care of the combat-injured and clinical differences between Beirut and Grenada casualties. In *Proceedings, Fourth Users' Workshop on Combat Stress: Lessons Learned in Recent Operational Experiences*. Fort Sam Houston, Tex: US Army Health Services Command; 1985: 180–206.

53. Department of Defense. *Selected Manpower Statistics, 1992*. DoD, Washington Headquarters Service. Washington, DC: GPO; 1993. GPO Stock No. 1993-720-091/80107.

54. Noy S. Personal Communication, 1983

55. El Sudany El Rayes M. Combat psychiatry in Arab-Israeli wars. Presented at Grand Rounds, Psychiatry Department, Walter Reed Army Medical Center; October 21, 1982; Washington, DC.

56. Harris P. Personal Communication, 1986.

57. Belenky GL. Varieties of reaction and adaptation to combat experience. *Bull Menninger Clin*. 1987;51(1):64–79.

58. Soloman Z, Benbenishty R. The role of proximity, immediacy and expectancy in frontline treatment of combat stress reaction among Israelis in the Lebanon War. *Am J Psychiatry*. 1986;143(5):613–617.

59. Haggerty JJ. Afghanistan—the great game. *Milit Rev*. 1980;60(8):37–44.

60. Krivosheyev GF. *Losses to the Armed Forces of the USSR in Battles, Combat Operations, and Military Conflicts: Statistical Investigations*. Moscow: Military Press; 1993: 402–404.

61. Klose K. Ex-Soviet's escape into a childhood dream. *Washington Post*. 16 November 1985: A-3.

62. Moore M. A post-Afghan syndrome? *Washington Post*. 1 October 1989: D-1, D-5.

63. O'Ballance E. Soviet tactics in Afghanistan. *Milit Rev*. 1980;60(8):45–52.

64. Mohair M, Mottaghi Y. Psychiatric war casualties in Iran: Presentations. Presented at American Psychiatric Association Annual Meeting; May 1985; Dallas, Tex.

65. Kadivar H, Adams SC. Treatment of chemical and biological warfare injuries: Insights derived from the 1984 Iraqi attack on Majnoon Island. *Milit Med*. 1991;156(4):171–177.

66. Mohajer M, Dekjam M, Moheb-Ali A. Psychosocial condition of war refugees of Iran after 4 years. Presented at American Psychiatric Association Annual Meeting; May 1986; Washington, DC.

67. Fisher M. Lessons of the Falklands: Prepare for surprises. *US Medicine*. 1983;19(5):3,16.

68. Pincus W. British got crucial data in Falklands, diary says. *Washington Post*. 23 December 1984: A1, A20.

69. Harmon JW, Llewellyn C. Lessons of the Falklands. *Med Bull US Army Europe*. 1984;41(2):11–13.

70. O'Connell MR. Psychiatrist with the task force. In: Pichot P, Berner P, Wolf R, Thau K, eds. *Psychiatry: The State of the Art*. Vol 6. New York: Plenum Press; 1985: 511–513.

71. Russell G. Falkland Islands: Explosions and breakthroughs. *Time*. June 7, 1982: 30–36.

72. Collazo C. Psychiatric casualties in Malvinas War: A provisional report. In: Pichot P, Berner P, Wolf R, Thau K, eds. *Psychiatry: The State of the Art*. Vol 6. New York: Plenum Press; 1985: 499–503.

73. Abraham P. Post-traumatic stress disorder. *J R Coll Gen Pract*. 1987;37(300):321–322. Letter.

74. Fullerton T. A soldier's view of combat medicine in Grenada. Presented at Psychiatric Grand Rounds, Walter Reed Army Medical Center; November 1984; Washington, DC.

75. Belenky GL. Talking with US casualties from Grenada. Presented at Chief's Roundtable, Neuropsychiatry Department, Walter Reed Army Institute of Research; December 1983; Washington, DC.

76. Marshall SLA. *Bringing Up the Rear: A Memoir*. San Rafael, Calif: Presidio Press; 1979: xiv.

77. Stokes J. Written Communication, 24 February 1994.

78. US Department of the Army. *Leaders' Manual for Combat Stress Control*. Washington, DC: DA; 29 September 1994. Field Manual 22-51.

79. US Department of the Army. *Combat Stress Control in a Theater of Operations*. Washington, DC: DA; 29 September 1994. Field Manual 8-51.

80. Selye H. The General Adaptation Syndrome and the diseases of adaptation. *J Clin Endocrinol* [now *J Clin Endocrinol Metab*]. 1946;6(2):117–230.

81. Miscellanea Medica. *JAMA*. 1991;266(15):2053.

82. Gunby P. Another war...and more lessons for medicine to ponder in aftermath. *JAMA*. 1991;266(5):619–621.

83. Campbell SJ, Engel CC. Combat psychiatry the "First Team" way: First Cavalry Division mental health operations during the Persian Gulf War. In: Belenky G, Martin J, Sparacino L, eds. *A Shield in the Storm: Mental Health Operations During the Gulf War*. Westport, Conn: Greenwood Press. In preparation.

84. Campbell SJ, Carter BS. Forward location of the combat stress control team contributing to the primary prevention of combat stress and battle fatigue in Operation Desert Shield/Storm. Paper presented at the 7th Military Medicine Conference, Uniformed Services University of the Health Sciences, Bethesda, Md. April 1992.

85. Mateczun J. Personal Communication, 1995.

86. Martin JA. Personal Communication, 1995.

87. Johnson LB, Cline DW, Marcum JM, Intress JL, Effectiveness of a stress recovery unit during the Persian Gulf War. *Hosp Community Psychiatry*. 1992;43(8):829–833.

88. Cody P. Military fails to follow own psychiatric guidelines in handling survivors of Dhahran Scud attack. *Psychiatric News*. 16 August 1991: 2, 5.

89. Persian Gulf vets, families expected to need mental health care at some future time. *Psychiatric News*. 16 August 1991: 2, 13.

90. Schneider RJ, Martin JA. Military families and combat readiness. In: Jones FD, Sparacino LR, Wilcox VL, Rothberg JM, eds. *Military Psychiatry: Preparing in Peace for War*. Part 1. In: *Textbook of Military Medicine*. Washington, DC: Office of The Surgeon General, US Department of the Army and Borden Institute; 1994: 19–30.

91. Graham B. Responsibilities of U.S. military expanded. *The Washington Post*. 9 March 1995. A36.

Chapter 2

TRADITIONAL WARFARE COMBAT STRESS CASUALTIES

FRANKLIN D. JONES, M.D., F.A.P.A.*

*Colonel (ret), Medical Corps, U.S. Army; Clinical Professor, Uniformed Services University of the Health Sciences, Bethesda, Maryland; Past President and Secretary and current Honorary President of the Military Section, World Psychiatric Association; formerly Psychiatry and Neurology Consultant, Office of The Surgeon General, U.S. Army

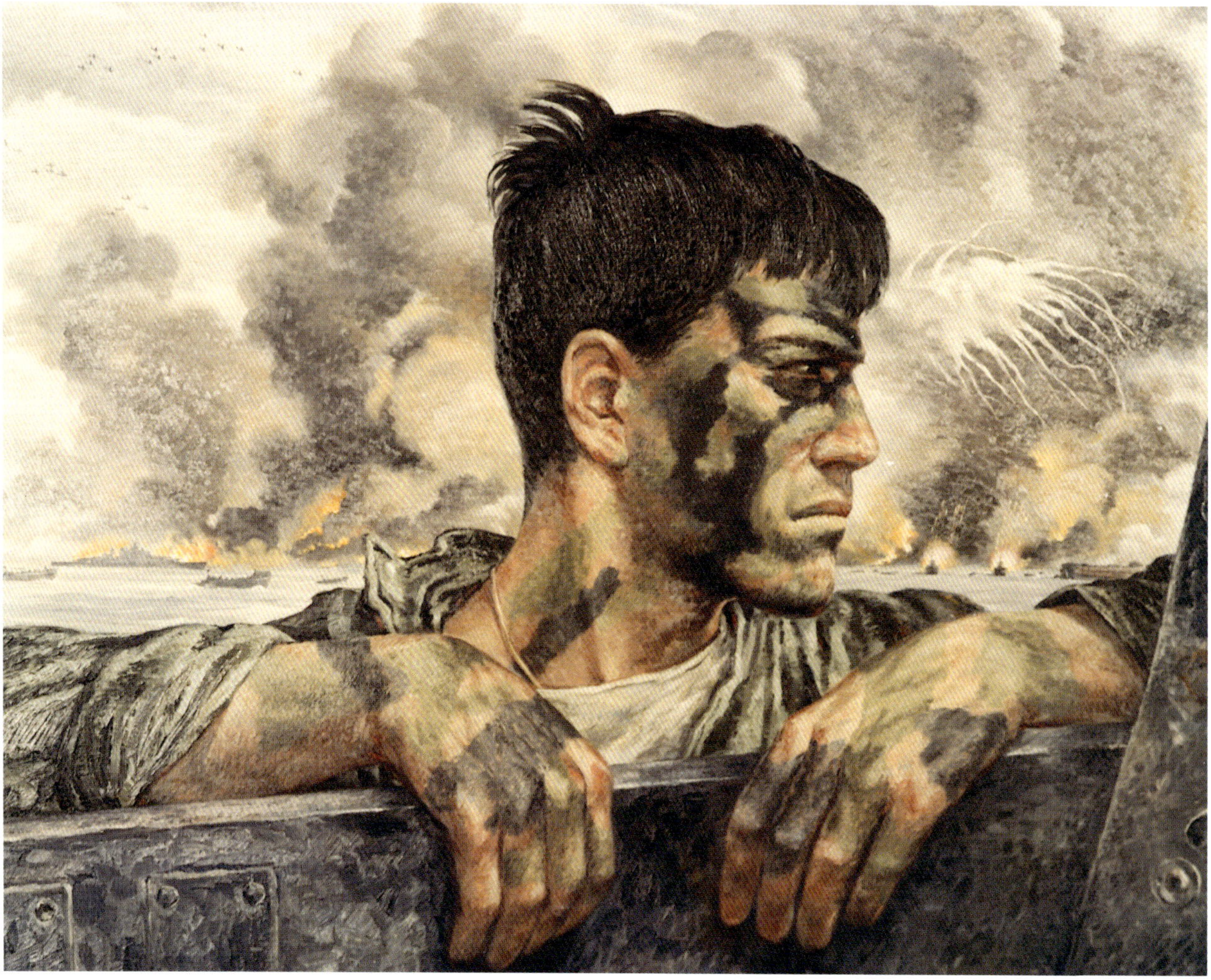

Tom Lea *Going In, Peleliu* 1944

Tom Lea was an artist correspondent for Life Magazine during World War II. He participated in the landing of U.S. Marine forces at Peleliu, hitting the beach 15 minutes after the troops. This painting was done from memory as he spent the first 36 hours after landing just trying to stay alive. The painting powerfully depicts the psychological mindset of a veteran going into combat yet again. The set of the jaw and the look of determination, against the background of ongoing death and destruction, was familiar to combat artists during World War II as they accompanied the fighting troops into "traditional warfare."

Art: Courtesy of US Center of Military History, Washington, DC.

INTRODUCTION

The diagnosis and treatment of combat stress casualties range from the easily accomplished to the highly difficult. Diagnosis may be apparent when a fatigued, anxious, otherwise intact soldier says, "Doc, I can't take it anymore." Diagnosis may be more difficult when the casualty is mute and unresponsive, or aggressive. Making the diagnosis is complicated not only by the heterogeneity of symptoms in the unwounded but also by potential wounding agents that can present with or mimic psychiatric symptoms. In addition to bullets, fragments, and burns, such wounding agents include biological and chemical agents, and radiation, both nuclear and microwave.

Treatment involving rest, nutrition, and expectancy, while generally easy in concept, may be difficult in application. During World War II, it was not unusual for sheer numbers of surgical casualties to overwhelm the forward treatment capabilities and result in evacuation rearward of stress casualties. High-intensity warfare, in addition to making forward treatment difficult because of the absence of a safe treatment area, will likely overwhelm the forward treatment facility with very large numbers of surgical and psychiatric casualties.[1] Low-intensity warfare can also produce psychiatric casualties and misconduct stress casualties (drug abuse, disciplinary infractions, venereal diseases) that may be difficult to treat—as was seen in Vietnam.

The types of casualties and their treatment depend on the type of war. It is, therefore, appropriate to discuss them in this context after first defining stress and psychiatric casualties.

DEFINITION AND MANIFESTATIONS

Historically, since late World War I, a combat psychiatric casualty has been defined as any militarily ineffective soldier (or organization) in whom the predominant factors producing ineffectiveness were of psychological (as opposed to physical) or neuropsychiatric origin. Although partly fulfilling this definition, disorders involving structural damage or major physiological disturbances of brain tissue were normally excluded from this category. Nonconflicted malingering was also excluded.

Current U.S. Army doctrine[2] distinguishes psychiatric from stress casualties. Psychiatric casualties are those with standard Diagnostic and Statistical Manual (DSM-IV)[3] diagnoses which are not simply the temporary consequence of the intense psychological and/or physiological stress of combat or other highly stressful missions. These latter are labeled "stress casualties," "battle fatigue," or "contingency fatigue." The U.S. Army classification also defines the "misconduct stress behaviors" as violations of regulation or law which require disciplinary action even though they are largely attributable to stressful conditions. It is recognized that psychiatric disorders, battle fatigue, and misconduct stress behaviors can coexist in the same soldier, with some grey areas where any of these labels can be used, based on the command's judgment of which will be best for the mission, the unit, and the individual soldier. This textbook will distinguish the psychiatric, stress, and misconduct categories except when making historical references and citations where "psychiatric" is historically accurate.

Manifestations of combat stress overlap at both ends of the psychobiological spectrum, and one role of the psychiatrist is to separate out particularly the neurological cases that require a different, sometimes surgical form of treatment. Sometimes it is important also to separate out the conscious malingerers, but this is not always the case because the treatment involving rest, expectancy, and strengthening the desire, however attenuated, of the soldier to return to his unit is generally the same in cases of combat fatigue and malingering. In the latter instance, however, a more coercive stance (threat of court-martial) may be required if early rest, expectation of recovery, and talking therapy do not produce willingness (however reluctant) to return to duty.

It is important to remember that most psychiatric casualties are soldiers who, because of the influence of negative psychological, social, and physiological factors, unconsciously seek a medical exit from combat. Most cases, therefore, will mimic features of other medical disorders that would be "legitimate" forms of escape from combat, thus becoming "evacuation syndromes."[4] Improperly treated through evacuation, the symptoms may persist or worsen, developing characteristics of traumatic neurosis (chronic post-traumatic stress disorder).

The symptoms displayed are those considered more acceptable by fellow soldiers, commanders, and medical personnel. The symptoms often have a neurological or psychophysiological flavor, which in the past led to their classification as neuroses (anxiety and somatoform disorders). The absence of "neurotic" personality patterns and the transience of the syndrome when properly treated indicate a more appropriate categorization as a transient or situational stress or adjustment disorder.

Based on World War II experience, Weinstein and Drayer[5] distinguished the anxiety states of combat from those of civilian life by the following characteristics of combat anxiety: (*a*) the extraordinary precipitating factors in the perils and hardships of the combat environment, (*b*) symptom plasticity, (*c*) the importance of hostility and guilt, which is more immediately apparent than in most neuroses in civilians, and (*d*) the fact that they are in large part group phenomena. The soldier is a member of a closely knit, interdependent group, and group effectiveness and attitudes as well as ability to identify with the group modify significantly the soldier's capacity to withstand the traumas to which he is subjected. Failure in group membership may result in symptom formation.

From this discussion it is obvious that the symptom complex may be quite heterogeneous and fluid. During the early years of World War I, when it was believed that many soldiers were suffering from concussion caused by exploding shells or bombs, a diagnosis of "shell shock" was given and the symptoms mimicked those of persons who had suffered from a blow to the central nervous system. In the words of Bailey, Williams, and Komora: "There were descriptions of cases with staring eyes, violent tremors, a look of terror, and blue, cold extremities. Some were deaf and some were dumb; others were blind or paralyzed."[6(p2)]

Later, after the use of poison gas had become widespread, many soldiers presented with respiratory symptoms, particularly "choking" and hyperventilation, and they were often labeled "gas hysteria." As the psychological nature of the syndromes became known and the term "war neurosis" came into vogue, soldiers would present themselves as suffering from neurosis and latch onto this label as a legitimate escape from combat, leading to a policy by medical personnel of using a cryptic label, "N.Y.D. (nervous)" which stood for "not yet diagnosed (nervous)," as described in Chapter 1, Psychiatric Lessons of War.

Similarly, in the early phases of U.S. involvement in World War II, medical personnel used the term "psychoneurosis." Soldiers abbreviated this unfamiliar term to "psycho," and the casualties frequently displayed bizarre and regressive symptoms similar to those often seen in psychotic patients.[7] With the rediscovery of the principles of treatment by Hanson in North Africa,[8] and the use of the term "exhaustion," the bizarre symptoms receded to be replaced by symptoms of fatigue.

Glass[7] explained the efficacy of the term "exhaustion" compared with the diagnosis of psychoneurosis. Psychoneurosis implied unresolved intrapsychic conflict with unconsciously derived symptoms. The linkage between the symptoms and the conditions of combat was lost, and such casualties would not be accepted by the soldier's combat reference group as a normal result of battle. Instead, such soldiers were considered weaker, predisposed persons who had not been properly screened out at induction. Exhaustion was selected because it best described the appearance of most psychiatric casualties and of most combat participants of the time. Exhaustion was readily accepted by the casualty and his combat reference group. They could appreciate that anyone could become exhausted by the stress and strain of continual combat. The psychiatric casualty became a rational consequence of battle conditions. The new terminology communicated that the casualty was afflicted with a temporary, situationally-induced disorder that only required rest for restoration of function.

Despite the variability of symptoms in combat breakdown, some groups of symptoms have predominated in various wars. Bar-On and colleagues, as cited in Belenky,[9] have reviewed the predominant symptoms described in U.S. and Israeli casualties in World War I, World War II, Vietnam, and the Arab-Israeli wars of 1973 and 1982. These symptoms were grouped by Jones[10] in Table 2-1. These listings are not actuarial and should be viewed as showing tendencies only. When the anxiety and fear categories are collapsed, these symptoms are found to predominate in all U.S. wars except the Vietnam conflict. Even in the Vietnam conflict, an examination of psychiatric syndromes among sol-

TABLE 2-1

SYMPTOM CLUSTERS IN VARIOUS WARS

Most Prevalent Symptoms	World War I	World War II	Vietnam	Arab-Israeli 1973	Arab-Israeli 1982
Depressive affect	X			X	X
Fear: diffuse, focused	X			X	X
Noise sensitivity, startle	X				
Tremors	X				
Psychomotor disturbances	X				
Conversive reactions	X	X		X	X
Confusion, aprosexia	X				
Dissociative states	X			X	
Anxiety		X		X	X
Disturbing dreams, memories		X		X	
Exhaustion, fatigue		X			
Decreased appetite		X			
Gastrointestinal discomfort		X			
Headaches		X			
Sleep disturbances		X		X	X
Constricted affect			X		
Social estrangement			X		X
Discipline problems			X		
Explosive aggressive behavior			X		
Substance abuse			X		
Delayed post-traumatic stress disorder (PTSD)			X		X

Adapted with permission from Jones FD. Psychiatric lessons of low-intensity wars. *Ann Med Milit Fenn* [Finland]. 1985;60:129.

diers seen at a rear-echelon care facility staffed by a mobile psychiatric detachment (KO Team) early in the war before drug abuse and disillusion became widespread reveals a large number of anxiety-type symptoms. This is evident in Exhibit 2-1. In nonwounded soldiers, Bowman[11] found a predominance of dissociative, anxiety, and conversion symptoms, and in wounded soldiers anxiety dreams and neurological symptoms.

Similarly, Jones[12] found that anxiety and fear symptoms predominated in combat soldiers in Vietnam. In contrast, combat-support soldiers were more likely to present with what Jones referred to as "disorders of loneliness," which may be the modern analog of the "nostalgia" of previous centuries. Copen described the psychiatric stresses of military advisory soldiers in Vietnam in 1962 before large-scale U.S. involvement:

> Support troops, although exposed to little physical danger or hardship, nevertheless were stressed by separation from family, boredom, and job frustration. These men were frequently seen because of excessive drinking, psychosomatic complaints, and behavioral problems. Such individuals from support units were contrasted with advisors to combat units in which there was constant physical danger and far less comfortable environmental surroundings. These stresses resulted in casualties referred to as combat fatigue, although this entity tended frequently to be disguised in the form of antisocial behavior or vague physical symptoms.[4(p50)]

Thus, it appears that some manifestations of psychiatric difficulty are related to frequency and intensity of exposure to combat. The relationship of breakdown and its psychiatric manifestations to combat conditions will now be examined.

EXHIBIT 2-1

STRESS SYMPTOMS IN WOUNDED AND NONWOUNDED SOLDIERS AT THE 93RD EVACUATION HOSPITAL, VIETNAM, JANUARY–JUNE 1966 (Not listed in order of prevalence)

A. Stress Symptoms Seen in Wounded Soldiers

The disabling symptoms of wounded soldiers usually developed after hospitalization, or if present when hospitalized, the symptoms persisted or became more severe, requiring neuropsychiatric consultation.

1. Persistent anxiety dreams.
2. Pain in wounded extremity following complete healing.
3. Sensory defects in which the patient claimed hypesthesia and weakness of an extremity but the neurological examination was negative.

B. Stress Symptoms Seen in Nonwounded Soldiers

1. Somnambulism.
2. Anxiety dreams with talking or shouting.
3. Syncope and vertigo.
4. Narcolepsy-like complaints.
5. Seizures—not proved to be grand mal or petit mal.
6. Musculoskeletal-type complaints, such as low back pain, where the orthopedic examination is negative.
7. Amnesia, especially following exposure to explosions (mortar, artillery, or mines) but having no concussion.
8. Blurred vision—when the ophthalmologist can find no visual defects.
9. Stuttering, expecially following exposure to loud noises or automatic weapons fire.
10. Aphonias or other speech disturbances, such as whispering.
11. Persistent nausea or abdominal pain in which no gastrointestinal disease could be demonstrated by the internal medicine service.
12. Headaches, atypical but severe, persistent, and disabling, most often diagnosed as "tension headache."
13. Loss of hearing—in which ear, nose, and throat examination could find no hearing loss.

Adapted with permission from Bowman J. Recent experiences in combat psychiatry in Vietnam. Presented at the Social and Preventive Psychiatry Conference. 1967; Walter Reed Army Medical Center. Washington, DC.

ETIOPATHOGENESIS

The etiopathogenesis (origin and process of disability) of the stress casualties of mid- to high-intensity combat was well known by the French and British during World War I and became the basis for Salmon's "forward treatment." Strecker describes Salmon's etiological concept as follows:

> His visualization of the concept of the emotional conflict underlying war conversion hysteria (the moving demands of the instinct of self-preservation stirring deep and strong affective currents vs. the conscious expectations, desires, and requirements of "soldierly-ideals" imbedded in an emotional matrix of discipline, patriotism, and the like) was so dynamic and stimulating that it served as a beacon light to every psychiatrist in France, no matter how dark the outlook.[13(p386)]

Appel and Beebe put it more starkly in describing psychiatric casualties of World War II:

> [T]he danger of being killed or maimed imposes a strain so great that it causes men to break down … Each man (up there) knew that at any moment he may be killed, a fact kept constantly before his mind by the sight of dead and mutilated buddies around him. Each moment of combat imposes a strain so great that men will break down in direct relation to the intensity and duration of their exposure. Thus psychiatric casualties are as inevitable as gunshot and shrapnel wounds in warfare.[14(p185)]

Psychiatric Casualties and Combat Intensity

Glass has described the relationship of intensity and breakdown as following a bell-shaped or Gaussian curve:

> Very obviously, if you raise the destructive power of the weapon so that the individual cannot cope with it, then non-effectiveness is enhanced. If you have a weapon that is of minor destructive power such as bows and arrows, or rifles, more people can cope with it. This is why men tell you in combat they don't mind small arms fire; what they detest is artillery fire or mortar or other high explosives. So if you diminish the destructiveness, your curve looks different; if you raise it, then you have more non-effective people.[15(p4)]

Marlowe[16] has discussed the concept that combat stress casualties occur as a function of various "battle ecologies" in which the most important variable is the lethality of the environment. The stress casualties more directly related to combat have been shown in numerous studies to occur in a direct ratio to combat intensity as measured by killed-in-action (KIA) or wounded-in-action (WIA) casualties.[17] This ratio usually is about one stress casualty per three or four WIA casualties; however, other factors related to morale, training, physical fatigue, prior exposure, and combat success can markedly change this ratio. It, therefore, becomes appropriate to group stress casualties according to combat intensity. Combat intensity has generally been measured by numbers of WIA and KIA per combat day (any day in which one or more soldiers per company was killed or wounded). Because some injuries are combat-related but not caused by wounding, statisticians often combine the rate of battle injury and wounding (BI & W), usually given per 1,000 troops per year. Based on BI & W rates, World War II and most of the Korean conflict may be considered mid-intensity combat, and much of the Vietnam conflict may be considered low-intensity combat,[18] as seen in Table 2-2.

Obviously, during some periods of engagement with the enemy, BI & W rates for the engagement may be quite high but may or may not reflect significant changes in the overall rate. For example, during the first 6 months of the Korean conflict, casualties were higher than in any other American war by a factor of two due to the surprise North Korean invasion, the retreat to Pusan, the amphibious U.S. counterattack at Inchon, and the surprise Chinese attack from Manchuria. Because of the large numbers of U.S. casualties and relatively small numbers of U.S. troops in Korea, the annual rate approaches that of a high-intensity conflict.[19]

Similarly, during much of the Vietnam conflict, battle intensity as measured by BI & W rates was low; however, during the several months of the Tet offensive of 1968, casualties were relatively high,

TABLE 2-2

BATTLE INJURY AND WOUNDING RATES/ 1,000 TROOPS/YEAR DURING VARIOUS U.S. WARS

War	Year	Nonbattle Injuries	Battle Injuries and Wounds
U.S. Civil War	1861–1865	—	97
World War I	1917–1918	—	238
World War II			
Pacific	1942–1945	122	39
Europe	1942–1945	101	108
Mediterranean	1942–1945	131	80
Korea	1950	242	460
	1951	151	170
	1952	102	57
Vietnam	1965	67	62
	1966	76	75
	1967	69	84
	1968	70	120
	1969	63	87

Data sources: [US Civil War, World War I, and World War II] Beebe GW, De Bakey ME. *Battle Casualties: Incidence, Mortality, and Logistic Considerations*. Springfield, Ill: Charles C Thomas; 1952: 21. [Korea] Office of the Surgeon General. Korea: A summary of medical experience July 1950–December 1952. In: *Health of the Army, January, February, and March 1953*. Washington, DC: US Department of the Army; 1953. [Vietnam] Neel S. *Vietnam Studies: Medical Support of the U.S. Army in Vietnam, 1965–1970*. Washington, DC: US Department of the Army; 1973: 33, 36.

resulting in an annual BI & W rate for 1968 of 120, above the World War II (1942–1945) European rate of 108. Despite some intense battles, U.S. Civil War (1861–1865) casualties among Union troops were only 97/1,000/y,[15(p6)] making it a low- to mid-intensity conflict, while the American Expeditionary Forces' World War I (1917–1918) rate of 238 would place it in the mid- to high-intensity range.[17(p6)]

Another factor in intensity is total number of casualties per unit of time. The suddenness and intensity of the 1973 Yom Kippur War resulted in the compression of the amount of casualties normally occurring in the first 20 days of combat in World War II battles into the first 24 to 72 hours of combat.[1]

To take into account this factor of large numbers of casualties in a brief period of time, combat intensity has also been measured by the numbers of "pulses" of fighting in a given time period. During most of the battles of World War II and the Korean conflict, the number of battle pulses per day of combat did not exceed 4 or 5, whereas during the 1973 Yom Kippur War there were 10 to 12 battle pulses per day for the first week.[1]

Battle pulses of high-intensity combat are accompanied not only by high rates of killing and wounding but also by high rates of stress casualties. In the 1973 Yom Kippur War, some units, for example, had as many stress casualties as surgical casualties among both the Israeli and Egyptian forces.[20,21] There is much overlap not only in combat environments but also in symptom complexes.

In general, however, when one compares the symptoms predominating in various wars during the past century, a clustering can be seen based to a degree on the intensity of combat. For example, in addition to venereal diseases and "voluntary casualties"—those caused by failure to take antimalarial pills, engaging in substance abuse, presenting discipline problems (including refusal to fight and assassination of superiors)—are the primary characteristics of low-intensity, unpopular wars: explosive aggressive behavior, social estrangement, and constricted affect. Depressive affect reported by Bar-On and colleagues[22] as occurring in World War I, the 1973 Yom Kippur War, and the 1982 Lebanon War psychiatric casualties may also fit into this low-intensity war symptom complex depending on how it is defined.

During World War I, stress casualties presented with hysterical syndromes, psychomotor disturbances, and fear, as well as depressed affect. The high-intensity combat of the 1973 Yom Kippur War produced similar casualties, and the roughly 2-week period of intense warfare during the 1982 Lebanon War also produced these casualties. Except for that 2-week period, which produced most of the "traditional" (anxiety and fear) stress casualties, engagements in Lebanon were more of a low-intensity, insurgency nature with snipers and booby traps accounting for many casualties.[9] In this situation the development of symptom overlap between Vietnam, overall a classic low-intensity conflict, and the 1982 Lebanon War (ie, social estrangement) is seen. In a review of follow-up studies, Belenky[23] has detected another similarity between Israeli casualties from the 1982 Lebanon War and U.S. casualties from the Vietnam conflict, namely, the development of delayed stress casualties, which are reported as high in both groups of veterans.

These low-intensity warfare casualties, who present with problems that suggest a depressive core and depressive symptoms, were the primary presentation of nostalgia in preceding centuries.[24] Unchecked, these casualties can significantly degrade the combat efficiency of a unit as was seen in the latter phases of the Vietnam conflict.[4]

The "short-timer's syndrome," the development of superstitious dread that one's chances of being killed are increased followed by phobic anxiety and attempts to avoid all risks even when called for by the military mission, was described as a frequent occurrence in most combat and many combat-support soldiers in Vietnam in the final weeks before rotation home.[25] This syndrome had been described in other situations in which exposure to combat is limited by length of time (9 mo of combat in the Korean conflict) or number of missions (a fixed number of bombing runs by aircrews during World War II). Its appearance in Vietnam was, therefore, not surprising; however, its widespread occurrence, affecting even those in minimal danger, may have reflected disaffection and a sense of hopelessness in fighting the war.

Stress casualties of low-intensity combat differ substantially from those of mid- to high-intensity combat, which present primarily with anxiety and conversion and dissociative symptoms. In contrast, low-intensity combat casualties tend to present with "nostalgic" symptoms such as alcohol and drug abuse, venereal diseases, and character and behavior problems of indiscipline. Nostalgic casualties, for the purposes of this chapter, will be defined as the psychiatric symptom clusters that predominated in the behavior leading to ineffectiveness in Vietnam (see Table 2-1). Venereal diseases may be included because, like failure to take malarial prophylaxis or to protect oneself from frostbite, psychological ineffectiveness is often manifested by their appearance.

Prediction of Psychiatric Casualties

From this discussion one may conclude that there is a certain degree of predictability of numbers and types of stress casualties when one knows the intensity of warfare (WIA rate) and composition of the soldier population (combat vs combat-support troops). In a general way this is true. In a mid- to high-intensity battle, soldiers will present with combat stress disorders, but in low-intensity or nonbattle conditions, "garrison neuropsychiatric" casualties will predominate. As combat intensity increases the number of combat stress casualties also increases. There are not yet enough data to predict with confidence the incidence of garrison stress casualties, but the subject is treated extensively in Chapter 3, Disorders of Frustration and Loneliness.

This generalization is, however, an oversimplification that does not take into account the numerous factors that protect a soldier from or predispose him to breakdown. The protective factors include unit cohesion, good leadership, experience with and confidence in one's weapons, absence of fatigue, and prior exposure to combat. Predisposing factors would be the negatives of these. The progress and type of battle also influence the rate of stress casualties. Advancing victorious and retreating defeated armies usually have few stress casualties. In static warfare, with much indirect fire from heavy artillery barrages or aerial attack, stress casualties are increased.[15]

A recently identified factor found to be significant in producing Israeli stress casualties in the 1973 Yom Kippur War is the presence of concurrent nonspecific stress.[26] The stress usually is a product of situations in the soldier's nonmilitary life; for example, pregnancy of spouse, birth of offspring, an ill relative, or financial adversity.

Many of these factors would be unknown to the clinician under usual battle conditions, and, even if they were known, it would be difficult to assign them a particular weight for prediction purposes. Their importance lies in preventive programs. Judging from historical review and recent experience of Israeli medical personnel in the 1982 Lebanon War (23% stress casualties despite attempts to prevent the influence of predisposing factors), the factor of combat intensity seems to outweigh most of the other factors in generating combat stress casualties. In future wars, therefore, the battle ecology can be expected to produce high or low stress casualty rates. A "Yom Kippur" (sustained, high-intensity) war may result in large numbers of combat stress cases, while a "Vietnam" (low-intensity, garrison) war may produce "nostalgic" disorders. Military psychiatry must have the flexibility to respond to either circumstance and to the possibility of nuclear, biological, and chemical (NBC) warfare. The latest U.S. Army neuropsychiatry doctrine[2,27–29] addresses the distribution of mental health resources to respond to all scenarios.

Both traditional combat stress casualties ("combat fatigue," "battle shock," or "combat reaction") and low-intensity combat casualties ("nostalgic") will occur in most protracted conflicts. The traditional casualties will occur proximate to the battles and the nostalgic will occur among rear-area troops or when combat troops rotate back to rear areas. The principles of combat psychiatry were developed during World War I and refined during World War II and the Korean conflict, but not until the Vietnam conflict were nostalgic casualties recognized as a serious cause of ineffectiveness in U.S. forces. It seems appropriate to address first the traditional combat stress casualties that predominate in mid- to high-intensity conflicts. Low-intensity combat stress casualties will be addressed in Chapter 3, Disorders of Frustration and Loneliness; NBC combat stress casualties in Chapter 4, Neuropsychiatric Casualties of Nuclear, Biological, and Chemical Warfare; and high-intensity combat stress casualties in Chapter 5, Psychiatric Principles of Future Warfare, of this textbook.

TREATMENT

The principles of forward treatment were developed and refined during the mid-intensity battles of World War I, World War II, and the Korean conflict. For the casualties of such conflicts they worked reasonably well. Treatment failures, when they occurred, were generally because the principles were not applied. This usually occurred when the conflict took on the characteristics of high-intensity battles, overwhelming forward medical resources and forcing evacuation of casualties, or the characteristics of low-intensity battles, making evacuation more feasible. With future battle circumstances uncertain, all medical personnel and unit leaders should become familiar with the traditional principles of combat psychiatry and be prepared to adapt them to a variety of evolving situations, ranging from low-intensity insurgency actions to high-intensity NBC actions.

The treatment of combat stress casualties depends on a variety of circumstances impossible to foresee until actual engagement with the enemy. These circumstances include the type of battle, the length and location of the war, the type of soldier, the manifestations of ineffectiveness, the type of treating person, and other unforeseen conditions.

The treatment setting depends on the type of war, the type of evacuation (if any), and the availability of resources. Possible treatment settings range from the active battle scene to a medical center in the United States, as shown in Table 2-3.

Treatment of battle fatigue cases begins with their identification. Battle fatigue casualties should never be referred to as psychiatric casualties. The term battle fatigue is more appropriate because it suggests a normal response to the extreme mental and emotional demands of combat.

Treatment of identified combat stress casualties begins with casualty sorting, as shown in Figure 2-1. Battle fatigue cases may be labeled to indicate where they are being treated, with labels such as light, heavy, duty, rest, hold, and refer. These labels do not indicate the presumed cause of the symptoms or the likely response to treatment; they merely designate where the soldier is being treated. While these labels can be useful, there are two compelling reasons to avoid making judgments early in treatment about the presumed etiology and prognosis of individual cases of battle fatigue. First, the initial appearance and symptoms of soldiers may reveal little about the cause or the course of their condition. Second, in time of battle and during the initial interviews, it may not be possible to obtain complete and accurate information about the casualty's personal history. Therefore, all battle fatigue casualties should receive immediate treatment guided by the expectation of rapid and full recovery, as far forward as possible without jeopardizing the mission. As the soldier improves or arrives at a new echelon of care, the label should be modified accordingly.

Casualties are labeled as light or heavy battle fatigue casualties to designate their initial treatment. Battle fatigue cases designated as "light" continue on duty or rest in the unit. Treatment can be provided through buddy aid, unit medics, or leader actions, or can be self-administered. Most soldiers exposed to combat will experience light battle fatigue at some time. Light battle fatigue includes the normal, common signs of battle fatigue, as shown in Exhibit 2-2. It also includes the warning or more serious symptoms, as shown in Exhibit 2-3, if the symptoms respond quickly to treatment. Even soldiers with relatively serious symptoms can often continue on duty and do not necessarily need immediate medical attention. If the symptoms continue despite rest, the soldiers should be sent to their unit surgeon or physician

TABLE 2-3

PSYCHIATRIC ECHELON CARE

Site	Level	Holding Time
Battle	1. Self/buddy	4 h
	2. Small unit leader	4 h
	3. Medical aidman	4 h
Forward area	4. Battalion aid station	8 h
	5. Brigade clearing station	3 d
Rear area	6. Division clearing station	4 d
	7. Special treatment hospital	1–2 wk
	8. Evacuation hospital	1–2 wk
Communication zone	9. Hospital outside combat zone	wk–mo
Continental United States	10. Medical center in United States	Indefinite

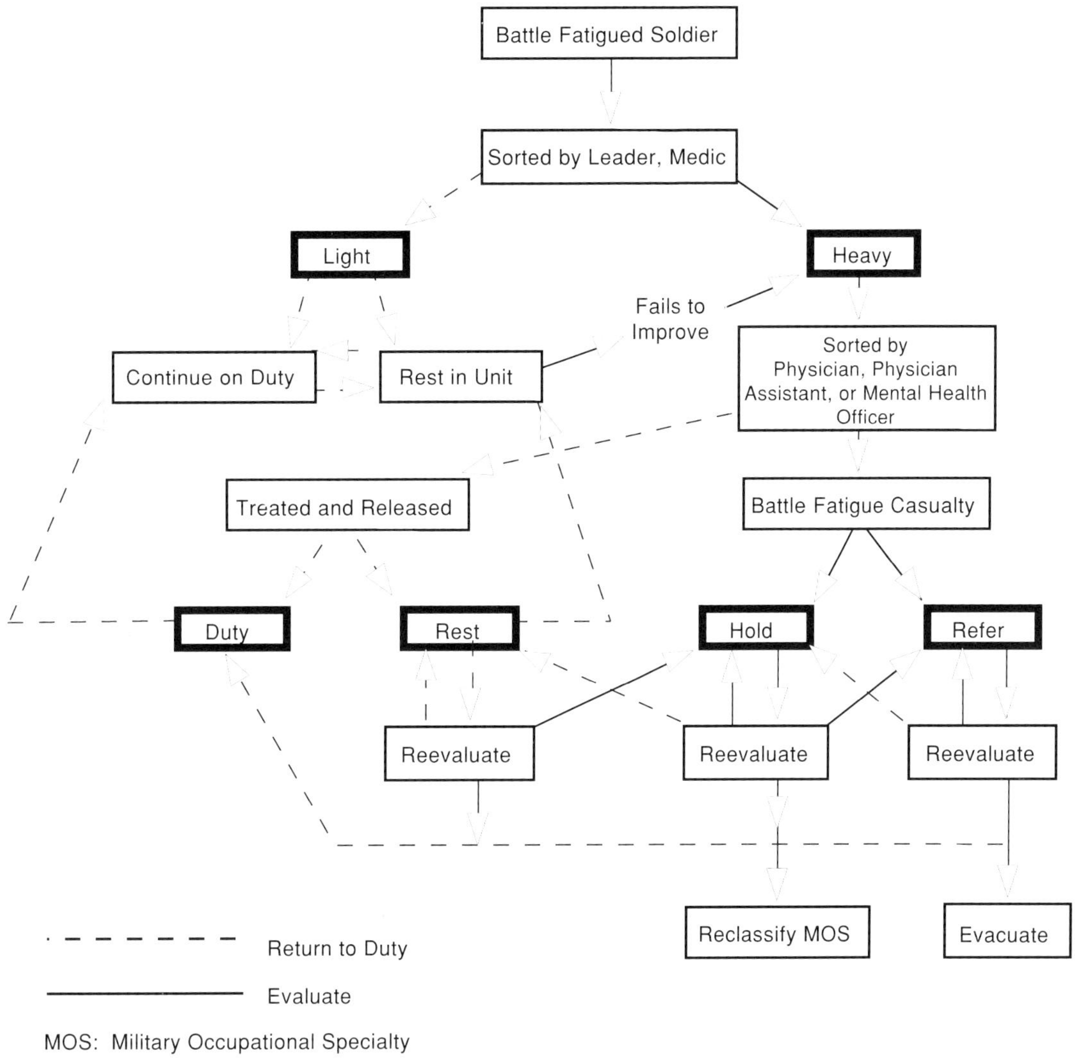

Fig. 2-1. Diagram of sorting choices and labels for battle fatigue cases according to severity of symptoms and unit situation. Reprinted from US Department of the Army. *Leaders' Manual for Combat Stress Control*. Washington, DC: DA; September 1994. Field Manual 22-51: 5-7.

assistant at routine sick call and treated as a heavy battle fatigue casualty.

In contrast to light battle fatigue, heavy battle fatigue requires immediate medical attention. In addition to failure to respond to initial treatment, the "heavy" label can indicate that the soldier's symptoms disrupt the mission of the unit, or that the casualty has a medical condition such as heat stroke that may require emergency treatment.

The triage medic sorts soldiers experiencing heavy battle fatigue based on where they can be treated, as indicated by the labels duty, rest, hold, and refer. Duty cases are heavy battle fatigue casualties who are treated immediately by a physician, physician assistant, or mental health officer and returned to duty. Rest cases do not require continual medical attention and are sent to their unit's nonmedical combat service support elements for brief rest and light duties. Hold cases are heavy battle fatigue casualties who are held for treatment at the triage medic's own medical facility if the tactical situation and the symptoms permit. Refer cases are those who must be treated at a medical facility that is more secure or better-equipped than the triage medic's own facility due to the tactical situation or the casualties' symptoms. Refer cases are relabeled as hold cases when they reach a medical facility where they can be treated.

The decision to label an individual soldier as a case of duty, rest, hold, or refer battle fatigue is not a simple one. Rather, it must be guided by a combination of factors, including the soldier's character-

EXHIBIT 2-2

NORMAL, COMMON SIGNS OF BATTLE FATIGUE

Physical Signs*

- Tension: aches, pains; tremble, fidget, fumble things.
- Jumpiness: startle at sudden sounds or movement.
- Cold sweat; dry mouth; pale skin; eyes hard to focus.
- Pounding heart; may feel dizzy or light-headed.
- Feel out of breath; may breathe too much until fingers and toes start to tingle, cramp, and go numb.
- Upset stomach; may throw up.
- Diarrhea or constipation; frequent urination.
- Emptying bowels and bladder at instant of danger.
- Fatigue: feel tired, drained; takes an effort to move.
- Distant, haunted ("1000 yard") stare.

Mental and Emotional Signs*

- Anxiety: keyed up, worrying, expecting the worst.
- Irritability: swearing, complaining, easily bothered.
- Difficulty paying attention, remembering details.
- Difficulty thinking, speaking, communicating.
- Trouble sleeping; awakened by bad dreams.
- Grief: tearful, crying for dead or wounded buddies.
- Feeling badly about mistakes or what had to be done.
- Anger: feeling let down by leaders and others in unit.
- Beginning to lose confidence in self and unit.

*Many soldiers have these signs, yet still fight well and do all their essential duties.
Source: US Department of the Army. Battle fatigue: Normal, common signs; What to do for self & buddy. US Army Training and Audiovisual Support Center, GTA 21-3-4, June 1986. GPO Stock No. 1991–303-121/49293.

istics, the stressors involved, the soldier's response to treatment, the tactical situation, and the resources available. Furthermore, once the decision is made, it may need to be modified to reflect changing conditions. Successful treatment of combat stress casualties prevents unnecessary evacuation and shifts battle fatigue casualties from refer to hold, from hold to rest, and from rest to duty. The lowest level of treatment likely to be effective should be administered, since holding or evacuating casualties may delay or prevent recovery.

Since World War I, the appropriate use of the principles of forward treatment has resulted in the return of 40% to 90% (optimal conditions) of combat stress casualties to combat duty within days.[7] Forward treatment consists of immediate, brief, simple interventions (immediacy, brevity, simplicity) such as rest and nutrition in a safe place as near the battle lines as possible (proximity), with an explicit statement to the soldier that he will soon be rejoining his comrades (expectancy). These measures create in the soldier a sense that he is only temporarily disabled by fatigue and further create the expectancy that he will quickly return to duty. This expectancy is strengthened when the casualty's small unit comrades can visit him and indicate that they need him and will welcome him back. Treatment is kept simple to foster this expectancy by giving the message that nothing is seriously amiss. Glass[30] has characterized Salmon's approach as a three-tiered (division psychiatrist, front-line specialized hospital, rear-area specialized hospital) related echelon treatment system that takes into account individual and battlefield hindrances to recovery and maximizes the return of the casualty to combat. A further aspect of this echelon approach to treatment calls for soldiers evacuated rearward to be screened at a central collecting point from which they may still be returned to duty if further rearward movement is inappropriate (centrality).

In practice this approach requires four essential elements: (1) a safe place near the battle area (refuge), (2) a treating person (therapist), (3) time for restoration of physiological needs (rest), and (4) a method for returning to one's unit (return). Each element is critical to the process; and each is potentially jeopardized by modern, high-intensity warfare.

EXHIBIT 2-3

MORE SERIOUS SIGNS OF BATTLE FATIGUE

Warning signs that deserve special action, but do NOT necessarily mean a "casualty" who must be evacuated.

Even the normal, common signs become "more serious" if:

- They still disrupt the mission after you take action.
- They don't improve somewhat after good rest.
- The soldier is acting very differently from the way he or she usually does.

More Serious Physical Signs

- Can't keep still; constantly moving around.
- Flinching or ducking at most sudden sounds and movement.
- Shaking (of arms or whole body); cowering in terror.
- Part of body won't work right, with no physical reason:
  - Can't use hand, or arm, or legs.
  - Can't see (or hear, or feel), partially or at all.
- Freezing under fire, or prolonged, total immobility.
- Physical exhaustion; slowed down, just stands or sits.
- Vacant stare, "spaced out"; staggers, sways when stands.

More Serious Mental and Emotional Signs

- Rapid talking; constantly making suggestions.
- Arguing, starting fights; deliberately reckless action.
- Inattention to self-care, hygiene; indifference to danger.
- Memory loss:
  - For orders; for military skills; for a bad event;
  - For time, place, what's going on; or for everything.
- Severe stuttering, mumbling, can't speak at all.
- Afraid to fall asleep for fear of terror dreams, danger; unable to stay asleep even in a safe area.
- Seeing or hearing things that aren't really there.
- Rapid emotional shifts; crying spells; wishing was dead.
- Social withdrawal; silent or sulking; prolonged sadness.
- Apathetic; no interest in food or anything else.
- "Hysterical" outburst, frantic or strange behavior.
- Panic running under fire.

Source: US Department of the Army. Battle fatigue: 'More serious' signs; Leader actions. US Army Training and Audiovisual Support Center, GTA 21-3-5, October 1983.

Both for historical reasons and because psychiatric interventions are most successful in handling the typical stress casualties of mid-intensity, conventional conflicts, they will be addressed first. Such casualties may be grouped roughly in order of increasing exposure to combat as follows: (1) normal battle reactions (not counted as a casualty), (2) acute anxiety syndromes, (3) precombat syndromes (hypochondriasis/following prior combat), (4) chronic anxiety-depressive syndromes (old sergeant syndrome), and (5) atypical syndromes (occurring at all levels of exposure).

Although these symptom constellations may appear at any level of combat intensity, they have been most apparent in World War I and World War II, now considered to be mid-intensity conflicts, based on frequency of battle pulses in a 24-hour period and levels of casualties sustained.

The bulk of combat stress casualties typically occur in the first week of exposure to combat (80%) and present with severe anxiety or with physical symptoms that reflect fear and anxiety.[31] Such symptoms may consist of one or more of the following: rapid heart rate (DaCosta's "soldier's heart" of the U.S. Civil War), profuse sweating, muscle tension, shaking and cramps, nausea, vomiting, diarrhea, and involuntary defecation and urination. At times the casualty may present with minimal anxiety but with complaints that render him unable to function such as loss of the use of muscles (paralysis or aphonia) or disturbances of sensory organs (blindness, deafness, anesthesia, or pain). As with the anxiety symptoms, the unstated but implicit meaning is clear: the soldier has a recognizable medical condition that, he believes, prevents him from further engagement in combat and is thus an honorable escape from battle.

Although malingering might be suspected in some cases, most soldiers present with unconsciously derived symptoms similar to those found in the neurotic conditions of civilian life. During World War I and thereafter, able clinicians have found that interpreting this temporary defection as malingering only forces the soldier to strengthen, usually unconsciously, the symptoms to disprove such an allegation, making restoration to duty less likely.

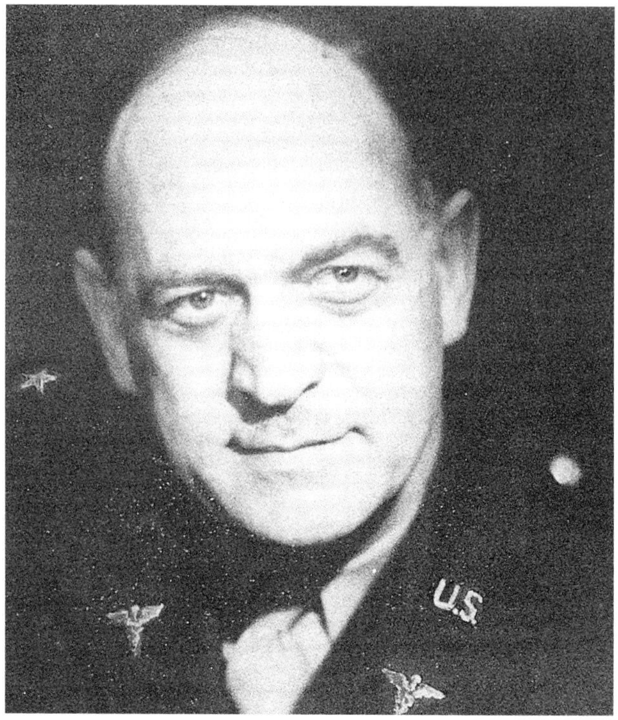

Fig. 2-2. William C. Menninger, from a family of famous psychiatrists, was Neuropsychiatry Consultant to the Army Surgeon General during most of World War II. Among many accomplishments, he arranged for appropriate treatment of psychiatric casualties and established a psychiatric nomenclature that formed the basis for the first Diagnostic and Statistical Manual of the American Psychiatric Association.

Normal Reactions to Combat

Transient fear reactions are universal and should not be considered pathological. In fact, such responses came to be called the normal battle reaction. During World War II a number of surveys were made of physical symptoms experienced by infantry soldiers in combat. According to several studies reviewed by Menninger,[32] (Figure 2-2) and summarized by the author, of infantry soldiers in combat for any length of time, approximately 50% would experience a pounding heart, 45% a sinking stomach, 30% cold sweat, 25% nausea, 25% shakiness and tremulousness, 25% stiff muscles, 20% vomiting, 20% general weakness, 10% involuntary bowel movement, and 6% involuntary urination. Menninger refers to this group of symptoms as the normal battle reaction. The author will detail a number of cases from his experience as a division psychiatrist in Vietnam to illustrate various kinds of stress reactions to combat. The following case illustrates physiological (involuntary urination) and psychological (mutism) responses to combat that led to psychiatric intervention.

Case Study 1: The Tunnel Rat

Corporal A, a 20-year-old single man who had come to Vietnam by troopship in late February 1966 was brought to the 25th Infantry Division Base Hospital in late March 1966 by his platoon sergeant and lieutenant in a mute and unresponsive, but tense and alert condition. On a "search and destroy" mission he had volunteered as a "tunnel rat" to enter part of the extensive Viet Cong underground tunnels near Cu Chi, where the 25th had its base camp. Jumping into an 8-foot hole, he found himself facing a Viet Cong (VC) soldier , who was lying in a side tunnel. The VC aimed a pistol at CPL A's head and pulled the trigger. The pistol misfired, and CPL A's platoon sergeant shot the VC in the head with several blasts from his M16 rifle, splattering CPL A with blood and brain tissue. Examination at the base hospital revealed no wound, other than a small facial scratch from a bone fragment, despite CPL A's gory appearance. The 25th Division psychiatrist (the author) was called to see a "catatonic" patient.

The psychiatrist saw CPL A alone in a shielded area of the hospital tent (the "Mental Hygiene tent" had not yet been erected), and a repeat physical exam was performed. During the examination the physician soothingly pointed out that CPL A was safe and that he had normally functioning body parts and the ability to cooperate in the examination. He was then told that his "vocal cords," which had been temporarily "stunned," were back to normal and that he could say anything he wished. After a brief hesitation CPL A broke into a long, pressured explosion of profanity, ending with, "Damn, I peed my pants." He was told that his reactions were completely normal and that after resting that night in his own bed, he would wake up fully able to return to his usual duties tomorrow.

Comment: The psychiatrist did not see CPL A again; however, informal follow-up with the corporal's platoon leader a few months later revealed that he became cheerful the following day when told that he would get a Purple Heart medal for the wound to his face. CPL A did not volunteer for "tunnel rat" duty again.

The labeling of such normal reactions to battle as abnormal can create psychiatric casualties who may become "evacuation syndrome" patients. Such soldiers are best handled by enlightened commanders and senior noncommissioned officers (NCOs) who can reassure them that their responses are normal for the situation. Should such soldiers come to medical attention, a brief but thorough physical exam (to rule out brain injury, internal hemorrhage, or spinal cord injury) followed by reassurance usually suffices. The following case illustrates the need for a physical exam.

Case Study 2: The Mortar Attack Victim

During the course of an all-night mortar attack on the 25th Infantry Division base camp by Viet Cong guerrillas, the author, as division psychiatrist, was assisting the headquarters surgeon in treating casualties presenting with minor injuries (most caused by small pieces of fragmentation devices or bruises and abrasions sustained when soldiers were hastily seeking shelter). A military policeman (MP) brought his youthful fellow MP for treatment of complaints of apprehensiveness. The two of them were driving across the compound when a mortar landed just behind their jeep, momentarily "stunning" the patient, who had been sitting in the back seat. The patient had been "jarred" by the concussion but was unaware of any injury.

Examination revealed a pale (even in the subdued light used to avoid targeting the dispensary tent), apprehensive young man who was sweating profusely. His muscles were tense, and his skin was cool and clammy ("cold sweat"). He had no complaints of pain and no apparent injury; however, his pulse was rapid and weak (low pulse pressure). He was allowed to rest, but his condition deteriorated with development of marked apprehensiveness. Reexamination in better light revealed a small tear in his field jacket, which had been covered by his MP belt. Removing the jacket and undershirt revealed a small puncture wound of the left lower back. A diagnosis of hemorrhagic shock was made, and the Division Psychiatrist accompanied the patient to the division surgical unit where the patient received blood transfusions. Subsequently he was evacuated to a field hospital where abdominal surgery revealed massive hemorrhage from a ruptured spleen.

Comment: This patient had typical symptoms found in acute anxiety or fear reactions in combat: apprehensiveness, sweating and peripheral vasoconstriction (producing the "cold sweat"), tachycardia, and increased muscle tension. The weak pulse, presumably due to impending hypovolemic shock with decreased pulse pressure, should have been a clue to the internal hemorrhaging. Had this patient been uninjured, reassurance and return to his unit would be the treatment procedure.

Ranson has described a spectrum of symptomatology in combat ranging from "the normal battle reaction" to "the pathologic battle reaction." He observes that:

> [T]he normal battle reaction is made up of a variable set of symptoms that arise from (1) moderate to extreme physical fatigue; and (2) extreme, repeated, and continued battle fear, with (a) marked psychosomatic symptoms resulting from this fear and (b) certain psychologic symptoms resulting therefrom.[33(p3)]

Ranson described normal psychosomatic response patterns to combat stress to include muscular tension, "freezing" or temporary immobility, shaking and tremors, excessive perspiration, anorexia or nausea, occasionally vomiting, abdominal distress, mild diarrhea and urinary frequency including incontinence of feces or urine, tachycardia and palpitation, hyperventilation to the point of giddiness and syncope, weakness and lassitude, and aches and pains. He also described special psychologic considerations in the normal battle reaction including combat sensitization with anticipatory anxiety, sensitization to combat noises, insomnia, diminished drive and initiative, irritability and increasing fear, including fear of showing fear.[33]

This normal reaction may be mislabeled as abnormal. This may have occurred in Israeli forces in the 1982 Lebanon War. Despite relatively low-intensity combat, 23% of Israel's total casualties were labeled as psychiatric. Israel, following the 1973 Yom Kippur War, had devised a system of early identification of psychiatric casualties with an increased expectancy that such casualties would occur.[10] Furthermore, by labeling such casualties "combat reaction," Israeli mental health personnel created an expectancy that combat alone would create such casualties. Early in World War II American medical personnel, by eliminating soldiers who exhibited symptoms of anxiety, had created a similar expectancy that was further compounded by the evacuation of such soldiers out of combat. Management, therefore, requires informing the soldier that his symptoms, while calling for rest, are not a reason for evacuation.

Inappropriate evacuation of the lightly wounded not only creates an evacuation syndrome but often results in a psychiatric casualty. Lightly-wounded Israeli soldiers in the 1973 Yom Kippur War were found to respond similarly to psychiatric casualties when evacuated from battle,[21] that is, they developed complaints that prevented them from returning to combat. These complaints were both physical (eg, pain, weakness) and psychological (eg, anxiety, fear, depression). As seen in Bowman's[11] listing of psychiatric casualties in Vietnam (see Exhibit 2-1), a significant number were wounded soldiers. Wounding always elicits psychological responses, though not always negative. During World War II, soldiers spoke with elation of receiving "the golden wound," one that would honorably excuse the soldier from battle but not produce permanent disability. Bowman's patients, for instance, developed symptoms as the time drew near for them to return to combat. Such symptoms were usually physical complaints—pain in healed wounds, weakness, and even frank conversion reactions.

In treating the lightly wounded, it is important to treat forward and attempt to avoid rearward evacuation. If evacuation has occurred, "forward evacuation" nearer the battle area with application of the principles of combat psychiatry was found effective by the Israelis in the 1982 Lebanon War.[9] The more seriously wounded who have recovered to the point of return to combat must be managed with the same expectancy approach utilized with recognized psychiatric casualties.

By contrast, severely disabled soldiers—those with amputations, severe thoracic or abdominal wounds, widespread burns, blindness, and brain or spinal cord injuries—generally cannot be returned to combat; thus early psychiatric treatment is often needed in long-term treatment centers to help the veteran adjust to the disability. A variety of psychological responses similar to those described by Kubler-Ross[34] in the dying patient will be encountered: denial, anger, bargaining, depression, and acceptance. Weinstein and Kahn,[35] in their study of brain-injured and amputee patients, found that denial remains the predominant, underlying mechanism in such patients with manifestations such as phantom limb, amnesia, confabulation, reduplication, and other often bizarre responses. These are discussed in Chapter 14, Disabling and Disfiguring Injuries.

In summary, it has been shown that the normal psychological reactions to combat when inappropriately labeled and evacuated lead to actual disability. Such inappropriate evacuation of the lightly wounded likewise often results in psychiatric decompensation.

Pathological Reactions to Combat

Ranson[33] argued that these normal responses to battle shade into pathological responses usually as prolonged or exaggerated normal responses. Examples include the immobilized soldier who remains so for several hours or when the immobility poses a danger to himself or his comrades; autonomic overactivity symptoms that persist long after the danger; noise sensitization that generalizes to innocuous noises; lassitude that becomes persistent apathy and depression; and fear that develops into panic. Such symptoms in response to the threat of death are normal and virtually universal. A variety of personal and interpersonal interactions can result in the transformation of the normal battle reaction into a pathological battle reaction. Also, if the soldier lacks the adaptive capacity to handle the anxiety, it may be expressed through mental defense mechanisms as conversion or dissociative reactions.

Acute Anxiety Syndromes

As suggested earlier, the symptoms in such cases are the same as those occurring in the normal battle reaction—basically exaggerated physiological responses of autonomic overactivity combined with mental states of fear or apprehension.

Conversion reactions generally involve interference with voluntary muscle (paralysis, convulsions, muteness, ataxia, movement disorders) or sensory (anesthesia, blindness, deafness, pain) function. Psychogenic loss of smell or taste is rare; however, complaints of smelling burning flesh, napalm, or other battle smells often occur in chronic post-traumatic stress disorders. The paralyses frequently involve organs important for combat functions, for example, paralysis of the trigger finger. Similarly, pain complaints may prevent combat function. Helmet headaches were briefly a problem in some units in Vietnam, because this equipment was required for soldiers on ambush or perimeter patrols. It was the author's experience that the symptom disappeared when soldiers were told that they would have to do such duty without head protection.

Conversion symptoms appear to occur more frequently in medically naive and medically sophisticated populations. In the latter cases symptoms often consist of pain and weakness that may be difficult to distinguish from neurological or musculoskeletal dysfunction. In the former cases, naive populations may present with classical hysteroepilepsy, hemipareses, and stocking and glove anesthesias. Such symptoms were observed, for example, in the Iraq-Iran War among Iranian soldiers.[36]

Because conversion reactions indicate a relative breakthrough of primary process thinking, though disguised, limited, and controlled, treatment may be more prolonged than with anxious and fatigued casualties unless corrected early. World War I U.S. Army psychiatrists reported substantial success with strong positive suggestion and simple explanation when given early and far forward (today called "immediacy, proximity and expectancy").[37] In some cases hypnotherapy and abreactive treatments may be indicated. The following case, known to the author, illustrates severe anxiety and stuttering in response to combat.

Case Study 3: The Stutterer

Following an all night mortar attack on the 25th Infantry Division base camp in which several soldiers died and nearly 100 were wounded, a 20-year-old radio operator for hospital communications complained of the sudden onset of severe stuttering as well as anxiety. On examination the soldier appeared as a lanky, blond youth wearing glasses, stuttering, and displaying startle reaction to outgoing artillery rounds. The soldier had a history of briefly suffering from stuttering at about age 5 years when he first left home to start school (kindergarten). Physical exam was normal.

The author, as division psychiatrist, arranged for the soldier to be temporarily relieved from radio operator duty but hinted that if symptoms persisted the soldier would have to revert to his primary specialty of general infantryman. After one day the soldier's symptoms began to abate: however, the division surgeon, a kindly and sympathetic man, evacuated the soldier from the division while the psychiatrist was away on a MILPHAP (Military Public Health Action Program) mission to a local Vietnamese hamlet. The soldier never reurned to the division.

Comment: This case reveals the failure of treatment because of a physician's humanitarian instincts' leading him to believe that he was alleviating suffering. No follow-up was available, but similar inappropriate evacuations during World War II led to chronic disability. The appropriate treatment was rest, reassurance, and return to duty.

Dissociative reactions classically consisted of somnambulism, amnesia, fugue, and multiple personality. The following example from Vietnam illustrates the manner by which somnambulism became an evacuation syndrome in the unit to which the author was assigned.[38]

Case Study 4: The Sleepwalkers

A brief "epidemic" of somnambulism occurred in 1966 during the early deployment of the 25th Infantry Division in Vietnam. The engineer battalion surgeon had sought the help of the division psychiatrist to treat soldiers who were developing sleepwalking (somnambulism). The battalion surgeon was surprised to find a rash of such cases in his relatively small unit. The initial case had presented with a history of sleepwalking during childhood with occasional episodes of falling and injuring himself. His family had been completely dominated by his symptoms, being forced to move to a one-story house, placing a high fence with locked gates around the house, and making other arrangements for his safety. His sleepwalking, however, had disappeared until arrival in Vietnam. Following the example of the soldier's parents, the battalion surgeon moved the patient's sleeping area to the center of the base camp to prevent him from wandering into the minefields that surrounded the base camp.

This environmental manipulation appeared to succeed; however, in the subsequent two weeks three more soldiers reported with complaints of sleepwalking. The battalion surgeon was running out of space in which to house these men. The division psychiatrist observed that the engineering battalion was located along one perimeter of the base camp on the side where a pro-Viet Cong village had been located and from which sniper fire was a regular occurrence at night. There had also been rumors of incidents in other camps during which "sappers" (infiltrators) had in nighttime forays cut the throats of sleeping soldiers. The perimeter area had been cleared of trees, had been heavily mined, and had nighttime perimeter guards (only subsequently was it learned that a very extensive tunnel system was the source of much of the sniper fire).

The division psychiatrist recommended that the sleepwalkers be told that the new policy was to place sleepwalkers on permanent nighttime perimeter guard duty (considered unsafe) or generator maintenance duty (considered undesirable) to protect them from wandering into the minefield at night.

Comment: This intervention consisted of preventing the sleepwalking from allowing the soldiers to escape hazardous duty. When this was accomplished, the "epidemic" abruptly ceased.

Multiple personality has rarely occurred in a combat setting, and current evidence suggests childhood sexual trauma as the etiologic agent in most cases. Soldiers presenting themselves as suffering from multiple personality in combat settings are most often malingering to escape punishment for being absent without leave (AWOL). Such presentations tend to wax and wane with mass media publicity of cases.

Amnesia is often attributed to concussion by the patient with more or less justification. Amnesia is sometimes used as an excuse to account for AWOL or other temporary dereliction from duty. Confronting the soldier with disbelief is generally not useful. The proper therapeutic stance in most cases is to reassure the soldier that his memory will return but, if not, that the amnesia will not prevent him from fulfilling some role in combat. A day might be spent teaching the soldier to load, aim, and fire a rifle, for example, with the clear implication that no matter what his original specialty was, he can be an infantryman. The following case illustrates the efficacy of such suggestion in soldiers with psychological amnesia.

Case Study 5: The Amnesiac

In 1968, a 19-year-old single male was evacuated to Walter Reed Army Medical Center in Washington, D.C. from a nearby post at which he was in training as a paratrooper. He was scheduled to graduate from "jump school" and had received orders for Vietnam. Following his final parachute jump, he was found unconscious, was hospitalized locally, and was found to have no neurological deficit other than amnesia for his entire life. He did not know his name and did not recognize friends and family members. At Walter Reed, where the author was supervising the case, the soldier underwent Amytal interview without remission. Collateral history including early development was not impressive of psychogenic trauma. The soldier was told that there would be another attempt at Amytal; but, that if it failed, he would have to return to basic training and then be sent to Vietnam. It was suggested during Amytal interview that his memory would begin returning and should be completely normal within a week.

Comment: Within a week his memory had returned, and he was sent on amended orders to Vietnam but not to an airborne unit. Although this is not a true combat breakdown, it does have characteristics of a precombat syndrome.

Fugue states in military settings are often accompanied by alcohol or drug abuse and licentious behavior, frequently in contrast with the soldier's usual personality.

Case Study 6: The Wild Week

In 1966, a 32-year-old staff sergeant with 12 years of active duty was brought to the attention of the Shore Patrol by prostitutes on Tu Do Street in Saigon because of his unresponsive behavior. In a confused state he was taken to the Third Field Hospital where it was established that physical examination was normal except for mental status. Mental status examination by the author revealed a thin, balding Caucasian man who was dressed in soiled civilian clothing. He smelled of urine but not alcohol. He appeared perplexed and asked where he was. He gave the date as November 5, 1965 (it was later established that he had left the United States on this date and that he was in the last month of his tour in Vietnam). He was oriented to person and, except for amnesia since coming to Vietnam, mental functions were essentially normal. He was sedated (Librium) and put to bed.

The following day his memory had returned up to about 1 week before. He stated that his last memories were of coming to Saigon with a convoy from a nearby village, Dian, where he was a mess sergeant with an infantry company. Although he was technically AWOL, the unit was tolerant of his absence because he was close to the end of his tour and his replacement had already arrived. The company commander merely thought that "he was having a good time in Saigon." The commander also stated that the staff sergeant was a devout, nondrinking, married man who attended chaplain's services regularly and that "sowing a few wild oats" might be helpful to him.

Although all of the details of the missing week were never discovered, it appeared that the staff sergeant, who had reportedly never been unfaithful in his 10 years of marriage, succumbed to the charms of a prostitute. Ensconced in a hotel room, he spent a month's pay with a succession of prostitutes accompanied by liberal intake of the local beer, "33" ("Bah moui bah" in Vietnamese). After an additional day of rest during which he was reassured that such an incident was unlikely to occur again if he avoided alcohol and prostitutes, he was discharged and returned to his unit where he remained an uneventful 2 weeks until returning to the United States.

Comment: It is sometimes difficult to determine how much intoxication contributes to the amnesia in such fugue cases. In addition to protecting him from guilt-inducing memories, the amnesia also protects the patient from having to recount embarrassing behavior.

Precombat Syndromes

Psychological adjustment to combat may begin long before an actual battle. It begins as soon as the possibility of going into combat is seriously entertained. It is even possible to conceive of those who burned their draft cards as engaging in a long-term avoidance maneuver. When the author arrived in Hawaii as the new 25th Infantry Division Psychiatrist, he found the topic of most immediate concern was whether the 25th Division would stay in Hawaii as a "strategic reserve" or go to Vietnam. Although no official confirmation was given until the day prior to departure, it became increasingly evident that the next assignment would be in Vietnam. The majority of soldiers began preparing for combat duty. Some took courses in the Vietnamese language or read books on tropical diseases, insects, and reptiles. Others purchased hunting knives, special water-repellent clothing, and enormous amounts of soap because there were rumors of a shortage. Exercising became fashionable. This somewhat compulsive behavior served its purpose. A soldier who is busy learning a language, practicing with a knife, or running to increase lung and leg power does not have as much time to think about being killed, crippled, or separated from loved ones.

A small minority of soldiers, however, consciously or unconsciously sought to evade combat duty. Some wives appeared at clinics describing medical conditions in themselves or their children for which they felt justified in having their husbands near. Some soldiers appeared in dispensaries or clinics having discovered physical defects in themselves that they thought would make them vulnerable in combat. These defects included decreased hearing, a childhood heart murmur, mild hypertension, a "trick knee," and even simple obesity. A few individuals inflicted wounds on themselves. In one incident, a medical corpsman anesthetized a friend's foot with the local anesthetic, Xylocaine, then shot it with an M-16 rifle. Several soldiers claimed to be homosexual because this condition called for separation from the military. Others committed military crimes (usually AWOL or insubordination) in an attempt to achieve medical or administrative separation from the service. Their usual comment in the stockade was, "I just want out. Any kind of discharge will do." These individuals were few in number, however. A more common response was for a soldier to express relief to finally know for sure that he was going to Vietnam and to begin preparing himself.

The term "precombat syndrome," however, has generally not included these attempts to evade altogether duty in a combat zone. Rather, this term has been reserved for combat veterans, often with lengthy exposure to battle conditions, who on the eve of combat report to medical officers with hypochondriacal or minor complaints.[39] Such persons usually believe that their symptoms are real and significant. Symptoms may include headaches, toothaches, indigestion, and worry over healed or nearly healed wounds. On a more conscious level, some individuals report with broken spectacles and dentures or, more rarely, with self-inflicted wounds.

Failing to understand the nature of these symptoms, some commanders have regarded such soldiers as malingerers and have taken a punitive approach to deterrence of "goldbricking." One support commander in the 25th Infantry Division ordered that sick call be held outside, exposed to the weather, which was often inclement, with daily rains and a hot tropical sun. Unable to gain the reassurance that nothing serious is wrong and the support from the physician, such soldiers may become demoralized and more subject to combat breakdown.

The proper approach to such soldiers is a thorough physical examination (especially because some illnesses, particularly hepatitis, are of insidious onset with vague complaints and exacerbation of characterological tendencies) followed by reassurance that all is well and expressions of gratitude to the soldier for adhering to duty, in spite of pain, for his comrades and country.

Chronic Anxiety-Depressive Syndromes

Continuous or long-term exposure to the lethal combat environment in which the emergency "fight-flight"[40] response is repeatedly invoked eventually results in performance decrements in virtually every combatant. Such repeated physiological arousal gradually has a conditioning effect on voluntary muscles (increased tension, tremors), involuntary or autonomic responses (tachycardia, increased blood pressure, increased perspiration and respiration), and cognitive responses (anxiety, fear). The loss of comrades not only provokes anxiety about one's own mortality but also represents a loss of social reinforcement with subsequent anger and depression. During World War II, Sobel[41] referred to such casualties as "the old sergeant syndrome."

In analyzing the factors leading to breakdown in "the old sergeant syndrome," Sobel traced the "progressive breakdown of the adaptive mechanisms of the normal soldier to the point at which his natural resources are exhausted in the struggle against his environment."[41(p145)] In the loss of his defenses against combat anxiety, the soldier successively lost his ideals about the war (the goals of freedom for Nazi-held peoples and "keeping the enemy out of the United States"), his hatred of the enemy (producing vulnerability to guilt), his short-term goal of being relieved from combat, his pride in himself (feeling of responsibility to be courageous and to endure), and, finally, loss of loyalty to the group (chiefly through actual physical depletion of the group from death, wounding, and illness).

When such repeatedly traumatized combat veterans emerge as psychiatric casualties, they usually present with some variant or mixture of anxiety or depressive symptoms. The "startle reaction," for instance, may represent conditioned muscle tension and other physiological arousal to loud noises (as from exploding mortar, artillery, or bomb attacks). Soldiers presenting with lethargy, decreased self-esteem, and insomnia may be responding with depression to repeated losses and fatigue from repeated arousal. In one model of depression,[42] the hormonal regulatory system of the hypothalamus has become disturbed from higher cognitive and limbic (emotional) inputs. The repeated physiological and cognitive arousal invoked by combat exposure would seem appropriate to such a model. The following cases illustrate some of the symptomatology in such casualties.

Case Study 7: The Fourth Ship

Laughlin[43] in his "case 184" describes a "severe combat reaction following maximal stress." Toward the end of World War II he came across a naval petty officer whom a physician described in disparaging terms as an inferior and unstable person because he had broken down in combat. On closer examination Laughlin recognized him as a fellow shipmate of several years before. His service on ship as quartermaster had included "all kinds of strenuous operational and combat conditions." Laughlin could barely recognize him: physically he had shrunk and aged unbelievably. When seen about 2 years earlier, he had been a young, strong, self-possessed person with a "rock-like quality" of strong leadership; but, now "he was an aged, palsied, defeated and pathetic figure, shriveled and shrunken to nearly half his former weight." Laughlin's colleague who espoused character deficits as the cause of breakdown could not have made a more unjustified case for his assumptions of the etiology of such breakdowns.

Laughlin had traveled with him from the North Atlantic on convoy duty through the North African landing operations finally to the Pacific for the final phase of the campaign for Guadalcanal and the Solomon Islands. In the Pacific, enemy air and naval engagements had occurred, and finally the ship was sunk during an engagement of great stress to the crew. Among the survivors "a fair number developed combat fatigue and various stress reactions." The patient, who had been "a tower of strength" throughout all these exigencies, continued outwardly unfazed and promptly returned to duty, volunteering for service on another destroyer. Laughlin did not see him again until the recently described meeting.

Intrigued by what could have rendered such a change, Laughlin spent time with him and gradually pieced together his history. After loss of the ship in early July 1943, "the tempo of stress" did not abate but actually increased. He continued an unusually extensive combat experience on two subsequent destroyers, each of which had sunk in turn. Not until after the second sinking did he have his first nervous symptoms (depression and anxiety), which gradually increased during service on the third destroyer and after its loss. The culminating traumatic experience occurred on ship number 4 about a month prior to his hospitalization. Scouting enemy shore battery positions that had previously been thought silenced on Southern Okinawa, the ship ran aground on a poorly charted ledge. At this point the "silenced" shore batteries had suddenly opened up at point-blank range. Hundreds of rounds were poured into the helpless ship, until the ship, riddled, dead in the water and sinking, was ordered abandoned. The patient got off the ship and into the water but was seized by the tide, drawing him, despite his strongest efforts, toward a large, burning oil slick from the stricken ship. For what seemed an eternity, he managed to stay clear of the fire until the batteries were in fact silenced and he could be rescued. The anorexic, apathetic, depressed patient resulted from what Laughlin calls "the Final Straw."[43(p11)]

Comment: Laughlin does not discuss treatment in this particular case; however, at that time hospitalization with rest, sedation, insight-oriented psychotherapy or group therapy, and sometimes abreaction, often assisted with hypnosis or intravenous barbiturates, would have been the usual treatment for chronic, fixed neurotic states.

Currently, group or individual psychotherapy with perhaps an abreactive technique might still be called for, but the emphasis in treatment would be "here and now" issues (ie, work, relations with others). Relaxation exercises involving deconditioning to noises or battle memories might be used as well; and, if nightmares and depression were prominent, an antidepressant such as phenelzine (a monoamine oxidase [MAO] inhibitor) or imipramine (a tricyclic) would probably be used, since they suppress dream sleep and hence prevent nightmares.

During World War II, return to a combat role was usually impossible; however, duty in noncombat roles was generally successful. Perhaps a primary factor in the inability to return "the old sergeant syndrome" patient to duty was the consensus that the soldier had done his part and deserved release from combat service. This is illustrated in Sobel's "Case 27":

Case Study 8: The "Old Sergeant Syndrome"

A 20-year-old technical sergeant with 30 months' service who had been overseas 21 months and had an aggregate of 310 days of combat was admitted during a rest period after the battle of the Gothic Line. He had been thrice wounded in action. He stated that he began to have abnormal battle reactions 60 combat days previously. He said: "Now if I get in a hole I just want to stay. It bothers me more now than it ever did before. This last battle my company was ordered to take a house, and within a few hundred yards of the place a couple of my boys got their feet blown off. We withdrew and I went to the commanding officer and told him I had a feeling that I was going to get it this time, and that I couldn't take it any more. He gave me a direct order to, and it was either do that or have a bad record, so I went."

This soldier had tried on three occasions to have his rank reduced to that of private. "You see," he said, "as a platoon sergeant, you are more often than not a platoon leader, and I couldn't lead the men like I did before. Under shelling I got jittery. A platoon sergeant is a leader. If he isn't out in front it affects the men."

This soldier was born on a ranch in Texas. He stated that his father was epileptic, but that he rarely worried about it and that it had not affected him in any way. His parents were harmoniously married. There were seven children, of which he was next to the oldest. He had a happy family life and had many friends on nearby ranches. No significant neurotic traits or conflicts were elicited in the history. Enuresis, nail biting, temper tantrums, running away from home, nightmares, and somnambulism were all denied. He left home to work on another ranch at the age of 14, after completing the eighth grade, and had been steadily employed as a rancher until induction. He had always been self-reliant and industrious. Single, he had no significant sexual conflicts.

His Army career was characterized by steady promotion after his arrival overseas. He stated that he had been held down in the States by a lack of T/O [Table of Organization] vacancies. A letter from his battalion commander stated: "It is my opinion, through observation, that he has reached the end of endurance as a combat soldier. Therefore, in recognition of a job well done I recommend that this soldier be released from combat duty and be reclassified in another capacity." This battalion commander, incidentally, was noted for his unyielding attitude toward psychiatric casualties.

Therapy was found to be surprisingly simple, but administratively difficult. The most effective single therapeutic tool was assigning these men within the army area, out of shellfire but close enough for them to feel that they were actually helping the men "up front." The usual psychotherapeutic procedures were necessary and valuable, but because the "old sergeant syndrome" is primarily a situational reaction, altering the environment by means of reassignment is the most important aid to readjustment and cure. At one time we had several of these men on the cadre of the divisional training and rehabilitation center. Their work over a four-month period was beyond reproach.[41(p145)]

[The divisional training and rehabilitation center was the facility in the rear of each division, in the late World War II European and Mediterranean theaters, responsible for returning soldiers with combat exhaustion to duty. It was located close to the division medical clearing station, was supervised by the division psychiatrist, but was staffed entirely by line officers and NCOs and maintained a strictly military atmosphere, including realistic combat drills.[44]—JWS, Ed.]

Comment: Given the efficacy of modern drugs in controlling anxiety and depression, it is possible that in extreme need such skilled soldiers might be returned to combat roles. The Israelis, always short of manpower, treated a few such casualties with tricyclic antidepressants during the 1982 Lebanon War. Belenky, Tyner, and Sodetz reported that five Israeli soldiers, representing 8% of the casualties treated in a third-echelon, longer-term treatment facility (total of 60 patients), received tricyclic antidepressants.[9] Although between one third and one half of the total patients returned to their original units, it is not known whether these men were among such returnees, or whether the units were still in combat. The risks of returning soldiers on medication to forward deployed duty include: side effects profiles which may interfere with psychomotor performance; impaired judgment in dangerous situations; medical risks from side effects in the field environment; problem with resupply; and adjusting dosage at far-forward medical aid stations.

Atypical Reactions to Combat

Atypical Anxiety/Depressive Cases

Men with "pseudopsychotic reactions," according to Weinstein,[45] appeared to be out of contact with their current physical environment, being "agitated, hallucinatory, and delusional, performing such stereotypes as digging foxholes with their fingers, taking shelter under their cots at any sudden sound and 'warning' others of the approach of shells."[45(p138)] In Italy most such cases occurred in troops new to battle and to the group who had been freshly called up before an offensive action. Group ties had not only been weakly established at the outset but also they rapidly dissolved when the group faced hostile enemy fire. Glass[7] reported that such casualties occurred early in World War II when the designation "psychoneurosis" (abbreviated "psycho" by the soldiers) was given to most psychiatric (stress) casualties. This illustrates the continuing importance of not calling these soldiers "psychiatric casualties" today.

The ambiguities of low-intensity, civil-war-type conflicts can produce atypical reactions. The following two cases illustrate the buildup of personal problems in a noncombatant in the first case and the issue of ethical conflicts in a new combatant in the second case.

Case Study 9: Shots in the Night

After several months in Vietnam, the author had begun taking sick call with the Headquarters (HQ) Company surgeon (who had been an "on-the-job-training" psychiatrist in Hawaii) due to the lack of significant numbers of psychiatric casualties. He and the surgeon bunked in the back of the dispensary, which was adjacent to the HQ supply tent where the supply sergeant slept. One night the two physicians were awakened by shots fired at close range. Dressed only in their underclothing and Colt .45 gunbelts, the two rushed next door to find the supply sergeant firing his M-16 rifle in the direction of the division commander's tent.

The HQ surgeon, who had been treating the sergeant for bursitis, was able to talk him into surrendering the rifle. Subsequently the sergeant's story came out. In his mid-40s, he had bitterly resented being sent to a combat zone in his last tour of duty after having already been in combat during the Korean conflict. Furthermore, he suffered from bursitis of the shoulder, which he felt should have kept him from a combat assignment. Except for some general complaining, however, he had hidden his feelings. The HQ surgeon had been treating his bursitis with periodic injections of hydrocortisone with only minimal relief of pain. Increasingly despondent, the sergeant began drinking to fall asleep at night. Finally on the night in question, mildly inebriated, he began firing at the general's tent in expectation that he would be shot: suicide by someone else's hands.

The following morning, the sergeant was remorseful about the event, expressed that he had no suicide intention, and asked to continue his assignment. He was closely followed by the HQ surgeon, steroid injections were replaced by large dosages of aspirin, he was given Librium for sleep (the only nonneuroleptic, nonbarbiturate sedative available) and he discontinued all alcohol intake. His mood gradually improved, and he was able to complete the remainder of his tour.

Comment: A number of confounding factors were present in this case. In the biological area is a chronic pain problem compounded by treatment with steroids, which are known to alter mood in many cases. In terms of intrapersonal variables, the sergeant had a basically obsessive-compulsive personality with passive-aggressive features. The situational variables included some isolation from his fellow soldiers by reason of age and temperament. In interpersonal contacts he frequently had to respond with negatives to demands for clothing and equipment. Also, the news from home was sometimes alarming with his wife's complaints about the rebellious behavior of their teenage children. Finally, a few weeks prior to this incident, the base camp had sustained an all night mortar attack with numerous wounded and a few killed.

One outcome of this incident was the development of a Standing Operating Procedure (SOP) for berserk soldiers.[38] There had been several prior incidents in which soldiers would "go berserk" and start firing indiscriminately or barricade themselves and threaten any approaching personnel. Following this incident, the commanding general asked the provost marshal and division psychiatrist to develop an SOP for dealing with such soldiers. The provost marshal suggested that the area be evacuated and sealed off from all but selected personnel, mostly military police, then the division psychiatrist be summoned to speak with him. If he continued to be a threat and waiting was not feasible, sharpshooters would shoot to wound or, if all else failed, to kill. The division psychiatrist agreed with most of the SOP but recommended that the person called to negotiate be either a known friend of the soldier or his commander if he were not hostile to the commander. The division psychiatrist would either accompany the negotiator or be in radiotelephone contact with him. After the SOP became known, very few such incidents occurred.

Case Study 10: The Atrocity

Several months after the 25th Infantry Division had been in Vietnam, the division chief of staff requested the division psychiatrist to evaluate an infantry second lieutenant, a West Point graduate, who had requested that his military occupational specialty (MOS) be changed to that of a chaplain's assistant. When questioned, the lieutenant, a single male in his early twenties, was found to have no evidence of schizophrenia, mood disorder, or any other significant mental affliction.

He had been in several "search and destroy" missions, including some exposure to combat; however, he attributed his change from a warrior to a "man of God" to a recent incident. His platoon had engaged in a firefight at a small Vietnamese village known to be sympathetic to the Viet Cong. After the shooting stopped, an elderly Vietnamese man was found killed with his rifle nearby. The soldiers tied his feet to the rear bumper of a jeep and repeatedly dragged his body up and down the main street of the village. This created a sense of revulsion in the lieutenant but he did not stop what he subsequently referred to as "the atrocity." The day after the incident he requested a change of MOS.

Background history revealed that although he had followed his father, now a general, into the military, he had always been somewhat ambivalent about doing so. Also, he was deeply religious, the legacy of his mother. He was a member of a Christian sect that did not require one to be a conscientious objector, but he stated that he had always felt that he could not kill another human being. The division psychiatrist recommended that the lieutenant be given his requested assignment change. In subsequent sessions the consequences of his choice were explored (one was that the chief of staff delayed his promotion because he had "failed the test of battle").

Comment: Although the psychiatrist suspected neurotic conflicts concerning his identity involving ambivalence toward his father and the army he represented, the lieutenant was determined to pursue his new career. When the division psychiatrist left the division, the lieutenant was still working as a chaplain's assistant.

With hindsight regarding the failure of the U.S. pacification and Vietnamization programs in the Vietnam conflict, and of the serious problems of indiscipline which continued to haunt the U.S. Army through the period of the "hollow Army" of the 1970s, it is apparent that this case was not dealt with appropriately by the chain of command. It must be noted that the lieutenant was morally and legally correct in his distress, and in labeling the event "the atrocity." Desecrating enemy dead (whether combatants or noncombatants) is a war crime, punishable under the Uniform Code of Military Justice (UCMJ). Officers who allow their subordinates to commit war crimes without intervening or subsequently bringing charges are also subject to disciplinary action. The severity of the disciplinary action may depend on the seriousness of the violation. Dragging the body of an enemy already killed in combat is not as serious an offense as killing a disarmed enemy after surrender or an unarmed civilian, but it cannot be allowed to pass without firm action by command which makes clear to all that such misconduct must never happen again or worse will happen.

It is unclear why the lieutenant did not (or was unable to) intervene at the time to stop the misconduct. It is likely that he had reason to doubt that his higher command would back him up in enforcing the Law of Land Warfare,[46] as they do not appear to have validated his sense of wrongness or assisted him in reestablishing discipline after the fact. The failure of the chain of command in Vietnam to clearly state and enforce the standards of conduct contributed to a serious breakdown of civilized behavior in U.S. soldiers. That, in turn, alienated the local populations and provided ammunition to the antiwar movement at home.

Shay[47] has pointed out the parallels between the behavior of the Greek hero Achilles in the Trojan War (as reported in Homer's Iliad) and Shay's Vietnam veterans now suffering from post-traumatic stress disorder. A common theme is that the loss of comrades in battle can lead to rage against the enemy and a "berserk state" in which the soldier performs feats of both heroism and moral depravity. Like the soldiers in this example, Achilles also dragged the body of his defeated foe, Hector, by the heels behind his chariot. Achilles did not survive his war, but the Vietnam veterans seen by Shay came home. Shay writes, "On the basis of my work with Vietnam veterans, I conclude that the berserk state is ruinous, leading to the soldier's maiming or death in battle—which is the most frequent outcome—and to life-long psychological and physiological injury if he survives. I believe that once a person has entered the berserk state, he or she is changed forever ... If a soldier survives the berserk state, it imparts emotional deadness and vulnerability to explosive rage to his psychology and a permanent hyperarousal to his physiology—hallmarks of post-traumatic stress disorder in combat veterans."[47(p98)]

Self-Inflicted Wounds

Glass and Drayer[44] reported that at the end of hostilities in Italy numerous incidents of self-inflicted wounds (SIW) occurred, presumably due to carelessness in handling small arms captured from the Germans and Italians, although there were some who felt that underlying guilt about war behaviors might have also played a role in these incidents. The solution adopted by the command structure involved ordering all captured arms turned over to ordnance, where they were tagged and not returned until time of departure for home.

AWOL from Battle

"AWOL from battle," the informal term, subsumes charges of desertion, refusal to obey orders, and misbehavior before the enemy or similar military offenses.[48] Such offenders are seldom found to have serious mental illness. In a survey of 200 such cases in the 85th Infantry Division in Italy from September 13 to November 22, 1944, Glass[48] found the following characteristics of such cases:

1. The AWOL from combat rate increases with the duration of offensive action, a cumulative effect of combat rather than a result of the intensity of battle and unlike the psychiatric casualty rate, which rises and falls with combat intensity.
2. The majority of offenders are veterans and have had relatively long exposure to combat (only 17 of the 200 were in their first combat period).
3. In two thirds of cases the offense was initiated at a safe rear area—returning from hospitalization, during a rear area detail, or when the unit was preparing to move forward into combat. In this respect the casualties are similar to self-inflicted wounds cases.
4. Age and intelligence seemed to play no role.

5. Three fourths admitted that fear of combat motivated their action.
6. Only one fourth sought medical or psychiatric care prior to the offense and were refused evacuation. Of this group, in retrospect, only one fourth (1/16 of the 200) should have received such medical care. The majority did not feel they were ill and saw AWOL as the only way to avoid combat.
7. There was no clear correlation between psychiatric and AWOL rates with regiments, with the highest and lowest psychiatric rates having similar AWOL rates, but the battalion with the highest number of AWOL had a high psychiatric rate and contained three of the five officer offenders, indicating a leadership element in the behavior of the offenders.
8. About one third of the offenders had been recently hospitalized, before AWOL, many for wounds, indicating an adverse effect of rearward evacuation even when surgically necessary, but only three of the 200 had received prior psychiatric treatment. [In 1973, the Israelis experienced similar losses due to psychiatric breakdown in lightly wounded, evacuated casualties.—Au.]

One may conclude from these findings that while both the psychiatric casualty and AWOL offender have a common etiology, the dangers of battle, quite different mental mechanisms are operating. The AWOL soldier consciously elects to avoid combat as a result of chronic anticipatory anxiety deriving from accumulated battle experiences and goes AWOL while away from the supportive or sustaining influence of the combat group or when support is no longer operative. Conversely, the psychiatric casualty arises during the intensity of battle and occurs when the individual is bereft of his own individual sustaining powers or group support by the traumatic and disruptive forces of combat.

Kirkland, a combat veteran and student of soldier stress, has commented on the different symptomatology between combat and rear-echelon troops: "In a unit in combat a soldier is torn between loyalty to his comrades and his identity as a soldier on the one hand and terror on the other. Fleeing and staying are both unacceptable ... unconscious ... symptoms occur [that remove him honorably from combat]. In the rear, however, the loyalty and identity factors are not present [but] terror is ... [the soldier] ... is less conflicted and can make a conscious choice—go AWOL."[49]

The salvage of some AWOL soldiers was considered feasible and, with the cooperation of the judge advocate general of the 85th Infantry Division, recommendations as to whether or not the offenders were reclaimable for combat duty were made.[48] Those without a chronic anxiety state who presented a favorable attitude to return to combat were so recommended. Such individuals were held in the division stockade and released to their units after several months of good conduct and work. No follow-up was available because the 85th Infantry Division did not have any further prolonged combat.

Enjoyment of Combat

Absenting oneself from the dangerous combat situation may be dishonorable but understandable to all; however, what is to be made of the occasional soldier who actually seems to enjoy immersion in combat? Are such men unconsciously suicidal? Does their pleasure stem from unleashing Freud's postulated Thanatos, the death instinct? Can such behavior be explained on the basis of powerful social reinforcement from peers and command? Like most human behavior, enjoyment of combat may be of multifactorial origin, resulting from several or all of these inputs. The following case is typical in that such men are often not well-regarded by their peers though command often regards them highly.

Case Study 11: Enjoyment of Combat

Major Glass, while resting in the Alpines after hostilities ended in Italy, was confronted by a jeepload of sergeants from the 85th Infantry Division. They described Sergeant X, a wonderfully resourceful, reliable, cool-in-combat soldier with several decorations including the Silver Star. But now, when there were no longer any hostilities, Sergeant X was restless. He was going on patrol every night, had shot out the light at their parties, and had been prowling around. They considered him a menace.

During the interview he appeared embarrassed and apologetic, stating he liked the fellows but was bored and restless and needed something exciting to do. He requested transfer to the Pacific Theater. He told Major Glass that he must avoid disciplinary problems because he had been paroled to the Army from State prison, where he had been serving a sentence for manslaughter; therefore, he must receive an honorable discharge. He admitted he enjoyed the thrill of combat and danger. He was easily angered and had no close friends, either civilian or military. No psychosis was present. He was evacuated to the 601 Hospital; there was no follow-up.[48(pp59-60)]

Comment: The author saw a few cases similar to this when directing a research ward for severe character disorders. Most of these men had severe personality distortions with prominent antisocial aggressive tendencies. Far from having been created by combat, these men had usually been delinquent and involved in aggressive behavior prior to military service. Their adjustment to civilian life was frequently poor. Persons who enjoyed combat rarely came for treatment; they seldom responded to psychotherapeutic attempts. It is possible that serotonergic antidepressants might be helpful because antisocial persons such as arsonists have been found to have decreased spinal fluid levels of breakdown products of serotonin.[50]

CONCLUSION

The diagnosis of psychiatric casualties is made difficult not only by the protean symptomatology and potential mimicry of "organic" conditions but also by the intentional vagueness of the nomenclature itself. At a time when psychiatrists are striving for increasing precision in diagnosis it may appear anomalous that the military is clinging to the nonspecific term "combat fatigue" to categorize the psychiatric casualties of combat. The glossary to DSM-III (published separately) even lists "combat fatigue" as "an obsolete term for post-traumatic stress disorder." That interpretation is plainly misinformed. Post-traumatic stress disorder, by DSM-IV's own criteria, cannot be diagnosed until 1 month after the traumatic event is in the past. Combat fatigue, by definition, applies to soldiers who are still in the traumatic (combat) situation. In prolonged combat, however, some traumatic events may have occurred more than 1 month ago. In general, "combat fatigue" corresponds more closely to the new DSM-IV classification of "acute stress disorder," which is used in the interval from 3 days after the traumatic event to 1 month (when post-traumatic stress disorder [PTSD] becomes appropriate). But even organized civilian psychiatry has not placed a diagnostic label on the distress and disturbed behavior which may occur within the first 3 days after an extremely traumatic (life-threatening) event. This is the period of time in which most battle fatigue symptomatology is detected and (ideally, with "immediacy") treated and resolved. This temporary disturbance can be described as the normal human response to very abnormal, threatening conditions. Using a "normalizing" label such as combat fatigue is an important therapeutic maneuver intended to impress the soldier with the idea that he is not mentally ill but just tired and can expect to recover with rest. As seen with the diagnostic label, expectancy is the critical psychological variable in the recovery of the combat stress casualty. Thus, diagnosis and treatment are inextricably intertwined.

REFERENCES

1. Gregory GA, Lawson TR, Brooks FR. *Behavioral Science Support in the Theater of Operations: Casualty Generation Study*. Fort Sam Houston, Tex: Academy of Health Sciences, US Army, 1979.

2. US Department of the Army. *Leaders' Manual for Combat Stress Control*. Washington, DC: DA; March 1994. Field Manual 22-51.

3. American Psychiatric Association. *Diagnostic and Statistical Manual of Mental Disorders*. 4th ed. (DSM-IV). Washington, DC: APA; 1994.

4. Jones FD, Johnson AW. Medical and psychiatric treatment policy and practice in Vietnam. *J Soc Issues*. 1975;31(4):49–56.

5. Weinstein EA, Drayer CS. A dynamic approach to the problem of combat-induced anxiety. Combat psychiatry. *Bull US Army Med Dept*. 1949;9:12–25.

6. Bailey P, Williams FE, Komora PO, eds. Introduction [Section I]. In: *Neuropsychiatry*. Vol 10. In: *The Medical Department of the United States Army in the World War*. Washington, DC: Office of The Surgeon General, US Army; 1929: 1–22.

7. Glass AJ. Lessons learned. In: Glass AJ, ed. *Overseas Theaters*. Vol 2. In: *Neuropsychiatry in World War II*. Washington, DC: Office of The Surgeon General, US Army; 1973: 989–1027.

8. Drayer CS, Glass AJ. Introduction. In: Glass AJ, ed. *Overseas Theaters*. Vol 2. In: *Neuropsychiatry in World War II*. Washington, DC: Office of The Surgeon General, US Army; 1973: 1–23.

9. Belenky GL. Military psychiatry in the Israeli Defence Force. In: Gabriel RA, ed. *Military Psychiatry: A Comparative Perspective*. Westport, Conn: Greenwood Press; 1986: 147–179.

10. Jones FD. Future directions of military psychiatry. In: Gabriel RA, ed. *Military Psychiatry: A Comparative Perspective*. Westport, Conn: Greenwood Press; 1986: 186.

11. Bowman J. Recent experiences in combat psychiatry in Vietnam. Presented at the Social and Preventive Psychiatry Conference. Walter Reed Army Medical Center, Washington, DC. 1967.

12. Jones FD. Psychiatric lessons of low-intensity wars. *Ann Med Milit Fenn* [Finland]. 1985;60:128–134.

13. Strecker EA. Military psychiatry: World War I 1917–1918. In: Hall JK, Zilboorg G, Bunker HA, eds. *One Hundred Years of American Psychiatry: 1844–1944*. New York: Columbia University Press; 1944: 385–416.

14. Appel JW, Beebe GW. Preventive psychiatry. *JAMA*. 1946;131(18):182–189.

15. Glass AJ. Leadership problems of future battle. Presented to The US Army War College, Carlisle Barracks, Pennsylvania. January 23, 1959.

16. Marlowe DH. Personal Communication, 1985.

17. Beebe GW, De Bakey ME. Incidence of hits and wounds. *Battle Casualties: Incidence, Mortality, and Logistic Considerations*. Springfield, Ill: Charles C Thomas; 1952: 16–73.

18. Neel S. *Vietnam Studies: Medical Support of the U.S. Army in Vietnam, 1965–1970*. Washington, DC: Department of the Army, 1973: 33,36.

19. Korea: A Summary of Medical Experience July 1950–December 1952. Reprinted from: *Health of the Army, January, February, and March 1953*. Washington, DC: Office of The Surgeon General, US Army; 1953.

20. El Sudany El Rayes M. 1982. Combat psychiatry in Arab-Israeli wars. Presented at Grand Rounds, Psychiatry Department, Walter Reed Army Medical Center; October 1982; Washington, DC.

21. Noy S. Arab-Israeli casualties. Presented at Combat Psychiatry Seminar, Walter Reed Army Medical Center; June 1981; Washington, DC.

22. Bar-On R, Solomon Z, Noy S, Nardi D. War related stress: An overview of the clinical picture in the 1982 conflict in Lebanon. Presented at the Third International Conference on Psychological Stress and Adjustment in Time of War and Peace; January 1983; Tel Aviv, Israel.

23. Belenky GL. Varieties of reaction and adaptation to combat experience. *Bull Menninger Clin*. 1987;51(1):64–79.

24. Rosen G. Nostalgia: A "forgotten" psychological disorder. *Psychol Med*. 1975;5:340–354.

25. Tischler GL. Patterns of psychiatry attrition and of behavior in a combat zone. In: Bourne PG, ed. *The Psychology and Physiology of Stress*. New York: Academic Press; 1969: 19–44.

26. Solomon Z, Flum H. Life events and combat stress reaction in the 1982 war in Lebanon. *Isr J Psychiatry Relat Sci*. 1986;23(1):9–16.

27. US Department of the Army. *Neuropsychiatry and Mental Health*. Washington, DC: DA; 10 August 1984. Army Regulation 40-216.

28. US Department of the Army. *Planning for Health Service Support*. Washington, DC: DA; 9 September 1994. Field Manual 8-55.

29. US Department of the Army. *Combat Stress Control in a Theater of Operations,*. Washington DC: DA; 29 September 1994. Field Manual 8-51.

30. Glass AJ. History of division psychiatry or the origin and development of related echelons of military psychiatric services. Presented at Army Medical Department Division and Combat Psychiatry Conference; April 28–May 2, 1980; Monterey, Calif.

31. Swank RL, Marchand F. Combat neuroses: Development of combat exhaustion. *Arch Neurol Psychiatry* [superseded in part by *Arch Neurol* and *Arch Gen Psychiatry*]. 1946;55:236–247.

32. Menninger WC. Reactions to combat. *Psychiatry in a Troubled World*. New York: Macmillan; 1948: 134–152.

33. Ranson SW. The normal battle reaction: Its relation to pathologic battle reaction. Combat Psychiatry. *Bull US Army Med Dept*. 1949;9:3–11.

34. Kubler-Ross E. *On Death and Dying*. London: Macmillan; 1969.

35. Weinstein EA, Kahn RL. *Denial of Illness*. Springfield, Ill: Charles C Thomas; 1955.

36. Mohajer M, Mottaghi Y. Psychiatric war casualties in Iran: Presentations. Presented at American Psychiatric Association Annual Meeting; May 1985; Dallas, Tex.

37. Salmon TW, Fenton N, eds. In the American Expeditionary Forces [Section 2]. *Neuropsychiatry*. Vol. 10. In: *The Medical Department of the United States Army in the World War*. Washington, DC; Office of The Surgeon General, US Army; 1929.

38. Jones FD. Experiences of a division psychiatrist in Vietnam. *Milit Med*. 1967;132(12):1003–1008.

39. Johnson AW. Combat psychiatry I: Historical view. *Med Bull US Army Europe*. 1969;26(10):305–308.

40. Cannon WB. *Bodily Changes in Fear, Hunger, Pain and Rage*. 2nd ed. New York: Appleton-Century; 1929.

41. Sobel R. Anxiety-depressive reactions after prolonged combat experience: The "old sergeant syndrome." Supplement on combat psychiatry. *Bull US Army Med Dept*. 1949;9:137–146.

42. Akiskal HS, McKinney WT. Overview of recent research in depression: Integration of ten conceptual models into a comprehensive clinical frame. *Arch Gen Psychiatry*. 1975;32:285–305.

43. Laughlin HP. *The Neuroses*. Washington, DC: Butterworths; 1967: 909–911.

44. Glass AJ, Drayer CS. Italian campaign (1 March 1944–2 May 1945), Psychiatry established at division level. In: Glass AJ, ed. *Overseas Theaters*. Vol 2. In: *Neuropsychiatry in World War II*. Washington, DC: Office of The Surgeon General, US Army; 1973; 47–109.

45. Weinstein EA. The Fifth US Army Neuropsychiatric Center—"601st." In: Glass AJ, ed. *Overseas Theaters*. Vol 2. In: *Neuropsychiatry in World War II*. Washington, DC: Office of The Surgeon General, US Army; 1973: 127–141.

46. US Department of the Army. *Treaties Governing Land Warfare*. Washington, DC: DA; 7 December 1956. Pamphlet 27-1.

47. Shay J. *Achilles in Vietnam: Combat Trauma and the Undoing of Character*. New York: Atheneum; 1994.

48. Glass AJ. Psychiatry at the division level. Supplement on combat psychiatry. *Bull US Army Med Dept*. 1949;9:45–73.

49. Kirkland F. Written Communication, 1991.

50. Virkkunen M, DeJong J, Bartko J, Goodwin FK, Linnoila M. Relationship of psychobiological variables to recidivism in violent offenders and impulsive fire setters: A followup study. *Arch Gen Psychiatry*. 1989;46:600–603.

Chapter 3

DISORDERS OF FRUSTRATION AND LONELINESS

FRANKLIN D. JONES, M.D., F.A.P.A.*

*Colonel (ret), Medical Corps, U.S. Army; Clinical Professor, Uniformed Services University of the Health Sciences, Bethesda, Maryland; Past President and Secretary and current Honorary President of the Military Section, World Psychiatric Association; formerly Psychiatry and Neurology Consultant, Office of The Surgeon General, U.S. Army

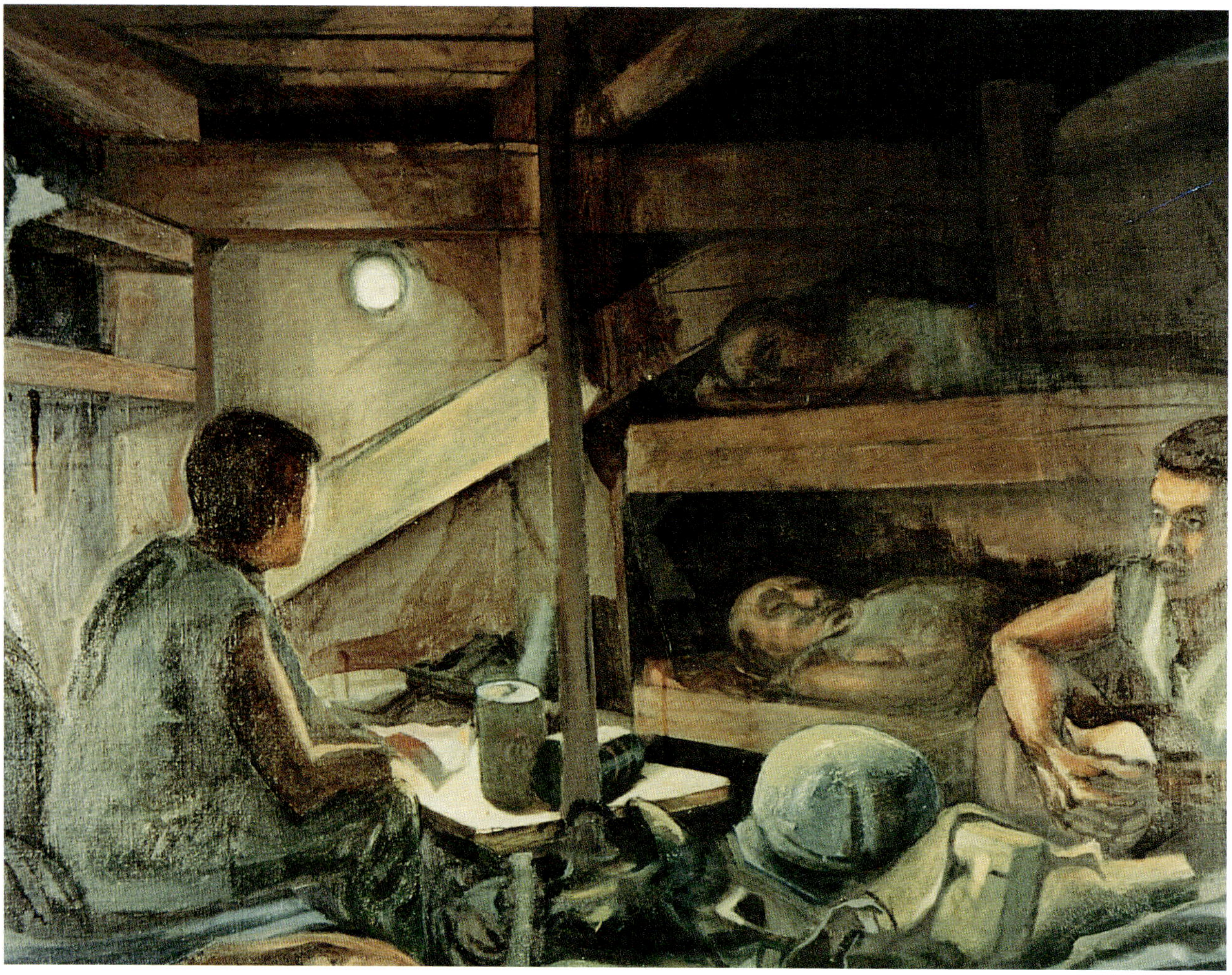

Edward J. Bowen *Bunker on Nuo Ba Dhn Mountain* 1969

Private Edward J. Bowen, a member of the U.S. Army Artist Program, depicts soldiers in their bunker in Vietnam. Low-intensity combat is characterized by significant lulls in the fighting, during which soldiers have time for a variety of activities, as shown in this painting. If not managed properly through constructive activity, such lulls can give rise to disorders of frustration and loneliness.

Art: Courtesy of US Center of Military History, Washington, DC.

INTRODUCTION

The future may produce many different types of war; however, because of the nuclear stalemate, modern wars involving industrialized nations are increasingly of the low-intensity, intermittent, but protracted type experienced by the French in Algeria and Indochina, by the United States in Vietnam, and by the Soviets in Afghanistan. Such conflicts range from low-frequency terrorist actions to full-scale but intermittent warfare. In mid-1986, 42 conflicts were occurring.[1] These ranged from World War II-type mid-intensity combat operations (Iraq-Iran) to low-intensity counter-terrorist/guerrilla operations. Conflicts of the latter type were occurring at that time in Afghanistan, Cambodia, Central America (Nicaragua and El Salvador), Chad, West Irian, Northern Ireland, India, Sri Lanka, Burma, and Angola. In 1992, the decline of Communism was accompanied by the emergence of factionalism or civil wars in Yugoslavia, Russia, Azerbaijan, Georgia, Moldavia, and Czechoslovakia. Also, Kurdish and Shiite minorities are at war in Iraq and Turkey and threaten other states. Virtually every large country and many small countries have the potential for such conflicts.

These conflicts are of low intensity in the sense that battles are interspersed with periods of inactivity and relative safety for the combatants. Overt combat is brief, and usually involves squads, platoons, companies, and rarely battalions, although at those levels casualties may be extremely high. There is often a civil-war quality. Guerrilla activity may be the predominant form of engagement, with small arms and booby traps accounting for most of the wounding and killing rather than artillery and other indirect fire weapons. Here, too, "low-intensity" does not necessarily mean low-casualty: one car bomb killed nearly 250 U.S. Marines in their barracks in Beirut.[2] Often the weaker military force will use terrorist activity to achieve political ends. Such conflicts and operations other than war are often ambiguous with no directly appreciable threat to the national interests of the more powerful country, which may be fighting a foreign, proxy war, or participating in a multinational peacekeeping or constabulary operation. As such they often do not enjoy full public support. The psychiatric casualties of operations other than war differ qualitatively and quantitatively from those of conventional wars involving prolonged or intense heavy (mechanized) combat. This chapter will describe these differences and propose methods of preventing and managing such casualties.

LOW-INTENSITY VS TRADITIONAL COMBAT STRESS CASUALTIES

The epidemiology of psychiatric casualties among troops in battle has been examined in numerous studies since World War I.[3–14] Such studies tended to emphasize the psychiatric casualties that resulted from battlefield stress even though casualties resulting from less dramatic causes had been recognized since World War I. These less dramatic casualties presented with problems of alcohol and drug abuse, disciplinary infractions, venereal diseases, and "self-inflicted" medical disorders (for example, malaria from failure to use prophylaxis). Not until the Vietnam conflict were these casualties recognized as potentially serious causes of ineffectiveness.

Although the casualties that occur during actual engagement with the enemy may present the traditional picture of battle fatigue (eg, anxiety, fatigue, and conversion and dissociative syndromes), the majority of neuropsychiatric cases in low-intensity combat present a picture similar to those that occur among rear-echelon troops in wartime and among garrison troops during peacetime (venereal diseases, alcohol and drug abuse, and disciplinary problems, often related to personality disorders). It is not surprising then that various authors have called such casualties "guerrilla neurosis,"[15] "garrison casualties,"[16] "disorders of loneliness,"[17] and "nostalgic casualties."[18,19] U.S. Army field manuals refer to them as "misconduct stress behaviors"[20–22] (Figure 3-1).

Jones[23] studied the features distinguishing psychiatric casualties among combat troops from those among combat-service-support troops not normally exposed to combat. ("Combat-service-support" in this context refers to soldiers whose primary mission is not to fight the enemy but to assist those

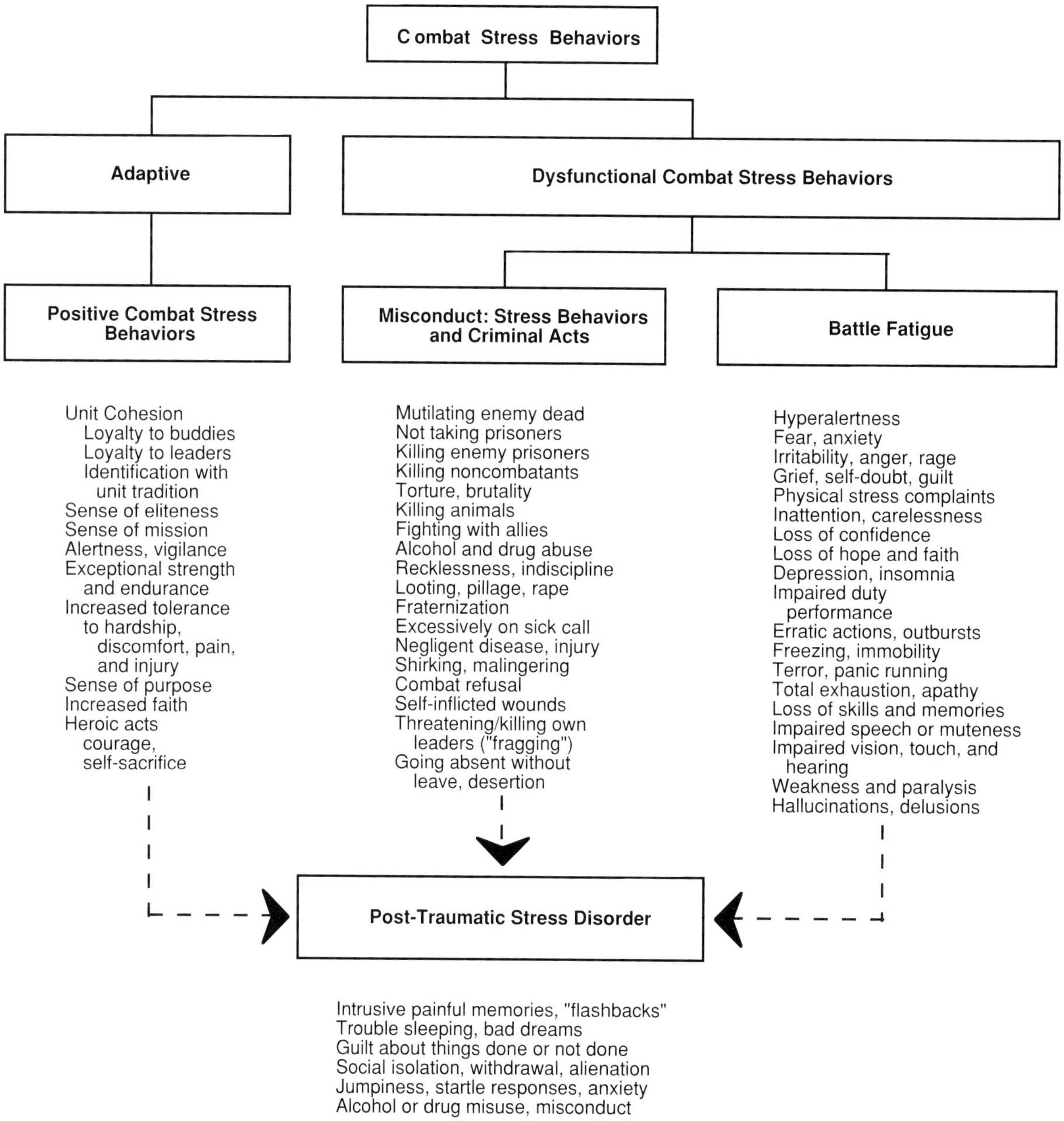

Fig. 3-1. Combat stress behaviors may be adaptive or dysfunctional. The most serious of these behaviors are those involving criminal acts. However, all stress behaviors can evolve into PTSD. Reprinted from US Department of the Army. *Leaders' Manual for Combat Stress Control.* Washington, DC: DA; September 1994. Field Manual 22-51: 2-12.

doing the fighting.) He concluded that such "garrison casualties" were found particularly among rear-echelon elements in Vietnam, a conflict in which each combat soldier was supported by about eight noncombat-arms troops. Such troops characteristically present with behavioral disorders related to separation from family and friends, boredom, and social and sometimes physical deprivation. Considering their source, Jones[17] had labeled these casualties as suffering from "disorders of loneliness"; however, since before the Napoleonic Wars, such disorders have been termed "nostalgia." Obviously, such disorders can and do occur in combat troops as well.

NOSTALGIA: REDISCOVERY OF A CONCEPT

Nostalgia was a medical concept recognized even before 1678, when the Swiss physician Hofer created this term to describe soldiers previously labeled as suffering from "Das Heimweh" or homesickness.[24] Earlier in the 17th century, soldiers in the Spanish Army of Flanders were stated to suffer from "mal de corazon" ("illness of the heart"), and Swiss mercenaries in France were said to suffer from "maladie du pays" ("homesickness"). Because the majority of such soldiers were mercenaries uprooted by financial exigencies from their farms in Switzerland, these soldiers were often described as suffering from "the Swiss disease." The critical variable was service, often involuntary, far from one's country, family, and friends. By the middle of the 18th century, nostalgia was a well-defined nosologic entity recognized as afflicting not just Swiss soldiers but potentially any soldier displaced from his milieu of origin, and generally was considered to be a mental disorder.

The symptomatology associated with nostalgia was consistently compatible with modern descriptions of depression, with complaints, for example, of "moroseness, insomnia, anorexia, and asthenia" in a report by Sauvages in 1768.[24] Even this early there were observations that nostalgia might be feigned as a method of avoiding duty. A French physician, De Meyserey, who published a treatise on military medicine in 1754, observed that war and its dangers always produced a fruitful crop of malingerers who must be discriminated from soldiers with "true nostalgia."

Baron Larrey, Napoleon's Chief Surgeon, prescribed a course of treatment which, while ostensibly biologically oriented, reveals a keen awareness of social factors and is surprisingly close to modern handling of combat psychiatric casualties, both preventively and curatively. He stated that it is necessary not to allow individuals who are predisposed to nostalgia more rest than is necessary, to vary their occupations, and after military exercises to subject them to regular hours, gymnastic recreation, and some mode of useful instruction. He also stated that they should have mutual instruction with troops of the line and that warlike music will contribute to preventing gloomy reflections which can lead to nostalgia. This would ensure physical bodily integrity, produce a conviction of health, give a sense of mastery of weapons, and integrate the unit. This regimen prevents evacuation home (the treatment approach of earlier physicians) and minimizes any secondary gain from illness.[24(p348)]

During the Civil War, Calhoun, reviewed in Deutsch,[25] ascribed a relationship between nostalgia and the recruiting methods of the Union Army that could have parallels with the "nostalgic casualties" of the Vietnam conflict. Calhoun described initially enthusiastic soldiers who had expected an early end to the conflict and who became disenchanted as the war dragged on. The statistics on desertion, draft dodging, and similar attempts to avoid duty were not much different during World War II, a more popular war, and the Vietnam conflict (in fact, these rates were generally lower during Vietnam than during World War II). This suggests that the disenchantment toward the end of the conflict in Vietnam may not have been as important a factor in generating nostalgic casualties as the loss of unit cohesion.

Nostalgic casualties occurred in soldiers separated from their home environment with attendant loss of social reinforcement. Rosen[24] has pointed out that one need not be a soldier for this to occur and that displaced persons and other groups often suffer from this "forgotten" psychological disorder. Situations such as the fighting of an unpopular war of indefinite duration are likely to increase these casualties, particularly in the absence of strong cohesive forces, which usually develop from shared hardship and danger. Hence, Calhoun cited battle action as a curative factor in nostalgia:

> Their thoughts were turned from home, and they felt they were men and soldiers, peers of the veterans with whom they associated; and from that day to this there has been but little or no sickness, and but one or two deaths...When men have passed through the baptism of fire together, they feel they have something in common. They have a common name, a common fame, and a common interest which diverts their thoughts away from home.[25(p376)]

Based on the recollections of Civil War veterans, Stephen Crane's *The Red Badge of Courage* eloquently described the development of cohesive bonds in response to the horrors of battle:

> There was a consciousness always of the presence of his comrades about him. He felt the subtle battle brotherhood, more potent even than the cause for which they were fighting. It was a mysterious fraternity born of the smoke and danger of death.[26(p31)]

Unit cohesion is group and self-preservative behavior that evolves from shared danger in an almost impersonal manner despite its very personal nature. This group cohesion evolves in almost any situation of shared hardship or danger. Belenky and Kaufman[27] found that vigorous training involving some danger produced cohesion in air assault trainees. In combat situations, cohesion needs little encouragement to flourish. Recognizing this, one company commander, when asked about cohesion in his unit in West Germany, commented, "I train my men to be skilled soldiers; I'll rely on the enemy to make them cohesive." Such a laissez-faire attitude ignores the possibility that noncohesive units may disintegrate in high-stress combat before cohesive bonds can develop.

Low-intensity combat, often characterized by long periods of idleness without the shared experience of cohesion-building danger, should produce more nostalgic casualties. This situation probably also accounts for the higher incidence of such casualties among support troops than among combat troops.[23]

During World War I, conditions of battle did not lend themselves to producing large numbers of nostalgic casualties; however, following the Armistice, the Third Army, which remained as an army of occupation, was in a garrison-type role. The casualties in this situation began to approximate those seen in low-intensity warfare. For example, from December 1918 to June 1919 at the hospitals at Coblenz and Trier, 1,022 psychiatric cases were evaluated.[28] In this garrison setting, the largest groups of casualties were those diagnosed as "defect" (presumably retarded) and "psychopathy" (36.8%). When these are added to alcoholism and drug states (6.8%), they account for nearly half of the psychiatric morbidity, and over half if epilepsy is excluded. There were many disciplinary problems in this occupation group. An attempt was made by commanders and medical officers to eliminate "misfits—defectives and psychopaths," which may have accounted for the identification of a relatively high number of mentally retarded and epilepsy patients; however, "Had not many been evacuated through other than hospital channels (replacement depots) the figures would be even higher."[28(p426)] (In a curious parallel with World War II, in the Vietnam conflict an attempt was made to utilize lower-functioning [though not retarded] men as soldiers in the U.S. Army, the so-called "McNamara's 100,000." Such soldiers performed more poorly as a group than normally selected soldiers but some were superior.)

At a time during World War I when the military population in France of U.S. soldiers averaged 200,000 persons, the incidence of hospitalized "psychopathic states" was 5 per 1,000, comparable with the overall rate for "character and behavior disorders" in overseas areas in World War II of about 4 per 1,000.[25] However, because diagnostic practices in World War I and World War II differed markedly, true comparability may not exist. The difference in types of casualties in garrison settings was observed by Salmon and Fenton, who commented that the cessation of hostilities did not reduce the need for psychiatric beds:

> A number of more recent cases showed simple depression...An intense longing for home was characteristic of this condition. It resembled a set of reactions to which the term "nostalgia" used to be applied and is common in all military expeditions when a period of intense activity is succeeded by an uneventful one.[28(p287)]

About one half of the U.S. psychiatric casualties of World War II were unrelated to combat and actually occurred during stateside service.[29] During World War II, "homesickness" was listed as a factor in the breakdown of 20% of psychiatric casualties among U.S. forces.[30] At that time, however, the relationship of these homesick casualties to combat situations was not explored.

The North Pacific Area (Alaska and the Aleutian Islands) during World War II was almost devoid of combat but was also a situation of extreme social deprivation. The ubiquitous state of "chronic depression" was not reflected in neuropsychiatric admissions because the overall neuropsychiatric admission rate was 10.5/1,000/y in the Alaskan Department, the lowest in any combat area. Of 325 neuropsychiatric admissions to the 186th Station Hospital at Umnak (Aleutians) from January 1942 through January 1945, 53% were for psychoneurosis, 14% for constitutional psychopathic state, 12% for dementia praecox, 1% for manic-depressive, 3% for mental deficiency, 1% for epilepsy, 3% for unclassified psychosis, and the remainder (13%) for miscellaneous, primarily situational reactions.[31(p723)] Despite a state of "chronic depression" that afflicted virtually everyone, hospital admission rates were low.[31] Perhaps the fact that alcohol and drugs were scarce in the theater had a salutary effect on these statistics.

In the Korean conflict, three fairly distinct phases are reflected in the varying types of casualties reported. The mid- to high-intensity combat from June 1950 until November 1951 was reflected in traditional anxiety-fatigue casualties and in the highest rate of combat stress casualties of the war, 209/1,000/y in July 1950.[32] Most of the troops were divisional, with only a small number being less exposed to combat. This was followed by a period of static warfare with maintenance of defensive lines until July 1953 when an armistice was signed. The gradual but progressive buildup of rear-area support troops was associated with increasing numbers of characterological problems. Norbury[33] reported that during active combat periods anxiety and panic cases were seen, while during quiescent periods with less artillery fire the cases were predominantly characterological. Following the armistice, obviously, few acute combat stress casualties were seen. The major difference in overall casualties other than surgical before and after the armistice was a 50% increase in the rate of venereal disease among divisional troops.[32]

Commenting on the observation that psychiatric casualties continued to present in significant numbers following the June 1953 armistice of the Korean conflict, Marren gives a clear picture of the reasons:

> The terrors of battle are obvious in their potentialities for producing psychic trauma, but troops removed from the rigors and stresses of actual combat by the Korean armistice, and their replacements, continued to have psychiatric disabilities, sometimes approximating the rate sustained in combat, as in the psychoses. Other stresses relegated to the background or ignored in combat are reinforced in the postcombat period when time for meditation, rumination, and fantasy increases the cathexis caused by such stresses, thereby producing symptoms. Absence of gratifications, boredom, segregation from the opposite sex, monotony, apparently meaningless activity, lack of purpose, lessened chances for promotion, fears of renewal of combat, and concern about one's chances in and fitness for combat are psychologic stresses that tend to recrudesce and to receive inappropriate emphasis in an Army in a position of stalemate...Sympathy of the home folks with their men in battle often spares the soldier from the problems at home. The soldier in an occupation Army has no such immunity ... Domestic problems at home are often reflected in behavior problems in soldiers, particularly those of immature personality or with character defects.[34(pp719–720)]

French experience in Indochina and Algeria[15] revealed characterological problems among French soldiers in these generally low-intensity campaigns. Because there is a several-hundred-year history of colonial wars and occupation forces for many European countries, it is surprising that reports of these casualties are sparse. It seems plausible that these were simply not considered medical, particularly psychiatric, problems but rather moral issues similar to earlier consideration of active combat stress breakdown as cowardice or lack of moral fiber. In the French Indochina War (1945–1954), such character disorders were reportedly responsible for a high number of evacuations, but no statistics are available. Crocq and colleagues[15] studied French psychiatric casualties of the French-Algerian War (1954–1962). They used statistics compiled by LeFebvre and colleagues for 1,280 cases of mental disorders at the military hospital at Constantine who were then evacuated to France between 1 July 1958 and 1 July 1962 (second half of the French-Algerian War). Diagnostically, 19.7% of the total cases were character disorders, and another 14.5% were organic psychoses, predominantly from alcoholism. Only 20% of all cases were related to a triggering event during combat. Functional psychoses accounted for 36.7% of cases with approximately one half of these being schizophrenia (224 of 464 cases). The remainder were mentally retarded (14.5%) and neurotic conditions (14.6%).[15] Because these are evacuation statistics, they only indicate in a general way relative prevalence because characterological problems usually are not handled by medical evacuation. It is unfortunate that actual behaviors cannot be examined to determine the comparability of problem behaviors among soldiers of this war and the Vietnam conflict; however, there is a strong suggestion of comparability in that only a small fraction of alcohol abusers will develop brain syndromes. The relatively high percentage of such cases among the French suggests that this type of substance abuse was widespread.

For the United States, Vietnam represented the epitome of a conflict in which nostalgic casualties occurred. During the early years of the war, the psychiatric casualty rate of about 12/1,000/y was lower even than that in noncombat overseas areas (Europe and Korea) at the same time.[9] The average psychiatric evacuation rate during the first year of the war was 1.8/1,000/y, lower than that from army posts in the United States.[9] The most intense fighting occurred in 1968 to 1969, with one half of those killed in action killed during this period. In June 1968, 1,200 were killed, close to the peak number.[9] As the war dragged on and the U.S. presence took on many of the characteristics of an occupation force, characterological problems began to surface. Racial incidents began to occur, beginning in the rear areas. Psychiatric problems initially took primarily the form of alcohol and drug abuse but later, as the unpopularity of the war intensified, disciplinary problems approaching the magnitude of mutiny in some cases occurred.

President Nixon announced withdrawal plans on June 9, 1969. Fragging incidents (the murdering or injuring of a fellow soldier with a fragmentation grenade) increased from 0.3/1,000/y in 1969 to 1.7/1,000/y in 1971.[35] Psychiatric evacuations rose from 4.4/1,000/y (4% of all evacuations) to 129/1,000/y (60% of evacuations) in April 1972. Several authors have described these casualties and factors in their causation.[9,23,35-39]

These problems were further aggravated by the "Vietnamization" policy in which U.S. soldiers were increasingly relegated to garrison settings and roles in the later phases of the conflict. The subsequent drug abuse epidemic may have played a decisive role in the abrupt withdrawal of U.S. troops and the ultimate loss of the war. The "garrison neuropsychiatric casualties" in fact accounted for most of the consumption of mental health resources during the Vietnam conflict. When a policy of medically evacuating soldiers if they were found to have heroin breakdown products in their urine went into effect, heroin abuse became an "evacuation syndrome."

Marlowe[40] pointed out that Vietnam was aberrant compared with World War II and most of the Korean conflict:

> [T]he soldier's future was as much controlled by the calendar (DEROS) [date of expected return from overseas station] as by the outcome of combat with the enemy. The Viet Nam war was particularly variant in that the enemy lacked a significant capacity in weapons of indirect fire, thus providing a battlefield ecology that was substantively different both from the past and the anticipated future.[40(p1)]

This battlefield ecology, however, was not new to other nations. The French forces preceding the United States in Vietnam fought a similar war until the decisive defeat at Dien Bien Phù where they were beaten by indirect fire weapons artillery. The author contends that the casualties of such low-intensity, intermittent campaigns are similar to nostalgic casualties of the Civil War and of prior wars.

The 1982 Lebanon War is an excellent example of the problems of a war unpopular at home. While the 1973 Yom Kippur War has been used as an exemplar of modern, high-intensity combat and Vietnam as an exemplar of low-intensity combat, Lebanon had elements of both. There were approximately 2 weeks of intense combat in early and late June 1982 with the remainder of the war being more of a static situation with Israel as an occupying force. The result in terms of casualties is revealing, showing casualties similar to those during the intense battles of World War I, World War II, and the 1973 Yom Kippur War but also symptoms of estrangement and delayed stress casualties found in Vietnam (see Figure 3-1). Recent studies[41] revealed that about two thirds of the psychiatric casualties from the 1982 Lebanon War presented during the postcombat period as chronic and delayed posttraumatic stress disorder cases.

LONELINESS AND FRUSTRATION CASUALTIES: PRECIPITANTS

In making a diagnosis of combat stress casualty, the clinician must strive for balance and avoid a "recipe" approach. A major failing in the psychiatric management of casualties in the Vietnam conflict was in not recognizing early enough that psychiatric casualties were taking new forms: alcohol and drug abuse, and venereal disease and malaria from failure to take prophylactic measures. Armed with a stereotypical model of combat fatigue and a recipe for its treatment, psychiatrists were slow to recognize that escape from battle (evacuation syndrome) had taken a new form. Even when the recognition occurred, the ability to adapt "forward treatment" to these casualties was hampered by moralizing and punitive regulations[42] and by stereotyping casualties as drug addicts, alcoholics, cowards, and malingerers. Lost amid a welter of negative reports were occasional successful interventions, particularly at the division level. Such approaches included medical screening of prostitutes, making malarial prophylaxis a command responsibility, and alcohol and drug abuse rehabilitation programs at the division level.[43]

Psychiatric casualties occurring in actual combat are qualitatively different from those occurring in soldiers less exposed to combat. Billings reported that 28% of all medical evacuees from the South Pacific Command during World War II were sent to the Zone of the Interior because of personality disorders during 1943.[44] Billings also described the stresses and personality symptoms of combat and combat-service-support troops. Writing of the men sent to the South Pacific during World War II and subsequently diagnosed as having personality disorders, Billings believed that certain characteristics of Americans helped produce this outcome. He recorded as follows:

> Men ... were products of our sociology and ideology. Individualism; the belief in a freedom for all men to compete on an equal basis; the tendency for the American to need tangible evidences of success at frequent intervals; the inclination to be too dependent on others for distraction, recreation, and maintenance of interest; the assumption that American business philosophy is a matter of "not what you do but what you are caught doing," with the unconscious realization that the one who does not or cannot do the job gets the benefits and escapes unpleasantness whereas the one who accomplishes the task only faces more work or loses his life—all stood out as dynamic factors in breakdowns in morale, occurrence of resentment reactions, aggressive tendencies, and hurt feelings. These in turn placed certain personalities in considerable jeopardy of psychiatric disability when they were subjected to special circumstances.[44(pp479–480)]

Precipitants for Combat Troops

Billings describes such "special circumstances" as a variety of precipitants for combat troops.[44]

1. Facing impending danger, especially for a period of time without specific happenings to break the tension or circumstances permitting the venting of physical effort. For example, remaining alert for a prolonged period of time in a concealed position or foxhole, subjected to the full effects of loneliness and jungle sounds; being pinned down by artillery or heavy mortar fire; or being caught in the open by strafing from the air, especially when immobilized by impediments or terrain.
2. Subjection to heavy artillery fire.
3. Occurrences of a lull, following a period of danger, which allowed for cogitation and a fuller intellectual realization of what was and might be experienced.
4. Occurrence of transitory, psychobiological disorganization in a particularly susceptible personality when subjected to fear-inducing circumstances.
5. Prolonged patrol and reconnaissance work in enemy-controlled jungle.
6. Promotion, in the field, to positions of great responsibility.
7. Grief over loss of "buddies," or loss of a tactical position taking the form of self-condemnatory thinking.
8. Inadvertent evacuation to a position of safety with that [cogitation] noted in paragraph 3 resulting.
9. Loss of confidence in leaders.
10. Mass psychological reactions.
11. "Snow jobs" or tall tales told often by the veteran combat soldier to the new replacement at, or before, a critical time.
12. Unwarranted or unexplained evacuation or transfer of psychiatric and minor medical and surgical casualties ... resulting in loss of the individual's security in his bodily or personality integrity, loss of identification with his unit, diminished esprit de corps, decreased desire or feeling of need to continue fighting—all being replaced by a conscious or "subconscious" appreciation that it might be possible to return home and thereby honorably escape further danger.
13. Ill-considered or poorly-timed statements to troops by visiting high-ranking officers, which lead to misinterpretation of policy, or promote loss of confidence in the administration.
14. Repeated dress parades for visiting dignitaries when the combat team is staging for a forthcoming operation.

Precipitants for both Combat and "Service" Troops

Billings also describes the "special circumstances" that act as precipitants for both combat and "service" (support) troops.[44]

1. Hypochloremia, dehydration, fatigue, and subclinical or clinical illness decreasing the efficiency and smooth psychobiological functioning of the individual, thereby often setting the stage for insecurity, tension, and anxiety with personally alarming symptomatology.
2. Enemy propaganda.
3. Rumors stemming from isolation, ignorance of facts, and inactivity.

4. Postponement of the promotion of enlisted men and officers, and the filling of position vacancies with new men in grade or rank.
5. Ill-advised promotion of men and officers to responsibility beyond their ability.
6. Discrepancy between War Department and politically announced policy and plans for rotation and redeployment of overseas personnel.
7. Knowledge of the unfair discrepancy in remuneration to and appreciation for the individual in military service and the one in the merchant marine and industry.
8. Seeming ignorance of the average commander and the officer in personnel work either of War Department policy or of how to comply therewith in regard to proper assignment and readjustment of military personnel.
9. Poor leadership, especially of high-ranking officers, as evident in the officer looking after his personal comfort and safety before acquiring them for his command.
10. Apparent "empire building" of general officers.
11. Work or combat under adverse conditions prolonged to the breaking point of the "average" man.
12. Failure to expedite the elimination of ineffectuals from a unit.
13. Disturbing news from home, such as of a wife's infidelity, business reversals, deaths, illness, and encouragement to forego continuance of further military responsibility.

LONELINESS AND FRUSTRATION DISORDERS: PRESENTATIONS

Soldiers less exposed to combat and presenting with personality problems may be called loneliness and frustration casualties. Huffman[45] reported that only 48 of 610 soldiers (8%) seen in Vietnam from 1965 to 1966 suffered combat-related stress, while Jones[23] found combat-related stress in 18 of 47 soldiers (38%) seen in a similar hospital setting (September–December 1966). These 18 cases, however, were given character and behavior disorder diagnoses. As the 25th Division psychiatrist, Jones[17] saw approximately 500 patients from March through October 1966, of whom about one third were awaiting legal or administrative action. Of the remaining two thirds, almost all were diagnosed as having character and behavior disorders including situational fright reactions. The term "combat fatigue" was misleading to the novice psychiatrist with its mistaken implication of prolonged combat and cumulative fatigue. In retrospect, some of these cases would more appropriately have been so diagnosed; however, the treatment approach was the same: rest, reassurance, and return to his unit.

The term "loneliness and frustration casualty," like "combat stress reaction," and "battle fatigue," is an intentionally vague term describing a variety of dysfunctional behaviors, although unlike "battle fatigue" it is not readily understood by the average soldier or his sergeant and junior officer, and so should not be used when talking to them. Nostalgic casualties require interventions much like those for managing combat fatigue. U.S. Army doctrine[21,22] terms many of these casualties "misconduct combat stress reactions." The term suggests that disciplinary action may be indicated. This may be a profitable approach; however, command-sponsored substance abuse programs, programs to strengthen morale, and hygiene/prophylaxis programs may be more profitable. These dysfunctional behaviors often cluster in patterns forming syndromes. Such syndromes typically have many overlapping behaviors; however, it is useful to divide them into the categories of substance abuse, sexual problems, and indiscipline.

These cases (misconduct combat stress reactions) are ones which violate unit regulations or the Uniform Code of Military Justice or the Law of Land Warfare. The manuals state that such cases require disciplinary action. They cannot simply be treated as battle fatigue, with reassurance, rest, physical replenishment, and activities to restore confidence. Depending on the seriousness or criminality of the misconduct, disciplinary action ranges from simple verbal correction through assignment of unpleasant duties and denial of special privileges; written reprimand; nonjudicial punishment (Article 15); judicial punishment (court-martial); less than honorable discharge; confinement and, for extreme misconduct, the death penalty. For criminal cases, psychiatric expertise may be called upon to establish the validity of an insanity defense. In all cases, mental health personnel can advise regarding potential for recurrence or rehabilitation, and treat any associated mental disorders.

Substance Abuse

During the Civil War, the liberal use of opium caused widespread dependence called the "soldier's disease."[46] In low-intensity combat and garrison settings in which the risks of being intoxicated are not as great as in higher-intensity combat, substance abuse flourishes.

Froede and Stahl[47] evaluated the 174 cases of fatal narcotism retrieved from over 1.3 million surgical and autopsy cases sent to the Armed Forces Institute of Pathology from 1918 through the first 6 months of 1970. Although the data were incomplete, some interesting trends were observed that strengthen the observation that drug abuse is associated with low-intensity combat situations in geographical areas in which abuse substances are available (about two thirds of the deaths occurred in the Far East). In terms of combat intensity, the majority of cases in World War II, Korea, and Vietnam occurred in the closing years of the wars and in the postwar periods when fighting had diminished and large numbers of troops were serving in support roles. Their findings are supported by Baker's[48] estimate that there were 75 opiate deaths in Vietnam from August 1, 1970 through October 18, 1970, 11 confirmed by autopsy and 64 suspected.

Alcohol was the first substance of abuse in Vietnam. Huffman[45] reported that of his 610 patients seen early in the war, 113 (18.5%) suffered from severe problems associated with alcoholic intoxication but there were only five cases of unquestionable nonalcohol substance abuse. As the war progressed, marijuana came to be preferred because of the absence of a "hangover." Roffman and Sapol[49] reported that in an anonymous questionnaire given to soldiers departing Vietnam in 1967, 29% admitted using marijuana during their tour. Similarly, a survey of 5,000 enlisted men at Fort Sill, Oklahoma who had not served in Vietnam from January through April 1969[50] revealed that 29% admitted to using drugs sometime in their lives, 83% of the users identifying marijuana. In the early years of the Vietnam conflict marijuana users apparently were reflecting the experiences of their stateside cohorts, but this began to change. In a review of studies of drug abuse in Vietnam, Stanton[51] found that from 1967 to 1971 the proportion of enlisted men who used marijuana "heavily" (20 or more times) in Vietnam increased from 7% to 34%, while the proportion of "habitual" users (200 or more times) *entering* Vietnam remained at 7% to 8% for the years 1968 through 1970 and the proportion of habitual users *in* Vietnam stabilized at 17% to 18% between 1969 and 1971. Thus, about 9% to 10% of the lower grades of enlisted men first *became* habitual smokers (daily usage) in Vietnam.

Heroin abuse became significant in early 1970 when 90% to 96% pure heroin derived from the "golden triangle" of Thailand, Burma, and Laos became available countrywide. This pure heroin was so cheap that a significant "habit" could be maintained for $8 to $10 a day.[51] The preferred route was "snorting" through the nostrils or smoking. Of the small percentage who injected at all, this was only occasionally. At a peak in October 1971, almost one half of all lower ranking enlisted men (E-1 to E-4) were using heroin and half of these may have been addicted.[52] Like venereal disease rates, drug abuse rates tend to increase when there are lulls in combat or when exposure to combat is decreased.

Heroin reportedly displaced cannabis because it had no characteristic strong odor allowing detection, made time seem to go faster rather than slower as with marijuana, and was compact and easily transportable. However, McCoy[53] argues that heroin did not so much replace marijuana as augment its use and that the real reason for the heroin epidemic was enormous profits that South Vietnamese officials could make by selling it to Americans.

These findings must be considered in the light of a nationwide epidemic of drug abuse in American youths at that time. The biggest difference between drug abuse in Vietnam and in the United States was the ready availability of very pure, inexpensive heroin in Vietnam.[54]

Treatment of substance abusers has varied considerably over time. Early approaches were to consider such casualties problems of a moral nature and later of a character defect with punishment as the primary intervention. It was only when such losses of manpower became significant in the Vietnam conflict that a nonpunitive, therapeutic approach was undertaken. By 1971, more soldiers were being evacuated from Vietnam for drug use than for war wounds.[51] The U.S. Army had adopted a countrywide voluntary treatment program in Vietnam in October 1969 aimed primarily at marijuana abusers. This was patterned on an amnesty program developed in the Fourth Infantry Division in May 1969. Army regulations tended to be slow in changing to accommodate the therapeutic perspective, sometimes resulting in paradoxical punishment of recovered abusers.[42]

The main lessons from the U.S. experience in managing substance abuse in Vietnam are that treatment should be in-country to prevent an evacuation syndrome and that the factors that prevent breakdown in general—cohesion, effective leadership, and good morale—may protect soldiers from substance abuse. For example, the Australians serving in Vietnam did not have significant personnel losses from substance abuse.[55,56] Their forces were based on a regimental system with unit rather than individual rotations, and officers and troops had usually served together for long periods of time. This may have produced greater unit cohesion, a crucial difference from U.S. troops that protected Australian troops from developing nostalgic problems of substance abuse and indiscipline.

Sexual Problems

The most common nostalgic behavior coming to medical attention is sexual intercourse with prostitutes leading to venereal diseases. The following case, known to the author, reveals that officers were not immune.

Case Study 1: The "No-Sweat" Pill

When the author was taking sick call in the headquarters company dispensary, he was approached by Major INF, who stated that he was going to Saigon overnight and wanted a "no-sweat pill." The author was slow to realize that the major wanted penicillin to prevent getting gonorrhea or syphilis. When he did understand, he refused and gave him a lecture on the dangers of incompletely treated syphilis leading to tertiary lues of the brain and absence of protection from viral venereal diseases. Later the author learned that the major purchased antibiotics over the counter in Saigon and indulged himself apparently without complications.

Comment: The availability of antibiotics in Vietnam (and Korea) without prescription may have hastened the development of resistant strains of gonorrhea that have been reported since the Vietnam conflict.

Low-intensity combat operations frequently show an increased incidence of drug abuse and sexual disorders. The following case from the early phases of the Vietnam conflict reveals both.

Case Study 2: Seductive Marijuana

Sergeant First Class (SFC) MC was the noncommissioned officer in charge (NCOIC) of a technical support battalion assigned to an infantry division. He was given a forensic psychiatric evaluation in the course of a court-martial proceeding. SFC MC was a kindly, friendly man, well-liked by the officers and enlisted men with whom he worked. In the combat setting he was unable to satisfy his homosexual feelings by "cruising." Finally he hit upon a method that took advantage of the nostalgia and fears of the young soldiers. He offered them friendship, alcohol, and marijuana to alleviate their homesickness and fear, then performed fellatio when they were intoxicated. Most victims kept silent from embarrassment or fear of disciplinary action until a soldier who wanted to be separated administratively was seduced. He reported the incident.

Comment: Examples such as this have been used to vindicate the military policy of eliminating homosexuals from the service; however, a study of homosexual college students who served in World War II[57] revealed that the great majority served adequately and some with distinction.

Sexually-transmitted diseases (venereal diseases or VD) have been a major cause of lost soldier strength in wars of the 20th century. While modern medicine has markedly reduced the time lost and complications of venereal diseases, it has not reduced the infection rates as seen in Table 3-1.

Although the venereal disease rate of the American Expeditionary Forces (AEF) in World War I was a relatively low 34.3/1,000/y,[58] there were over 6.8 million lost man-days and 10,000 discharges.[59] Each

TABLE 3-1

VENEREAL DISEASE RATES BY WAR/1,000 TROOPS/YEAR

War	Years/Location	Rate
World War I	Expeditionary Force	34.3
	Continental USA	127.4
World War II	1941–1945	42.9
Post-World War II	1946–1950	82.3
Korea	1951–1955	184.0
Vietnam	1963–1970	261.9
	Peak Jan–Jun 1972	698.9
	Continental USA	31.7

Data sources: [World War I] Michie HC. The venereal diseases. In: Siler JF, ed. *Communicable and Other Diseases*. In: *The Medical Department of the United States Army in the World War*. Vol 9. Washington, DC: Medical Department, US Army, Office of The Surgeon General; 1928: 263–310. [World War II, post-World War II, Korea, Vietnam] Deller JJ, Smith DE, English DT, Southwick EG. Venereal diseases. In: Ognibene AJ, Barrett O Jr, eds. *General Medicine and Infectious Diseases*. In: Ognibene AJ, ed. *Internal Medicine in Vietnam*. Vol 2. Washington, DC: Medical Department, US Army, Office of The Surgeon General and Center of Military History; 1982: 233–255.

case resulted in over a month of lost duty time (from 1929–1939, lost days per case ranged from 38–50).[59] By the time of the Vietnam conflict, 9 of 10 cases were for gonorrhea (lymphogranuloma venereum, chancroid, and syphilis accounted for most of the rest), and lost duty time averaged only a few hours per case. Deller and colleagues[59] echo the observation of Jones[23] that rates were greatest in support troops with little combat exposure, and they add that such troops were most often near population centers. The peak incidence of nearly 700/1,000/y occurred in the period January to June 1972 when almost all U.S. troops were in support roles in accordance with the "Vietnamization plan" of using South Vietnamese forces in combat.

Prevention through education is a valid approach to venereal disease even though some soldiers will risk infection no matter what the threat. Prevention should not be directed at preventing sexual intercourse, which is an unrealistic goal, but toward the avoidance of high risk ("off limits") partners and the use of condoms, which should be made readily available. A study[60] that revealed that 50% of all prostitutes who have been randomly tested in the United States carry the HIV (human immunodeficiency virus) antibody suggests that this retrovirus, which is thought to cause the currently incurable and usually fatal acquired immunodeficiency syndrome (AIDS), may be a problem in future wars. In battlefield conditions, soldiers may have to donate blood to each other, and the presence of a soldier who is HIV positive could prove hazardous not only to the health but also to the morale of troops.

Although unlikely to have immediate effects on combat efficiency, the HIV virus poses severe problems in long-term prevention. Many of the world social tensions and ongoing wars are occurring in Africa, where the HIV infection is reaching epidemic proportions. Unlike in the United States, where the populations at risk are mainly homosexuals and intravenous drug abusers, the spread of HIV in Africa is primarily through heterosexual intercourse. In South America, another politically troubled area with insurgencies and narcotics production in several countries, AIDS is emerging as a difficult public health problem. Because urban areas in these third-world countries are being hit hardest by AIDS, there is concern that the professional and leadership classes of African, and to a lesser extent South American, countries could experience severe setbacks in goals of industrialization and democratic reforms. Internal unrest in Latin America frequently has led to U.S. deployment beginning before 1900.

Indiscipline

Indiscipline is a psychiatric issue in the sense that sociopsychological factors play a paramount role in its emergence. Furthermore, indiscipline and psychiatric breakdown merge almost imperceptibly as evacuation syndromes. For example, failure to take preventive hygiene measures in Korea allowed the development of frostbite in some cases. Similarly, failure to take the prophylactic chloroquine-primaquine pill in Vietnam allowed the infestation of malarial protozoans. In both cases, indiscipline rendered the soldiers unfit for duty.

Indiscipline may range from relatively minor acts of omission to commission of serious acts of disobedience (mutiny) and even murder (fragging). In an analysis and historical review, Rose[61] indicated that combat refusal has been a relatively frequent occurrence in most significant wars for which there is adequate data. The military has often colluded with the perpetrators in hiding the true nature of collective disobedience (mutiny) by using various euphemistic phrases ("unrest," ..."incident," "affair," "collective protest," "insubordination," "strike," and "disaffection").[61(p562)] Rose indicates that there are compelling reasons for command to do this: "...mutiny is the antithesis of discipline,"[61(p562)] and a commander who "allows" a mutiny to occur jeopardizes his career and those of his "commanding officers up and down the line."[61(p563)]

Most indiscipline, of course, is more subtle than combat refusal and does not appear to be related to it. However, unavailability for combat is a frequent consequence of indiscipline. The main role of the psychiatrist is in prevention because the same conditions that give rise to combat stress casualties may produce indiscipline as another evacuation syndrome. This section will address primarily clinically observed situations involving indiscipline actions.

The following examples of indiscipline, provided by the author, were fairly typical of conditions in Vietnam.

Case Study 3: The Major's Bullets

During the early phases of the Vietnam conflict Major MSC was the executive officer in the headquarters of a support battalion of an infantry division. Prior to deployment to Vietnam he had earned a reputation as a strict disciplinarian, once having demoted a soldier for having a pocket unbuttoned. The battalion commander, an alcoholic, stayed sequestered in his "hooch" leaving the major to run the unit despite his lack of expertise in the highly technical field in which most of his subordinates were far more skilled than he was. Feeling threatened by lack of proper technical background, the major became increasingly authoritarian, producing impaired morale in his unit. His authoritarian approach to leadership was not appreciated by the troops: he began finding bullets with his name written on them. This physical threat did not change his behavior. The appropriate intervention would have been to make higher command aware of the adverse effect on morale of Major MSC; however, he was well-regarded by command for taking over for the incompetent battalion commander and higher command turned a deaf ear. Eventually, Major MSC made a serious error leading to the death of a prisoner of war and he abandoned his authoritarian approach.

Comment: Early in the Vietnam conflict the majority of U.S. soldiers were volunteers who served together prior to deployment to Vietnam. Morale was generally high. In the later phases of the war an officer as unpopular as Major MSC would have been a likely fragging victim.

Linden[62] reported that there was a progressive rise in the number of courts-martial for insubordination and assaults (including murder) on officers and senior noncommissioned officers (NCOs) during the Vietnam conflict. He attributed these incidents to disaffection and poor morale because the war was increasingly seen as useless by the soldiers who were unwilling to risk their lives in a lost cause. The specificity of circumstances and the importance of leadership surrounding that form of indiscipline called combat refusal is seen in the following case.

Case Study 4: The Silver Star Medic

Specialist 4th Class (SP4) MC was the medical aidman ("medic") attached to an infantry company. In several battles he had performed with great valor, risking his life to treat wounded comrades, resulting in his being recommended for award of the Silver Star. He was referred for psychiatric evaluation when he refused to go out on a combat mission. The author found no evidence whatever of psychiatric impairment or personality disorder. The young soldier stated that he would not go into combat with a "green lieutenant" who had replaced the company commander, a captain, with whom the medic had deployed. The captain had been wounded and was currently performing light duties in the division headquarters. The medic stated that on the first engagement with the enemy the new lieutenant had foolishly risked his troops, resulting in several wounded soldiers. As much to protect his comrades as himself (because the unit could not go out without a medic), SP4 MC refused to go on a combat mission.

Comment: This young soldier was actually sent to the psychiatrist as a ploy on the part of command in hopes that a medical solution could be found for a leadership problem. When the psychiatrist refused to label the soldier psychiatrically ill, the medic was transferred to another company. The appropriate solution is a consultation with the lieutenant's commander in which assignment manipulations are recommended.

Indiscipline is not limited to subordinate ranks. Perhaps the most notorious example of collective indiscipline during the Vietnam conflict occurred in the My Lai atrocity, in which over 100 men, women, and children were killed in a village by U.S. forces.

Case Study 5: Lieutenant Calley

[Although the author was one of three U.S. Army psychiatrists who examined First Lieutenant William Calley and testified at his court-martial, the information given in this case comes from public records of the trial.—Au.] Calley testified that he had been ordered to go to My Lai and "kill the enemy"; however, the major who had allegedly given the order was killed before the trial began. Several factors are important in understanding this incident. First, prior to assignment in Vietnam, Calley was stationed in Hawaii where he was exposed to numerous "after-action" and "lessons learned" reports coming from Vietnam. Many of these emphasized the dangers from civilians who were secretly Viet Cong. Many reports included descriptions of Vietnamese women and children unexpectedly killing and wounding Americans with grenades and satchel bombs. While this intelligence justified heightened awareness and precaution to protect against such attack, it in no way justified the rape and murder of unarmed women and children, not even ones taken prisoner after committing such an attack, let alone ones rounded up in a village without resistance.

Secondly, Calley identified strongly with his men and was quite upset when his company incurred large numbers of casualties in the My Lai region (thought to be pro-Viet Cong) not long before the killings in My Lai. He was even more upset because he had been away when this occurred. This concern for his troops is to his credit, and qualifies his action as a misconduct stress behavior, rather than as simple criminal misconduct. It does not, however, excuse it or justify it.

Finally, Calley tended to see things in a black or white, all-or-none fashion. If the enemy included women and children and the enemy were supposed to be killed, so be it. Had the villagers (men, women, or children) been firing at the American troops, it would have been entirely correct to shoot and kill them, but only up until the point where they surrendered. If noncombatants had been killed in such a firefight, that would have been regrettable but justified. But Calley was convicted of having ordered and participated in the deliberate massacre of about two dozen unarmed Vietnamese men, women, and children. Evidence in the Peers Investigation Report suggested that over a hundred persons were in fact murdered.[63]

One of the soldiers at the My Lai atrocity, rather than participate in killing women, children, and old men, shot himself in the foot. Although self-inflicted wounds are usually intended to escape combat (in Vietnam this evasion was often thwarted by orthopedic surgeons who put some of these soldiers in "walking casts"), in this case an altruistic outcome was effected. When the author reviewed the testimony of all the U.S. Army participants at My Lai in preparation for his testimony at Calley's court-martial, he found most of the soldiers were deeply conflicted and some approved the self-inflicted wound solution to the conflict. Others, however, felt that this soldier was cowardly. His "indiscipline," via his self-inflicted wound, prevented worse indiscipline on his part.

Comment: Testimony[63] indicated that some of the U.S. soldiers committed unspeakable acts of sexual assault in committing the murders. The fact that presumably previously normal and moral human beings can commit such atrocities under the influence of uncontrolled combat stress makes clear why it is so important that leadership not let such misconduct begin. Calley's argument that he was just obeying the major's orders is irrelevant. The Uniform Code of Military Justice requires each soldier to refuse to obey a clearly illegal order such as the murder of unarmed prisoners or noncombatants. The command climate in Vietnam, and the training prior to the My Lai atrocity, may have failed to make that clear. No soldier appears to have overtly tried to get Calley to rescind his illegal order. Forms of indiscipline in which not only military but also international rules for handling prisoners and noncombatants are disregarded may be more common in low-intensity conflicts. Following the recapture (by U.S. and South Vietnamese forces) of Hue during the Viet Cong and North Vietnamese Tet Offensive, a mass grave was found containing the bodies of about one thousand men, women, and children presumably slaughtered by the North Vietnamese. Similarly, torture and killing of prisoners of war (POWs) occurred in the French-Algerian War, in the guerrilla warfare in Central America (El Salvador and Nicaragua) and South America (Argentina), and in 1992 reports of POWs in the former Yugoslavia.

"Indiscipline" by a high-ranking officer occurred in the 1982 Lebanon War when Colonel Eli Geva (commander of the Israeli tank force outside Beirut) refused to lead his troops into Beirut, which he expected to entail killing civilians. Geva urged that Beirut not be attacked and asked to be demoted to tank crew member if the city were attacked. Geva's courageous act resulted in rapid decisive action (Geva's prompt removal and isolation from other military personnel) coupled with the decision to launch a more discriminating attack that would minimize civilian casualties. This prevented other commanders from following suit.[64] Calley showed no concern for civilians; by contrast, Geva was criticized for showing too much concern.

Stress Disorders

To the heterogeneous syndromes found in low-intensity wars that have been labeled loneliness and frustration casualties ("nostalgic casualties") should be added acute stress disorders and chronic and delayed post-traumatic stress disorders (chronic and delayed PTSD). PTSD is usually and appropriately thought of in the context of acute overwhelming stress; however, the frequent morale problems of low-intensity, ambiguous wars may carry over into the postwar lives of the former combatants. The current discontents of these war veterans may find expression in the reappearance or new appearance of symptoms associated with combat: anxiety and fears, autonomic hyperactivity, reliving of psychologically traumatic events, and a variety of other malaises. Such symptoms often follow service in wars of high intensity as well, particularly when the outcome was unsatisfactory or there is psychological or financial gain from such symptoms. This was seen, for example, in the large numbers of German veterans of World War I who developed chronic war neuroses (many of whom would now be labeled chronic post-traumatic stress disorder) compared with the small numbers of such cases following World War II.[65] In both cases Germany lost the war, but one difference was that after World War II veterans were not given pensions for neurotic (nonpsychotic or nonorganic) conditions due to the experience of German psychiatrists who knew of the World War I findings, and due to the general opprobrium earned by the military because of Nazi atrocities.

Post-traumatic stress disorders evolved from the Freudian concept of "traumatic neurosis" and technically are part of the combat stress disorders spectrum, of the acute, chronic, or delayed type. The chronic and delayed forms of PTSD have assumed considerable importance as sequelae of combat in Vietnam and in the 1982 Lebanon War. PTSD is explored at length in Chapter 16, Chronic Post-Traumatic Stress Disorder. Here it is important to recognize that PTSD symptoms can follow any serious psychological trauma, such as exposure to combat, accidents, torture, disasters, criminal assault, and exposure to atrocities or to the sequelae of such extraordinary events. POWs exposed to harsh treatment are particularly prone to develop PTSD. In their acute presentation, these symptoms, which include subsets of a large variety of affective, cognitive, perceptual, emotional, and behavioral responses delineated in Exhibit 3-1, are

EXHIBIT 3-1

APA DIAGNOSTIC CRITERIA FOR 308.3 ACUTE STRESS DISORDER

A. The person has been exposed to a traumatic event in which both of the following were present:
 (1) the person experienced, witnessed, or was confronted with an event or events that involved actual or threatened death or serious injury, or a threat to the physical integrity of self or others
 (2) the person's response involved intense fear, helplessness, or horror

B. Either while experiencing or after experiencing the distressing event, the individual has three (or more) of the following dissociative symptoms:
 (1) a subjective sense of numbing, detachment, or absence of emotional responsiveness
 (2) a reduction in awareness of his or her surroundings (eg, "being in a daze")
 (3) derealization
 (4) depersonalization
 (5) dissociative amnesia (ie, inability to recall an important aspect of the trauma

C. The traumatic event is persistently reexperienced in at least one of the following ways: recurrent images, thoughts, dreams, illusions, flashback episodes, or a sense of reliving the experience; or distress on exposure to reminders of the traumatic event.

D. Marked avoidance of stimuli that arouse recollections of the trauma (eg, thoughts, feelings, conversations, activities, places, people).

E. Marked symptoms of anxiety or increased arousal (eg, difficulty sleeping, irritability, poor concentration, hypervigilance, exaggerated startle response, motor restlessness).

F. The disturbance causes clinically significant distress or impairment in social, occupational, or other important areas of functioning or impairs the individual's ability to pursue some necessary task, such as obtaining necessary assistance or mobilizing personal resources by telling family members about the traumatic experience.

G. The disturbance lasts for a minimum of 2 days and a maximum of 4 weeks and occurs within 4 weeks of the traumatic event.

H. The disturbance is not due to the direct physiological effects of a substance (eg, a drug of abuse, a medication) or a general medical condition, is not better accounted for by Brief Psychotic Disorder, and is not merely an exacerbation of a preexisting Axis I or Axis II disorder.

Reprinted with permission from American Psychiatric Association. *Diagnostic and Statistical Manual of Mental Disorders,* 4th ed. (DSM-IV). Washington, DC: American Psychiatric Press; 1994: 431–432.

relatively normal responses to gross psychological trauma. If persistent, however, they develop a life of their own and may be maintained by inadvertent reinforcement. Early intervention and later avoidance of positive reinforcement (which may be subtle) for such symptoms are critical preventive measures.

Current doctrine[22] emphasizes the importance of routine debriefing after any traumatic action to minimize subsequent post-traumatic stress. These debriefings may involve just the small unit itself, as leader-led after-action debriefings. These sessions review lessons learned while clarifying the facts of the event, by getting everyone to describe what he saw and did. Misperceptions and misunderstandings are corrected in the process, and feelings and reactions are shared openly. After an especially traumatic event, the small units should receive a formal critical event debriefing. These sessions should occur within several days of the event, and are led by trained debriefing teams. Critical event debriefings also get everyone to describe the facts of the event, and deliberately help everyone verbalize and process their thoughts, emotional reactions, and physical stress symptoms. The debriefing team must emphasize the normality of those reactions, and the value of talking them out now as wise preventive maintenance. Units should also conduct routine end-of-tour debriefings as part of prehomecoming activities. Chapter 11, Debriefing Following Combat, explores these issues in greater detail.

The only units in which psychiatric casualties of either the high-intensity combat stress or of the low-intensity combat stress type appear minimal are highly cohesive, usually elite units. Thus, the building of cohesive, well-led units is as important in this form of warfare as in higher-intensity combat. The dynamics of cohesive units are discussed at length by Manning.[66] The level of material support does not appear to be a factor in such units and, by giving an appearance that sacrifice is unnecessary, may even be detrimental. While some soldiers benefit from abundant material support and close communication with loved ones, many soldiers may paradoxically benefit from a more austere situation.

LOW-INTENSITY COMBAT STRESS CASUALTIES: PREVENTION AND TREATMENT

Although successful treatments for low-intensity combat stress casualties were developed as early as the Napoleonic Wars, circumstances can prevent the application of remedies. For example, during the Vietnam conflict the 1-year rotation policy, ostensibly for the purpose of preventing psychiatric casualties due to cumulative stress, the policy of rotating commanders out of combat units after 6 (and later only 3) months in order to give more officers combat experience, and the policy of individual replacement of losses rather than unit replacements, all interacted to impair unit cohesion, which might have prevented at least some of the nostalgic casualties. Most combat soldiers and marines left the combat zone by commercial air, without any combat comrades with whom to talk out (debrief) the memories of the tour. Their reception in the United States also usually discouraged further sharing and validation of their (and their dead comrades') experiences, accomplishments, and sacrifices.

Some aspects of treatment have been exemplified in the foregoing cases and in preceding chapters. It may be summarized as treatment of acute combat-induced stress disorder following combat psychiatric principles, not reinforcing symptoms associated with chronic and delayed post-traumatic stress disorder, use of evocative therapies emphasizing correcting current maladaptive behaviors, and judicious use of pharmacotherapy in some cases.

A critical component of treating chronic post-traumatic stress disorder is determining associated conditions, especially drug and alcohol abuse, and treating them as well. The use of a relaxation technique such as one of those described by Benson[67] can be critical in managing anxiety symptoms without resorting to medications or may be adjunctive to their use.

SUMMARY AND CONCLUSION

This chapter has described the emergence of symptoms more often encountered in garrison settings—various character and behavior disorder problems—as the primary nosologic entities in low-intensity combat. The resurrection of the ancient entity "nostalgia" seems appropriate as a generic approach to conceptualize and treat these casualties. The postwar emergence of large numbers of veterans suffering from chronic and delayed post-traumatic stress disorder following the Vietnam conflict and the 1982 Lebanon War is explored in Chapter 16, Chronic Post-Traumatic Stress Disorder, in terms of the evolution of the post-traumatic stress disorder concept and approaches to prevention and treatment. Studies from World War II reveal that improperly treated cases of acute combat-induced stress disorder (combat fatigue) account for most of the subsequent postwar disability from chronic post-traumatic stress disorder (formerly called war neurosis). Studies of American prisoners of war held by the Japanese and North Koreans reveal that harshly treated prisoners of war are at high risk for developing chronic post-traumatic stress disorder.

In the future, U.S. forces are far more likely to encounter low-intensity combat than high-intensity combat. The psychiatric casualties, which undoubtedly will be unique to the situation, are still likely to resemble in some fashion those of previous low-intensity wars. The human organism is amazingly adaptable, and responds to threats to its existence by calling forth the maximum adaptive strategies to escape from the perceived danger. When effective methods for returning combat fatigue cases to battle were developed, is it possible that newer symptom complexes to avoid danger occurred as an adaptive function? Failure to take malarial prophylaxis, drug abuse, and misconduct defy the application of traditional combat psychiatric principles but may reflect the same psychodynamic processes seen in combat fatigue. Given this difficulty, treatment and preventive psychiatric procedures must be flexible to optimize the return of such casualties to normal functioning.

REFERENCES

1. Omang J. "What do 42 wars add up to?" *Washington Post,* 27 April 1986: C5.

2. Hammel EM. *The Root: The Marines in Beirut, August 1982–February 1984.* San Diego, Calif: Harcourt Brace Jovanovich; 1985.

3. Adelaja O. The changing patterns of psychiatric incidence during and after a war: The Nigerian experience. In: Adelaja O, Jones FD, eds. *War and its Aftermath.* Lagos, Nigeria: John West; 1983: 34–42.

4. Collazo CR. Psychiatric casualties in Malvinas War: A provisional report. In: Pichot P, Berner P, Wolf R, Thau K, eds. *Psychiatry: The State of the Art.* Vol 6. New York: Plenum Press; 1985: 499–503.

5. Crocq L. Les nevroses de guerre. *La Revue De Medecine.* 1969;2:57–188.

6. Glass AJ. Psychotherapy in the combat zone. *Am J Psychiatry.* 1954;110(10):725–731.

7. Glass AJ, Bernucci RJ, eds. *Zone of Interior.* Vol 1. In: *Neuropsychiatry in World War II.* Washington, DC: Office of The Surgeon General, US Army; 1966.

8. Hanson FR. The factor of fatigue in the neuroses of combat. Combat Psychiatry. *Bull US Army Med Dept.* 1949;9:147–150.

9. Jones FD, Johnson AW. Medical and psychiatric treatment policy and practice in Vietnam. *J Soc Issues.* 1975;31(4):49–56.

10. Mansour F. Manifestations of maladjustment to military service in Egypt after prolonged stress. *Int Rev Army Navy Air Force Med Serv.* 1982;55:291–294.

11. Menninger WC. *Psychiatry in a Troubled World.* New York: Macmillan; 1948.

12. Ponteva M. Psychiatric disorders in conventional war. *Ann Med Milit Fenn* [Finland]. 1985;60(4):111–114.

13. Salmon TW, Fenton N. Neuropsychiatry in the American expeditionary forces. In: Bailey P, Williams FE, Komora PA, Salmon TW, Fenton N, eds. *Neuropsychiatry.* In: *The Medical Department of the United States Army in the World War.* Vol 10. Washington, DC: Office of The Surgeon General, US Army; 1929; 271–474.

14. Solomon Z, Schwarzwald J, Weisenberg M. *Mental Health Sequelae Among Israeli Soldiers in the 1982 Lebanon War.* Tel-Aviv: Medical Corps, Department of Mental Health, The Israeli Defence Forces; June 1985.

15. Crocq L, Crocq MA, Barrois C, Belenky GL, Jones FD. Low intensity combat psychiatric casualties. In: Pichot P, Berner P, Wolf R, Thau K, eds. *Psychiatry: The State of the Art.* Vol 6. New York: Plenum Press; 1985: 545–550.

16. Jones FD. Combat psychiatry in modern warfare. In: Adelaja O, Jones FD, eds. *War and its Aftermath.* Lagos, Nigeria: John West; 1983: 63–77.

17. Jones FD. Experiences of division psychiatrist in Vietnam. *Milit Med.* 1967;132:1003–1008.

18. Jones FD. Combat stress: Tripartite model. *Int Rev Army Navy Air Force Med Serv.* 1982;55:247–254.

19. Jones FD. Psychiatric lessons of low-intensity wars. *Ann Med Milit Fenn* [Finland]. 1985;60(4):128–134.

20. US Department of the Army. *Planning for Health Service Support*. Washington, DC: DA; 9 September 1994. Field Manual 8-55.

21. US Department of the Army. *Combat Stress Control in a Theater of Operations*. Washington, DC: DA; 29 September 1994. Field Manual 8-51.

22. US Department of the Army. *Leaders' Manual for Combat Stress Control*. Washington, DC: DA; 29 September 1994. Field Manual 22-51.

23. Jones FD. Reactions to stress: Combat versus combat-support psychiatric casualties. Presented at VI World Congress of Psychiatry; August 28—September 3, 1977; Honolulu, Hawaii.

24. Rosen G. Nostalgia: A "forgotten" psychological disorder. *Psychol Med*. 1975;5:340–354.

25. Deutsch A. Military psychiatry: The Civil War 1861–1865. In: Hall JK, Zilboorg G, Bunker HA. *One Hundred Years of American Psychiatry: 1844–1944*. New York: Columbia University Press. 1944: 367–384.

26. Crane S. *The Red Badge of Courage: An Authoritative Text, Backgrounds and Sources, Criticisms*. 2nd ed. New York: WW Norton; 1976: 31.

27. Belenky GL, Kaufman LW. Cohesion and rigorous training: Observations of the Air Assault School. *Milit Rev*. 1983;63:24–34.

28. Salmon TW, Fenton N. In the army of occupation. In: Bailey P, Williams FE, Komora PA, Salmon TW, Fenton N, eds. *Neuropsychiatry*. Vol 10. In: *The Medical Department of the United States Army in the World War*. Washington, DC: Office of The Surgeon General, US Army; 1929: 423–428.

29. Appel JW. Preventive psychiatry. In: Glass AJ, Bernucci RJ, eds. *Zone of Interior*. Vol 1. In: *Neuropsychiatry in World War II*. Washington, DC: Office of The Surgeon General, US Army; 1966: 373–415.

30. Brill NQ, Beebe GW. *A Follow-up Study of War Neuroses*. Washington, DC: US GPO; 1955: 329–333.

31. Frank RL. Alaska and the Aleutians (North Pacific area). In: Glass AJ, ed. *Overseas Theaters*. Vol 2. In: *Neuropsychiatry in World War II*. Washington, DC: Office of The Surgeon General, US Army; 1973: 681–737.

32. Reister FA. *Battle Casualties and Medical Statistics: US Army Experience in the Korean War*. Washington, DC: Office of The Surgeon General, US Army; 1973: 117.

33. Norbury FB. Psychiatric admissions in a combat division. *US Army Med Bull Far East*. July 1953:130–133.

34. Marren JJ. Psychiatric problems in troops in Korea during and following combat. *US Armed Forces Med J*. 1956;7(5):715–726.

35. Camp NM. 1982. Vietnam military psychiatry revisited. Presented at the annual American Psychiatric Association meeting. Toronto, Canada: May 15–21, 1982.

36. Fleming RH. Post Vietnam syndrome: Neurosis or sociosis? *Psychiatry*. 1985;48:122–139.

37. Holloway H, Ursano R. The Vietnam veteran: Memory, social context and metaphor. *Psychiatry*. 1984;47:103–108.

38. Renner JA. The changing patterns of psychiatric problems in Vietnam. *Compr Psychiatry*. 1973;14(2):169–180.

39. Silsby HD, Cook CJ. Substance abuse in the combat environment: The heroin epidemic. In: Adelaja O, Jones FD, eds. *War and its Aftermath*. Lagos, Nigeria: John West; 1983: 23–27.

40. Marlowe DH. Cohesion, anticipated breakdown, and endurance in battle: Considerations for severe and high intensity combat. Walter Reed Army Institute of Research, Neuropsychiatry Division. Washington, DC: Monograph; 1979.

41. Belenky GL. Varieties of reaction and adaptation to combat experience. *Bull Menninger Clin.* 1987;51(1):64–79.

42. Poirier JG, Jones FD. A group operant approach to drug dependence in the military that failed: Retrospect. *Milit Med.* 1977;142(5):366–369.

43. Tischler GL. Patterns of psychiatry attrition and of behavior in a combat zone. In: Bourne PG, ed. *The Psychology and Physiology of Stress.* New York: Academic Press; 1969: 19–44.

44. Billings EG. South Pacific base command. In: Glass AJ, ed. *Overseas Theaters.* Vol 2. In: *Neuropsychiatry in World War II.* Washington, DC: Office of The Surgeon General, US Army; 1973: 473–512.

45. Huffman RE. Which soldiers break down: A survey of 610 psychiatric patients in Vietnam. *Bull Menninger Clin.* 1970;34:343–351.

46. Cohen S. *The Drug Dilemma.* New York: McGraw-Hill; 1969: 76.

47. Froede RC, Stahl CJ. Fatal narcotism in military personnel. *J Forensic Sci.* 1971;16(2):199–218.

48. Baker SL. Drug abuse in the United States Army. *Bull NY Acad Med.* 1971;47(6):541–549.

49. Roffman RA, Sapol E. Marijuana in Vietnam. *Int J Addict.* 1970;5(1):1–42.

50. Black S, Owens KL, Wolff RP. Patterns of drug use. *Am J Psychiatry.* 1970;4:420–423.

51. Stanton MD. Drugs, Vietnam, and the Vietnam veteran: An overview. *Am J Drug Alcohol Abuse.* 1976;3(4):557–570.

52. Robins LN, Helzer JE, Davis DH. Narcotic use in Southeast Asia and afterward. *Arch Gen Psychiatry.* 1975;32:955–961.

53. McCoy AW. *The Politics of Heroin in Southeast Asia.* New York: Harper & Row; 1972.

54. Frenkel SI, Morgan DW, Greden JF. Heroin use among soldiers in the United States and Vietnam: A comparison in retrospect. *Int J Addict.* 1977;12(8):1143–1154.

55. Spragg G. Psychiatry in the Australian military forces. *Med J Aust.* 1972(1):745–751.

56. Spragg G. Australian forces in Vietnam. Presented at Combat Stress Seminar, Department of Military Psychiatry, Walter Reed Army Institute of Research, Walter Reed Army Medical Center. July 10, 1983; Washington, DC.

57. Fry CC, Rostow EG. *National Research Council, Interim Report.* Washington, DC: GPO; April 1, 1945.

58. Michie HC. The venereal diseases. In: Siler JF, ed. *Communicable and Other Diseases.* In: *The Medical Department of the United States Army in the World War.* Vol 9. Washington, DC: Office of The Surgeon General, US Army; 1928: 263–310.

59. Deller JJ, Smith DE, English DT, Southwick EG. Venereal diseases. In: Ognibene AJ, Barrett O Jr, eds. *General Medicine and Infectious Diseases.* In: Ognibene AJ, ed. *Internal Medicine in Vietnam.* Vol 2. Washington, DC: Office of The Surgeon General, US Army; 1982: 233–255.

60. MH staffs need more AIDS education, Pasnau advises. *Psychiatr News.* 4 July 1986;21(3):1,12.

61. Rose E. The anatomy of mutiny. *Armed Forces Society.* 1982;8(4):561–574.

62. Linden E. The demoralization of an army: Fragging and other withdrawal symptoms. *Saturday Review.* 8 January 1972:12.

63. United States. Department of the Army. *The My Lai Massacre and its Coverup: Beyond the Reach of Law? The Peers Commission Report.* New York: Free Press; 1972.

64. Gal R. Commitment and obedience in the military: An Israeli case study. *Armed Forces Society*. 1985;2(4):553–564.

65. Kalinowski LB. War and post-war neuroses in Germany. *Med Bull US Army, Europe*. 1950;7(3). [Reprinted *Med Bull US Army, Europe*. 1980;37(3):23–29.]

66. Manning FJ. Morale and cohesion in military psychiatry. In: Jones FD, Sparacino LR, Wilcox VL, Rothberg JM, eds. *Military Psychiatry: Preparing in Peace for War*. Part 1. In: *Textbook of Military Medicine*. Washington, DC: Office of The Surgeon General, US Department of the Army and Borden Institute; 1994: 1–18.

67. Benson H. *The Relaxation Response*. New York: William Morrow; 1975.

Chapter 4

NEUROPSYCHIATRIC CASUALTIES OF NUCLEAR, BIOLOGICAL, AND CHEMICAL WARFARE

FRANKLIN D. JONES, M.D., F.A.P.A.*

*Colonel (ret), Medical Corps, U.S. Army; Clinical Professor, Uniformed Services University of the Health Sciences, Bethesda, Maryland; Past President and Secretary and current Honorary President of the Military Section, World Psychiatric Association; formerly Psychiatry and Neurology Consultant, Office of The Surgeon General, U.S. Army

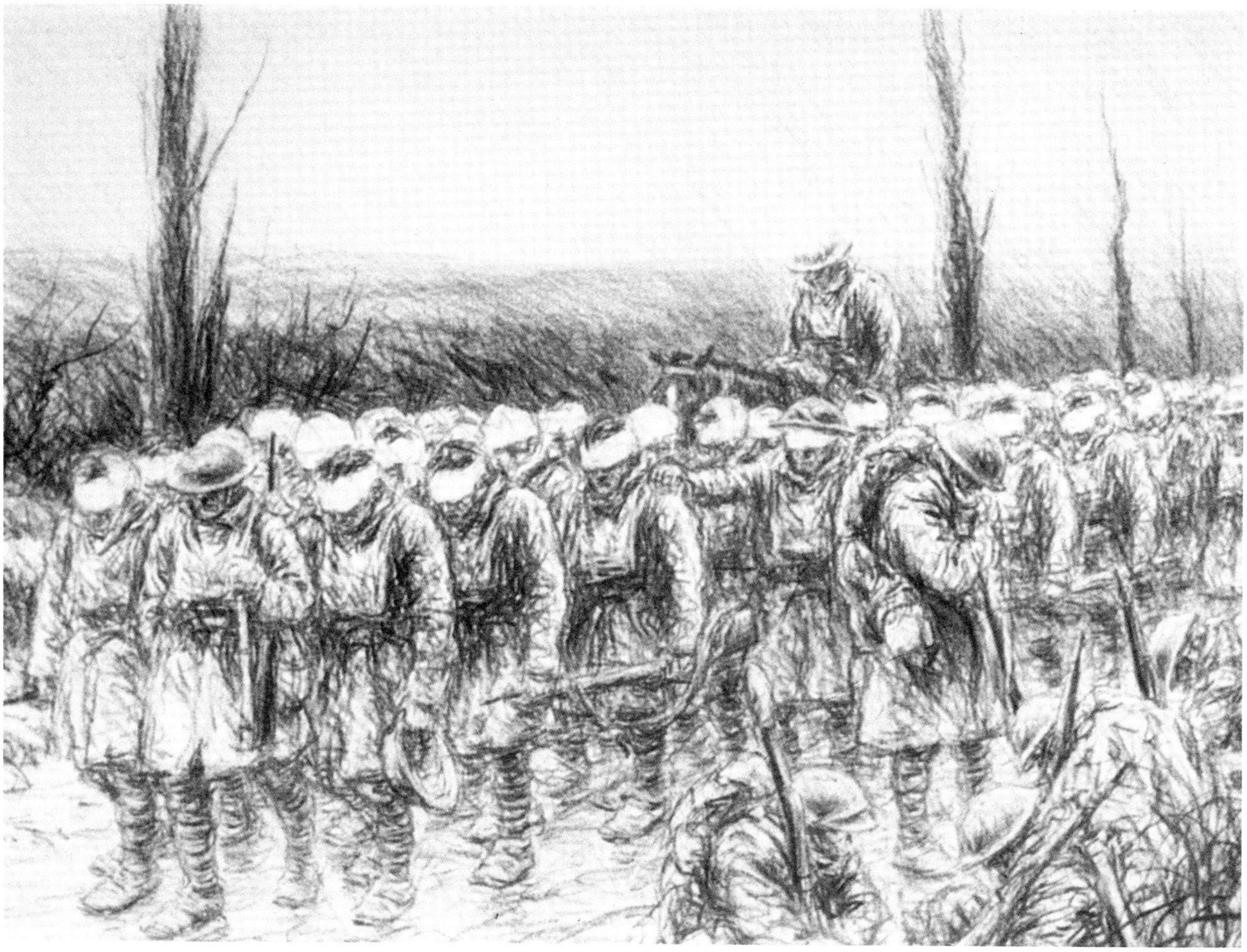

Kerr Eby *Match Sellers, Class of '17* 1918

Kerr Eby was initially a member of the Ambulance Corps in the U.S. Army in World War I, then transferred to the Engineers, and went to the front lines in France. His painting depicts a group of soldiers blinded during a gas attack. Whereas the neuropsychiatric casualties of other forms of warfare may present as individuals, the casualties of nuclear, biological, and chemical warfare are most often seen as groups because the agent, whatever it may be, is delivered in a dispersed form to affect as many troops as possible. The title, *Match Sellers*, refers to a possible occupation, from a previous era, for these soldiers when they return home.

Art: Courtesy of US Center of Military History, Washington, DC.

INTRODUCTION

Although outlawed by both the Hague Convention[1] and the Geneva Convention,[2] chemical warfare continues to exist along with potential use of nuclear and biological warfare. In recent wars it has been alleged that the former Soviets used mycotoxins against Afghan guerrillas and that Vietnam used "yellow rain" (mycotoxins) in Cambodia and Laos. Iraq used chemical agents against Iranian soldiers and Kurdish rebels, and had the ability to use them against coalition forces in the Persian Gulf War. The long history of the use of such agents is likely to continue. This usage has usually occurred when one side has, or believes that it has, superiority in such weaponry. During World War II, the Germans had a superior capability in the form of nerve agents; but, believing the Allies to have a similar capability, they did not use them. There is, therefore, a compelling argument in favor of the deterrent effect of parity in chemical warfare capability. Tear gas and nausea-producing agents, which were not designated as prohibited agents by the Hague[1] and Geneva[2] conventions, were used by U.S. forces in Vietnam.[3–5] Exhibit 4-1 reveals the frequency of alleged usage of chemical and biological weapons since World War I. This review indicates that the U.S. armed forces or modern armies must be prepared for the possible use of such agents in future wars.

The use of tactical (battlefield) nuclear weapons is possible not only between the major powers but also between smaller industrialized and nonindustrialized nations. In addition to the nations known to have nuclear arsenals in 1992 (United States, Russia, Ukraine, Khazakstan, Great Britain, France, China, and India), a number of countries had nuclear weapons or were developing them (South Africa, Israel, Pakistan, Iraq, and possibly North Korea, Iran, and Brazil). Most industrialized European nations are capable of developing such weapons if they choose to do so. Furthermore, the potential for terrorists to steal nuclear weapons or to make primitive devices also exists. Mental health workers must plan for tactical and strategic nuclear exchanges.[6] Strategic nuclear exchanges will be addressed in terms of disaster planning. This chapter will address the psychiatric aspects of tactical nuclear weapons and nonnuclear radiation threats after first discussing chemical and biological warfare which appear more likely to exist on the battlefield than nuclear warfare.

CHEMICAL WARFARE

Ancient artwork and documents reveal the use of chemical agents. Three-thousand-year-old Assyrian bas reliefs depict the use of liquid fire. Irritant or toxic smoke or fumes were used at the sieges of Syracuse (413 BC) and Rhodes (304 BC). Such agents were used for both their asphyxiating and incendiary effects but were not very effective.[7]

At the Hague Congress in 1899, all countries represented, except the United States, pledged to refrain from using suffocating or poisonous gases. The U.S. delegate felt that it was illogical to say that gas was inhumane while bombs, bullets, and other methods of warfare were more humane.[7]

Just 15 years later, the modern use of poison gas began in earnest during World War I. In August 1914, the French used tear gas against German troops. On the pretext that this was chemical warfare, in April 1915, the Germans attacked French troops by releasing 180 tons of chlorine in a cloud north of Ypres. This attack was devastating. In December 1915, the Germans introduced phosgene and in July 1917, mustard gas. Other gases were tried, including arsenic compounds and cyanide, but with limited success. Mustard gas was the most successful. During World War I, chlorine and mustard gas killed or injured more than a million soldiers and civilians.

Although the U.S. Army entered late in the war, 31% of all American battle casualties were due to gas.[7] Russian gas casualties amounted to half a million, of which 10% were fatalities. The Russian Army suffered twice the number of casualties and 5-fold the number of deaths secondary to gas than any other combatant.[8]

The forerunners of modern chemical nerve agents were developed by German chemists during the 1930s as a by-product of insecticide research. By the end of World War II, about 12,000 tons of Tabun (Ga) and small amounts of Sarin (Gb) and Soman (Gd) were synthesized, most of which fell into Soviet hands. As mentioned, the Germans did not use these weapons because they

EXHIBIT 4-1

CHRONOLOGY OF CHEMICAL AND BIOLOGICAL WARFARE ALLEGATIONS

1899: Hague Council outlawed use of chemical warfare (CW)

1915–1918: World War I—Both sides used chemical agents extensively

1919–1921: Russian Civil War—Both sides perhaps, Whites definitely, used CW

Early 1920s: British forces in Middle East—Both sides allegedly used CW

Mid 1920s: Morocco—Spanish used mustard gas in 1925; French allegedly used it

Early 1930s: China—Governor of Manchuria used CW against insurgents

1935–1936: Ethiopia—15,000 of total 50,000 Ethiopian casualties were from CW agents used by Italy

1936: Spain—Probably only tear gas used by Fascists

1937–1945: China—CW used by Japanese but probably irritants initially, mustard later; Japanese experimented with bacteria on human prisoners

1939–1945: World War II—Poles in 1939 used mustard gas defensively; Germans used chemical and bacterial agents in crimes against civilians in concentration camps; Japanese used cyanide hand grenades on U.S. forces in Pacific; U.S. forces had mustard gas available but the only casualties from its use were Americans accidentally exposed.

1945–1949: China—Civil War—Alleged use of CW by Nationalists

1947: Indochina—Alleged use of CW by French

1949: Greece—Civil War—Sulfur dioxide allegedly used by government (first military use of sulfur dioxide was in the same area 2300 years earlier when the Peloponnesians besieged Platea)

1951–1952: Korea—United States allegedly used CW and biological warfare, admits only to tear gas

1957: Cuba—Castro forces allegedly used mustard gas

1958: Rio de Oro—French and Spanish allegedly used CW in Sharan, Morocco, area

1958: China—Nationalists allegedly used CW from Quemoy against the mainland

1963-1967: Yemen—Egyptian forces allegedly used CW (multiple gases) in Yemeni Civil War

1965–1971: United States used tear gas in Vietnam; others were alleged

1968: Guinea and Bissau—Portugal allegedly used gas

1969: Palestine—Palestine Liberation Organization accused Israel of using gas warfare

1970: Angola—Portugal was accused of gas warfare

1970: Rhodesia (now Zimbabwe)—Government was accused of poisoning a rebel water supply

1980s: Afghanistan—Soviets allegedly used CW, particularly mycotoxins, especially early in the war

Early 1980s: Cambodia and Laos—Vietnam allegedly used mycotoxins in "yellow rain"

1980s: Iraq used several chemicals, including mustard gas and nerve agents, against Iranian ground troops. In 1988, hundreds of Kurdish civilians and Iranian soldiers were killed by Iraqi mustard and cyanide gas in territory captured by Iran; Iran allegedly retaliated with CW

1991: Iraq had chemical agents but did not use them during the U.N. attack on Iraq. Iraq was close to developing a nuclear capability.

Data sources: [1899–1970] Stockholm International Peace Research Institute. *The Problem of Chemical and Biological Warfare. Vol 1: The Rise of CB Weapons.* New York: Humanities Press; 1971: 1–5, 141–212, 212–230. [1980–1991] Author research.

mistakenly believed that the Allies also possessed them.

Many armies expect that chemical weapons will be used in any major conflict. Modern military doctrine assumes that combat operations will continue in the presence of toxic chemicals. As of 1990, training in the use of protective masks and clothing started at the grade school level in schools in the former Soviet Union and continued through adolescence and into the military service. Soviet troops were routinely trained to fight while wearing protective masks and clothing, and chemical defense personnel were integral to Soviet fighting units down to the company level.[9] Training of Soviet troops included exposure in protective gear to active diluted nerve agents. Psychological conditioning to fighting in a chemical environment was also heavily stressed.[8] Soviet chemical weapons were believed to consist predominantly of the nerve agents (particularly Soman), cyanide and mustard,[10,11] and possibly mycotoxins. With the demise of the Soviet Union and Warsaw Pact, the threat of major warfare and use of NBC warfare is lessened; however, terrorist use of such weapons remains a real threat. This is exemplified by the March 1995 use of Sarin in the Tokyo subway system terrorist attack, reportedly by the religious cult Aum Supreme Truth. The attack resulted in 10 deaths and over 1,000 injuries.[12]

Iraq used mustard and nerve agent[13] in its war against Iran after the tide of the war had turned in Iran's favor. Iraqi Republican Guard units, which had been trained to fight on the contaminated battlefield, enabled Iraq to win the limited counteroffensive which finally brought Iran to accept a grudging cease-fire. The threat of Iraqi chemical weapons was taken seriously during the 1991 Persian Gulf War. Many troops were given prophylactic pyridostigmine as pretreatment for nerve agent exposure. The U.S. units were frequently in mission-oriented protective posture (MOPP) gear. No cases of Iraqi chemical weapons' use were documented, although there were numerous chemical alarms sounded.

Since the Persian Gulf War, the media have reported that several thousand veterans have complained of miscellaneous symptoms including fatigue, trouble concentrating and remembering, paresthesias, hair loss, joint pains, skin rashes, respiratory and gastrointestinal problems, and caustic (irritating) semen.[14] Many show severe emotional distress as they testify before Congress or the news media that similar symptoms are affecting their spouses and children (who they also fear are subject to birth defects). Many of the sufferers (and one congressman) attribute this "Persian Gulf Syndrome" (which is perhaps more appropriately labeled "Possible Persian Gulf Illnesses") on either trace quantities of Iraqi chemical or biological agents, or on the U.S. pretreatment drug pyridostigmine or the vaccinations against anthrax. Another suspect is radiation from the depleted uranium used as antitank ammunition or additional armor for tanks. The difficulty of confirming or excluding any of these hypotheses illustrates the high ambiguity of the NBC threat and the severe stress that ambiguity causes.

Physiological Effects of Nerve Agents

The "nerve agents" are derived from organophosphorus compounds related to commercially available insecticides such as parathion and diazinon. They are extremely toxic. For example, 0.8 mg of Soman or 0.4 mg of agent VX can be lethal. Other nerve agents include Sarin and Tabun, which can penetrate ordinary clothes with ease, making special suits necessary for protection. Nerve agents in the liquid state can penetrate unbroken skin, and one or two droplets on the skin can be fatal if not removed immediately.[15] The addition of thickening compounds to these agents can increase persistence, resulting in a contact hazard that may last for weeks.[11]

Nerve agents are irreversible inhibitors of acetylcholinesterase, an enzyme that is present throughout the central nervous system, the skeletal muscles, numerous glands, and other cholinergically innervated organs. Poisoning with these agents leads to an inability to break down acetylcholine. An excess of acetylcholine in the synapses results, leading to a functional denervation state or subsensitivity of the post-synaptic receptor in response to overwhelming stimulation.[16] The resulting symptoms of cholinergic overstimulation include lacrimation, salivation, nausea, hyperpnea, rhinorrhea, bronchoconstriction, vomiting, muscle twitching, progressive respiratory paralysis, and death. The usual cause of death is respiratory paralysis, which may be central in origin.[17] Autopsy studies of animals who survived exposure to nerve agents revealed extensive damage to limbic neurons.[18] This suggests that human survivors of nerve agent poisoning may suffer serious, permanent personality changes.

The detailed treatment of acute poisoning with nerve agents is beyond the scope of this book; however, the mainstay of treatment is atropine. Currently U.S. soldiers are provided with three autoinjectors, each with 2 mg of atropine, for self-administration in the field. As further therapy, atropine is administered until significant side effects appear. Atropinization is usually maintained for at least 24 to 48 hours. As much as 10 to 40 mg of atropine may be necessary in the first 24 hours.[19,20] Some studies[21] indicate that scopolamine, which apparently enters the brain more readily than atropine, may be more effective than atropine in treating the central nervous system effects of nerve agent poisoning.

Treatment protocols[20,22–24] and military manuals[25–28] all call for treatment with pralidoxime (Protopam or 2-PAM chloride), which, by removing the bound agent from the enzyme, reactivates the enzyme.[23,24] While oximes are effective antagonists to many cholinesterase inhibitors, they also produce side effects. Furthermore, some nerve agents are refractory to currently available oximes; this is particularly true of Soman, the predominant nerve agent in the former Soviet Union arsenal.[29] The current standard oxime of the U.S. Army, pralidoxime chloride, is administered by the slow intravenous route along with atropine in the Mark I autoinjector.

Plans now include pretreatment with pyridostigmine 30 mg every 8 hours prior to anticipated exposure. This does not prevent symptoms but greatly increases the efficacy of atropine and pralidoxime. Pyridostigmine is itself a "nerve agent" which temporarily protects some acetylcholinesterase enzyme from deactivation by the enemy's nerve agents. Diazepam 10 mg is also issued as an anticonvulsant to be administered with the third autoinjector or if the casualty is convulsing, with the goal of decreasing the chances of lasting brain damage. Genetic engineering may allow the development of a more effective antidote in the future. This is suggested by the discovery of an enzyme in squid nerves that hydrolyzes and detoxifies Soman.[30]

If a nerve agent is used, many soldiers will receive only low doses by virtue of location or protective measures; this low-level poisoning may be accepted as a calculated risk or may even go undetected. If a nerve agent is used, many more soldiers will receive only very low doses than will receive high doses, by virtue of their location or protective measures. Some low-dose exposure may be accepted as a calculated risk. The first symptom of minimal exposure of the eyes to nerve agent vapor (at 1/30th to 1/50th of the lethal dose) is pinpoint pupils.[25] This does not grossly impair vision in bright light, but causes dimming of vision and may impair performance in the low levels of artificial illumination inside vehicles or tents (tactical operations centers) and/or at the critical times of predawn and dusk. Soldiers with pinpoint pupils would be seriously impaired and at a dangerous disadvantage in night operations under blackout conditions. At slightly higher doses, the soldiers also have eye discomfort on focusing, blurred vision, headaches, jitteriness, and runny noses to further distract them.[25] These symptoms could involve all members of a squad, platoon, or company, to greater or lesser degree. The pinpoint pupils remain marked for 24 hours, before gradually improving over several days. The soldiers may well be fearful of further NBC or conventional attack, unwilling to venture out after dark, and prone to overreact to threats until adequate vision returns.

Experience with human exposure to the chemically related organophosphate insecticides suggests that, in cases of *chronic* exposure to low concentrations, psychiatric symptoms may predominate over physical ones. Impaired thinking, judgment, attention, and short-term memory are likely, but toxic delirium may also be present. The cognitive deficits may persist many months, even after treatment, along with irritability, mood changes, depression, and insomnia with nightmares. Acetylcholinesterase inhibitors have been found to precipitate psychotic symptoms in predisposed individuals.[31]

Behavioral manifestations of nerve agent poisoning that antedate, follow, or occur independently of somatic symptoms[19] may be most prominent in individuals who have been exposed to sublethal doses or in those who have recovered from the somatic effects of poisoning. Acute organophosphorus intoxication produces cognitive impairment with difficulty in concentration, confusion, and drowsiness.[31,32] Airplane crashes of crop-duster pilots may be due to acute intoxication with organophosphorus compounds.[33] Chronically-exposed agricultural workers have complained of forgetfulness, difficulty in thinking, visual impairment, and drowsiness. These deficits were quantified by sophisticated testing.[34] Another study[32] showed that chronically-exposed workers had higher levels of anxiety than matched controls. Chronic exposure has also been associated with increased anxiety, possibly causing misdiagnosis of combat stress reactions.[35] Memory also appears to be impaired by organophosphate poisoning.[20] Significant impairment of cognition, vigilance, and memory may make it difficult for a minimally-exposed soldier to perform the often complex tasks that will be required.

Poisoning with nerve agents may cause other psychiatric disturbances that mimic psychological as opposed to organic disorders. Depression has been observed as a prominent symptom in accidental poisoning.[22,31,36] The severity of depression seems to be related to the severity of poisoning and the degree of acetylcholinesterase inhibition. This depressogenic effect of nerve agents is suggested by the observation that the reversible cholinesterase inhibitor, physostigmine, can normalize mood in manic patients and can cause depression in normal persons.[37,38] Could the same be true for the pretreatment drug, pyridostigmine, in some soldiers? Nerve agent toxicity has also been associated with complaints of "excessive" dreaming, nightmares, insomnia, and delirium.[22,32] Treatment with anticholinergic agents seems to reduce these symptoms.[22] Nerve agents may also lower the threshold for convulsive seizures. These could be mimicked by pseudoseizures in tense, anxious persons, creating a problem for differential diagnosis.

It is possible that nerve agents can cause psychosis, by altering the dopaminergic-cholinergic balance in mesolimbic structures. Anticholinesterases reportedly activate symptoms in schizophrenic patients.[36] One study[39] reported that a higher percentage of agricultural workers exposed to toxic agents developed psychotic illnesses than would have been expected. These results have not been confirmed, however.

In summary, the data on the subacute and chronic physiological effects of exposure to organophosphorus poisons reveal substantial risk of depression and sleep disturbances, decreased cognitive abilities, and a slight risk of psychosis and anxiety disorders.[40]

Added to the dangers of nerve agent poisoning are effects of antidotes, which may outweigh the danger of potential exposure to nerve agents. Self-injection of atropine by the soldier after exposure to nerve agents may be lifesaving, but inappropriate self-injection may lead to a central anticholinergic syndrome with delirium. If a false alarm (or a deliberate attempt to make oneself a casualty) leads to the administration of chemical warfare antidotes in the absence of the appropriate agent, serious psychological symptoms are likely. Atropine in low doses produces blurred vision, tachycardia, dry mouth, sweat suppression with increased risk of heat stroke, urinary retention, and perhaps impaired thinking, judgment, insight, and short-term memory. Even in the 2 to 6 mg range available for early self-administration, atropine may give some individuals a toxic anticholinergic delirium with disorientation, agitation or stupor, paranoid delusions, and visual and tactile hallucinations lasting 8 to 16 hours. TAB (TMB-4 [an oxime], atropine, and benactyzine), an antidote combination formerly used by the U.S. Air Force and U.S. Navy/Marine Corps, was virtually guaranteed to produce psychosis with visual hallucinations in its standard dose.[30] While the presence of anticholinesterase nerve agents in the body may partially counteract such psychiatric side effects, it is unlikely that agent and antidote will exactly cancel each other.

Studies conducted at the U.S. Army Aeromedical Research Laboratory demonstrated that experienced helicopter pilots can fly helicopters, although seriously impaired, after receiving 4 mg of atropine. "Effects were seen most often ... in terms of aircraft control problems, vision disturbances, impaired tracking, reduced cortical activation, and decreased cognitive skills. These problems indicate helicopter tactical flight is dangerous after an unchallenged 4 mg dose. Other types of flight should also be avoided for at least 12 hours after atropine."[41(p.857)]

Following the administration of large doses of atropine, symptoms progress from tachycardia and dryness of the mouth to ataxia, hallucinosis, and confusion. In a study performed at Edgewood Arsenal,[42] subjects administered large doses of atropine became unable to pay attention, carry out instructions, speak coherently, or perform calculations. Significantly, soldiers who had impaired judgment failed to recognize their degree of general impairment and resented assistance. In this study, chlorpromazine, strongly anticholinergic itself, potentiated the adverse mental effects of anticholinergic agents. This takes on added significance in view of the widespread use of phenothiazines to treat anxiety symptoms in Vietnam.[43,44]

Treatment of atropine-type psychoses should *not* include phenothiazines, which produce anticholinergic side effects of their own, although haloperidol may be used. Current definitive treatment is with the carbamate, physostigmine, but this requires careful and prolonged intravenous titration.

The effects of atropine resemble those of another class of chemical agents, the incapacitants. Agent BZ (3-quinuclidinyl Bensylate) is a strong antimuscarinic compound that for some time was kept in the arsenal of U.S. chemical weapons. It produces hallucinations and psychological incapacitation similar to that produced by atropine, but is more specific and longer lasting (24–48 h) than atropine.

The burden of self-diagnosis is formidable, particularly considering the fact that other agents or even anxiety may mimic early symptoms of nerve agent poisoning. Under battle conditions, with oncoming shells producing smoke or spreading tear gas, with troops dispersed and communications strained, the apprehension and ambiguities may unavoidably lead to individual or group decisions to administer antidotes when exposure to nerve agents has not, in fact, occurred.[45]

Whether due to mistaken self-administration of antidotes or exposure to antimuscarinic agents, the possibility of significant numbers of casualties with anticholinergic poisoning must be considered. One example of troops thus exposed was in 1676, when British troops in Jamestown, Virginia, ingested Jimson ("Jamestown") Weed (*Datura stramonium*) and suffered mass anticholinergic poisoning.[46] Bizarre behavior and amnesia allegedly lasted for 11 days. The soldiers, who had to be confined to prevent them from injuring themselves, were very negligent of personal hygiene. More recently, combativeness or hyperactivity was noted in 10% of a series of 212 cases of stramonium intoxication.[47] Hallucinations occurred in 99 of the 212 cases, and 5 deaths were directly attributable to psychosis.

The failure to maintain adequate self-care behavior such as keeping dry, maintaining adequate hydration, and attending to personal hygiene has been noted as a cause of soldier ineffectiveness.[48,49] Reported effects of high doses of anticholinergic agents on soldiers include impaired performance in timing and vigilance tasks, in firing rifles or running an obstacle course; ataxia; blurred vision; inability to perform calculations; and disruption of communication between individuals.[42] Possible effects in the field might include failure to observe discipline, failure to conserve drinking water, failure to wear protective clothing, misinterpretation of visual or auditory signals, misidentification of individuals, failure to maintain silence, and increased risk of heat stroke. Anticholinergic syndromes can be reversed with physostigmine,[50] but this drug is not easy to use in the field. There are storage problems and it requires careful titration in use. Furthermore, as mentioned earlier, physostigmine can produce serious depression in normal persons, and the same problem of inappropriate use described with atropine exists.

In summary, nerve agents present numerous problems in practical therapeutics for the psychiatrist. Both the agents themselves and their antidotes may have significant behavioral effects, and the military psychiatrist may be called upon to treat, and to advise other physicians on how to treat, these problems.

Physiological Effects of Other Agents

Cyanide

Other chemical agents also may be encountered. Cyanide gas, a nonpersistent agent, is especially dangerous because it may saturate the active material in gas mask filters and render them useless. A combination of cyanide and a nerve agent would be particularly deadly. The early symptoms of cyanide exposure are anxiety, confusion, giddiness, and hyperventilation. These symptoms can also be caused by stress, and could lead to unnecessary medication with cyanide antidotes. In civilian situations, antidotes to cyanide have often been administered inappropriately.[51,52] Chronic exposure to low levels of cyanide could lead to mental changes as was seen when cyanide compounds were used therapeutically.[53] The effects of administration of large doses of anticholinergic agents to soldiers who have been poisoned with cyanide is unknown. Atropinization may conceal the symptoms of cyanide poisoning or may increase its lethality.

Incapacitating Agents

Tear-gas agents have been extensively used in war as most countries have interpreted the Hague and Geneva accords against gas warfare as not applying to these agents. Intended to be used as harassing agents, their lethality is very low.

Nonlethal incapacitating agents may exert their own direct effects on psychological functioning (like the anticholinergic BZ). Those reportedly used in Afghanistan appear to cause temporary unconsciousness or immobilization. Incapacitants may also provoke inappropriate responses by mimicking the early symptoms of more lethal agents. The tear gases may be confused with the lacrimation-producing nerve gases. Vomiting agents may stimulate fears of having been irradiated or exposed to biological agents. Adamsite, in this class, reportedly also may cause depression.[11]

Mustard

Mustard gas was responsible for the majority of gas casualties during World War I. It is considered an obsolete agent by the U.S. but the former Soviets were believed to have stockpiles of it,[8] and it was used by Iraq against Iran. Mustard gas is unique for its insidious method of action and its latency of several hours before burns and blisters appear. It can present a contact hazard for weeks. Sulfur mustard (bis[2-chloroethyl] sulfide) is a powerful alkylating agent that can produce severe skin burns and pulmonary injury if inhaled. Very low doses of mustard produce painful conjunctivitis of the eyes which lasts for days to weeks, severely impairing vision.[54] As with nerve agent, blindness on the battlefield, even if known to be temporary, can produce anxiety, dependency, and other psychological as well as management problems. Higher-dose contact burns the eyes and causes permanent blindness as well as disfiguring facial burns. The potential psychological impact of these is discussed in Chapter 14, Disabling and Disfiguring Injuries. Blistering of exposed hands could also leave long-term physical and emotional scars. In soldiers without protective overgarments, mustard tends to produce blisters at the moist creases of the body, notably the genital region. Psychological reactions to genital injuries are also discussed in Chapter 14.

Blister agents (mustard gas, Lewisite) have been noted to produce chronic psychological symptoms of apathy and depression[55] in addition to their severe and delayed dermatologic, pulmonary, and systemic lesions. Phosgene, a suffocant gas, keeps active the traditional World War I terror of gas attack as producing a horrible sensation of the lungs filling with fluid, with the added threat that it permanently inactivates the charcoal in one's mask or overgarment. Phosgene's delay of several hours before the first symptoms, and the dangerous worsening of symptoms by physical exercise, was especially unnerving, even to those not actually exposed.[56]

Mycotoxins

The mycotoxins (thought to have been used by the Soviets and their allies in Southeast Asia and Afghanistan) produce terrifyingly rapid symptoms of vomiting, tissue necrosis, and failure of blood coagulation. Psychotic symptoms and bizarre behavior have not been mentioned prominently in current accounts; however, such psychiatric symptoms have been prominent in historical natural outbreaks of "St. Vitus' Dance" and "tarantism," which are now attributed to contamination of food grains by ergot derivatives from other fungal toxins. Mental symptoms may also become significant if mycotoxin patients are kept alive by treatment of the otherwise rapidly fatal symptoms.

Neuropsychiatric Syndromes Associated With Chemical Warfare

Large-scale gas warfare during World War I presented special problems. In addition to the "physical" casualties of chemical warfare, there were "psychological" casualties and syndromes. One of these was "gas hysteria," which usually occurred in small epidemics, threatening the integrity of entire units until remedial measures were taken.[57,58] This "epidemic" effect is seen in the following World War I episode:

> One morning a large number of soldiers were returned to the field hospital diagnosed as gas casualties. The influx continued for about eight days and the number of patients reached about 500. The divisional gas officer failed to find any clinical evidence of gas inhalation or burning.... Most of the patients had the fixed conviction that they had been gassed and would usually describe all the details with convincing earnestness and generally with some dramatic quality of expression.... It was obvious on examination that they were not really gassed. Further, it was inconceivable that they should be malingerers.[57(pp318–319)]

Acute symptoms of gas hysteria often mimicked some of the symptoms of gas poisoning and included dyspnea, coughing, and burning of the skin. Aphonia was also seen prominently.[59] For those in whom the symptoms persisted, the term "gas neurosis" was applied.[60] The degree of exact exposure to gas was unrelated to the symptoms presented. Dramatic symptoms were seen, such as tics and blepharospasm,[59] as well as "unconscious movements of the hands like clawing at the throat or removing a mask."[60(p214)] The patients presented with signs of air hunger and anxiety with alterations of consciousness, but no organic basis for the symptoms was found. One author suggested that gas neurosis patients "are particularly amenable to suggestion and rest. Optimism based on exact diagnosis and sincere faith in ultimate recovery is excellent therapy."[60(p214)] However, some of the gas neuroses continued until long after the war and were rewarded with compensation.[57] It should be remembered that during World War I there were approximately twice as many gas neurosis cases as there were gas exposure cases.[57]

Chemical warfare is still perceived as choking off one's breath. In spite of the complicated chemical properties of modern agents, respiratory symptoms are likely to predominate in conversion reactions.

This is reinforced by current military training requiring wearing protective clothing while tear gas agents are used to simulate poison gases.

More recently, similar conversion symptoms have been reported in the aftermath of chemical attacks in Afghanistan and Cambodia,[8] with aphonia and catatonic symptoms predominating. More generally, the mere act of donning protective gear will increase the soldier's sense of isolation from peers and decrease intragroup communication and support, factors that have been shown to be important in maintaining morale and probably in decreasing the incidence of psychiatric casualties.[61]

Gas warfare is perceived much as it was in 1918, as "awe inspiring" with "unbelievable horrors."[60] During World War I, units that were otherwise stressed, having spent long periods in combat under arduous conditions, were at much higher risk for "gas hysteria." This risk increased still further if relief was anticipated but did not arrive on schedule.[57] This aspect will loom large in any future mid- or high-intensity conflict, with the extremely high-pressure, continuous combat operations that are expected.[48,61]

As long as the nuclear, biological, and chemical (NBC) threat is an active, serious threat, protective masks and overgarments must be worn, certainly for brief periods and perhaps for prolonged ones. The protective gear distorts visual, auditory, and tactile perception; impairs fine motor coordination; increases physical effort, frustration, and fatigue; and increases psychiatric casualties in simulation exercises.[62,63] These effects may be especially disruptive to the performance of medical functions; however, modifications of protective gear for medical treatment[64,65] as well as approaches to triage have been proposed.[66] The protective ensembles retain body heat and increase the risk of heat exhaustion and heat stroke, which may present with mental symptoms and be difficult to diagnose in full MOPP (mission-oriented protective posture) gear. During a Scud missile attack by Iraq on Israel in January 1991, several elderly persons died of heart attacks while in gas masks.

The restrictions on eating, drinking, elimination, and hygiene functions, along with other discomforts and interference with sleep, can affect morale as well as physiological well-being. Decreased ability to recognize comrades and gauge their mood or resolve may lessen unit cohesion and increase the sense of helpless isolation (a prime factor in battle fatigue). Claustrophobic panic, premature unmasking (which may be imitated by others), spatial disorientation, and paranoid reactions to impaired sensory functioning may also occur. Such adverse reactions are exacerbated when visibility is further restricted by darkness, smoke, or vegetation. Gas mask phobia proved to be a significant problem in the Allied invasion of Iraq in 1991.[67]

Field studies and training exercises which test troops in force-on-force battles using the MILES (multiple integrated laser engagement system) to score who "shoots" whom have shown an alarming increase in friendly fire casualties ("fratricide") by insufficiently trained troops in the protective ensemble. Whereas only about 1 in 20 soldiers or vehicles is "shot" by their own side in conventional battles, the rate rises as high as 1 in 5 in full mission-oriented protective postures.[68,69] This is attributable to the combination of impaired vision and hearing plus the jumpiness this provokes. Fratricide, of course, is very disruptive of morale. Rigorous training is needed to reduce the risk.

Factors that predispose to psychiatric casualties include the rates of wounding in the unit, lack of sleep, and lack of prior combat experience.[70–72] Chemical attacks might increase psychiatric casualties by exacerbating all three of these factors.[45,73] Chemical weapons create fear of the unknown, a potent effect in inexperienced troops. Usually, troops entering combat will be, for the most part, untested in battle. Lack of sleep has produced hallucinations in troops during extended training exercises[74–76] and is a factor predisposing to combat psychiatric reactions.

With the possibility of high-intensity, continuous combat, psychiatric services will be strained to the limit. Because this country is committed against the initial use of chemical weapons, U.S. forces would be the first to suffer from chemical attacks, with the concomitant psychiatric casualties. Lack of experience in chemical warfare and the psychiatric syndromes arising from the physiological effects of chemical agents and their antidotes may lead to misdiagnosis and mistreatment. This may lead to decreased unit effectiveness at critical times. The difficulties in decontaminating large numbers of exposed soldiers may lead to removing them to centralized decontamination stations well to the rear. Many soldiers who might be medically fit to return to their units might develop an evacuation syndrome that would increase their resistance to returning to combat. In the 1982 Israeli incursion into Lebanon, some Israeli combat stress casualties were evacuated by air to Israel, while others were appropriately treated in forward areas. Almost all of the forward-treated cases, but few of the rear-evacuated cases, returned to combat.[77]

In summary, the psychological casualties of chemical warfare may well outnumber and prove more costly in personnel losses than the physical casualties, as occurred in World War I.[78] However, it should be noted that most veteran soldiers in World War I adapted to the threats and discomforts of chemical warfare. They often "preferred" this risk of chemical attack to those of high explosive shells and machine gun bullets because the protective equipment and good training allowed them to improve their odds of survival better.[79]

BIOLOGICAL WARFARE

Reports of biological warfare go back many centuries. One example is the introduction of smallpox to the American Indians by early settlers who gave or sold them infected blankets or trinkets.[80] However, in modern times the use of biological warfare agents appears to have been rare.

The United States did not have an offensive or defensive biological warfare capability until toward the end of World War II.[80] The nascent program focused on anthrax and botulinus toxins primarily. An anthrax plant received authorization to produce a million bombs and progress was being made in short-range dispersal techniques for botulin in paste form. Figure 4-1 shows a probable descendent of the World War II anthrax dispersal bomb. Moreover, there is evidence that research was conducted with brucellosis, psittacosis, tularemia, and the respiratory disease, glanders. In addition, botanical toxins and viruses were being explored with the aim of destroying Japanese vegetable gardens and rice crops. Tactical, rather than moral, considerations prevented the use of defoliants in World War II. They were later used in Vietnam, in the form of Agent Orange.

Rumors that a 1979 mishap with anthrax in the former Soviet Union produced scores of casualties at Sverdlovsk have been replaced by verified accounts that such a mishap actually occurred.[81] Iraq was suspected of working towards developing anthrax as a weapon. That led to the decision of the United States to vaccinate many personnel in the Persian Gulf campaign with an experimental anthrax vaccine. Many of the same considerations of chemical warfare apply to biological warfare; however, a major difference is the self-perpetuating effect of live biological agents. This can produce fear of contagion, which may severely impair relationships among troops and interfere with proper care of casualties. The near-panic responses of some persons in casual contact with victims of the practically noncontagious (except through sexual contact and shared needles) acquired immunodeficiency syndrome (AIDS) illustrate the validity of this factor.

Physiological Effects of Biological Agents

A number of viral, bacterial, and rickettsial agents have been identified as potential weapons, both for their psychological effects and the terror those effects produce in exposed troops. Anticipated psychiatric casualties of biological warfare will be included in a general discussion. It is, however, possible that an enemy could develop neurotropic viral agents that could produce primarily psychiatric symptoms.[82] Tables 4-1, 4-2, and 4-3 show agents considered by Malek[80] to have a biological warfare potential.

Neuropsychiatric Casualties of Biological Agents

Contagious biological organisms, like persistent transmissible chemical agents, would require quarantine and special handling. This would surely have widespread psychological effects on buddy-care and attitudes toward strangers, stragglers, and refugees. Within the medical system, the impact of invisible, patient-borne threats to other patients and to the treating personnel would reintroduce an old but now rarely encountered psychological as well as occupational stress, which may be difficult to cope with under field conditions. In World War I, entire medical/surgical teams were temporarily incapacitated by eye damage from mustard vapor brought into the operating room on wounded patients who had not yet shown any effects of their own exposure.

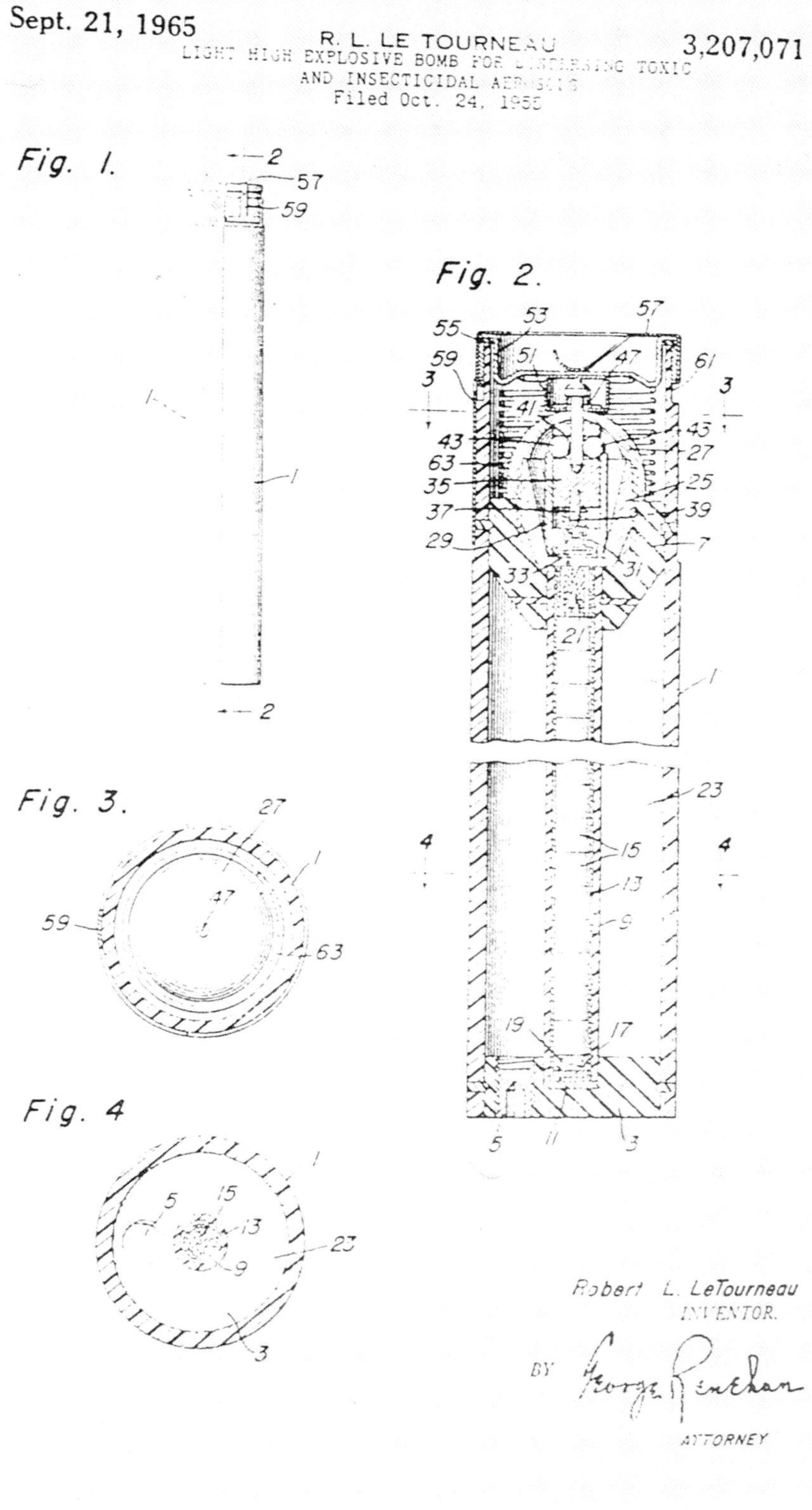

Fig. 4-1. Patent application of R. L. Le Tourneau for a light high-explosive bomb for dispersing toxic and insecticidal aerosols, 1955. Le Tourneau's patent application reveals the technological ingenuity he employed in continuing the production of gas warfare mechanisms. This technological interest continued for the next several decades with the development of safer binary weapons (ie, chemicals were inactive until combined at the time of actual use). Photograph: U.S. Patent and Trademark Office, Arlington, Va.

TABLE 4-1

POSSIBLE BIOLOGICAL WARFARE AGENTS—BACTERIAL

Disease	Transmission	Infectivity	Effects	Epidemicity	Therapy
Anthrax	Inhalation	Moderate	Respiratory Death	Low	Antibiotics
Brucellosis	Inhalation Ingestion	High	Fever Rarely die	Low	Antibiotics
Cholera	Ingestion	Low	Intestinal Can die	High	Difficult
Glanders	Inhalation Ingestion	High	Fever Often die	Low	Antibiotics
Melioidosis	Inhalation Ingestion	High	Fever Death	Low	Difficult
Plague	Inhalation Ingestion Fleas	High	Often die	High	Antibiotics
Tularemia	Inhalation Ingestion Insects	Very high	Fever 5%–8% die	None	Antibiotics

Adapted with permission from Malek I. Biological weapons. In: Rose S, ed. *CBW: Chemical and Biological Warfare*. Boston, Mass: Beacon Press; 1969: 60–61.

TABLE 4-2

POSSIBLE BIOLOGICAL WARFARE AGENTS—VIRAL

Disease	Transmission	Infectivity	Effects	Epidemicity	Therapy
Dengue	Mosquitoes Inhalation	High	Fever Rarely die	Low	Vaccine
Mumps	Inhalation	High	Not severe	High	Vaccine
Polio	Ingestion Inhalation	Low	Neurological Can die	Low	Vaccine
Psittacosis	Inhalation Ingestion Insects	High	Fever Can die	High	Antibiotics
Smallpox	Inhalation Ingestion	High	Often die	High	Vaccine
Yellow fever	Mosquitoes Inhalation	High	Jaundice 30% die	None	Vaccine

Adapted with permission from Malek I. Biological weapons. In: Rose S, ed. *CBW: Chemical and Biological Warfare*. Boston, Mass: Beacon Press; 1969: 60–61.

TABLE 4-3

POSSIBLE BIOLOGICAL WARFARE AGENTS—RICKETTSIAL, FUNGAL, TOXIC

Disease	Transmission	Infectivity	Effects	Epidemicity	Therapy
Rickettsial					
Q fever	Inhalation Ingestion Ticks	High	Fever 1% die	None	Antibiotics Vaccine
Typhus	Lice	High	Severe Often die	High	Vaccine Antibiotics
Fungal					
Coccidioidomycosis	Inhalation	High	Fever Rarely die	Low	Antibiotics
Toxin					
Botulism	Inhalation Ingestion	——	Severe 60%–70% die	None	Vaccine
"Yellow rain" (trichothecene mycotoxins)	Inhalation	——	Shock Often die	None	Difficult

Adapted with permission from Malek I. Biological weapons. In: Rose S, ed. *CBW: Chemical and Biological Warfare.* Boston, Mass: Beacon Press; 1969: 60–61.

NUCLEAR WARFARE AND DISASTERS

In some countries the use of nuclear weapons is a practical rather than a moral issue. An attack could be launched by tactical missile forces and fighter bombers.[73] There is concern that portable tactical nuclear weapons from the stockpiles of the former Soviet Union or from unstable states might fall into the hands of terrorists who could use them against cities. Industrial disasters like that at Chernobyl could release nuclear radiation to contaminate large areas and require military intervention to minimize the damage, evacuate the population, and maintain order.

Physical Effects of Nuclear Warfare

The energy generated by a typical tactical nuclear explosion consists of blast and shock waves (45% of the energy produced), light and heat (35%), initial radiation (5%), and residual fallout radiation (about 15%).[83] A ground detonation, vaporizing soil and melting granite and clay, results in large amounts of debris drawn by vacuum into the fireball, where it is mixed with radioactive bomb debris and subsequently falls to earth to contaminate it (fallout). While an air detonation produces the greatest blast damage, few particles are drawn into the atmosphere to mix with radioactive bomb debris so there is little residual contamination from fallout. Nuclear explosions over water produce massive vaporization and an intensely radioactive rainfall as well as a 50- to 100-foot tidal wave capable of drowning a coastal city.

Electromagnetic Pulse Effects of Nuclear Warfare

A high altitude electromagnetic pulse (EMP) is a radiated electromagnetic wave caused by the detonation of a nuclear weapon above the earth's atmosphere. A 3.3 megaton nuclear weapon, detonated 400 km above the center of the United States, can produce sufficient electromagnetic radiation to cover the entire country; and, if detonated over Europe, most of the continent would be affected.[84] Vandre, et al,[84] in simulated EMP tests, showed that by creating power surges in standard field medical equipment, an EMP would render about 65% of such equipment useless. The more modern and integrated the equipment, the greater the vulnerability to an EMP power surge.

An American Medical Association (AMA) report of the Board of Trustees indicated that civilian medical facilities would be equally devastated.[85] The AMA noted that in addition to medical equipment, telephone and other telecommunication equipment, computers and electronic equipment involved in life support systems, and diagnostic testing and other equipment utilizing solid state components are particularly vulnerable.

In a related paper, Vandre, et al,[86] described methods to minimize the vulnerability of equipment to EMP effects by keeping wiring near the ground, keeping it short, unplugging unused power equipment, running power cabling and tents in a north-south direction (thereby avoiding running power cabling in an east-west direction), and placing sensitive equipment in standardized shelters. By following such procedures Vandre, et al[86] estimated that 88% or more of unplugged field medical equipment could be kept functional in the event of EMP. The AMA noted that the increasing use of fiber optic components would decrease the effects of EMP because they are not vulnerable to the EMP surge. They recommended use of standby diesel generators to provide emergency power.[85]

Physiological Casualties of Nuclear Warfare

Studies of the effects of nuclear weapons on humans, with the exception of a few accidental radiation victims (particularly in Chernobyl), focus on the effects of the Hiroshima and Nagasaki bombings. A useful bibliography has been prepared by the Atomic Bomb Casualty Commission.[87]

Initial physical casualties are due to the blast and shock, heat, and nuclear radiation. Later, casualties are primarily from nuclear radiation. The initial effects are most closely related to the proximity and size of the fireball. At Hiroshima and Nagasaki more than 80% of the population within 0.6 of a mile of ground zero were casualties, and over 90% of these casualties were killed. In contrast, of individuals who were beyond approximately 1.6 miles from ground zero, less than 5% were killed.[88] These findings suggest that troop dispersal will be the primary defensive strategy in nuclear war. Burns accounted for two thirds of the initial deaths at Hiroshima and for one half of the total deaths. About 30% of those who died in Hiroshima had received lethal doses of radiation; however, this was not always the immediate cause of death.

There are two major biological effects of radiation in excess of 100 rad (a measure of the dose absorbed from ionizing radiation equal to 100 ergs per gram): (1) cell membrane damage leading to cellular and vascular leakage affecting especially brain and lungs, and (2) loss of reproductive capacity in stem cells.[87] Different tissues of the body show different sensitivities to ionizing radiation. In general, the radiosensitive cells are found in lymphoid tissue, bone marrow, spleen, organs of reproduction, and gastrointestinal tract. Of intermediate sensitivity are skin, lungs, and liver. Muscle, nerve, and adult bones are least sensitive.[88]

The medical manifestations of radiation damage can be conveniently divided into three time phases: initial, latent, and final.[88] During the *initial phase,* exposed persons may experience nausea, vomiting, headache, dizziness, and malaise. The onset time decreases and the severity of these symptoms increases with increasing dose. During the *latent phase,* exposed persons will experience few, if any, symptoms and will be able to carry on normal functions. The *final phase* is characterized by illness that requires hospitalization of people who have received the higher doses. The symptoms experienced in the initial phase will recur and be accompanied by skin hemorrhages, diarrhea, and sometimes loss of hair. At higher doses, seizures and prostration may occur. The final phase is ended by either recovery or death. These effects are summarized in Table 4-4 and Figure 4-2.

Persistent radioactive contamination is quite similar to persistent mustard gas in many of its effects. Presumed "psychological fallout" is an unseen hazard that produces delayed illness in all bodily systems that involve rapid cellular reproduction (ie, distressing gastrointestinal symptoms, impaired wound healing, and increased susceptibility to infection and hemorrhage). Early death may occur unless sophisticated medical support is given. Survivors are at increased risk of death from cancer.

Acute irradiation from a nuclear explosion (without concurrent disabling burn or blast injury) puts the military medical-ethical dilemma of these conditions into even starker relief. In the absence of quantitative dosimetry for each exposed patient (a difficult task in itself), how are the massed casualties to be triaged into those who are expected to die ("expectant") and those who can reasonably be saved with the over-used resources that remain? What is to be done with those fatally exposed who can still function? Should they be told the prognosis? Should they be discharged "RTDTD" ("Return To Duty To Die"), perhaps to carry out high-risk delaying ac-

TABLE 4-4

SUMMARY OF POTENTIAL MILITARY EFFECTIVENESS OF RADIATION CASUALTIES

Radiation in rems	Onset of initial incapacity from vomiting, etc.	Duration of effectiveness (latency)	Later incapacity (onset to duration)	Incidence of Death (time)
0–100	None	100%	None	None
100–200	3–6 h to 1 d	1 d to 2 wk	10–14 d to 4 wk	None
200–600	½–6 h to 2 d	1–2 d to 4 wk	1–4 wk to 1–8 wk	0%–90% 2–12 wk
600–1,000	15–30 min to 2 d	2 d to 5–10 d	5–10 d to 1–4 wk	90%–100% 1–6 wk
1,000–5,000	5–30 min to 1 d	0 to 7 d	2 to 10 d	100% 2–14 d
Over 5,000	Almost immediately	None	Almost immediately	100% 1–2 d

Adapted from Glasstone S, Dolan PJ. *The Effects of Nuclear Weapons*. 3rd ed. Washington, DC: US GPO; 1977: 580–581.

tions, "kamikaze" attacks, and operations in contaminated areas? What medications should they be given for symptom relief to improve their efficiency? Could those who cannot be discharged provide the answer to the shortage of whole blood in the combat zone? Will there be a place for euthanasia on the battlefield to end suffering and preserve other lives through allocation of medical resources, as suggested by Swann?[89] Such mind-chilling questions convey some of the moral and psychological implications that the Army Medical Department (AMEDD), the line military, and the exposed individuals themselves would have to deal with.

Triage by scarce medical resources is obviously the best way to preserve lives. This is critical in an operational sense in that the medical resources should be expended in helping those who are most likely to be able to return to duty.

Organs Affected by Ionizing Radiation

Range	0–100 rems Subclinical range	100–1,000 rems Therapeutic range			Over 1,000 rems Lethal range	
		100–200 rems	200–600 rems	600–1,000 rems	1,000–5,000 rems	Over 5,000 rems
Role of therapy		Clinical surveillance	Therapy effective	Therapy promising	Therapy palliative	
Leading organ	Hematopoietic tissue				Gastrointestinal tract	Central nervous system
Characteristic signs	None below 50 rems	Moderate leukopenia	Severe leukopenia; hemorrhage; infections; epilation above 300 rems		Diarrhea, fever, disturbance of electrolyte balance	Convulsions, tremor, ataxia, lethargy
Critical period postexposure	—		1–6 wk		2–14 d	1–48 h

Fig. 4-2. Summary of clinical effects of acute ionizing radiation. Adapted from Glasstone S, Dolan PJ. *The Effects of Nuclear Weapons*. 3rd ed. Washington, DC: US GPO; 1977: 580-581.

Neuropsychiatric Casualties of Nuclear Warfare

Although nuclear devices have been used twice in warfare, no one has actually fought a nuclear war. Neuropsychiatric casualties of nuclear warfare, therefore, must be inferred from studies of the primarily civilian victims of the nuclear explosions at Hiroshima and Nagasaki; from the disasters in Goiânia, Brazil, and Chernobyl, Ukraine; from a small number of imperfect simulations, such as the Desert Rock I, IV, and V studies; and from extrapolations from situations of extreme stress such as that during disasters or combat. The following sections will briefly review some of these studies.

Hiroshima and Nagasaki

There have only been about 20 useful studies of the psychological reactions to nuclear explosions; many of these are autobiographical accounts. Although retrospective, one of the best reviews of the physical, social, and psychological toll of nuclear devices is that of a Japanese committee commissioned by the cities of Hiroshima and Nagasaki. This report was first published in Japan in 1979; an English translation was published in 1981.[90] This review concluded that organic forms of mental illness among survivors were not prominent.

In one study[91] of 50 survivors at Omura Hospital in Japan, psychoneurological observations were made 2 to 3 weeks after exposure, the following month, and about 3 to 4 months after exposure. Only 4 of the 50 patients were diagnosed as having mental disorder in the initial stage. In the intermediate stage, some patients, especially those suffering thermal burns, showed neurasthenia-like symptoms. In the later stage, those suffering a specific diathesis tended to develop neuroses. These were considered indirect effects of physical deterioration. Acute radiation illness was considered to be the only direct effect of the atomic bomb on the human psychoneurological system. Konuma[91] has argued that complaints of "agony," lassitude, fatigability, and other symptoms constitute a "diencephalic syndrome," which can be diagnosed even in the absence of physical examination signs or abnormal laboratory findings. The presumption is that hematologic or other direct radiation effects on nerve cell membranes have damaged the vegetative nervous system. However, the severe losses (of relatives, physical capacities, and material resources) experienced by many of the victims could readily produce a depressive syndrome with many of these characteristics, particularly in a vulnerable personality.

Psychological studies were not conducted until years or decades after the event. Furthermore, disability compensation, social ostracism, and other factors colored the survivors' remembrances. Nevertheless, a fairly common response pattern was described in the 1952 study by Kubo,[90] who studied 54 victims from 1949 to 1952. Most of them had been 1 to 3 km from the bomb hypocenter. Kubo found that most were "startled" by the initial flash and fell down and covered their eyes in an "instinctive" withdrawal from the stimulus, while some turned to face the flash.

The blast, causing widespread damage, produced a feeling of "mental blankness" lasting for a few minutes. This was followed by attempts to escape the area of destruction and an inability to make clear judgments. Many of the victims aimlessly followed fleeing crowds until eventually they reached places where they felt safe; there they were given food and shelter. Most experienced a degree of recovery by the second day, but from 1 to 3 weeks later radiation sickness began to appear. This was, to most, a totally mysterious illness with high fever; bleeding from gums, throat, nose, and uterus; loss of hair; and fatigue. This produced high levels of anxiety, particularly as apparently uninjured persons began to die from intercurrent illness or other causes. The need for early treatment to prevent irreversible damage and death has been expressed.[92]

Goiânia and Chernobyl

Although the focus here is on short-term radiation effects, recognition of the longer-term effects of increased risk for cancer, sterility, and diminished life span may play an acute role in demoralizing the combatants. The Goiânia, Brazil, tragedy in which a small town was exposed to cesium isotopes from a medical device, reveals the potential for social disruption from radiation exposure. Many of the exposed individuals were shunned by friends and neighbors. Exports of produce from Goiânia dropped precipitously.

Similar effects were reported in the Chernobyl disaster in the Ukraine. Of 148 persons subjected to radiation effects of the Chernobyl atomic energy electrical plant accident and treated at Kiev Mental Hospital from 1986 through 1990, reactive psychoses were observed in only 11 cases and this was mainly during the 2 to 4 months after the disaster when the production of stress was maximal. It appears that stress, resulting in various psychopathological conditions including, rarely, psychosis, is paramount in producing psychiatric symptoms, rather than biological effects of ionizing radiation on central nervous system tissue.[93]

Extrapolation Studies

William James[94] appears to have been the first psychologist to systematically document the reactions of persons to disasters in his report of responses to the 1906 San Francisco earthquake and fire. It was not, however, until the late 1940s that Tyhurst[95] did field studies of two apartment house fires, a marine fire, and a flash flood from which detailed clinical and actuarial reports could be made. He formulated reactions during three overlapping phases: (1) impact, (2) recoil, and (3) post-trauma. During impact, reactions are automatic and can be separated into three main groups. The first of these is an "effective" group of about 12% to 25% who remain "cool and collected," and who appreciate and respond appropriately to the situation. The second group is characterized as a "normal" group, because this is the largest number (three fourths of the survivors), who are stunned and bewildered. Individuals in this group show a restricted field of attention and lack of awareness of subjective feelings or emotion; however, they display the physiological concomitants of fear, and automatic or reflex behavior. The last group of 10% to 15%, the "ineffectives," display manifestly inappropriate responses: confusion, paralyzing fear, inability to move or "freezing," and "hysterical" crying or screaming. During recoil there is a gradual return to normalcy; however, excessive dependency is common during the first day or two. The post-trauma reactions usually involve withdrawal, nightmares, anxiety, and pressured, repetitious recounting of the traumatic event. These responses are well known to psychiatrists and will not be addressed here.

Caldwell, Ranson, and Sacks[96] discussed potential reactions of a civilian population under atomic attack and applied Tyhurst's[95] formulations of the impact of disasters on communities. High among their considerations were expectations of group panic. Panic, however, occurs only rarely and in circumstances such that an overwhelming trauma is experienced or expected and all avenues of possible escape but one are closed.

Simulation Studies: Desert Rock I, IV, V

In Desert Rock I[97] an augmented airborne battalion combat team experienced an atomic bomb burst from a position in the open about 7 miles from the aerial explosion in October 1951. Attitude assessment, factual information questionnaires, and polygraph examinations at various times before and after the explosion were given to the participants and to control populations at the same base (Fort Campbell, Kentucky) and at another distant base (Fort Lewis, Washington).

The most significant finding was that anxiety concerning some of the bomb's effects persisted at a high absolute level throughout the entire experiment. It was also found that the better-educated were better informed, expressed more self-confidence, and experienced less anxiety. A disproportionate number of soldiers who experienced physiological disturbances on the day of the maneuver were in the lower-educated group. The few higher-educated men with physiological reactions differed from other higher-educated men only in having had greater difficulty adjusting to their roles in the U.S. Army.[97]

Desert Rock IV,[98] staged in May 1952, differed from Desert Rock I in that the participants were armored infantry troops who were stationed 4 miles from ground zero in trenches, and they witnessed the explosion of an atomic bomb emplaced on a tower rather than an aerial bomb. In all, the reactions of about 1,200 men from the 1st Armored Division, including those not involved in the maneuver, were tested from mid-May to mid-June 1952. Findings included the following:

1. Troops showed marked improvement in knowledge about atomic effects as the result of a 4-hour indoctrination at Desert Rock on the day before the atomic bomb explosion.
2. The soldiers were most successful in learning the kind of information that had to do with personal injury (eg, blindness, sterility, impotence). They tended, just after the indoctrination, to overestimate the potential dangers of the atomic bomb more than they did earlier or later.
3. The indoctrination appeared to lessen the fear the troops felt about being on an atomic bomb maneuver.
4. In contrast to the changes noted above, soldiers' attitudes other than fear toward atomic maneuvers and the U.S. Army were not appreciably altered as a result of the indoctrination.
5. There was no evidence that fear made any troops incapable of carrying out their duties just after the detonation; in fact, no

grossly disorganizing fear was observed at any time during the research. The spectacle of the blast apparently had complex effects upon soldiers' fears: In comparison to the previous night, less fear was expressed by the soldiers in answer to direct questions 15 minutes after the explosion, whereas more fear was revealed at this time by indirect (projective) tests.

6. The troops apparently were neither more nor less afraid of the effects of the bomb after they had seen the damage it had done in the forward area.
7. A material increase in the proportion of troops who would volunteer to go on another atomic bomb maneuver, and to occupy a position as close or even closer to ground zero, was recorded just after the bomb explosion.
8. The high point of troops' confidence in themselves and their outfits and in the experts' ability to use the atomic bomb safely apparently was reached just after they had completed the maneuver.

Desert Rock V found similar responses among officers.[99]

Vineberg Report

The Vineberg Report"[100] has remained the standard reference concerning potential psychiatric casualties in a nuclear war. Vineberg reviewed the relevant literature from a number of stressful situations including aerial bombing of cities (including Hiroshima and Nagasaki), the disasters' literature, the behavior of personnel in combat, and psychological mechanisms involved in coping with extreme stress such as major surgery or terminal illness. Based on these studies he formulated a model for nuclear combat.

Vineberg was reasonably optimistic about the ability of a well-trained, highly-motivated soldier to hold up, even when facing inevitable death. His general conclusion was that a soldier would act in tactical nuclear combat much as he had always acted in combat. He did feel that because of the greater stress there would be greater numbers of psychological casualties, but he did not foresee a sharp quantitative change in responses to such stress. As in conventional warfare, psychiatric casualties would arise as a function of cumulative stress related to the duration of exposure to combat and the intensity of combat. Vineberg did not believe that nuclear warfare would result in a breakdown of authority relationships resulting in amoral, lawless, and asocial behavior in civilian or military populations. Altogether, the Vineberg Report was reassuring to military commanders. This optimism had been reflected in the earlier "Clark Report,"[101] in which Clark had estimated total casualties of enlisted men in a unit to range from 4% to 23% in an infantry battalion under atomic attack and concluded that losses ranging from 40% to 70% would have to occur before the unit would be completely demoralized. Perhaps in keeping with this optimism, the NATO handbook, *Emergency War Surgery*,[102] while addressing mass casualties in thermonuclear warfare, was silent about psychiatric casualties.

The author does not share the optimism of Vineberg and others that while psychiatric casualties must be considered, they will not prove decisive in nuclear warfare. Such factors may well have been decisive in the defeat of France early in World War II.[103] Since 1965, neutron weapons capable of surgically killing living beings in precisely designated targets have been developed by the United States. Conventional weapons of near-nuclear capability in terms of blast and overpressure effects now exist, and these may be mistaken for nuclear devices.

Furthermore, it would be naive to believe that nuclear weapons would not be accompanied by chemical and biological warfare. A particularly horrible dilemma might face the irradiated soldier in a chemical environment who must remove his protective mask or die from aspiration of his own radiation-induced vomitus.

Laser and Microwave Radiation

One other form of radiation injury deserves mention because it will be encountered today on any conventional battlefield. The nonionizing electromagnetic radiation of current laser range finders and designators (U.S. forces' as well as the enemy's) will produce injuries ranging from covert retinal burns to sudden catastrophic blindness at distances of several kilometers in unprotected eyes (and further in those using optical instruments). Lasers of great power may be developed as direct weapons as well. This invisible threat with its especially frightening consequences could affect the willingness of troops to look toward the enemy and use weapons' sights, and might stimulate conversion reactions of hysterical blindness as an expression of battle fatigue.

Treatment of Neuropsychiatric Casualties of Nuclear Warfare

The nature of modern combat with its high noise levels, burning flesh, random death, and sleep and sensory deprivation suggests the kinds of psychiatric casualties to expect even in the absence of nuclear weapons.[104] The largest group, unless evacuation is possible, is likely to be the "psychological shock" or "disaster-fatigue" cases encountered in mass casualty incidents. The disaster-fatigue casualties will probably occur primarily in the first few hours and days of the initiation of hostilities. Glass and colleagues[105,106] applied Tyhurst's formulations to the atomic battlefield and established the concept of treating such casualties similarly to combat fatigue; hence, their use of the term "disaster fatigue." This treatment consists of replenishing physiological needs (rest, nutrition, sleep) as necessary, and giving the individuals simple tasks to perform. In this setting, the expectancy that they are "normal" and effective is just as important as on the nonnuclear battlefield.

The treatment of disaster-fatigue casualties must emphasize education and preparation as the critical elements in minimizing these casualties. Obviously, the main target of psychiatric intervention should be the 50% to 80% of "normal" dazed persons who can be given simple tasks to aid their recovery from the psychological shock. The small hysterical group may require sedation; however, this may fixate symptoms. Glass[105] has pointed out the need in these cases for a positive expectancy just as in traditional combat fatigue. The most important element in minimizing these casualties, however, is prevention. It is well known that psychological trauma can be minimized by decreasing the suddenness of the traumatic event; for example, a sudden bereavement, as in the death of a spouse in an accident, is more likely to produce psychiatric morbidity than death of the spouse following a long illness. It is as if time were available for a cognitive desensitization. To prevent these casualties, repeated exposure to as realistic a battle experience as possible must be part of the soldier's training.

Aside from their destructive potential both from blast and radiation effects, nuclear weapons produce in most people a not unwarranted fear verging on hysteria, a fear conditioned by hundreds of media exposures to nuclear holocaust. The mere threat, therefore, of nuclear weapons may result in psychiatric casualties with a primarily psychological etiology. Cataclysmic, unconventional warfare introduces new forms of psychopathology. Long periods of anxious waiting in shelters or in hermetic tanks, and long wearing of masks and NBC protection cause psychic vulnerability[106–109] as reported in the Persian Gulf War.[67,110]

In the event of actual nuclear attack, the direct effect of nuclear flash and blast would have a terrorizing psychological consequence. The extended material destruction and numerous victims create a sense of helplessness and vulnerability that undermines the fighter's morale. Observations of Hiroshima and Nagasaki survivors reveal a collective behavior of "shock-inhibition-stupor" followed by attempts to escape.[111] This is similar to behaviors in earthquakes and similar catastrophes.

Even in the case of threatened use of unconventional weapons, psychopathological behaviors should be expected. The terror of an unknown death with the mythic fantasy of disappearing in the nuclear flash (like the man from Hiroshima reduced to his shadow) and the conviction that one can neither be protected nor cured from radiation sickness are powerful psychological factors. The normal ambiguity of the battleground will be magnified by dispersal and loss of communications due to the destruction of all but hard-wire communications by the nuclear EMP. In such circumstances rumors may magnify in a contagious manner leading to collective panic. Even well-controlled fighters will experience increased levels of anxiety, leading at the minimum to increased numbers of combat fatigue casualties, already expected to be as high as one-to-one, that is, one combat fatigue to one wounded in action, due to the stress of modern continuous warfare. Added to this stress would be concern about family (especially when accompanying U.S. forces in Europe and Korea), a factor found to be important in Israeli casualties during the 1973 Yom Kippur War, increasing the likelihood of breakdown.

While realistic training and strong unit cohesion fostered by good leadership leading to high levels of fitness and morale will minimize psychiatric casualties in even this hellish combat environment, concrete steps should be undertaken now to minimize such casualties and make best use of all resources in the event of nuclear war. Information on the diagnosis and management of neuropsychiatric casualties of NBC warfare should be widely disseminated. Realistic training in a partially contaminated NBC environment should continue. This training should involve not only combat arms troops but also combat-support troops, who may be even more likely than combat troops to suffer chemical and nuclear attacks as the enemy attempts to disrupt logistical support. Education to combat rumors and fear of the unknown must be emphasized.

Fatally irradiated soldiers should receive every possible palliative treatment, including narcotics, to prolong their utility and alleviate their physical and psychological distress. Depending on the amount of fatal radiation, such soldiers may have several weeks to live and to devote to the cause. Commanders and medical personnel should be familiar with estimating survival time based on onset of vomiting (see Table 4-4). Physicians should be prepared to give medications to alleviate diarrhea, and to prevent infection and other sequelae of radiation sickness in order to allow the soldier to serve as long as possible. The soldier must be allowed to make the full contribution to the war effort. He will already have made the ultimate sacrifice. He deserves a chance to strike back, and to do so while experiencing as little discomfort as possible.

SUMMARY AND CONCLUSION

In summary, a wide range of chemical, biological, and nuclear threats exist. Many are invisible, persistent, have delayed effects, or are contagious. Delivery means may be nonspecific, ubiquitous, or covert. Detection methods are often inadequate. Early signs and symptoms of exposure may be nonspecific and common. The consequences of delaying treatment may be irreversible and fatal. Since Pavlov's studies with dogs, scientists have known that a requirement to discriminate between ambiguous stimuli typically produces severe anxiety, stereotyped, sometimes bizarre behavior, or both. This behavior must be expected to some extent in any combat against a foe known to be capable of using NBC weapons, even if those weapons are not actually employed.

A variety of maladaptive psychological reactions may be evoked by the threat of NBC warfare. Anxiety may lead to heightened susceptibility to rumors of the use of NBC warfare. This, in turn, could provoke undue concern, not only for self and unit, but also for the safety of dependent families if they are in the area at risk. Preoccupation with early warning symptoms may encourage individual hypochondriasis and increase the baseline demand for medical attention. Group amplification of stress and hyperventilation symptoms may cause epidemics of "gas hysteria," as seen in World War I. Even panic flight may occur if units feel completely unprepared or if protective measures seem inadequate (as they may in a hysterical epidemic). There may also be excessive concern with decontamination (perhaps leading to dermatologic problems), and overavoidance of possible sources of exposure (possibly causing dehydration, malnutrition, or even refusal to obey orders). On the other hand, there may be inappropriate fatalism or overconfidence leading to abandonment of NBC protective equipment and of sensible precautions.

Even without "gas hysteria," the added fear and uncertainty about NBC use will probably increase the incidence of acute stress reactions ("battle fatigue"). Rates as high as one case of transitory battle fatigue per one wounded in action have been projected based on historical data. Medical personnel are not immune to battle fatigue and must become familiar not only with its various presentations and basic treatment but also with its prevention.

Psychological stresses that seem unendurable have been described, but history proves that well-trained, cohesive units can come to accept such horrors as commonplace. Effective deterrence requires not only thinking about the unthinkable but obviously being prepared to deal with it. The psychological threats of NBC warfare have implications for psychological preparation that are especially relevant to the medical departments of the armed services, and to National Guard and reserve units. For example, training should avoid the traditional one-shot CS (tear gas) exposure exercise, which classically conditions somatic and anxiety symptoms to the protective mask. Such training resulted in significant gas-mask phobia cases in the Persian Gulf War. Instead, frequent practical exercises are needed to foster familiarity, confidence, and the special skills required to function in an NBC battlefield. Future warfare has aspects similar to mass-casualty disasters, which produce large numbers of psychological casualties among uninjured witnesses. Perhaps military units should train in naturally occurring disaster incidents. NBC warfare is an exceedingly unpleasant prospect to consider; however, failure to prepare for it only increases the risk of its use.

ACKNOWLEDGEMENT

The author wishes to acknowledge the assistance of Paul Newhouse, M.D., Department of Psychiatry, College of Medicine, University of Vermont; James Stokes, M.D., Colonel, Medical Corps, U.S. Army, Chief, Combat Stress Actions Office, Academy of Health Sciences, Army Medical Department Center and School, Fort Sam Houston; and Gregory Belenky, M.D., Colonel, Medical Corps, U.S. Army, Director, Division of Neuropsychiatry, Walter Reed Army Institute of Research, in portions of this chapter.

REFERENCES

1. Hague Convention IV Respecting the Laws and Customs of War on Land. 18 October 1907. The Hague, The Netherlands. Section 2, Chapter 1, Article 23A.

2. Geneva Convention for the Amelioration of the Condition of the Wounded and Sick in Armed Forces in the Field. 12 August 1949. Geneva, Switzerland. April 21–August 12, 1949.

3. Nielands JB. *Harvest of Death*. New York: The Free Press; 1972.

4. Bestwick FW. Chemical agents used in riot control and warfare. *Hum Toxicol*. 1983;2:247–256.

5. Vien NK. *Chemical Warfare, Vietnamese Studies*. Hanoi, Vietnam: Xunhasaka; 1971: 175–178.

6. Jones FD, Stokes JW, Newhouse PA, Belenky GL, Crocq L. Neuropsychiatric casualties of chemical, biological and nuclear warfare. In: Pichot P, Berner P, Wolf R, Thau K, eds. *Psychiatry. The State of the Art*. Vol 6. New York: Plenum Publishing; 1985: 539–543.

7. Vedder EB. *Medical Aspects of Chemical Warfare*. Baltimore, Md: Williams & Wilkins; 1925.

8. Westerhoff SH. *CBR Protection of Soviet Ground Forces*. [Defense Intelligence Report DDB-1600-5-80] Washington, DC: Defense Intelligence Agency; 1980.

9. US Department of State. *Reports of the Use of Chemical Weapons in Afghanistan, Laos and Kampuchea*. Washington, DC; August 1980.

10. Meselson M, Robinson JD. Chemical warfare and chemical disarmament. *Sci Am*. 1980;242(4):38–47.

11. *Medical Manual of Defense Against Chemical Agents*. 5th ed. London: Her Majesty's Stationery Office; 1972.

12. Reid TR. New cults flourish in a changed Japan. *Washington Post*. 27 March 1995. Vol 112: A1, A16.

13. United Nations, Security Council. Report of the mission dispatched by the Secretary-General to investigate allegations of the use of chemical weapons in the conflict between the Islamic Republic of Iran and Iraq. S/17911, March 12, 1986.

14. Why are we sick: Persian Gulf War leaves legacy of illness and broken faith. *Army Times*. 25 April 1994: 16–17.

15. Cookson J, Nottingham J. *A Survey of Chemical and Biological Warfare*. London: Sheep and Ward; 1969.

16. Heath DF. *Organophosphorus Poisons*. New York: Pergamon Press; 1961.

17. Gonsalves SF, Borison H. Atropine resistant central respiratory stimulants by bethanechol in cats. *J Pharmacol Exp Ther*. 1980;214:297–305.

18. Petras JM. Soman neurotoxicity. *Fundam Appl Toxicol.* 1981;1:242.

19. Grob D, Harvey AM. The effects and treatment of nerve gas poisoning. *Am J Med.* 1953;14:52–63.

20. Nambu T, Nolte CT, Jackrel J, Grob D. Poisoning due to organophosphorus insecticides. *Am J Med.* 1971;50:475–92.

21. Janowsky D, Ziegler M, Risch SC, Gillin JC. Antagonistic effects of scopolamine and atropine on the physostigmine response in man. *Milit Med.* 1987;152(11):579–581.

22. Sidell FR. Soman and sarin: Clinical manifestations and treatment of poisoning by organophosphates. *Clin Toxicol* [now *J Toxicol Clin Toxicol*]. 1974;7(1):1–17.

23. Wills JH. Pharmacology of anticholinesterases: CSW special publication 2-14. Army Chemical Center, Md: US Army Chemical Warfare Laboratories, Physiology Division, Directorate of Medical Research; 1958.

24. Sidell FR, Groff WA. Intramuscular and intravenous administration of small doses of 2-pyridinium aldoxime methochloride to man. *J Pharm Sci.* 1971;60:1224–1228.

25. US Department of the Army. *Treatment of Chemical Agent Casualties and Conventional Military Chemical Injuries.* Washington, DC:DA; February 1990. Field Manual 8-285: 2-2, 2-3.

26. US Department of the Navy. *Treatment of Chemical Agent Casualties and Conventional Military Chemical Injuries.* Washington, DC: Naval Medical Command; February 1990. NAVMED P-5041.

27. US Department of the Air Force. *Treatment of Chemical Agent Casualties and Conventional Military Chemical Injuries.* Randolph Air Force Base, Tex: Air Force Management Engineering Agency; February 1990. Air Force Manual 160-11.

28. US Department of the Army. *Clinical Notes on Chemical Casualty Care.* Aberdeen, Md: US Army Medical Research Institute of Chemical Defense; 14 August 1990. Technical Memorandum 90-1.

29. Chipman M, Sidell FR. *A Review of the Efficacy and Clinical Pharmacology of the Chloride and Methanesulfonate Salts of Pyridium 2-Aldoxime.* Edgewood Arsenal, Md: US Army Biomedical Laboratory; 1980.

30. Hoskin FCG, Roush AH. Hydrolysis of nerve gas by squid-type diisopropyl phosphoroflouridate hydrolyzing enzyme on agarose resin. *Science.* 1982;215:1255–1257.

31. Bowers MB, Goodman E, Sim VM. Some behavioral changes in man following anticholinesterase administration. *J Nerv Ment Dis.* 1964;138:383–389.

32. Levin HS, Rodnitzky RL. Behavioral effects of organophosphate pesticides in man. *Clin Toxicol* [now *J Toxicol Clin Toxicol*]. 1976;9(3):391–405.

33. Wood W, Gabrica J, Brown HW, Watson M, Benson WW. Implication of organophosphate pesticide poisoning in the plane crash of a duster pilot. *Aerosp Med* [now *Aviat Space Environ Med*]. 1971;42:1111–1113.

34. Metcalf DR, Holmes HH. EEG, psychological and neurological alterations in humans with organophosphorus exposure. *Ann N Y Acad Sci.* 1969;160:357–365.

35. Levin HS, Rodnitzky RL, Mick DL. Anxiety associated with exposure to organophosphate compounds. *Arch Gen Psychiatry.* 1976;33:225–228.

36. Rountree DW, Nevin S, Wilson A. The effects of diisopropyl flourophosphonate in schizophrenia and manic depressive psychosis. *J Neurol Neurosurg Psychiatry.* 1950;13:47–59.

37. Davis KL, Berger PA, Hollister LE, Defraites E. Physostigmine in mania. *Arch Gen Psychiatry.* 1978;35:119–122.

38. Janowsky DS, El-Yousef MK, Davis JM, Sekerke HJ. Parasympathetic suppression of manic symptoms by physostigmine. *Arch Gen Psychiatry*. 1973;28:542–547.

39. Gershon S, Shaw FH. Psychiatric sequelae of chronic exposure to organophosphorus insecticides. *Lancet* 1961;1:1371–1374.

40. Meyerhoff JL. *Neurochemical and Behavioral Effects of Anticholinergic Drugs*. Washington, DC: Medical Neurosciences Department, Walter Reed Army Institute of Research. Manuscript. 1980.

41. Caldwell JA Jr, Stephens RL, Carter DJ, Jones HD. Effects of 2mg and 4mg atropine sulfate on the performance of US Army helicopter pilots. *Aviat Space Environ Med*. 1992;63(10):857–864.

42. Ketchum JS, Sidell FR, Crowell EB Jr, Aghajanian GK, Hayes AH Jr. Atropine, scopolamine, and ditran: Comparative pharmacology and antagonists in man. *Psychopharmacology (Berlin)*. 1973;28:121–145.

43. Datel WE, Johnson AW Jr. *Psychotropic Prescription Medication in Vietnam*. Available from Defense Technical Information Center, Alexandria, Va. No. ADA097610. 1978.

44. Jones FD, Johnson AW. Medical and psychiatric treatment policy and practice in Vietnam. *J Soc Issues*. 1975;31(4):49–65.

45. Jones FD. Combat psychiatry in modern warfare. In: Adelaja O, Jones FD, eds. *War and its Aftermath*. Lagos, Nigeria: John West; 1983: 63–77.

46. Beverley R. *History and Present State of Virginia, Book 2*. Chapel Hill, NC: North Carolina University Press; 1947: 24.

47. Gowdy JM. Stramonium intoxication—review of symptomatology in 212 cases. *JAMA*. 1972;221(6):585–587.

48. Belenky GL, Jones FD. The evacuation syndrome in military exercises: A model of the psychiatric casualties of combat. In: Mangelsdorff AD, Furukawa PT. *Proceedings: Users' Workshop on Combat Stress*. Washington, DC: Defense Technical Information Center, Alexandria, VA. No. ADA 152464. September 1981: 140–142.

49. Jones FD. Lessons of war for psychiatry. In: Pichot P, Berner P, Wolf R, Thau K, eds. *Psychiatry: The State of the Art*. Vol 6. New York: Plenum; 1985: 515–519.

50. Duvoisin RC, Katz R. Reversal of central anticholinergic syndrome in man by physostigmine. *JAMA*. 1968;206(9):1963–1965.

51. Bryson DD. Cyanide poisoning (Letter to the editor). *Lancet*. 1978;1(8055):92.

52. Gosselin RE, Hodge HC, Smith HP, Gleason MN, eds. *Clinical Toxicology of Commercial Products*. 4th ed. Baltimore, Md: Williams & Wilkins; 1976: 105–112.

53. Barnett HOM, Jackson MV, Spaulding WB. Thiocyanate psychosis. *JAMA*. 1951;147(16):1554–1558.

54. Willems JL. *Clinical Management of Mustard Gas Casualties*. Ghent, Belgium: University of Ghent Medical School; 1989: 11. Vol 3: Supplement to Annales Medicinae Militaris Belgicae.

55. Grinstad B, ed. *BC Warfare Agents*. Stockholm: Forsvarets Forskningsanstalt; 1964.

56. Fisher GJB. *Chemicals in War: A Treatise on Chemical Warfare*. New York: McGraw-Hill; 1937: 156.

57. Salmon TW, Fenton N, eds. In the American Expeditionary Forces [Section 2]. *Neuropsychiatry*. Vol. 10. In: *The Medical Department of the United States Army in the World War*. Washington, DC; Office of The Surgeon General, US Army; 1929.

58. Miller E. *Neurosis in War*. New York: Macmillan. 1944.

59. Mott FW. *War Neuroses and Shell Shock*. London, England: Oxford University Press; 1919: 105.

60. Hulbert HS. Gas neurosis syndrome. *Am J Insanity* [now *Am J Psychiatry*]. 1920;77:213–216.

61. Ingraham LH, Manning FJ. Psychiatric battle casualties. *Milit Rev*. 1980;60(8):19–29.

62. Brooks FR, Xenakis SN, Ebner DG, Balson PM. Psychological reactions during chemical warfare training. *Milit Med*. 1983;148(3):232–235.

63. Fullerton CS, Ursano RJ. Health care delivery in the high-stress environment of chemical and biological warfare. *Milit Med*. 1994;159:524–528.

64. Bennion SD. Designing of NBC protective gear to allow for adequate first aid. *Milit Med*. 1982;147(11):960–962.

65. Burgin WW, Gehring LM, Bell TL. A chemical field resuscitation device. *Milit Med*. 1982;147(10):873–876.

66. Xenakis SN, Brooks FR, Burgin WW, Balson PM. A model for training combat medics for chemical warfare. Fort Sam Houston, Tex: US Academy of Health Sciences. Unpublished manuscript. 1983.

67. Took KJ, Ritchie EC, Sandman LM. Letters to the editor on gas mask phobia. *Milit Med*. 1992;157(8):A10–A11.

68. Draper ES, Lombardi JJ. Combined arms in a nuclear/chemical environment. In: Force Development Testing and Experimentation, CANE FDTE: Summary evaluation report, phase 1. Fort McClellan, Ala: US Army Chemical School; 1986.

69. Taylor HL, Orlansky J. The effects of wearing chemical warfare combat clothing on human performance. Alexandria, Va: Institute for Defense Analysis, IDAP 2433; August 1991: iii-3.

70. Glass AJ. Observations upon the epidemiology of mental illness in troops during warfare. Presented at the Symposium on Social Psychiatry, Walter Reed Army Institute of Research; April 1957; Washington, DC.

71. Jones FD. Combat stress: Tripartite model. *Int Rev Army Navy Air Force Med Serv*. 1982;55:247–254.

72. Noy S. Division-based psychiatry in intensive war situations. *J R Army Med Corps*. 1982;128:105–116.

73. Belenky GL, Newhouse P, Jones FD. Prevention and treatment of psychiatric casualties in the event of a war in Europe. *Int Rev Army Navy Air Force Med Serv*. 1982;55:303–307.

74. Belenky G. Unusual visual experiences reported by subjects in the British Army study of sustained operations, Exercise Early Call. *Milit Med*. 1979;144(10):695–696.

75. Haslam DR. The effects of sleep loss and recovery sleep upon the military performance of the soldier. *Int Rev Army Navy Air Force Med Serv*. 1981;54:103–116.

76. Sodetz FJ. Some constraints on the management of sleep and fatigue. *Revue Internationale des Services de Sante*. 1981;54:97–100.

77. Belenky GL, Tyner CF, Sodetz FJ. *Israeli Battle Shock Casualties: 1973 and 1982* [Report WRAIR NP-83-4]. Washington, DC: Walter Reed Army Institute of Research; 1983.

78. Cadigan FD. Battleshock, the chemical dimension. *J R Army Med Corps*. 1982;128:89–92.

79. Marshall SLA. *Bringing Up the Rear: A Memoir*. San Rafael, Calif: Presidio Press; 1979: 15.

80. Malek I. Biological weapons. In: Rose S, ed. *CBW: Chemical and Biological Warfare*. Boston, Mass: Beacon Press; 1969: 48–61.

81. Abramova FA, Grinberg LM, Yampolskaya OV, et al. Pathology of inhalational anthrax in 42 cases from the Sverdlovsk outbreak of 1979. *Proc Natl Acad Sci USA*. 1993;90:2291–2294.

82. Meyerhoff JC. Personal Communication, 1984.

83. Eastwood M. The medicine of nuclear warfare: A clinical dead end. *Lancet*. 1981:1(8232):1252–1253.

84. Vandre RH, Tesche FM, Kleber J, Blanchard JP. Electromagnetic pulse (EMP), Part 1: Effects on field medical equipment. *Milit Med*. 1993;158(4):233–236.

85. AMA Board of Trustees, Electromagnetic pulse and its effects. *JAMA*. 1992;268(5):639–641.

86. Vandre RH, Tesche RM, Klebers J, Blanchard JP. Electromagnetic pulse (EMP), Part 2: Field-expedient ways to minimize its effects on field medical treatment facilities. *Milit Med*. 1993;158(5):285–289.

87. Atomic Bomb Casualty Commission. *Bibliography of Publications Concerning Effect of Nuclear Explosions 1945—1960*. Washington, DC: US GPO; 1961.

88. Glasstone S, Dolan PJ. Biological effects. *The Effects of Nuclear Weapons*. 3rd ed. Washington, DC: US GPO; 1977: 541–559.

89. Swann SW. Euthanasia on the battlefield. *Milit Med*. 1987;152(11):545–549.

90. Committee for the Compilation of Materials on Damage caused by the Atomic Bombs in Hiroshima and Nagasaki, eds. *Hiroshima and Nagaski: The Physical, Medical and Social Effects of the Atomic Bombings*. Ishikawa E, Swain DL, Trans. New York: Basic Books; 1981.

91. Konuma M. Neuropsychiatric case studies on the atomic bomb casualties at Hiroshima. In: *Research in the Effects and the Influences of the Nuclear Bomb Test Explosions*. Vol 2. Tokyo: Japan Society for the Promotion of Science; 1956.

92. Stokes JW. Neuropsychiatric casualties of NBC and conventional warfare. Presented at Division and Combat Psychiatry Course, Army Medical Department; April 1982; Colorado Springs, Colo.

93. Revenok AA. Structural-dynamic characterization of reactive psychoses in persons subjected to the effect of ionizing radiation as a result of the Chernobyl AES disaster. *JAMA*. 1991;268(11):1406.

94. James W. On some mental effects of the earthquake. In: *Memories and Studies*. New York: Longmans, Green; 1911: 207–226.

95. Tyhurst JS. Individual reactions to disaster: The natural history of psychiatric phenomena. *Am J Psychiatry*. 1951;107:764–769.

96. Caldwell JM, Ranson WW, Sacks JG. Group panic and other mass disruptive reactions. *US Armed Forces Med J*. 1951;2(4):541–567.

97. Bordes PA, Finan JL, Hochstim JR, McFann HH, Schwartz SG. *Desert Rock I: A Psychological Study of Troop Reactions to an Atomic Explosion*. Washington, DC: Human Resources Research Office, George Washington University. TR-1. February 1953.

98. *Desert Rock IV: Reactions of an Armored Infantry Battalion to an Atomic Bomb Maneuver*. Washington, DC: Human Resources Research Office, George Washington University. TR-2. August 1953.

99. White BW. *Desert Rock V: Reactions of Troop Participants and Forward Volunteer Officer Groups to Atomic Exercises*. Washington, DC: Human Resources Research Office, George Washington University; August 1953.

100. Vineberg R. *Human Factors in Tactical Nuclear Combat*. Human Resources Research Office, George Washington University, Washington, DC. TR 65-2. April 1965.

101. Clark DK. *Casualties as a Measure of the Loss of Combat Effectiveness of an Infantry Battalion*. Chevy Chase, Md: Operations Research Office, Johns Hopkins University. ORO-T-289. August 1954.

102. *Emergency War Surgery: First United States Revision of the Emergency War Surgery, NATO Handbook*. Washington, DC: US GPO, Department of Defense; 1975.

103. Cline WR, Rath FH. The concept of the army as a psychiatric casualty. *J R Army Med Corps*. 1982;128:79–88.

104. Romo J, Schneider RJ. Disaster, psychiatric casualties and implications for future war. *J R Army Med Corps*. 1982;128:93–99.

105. Glass AJ. Management of mass psychiatric casualties. *Milit Med*. 1956;118(4):335–342.

106. Glass AJ, Drayer CS, Cameron DC, Woodward WD. Psychological first aid in community disasters. *JAMA*. 1954;156:36–41.

107. Crocq L, Lefebvre P, Girard V. Considerations sur l'evolution des conceptions en psychopathologie de guerre. *Revue de Medecine Psychosomatique*. 1965;7(3):253–262.

108. Crocq L. Guerre NBC et panique collective. *Revue des Corps de Sante des Armees*. 1970;11(4):483–497.

109. Doutheau C, Crocq L, Sailhan M. Panic and catastrophe behaviour. In Pichot P, Berner P, Wolf R, Thau K, eds. *Psychiatry: The State of the Art*. Vol 6. New York: Plenum Press; 1985: 471–478.

110. Ritchie EC. Treatment of gas mask phobia. *Milit Med*. 1992;157:104–106.

111. Gregory GA, Lawson TR, Brooks FR. *Behavioral Science Support in the Theater of Operations: Casualty Generation Study*. San Antonio, Tex: Behavioral Sciences Division, Directorate of Training, Academy of Health Sciences; 1979.

Chapter 5

PSYCHIATRIC PRINCIPLES OF FUTURE WARFARE

FRANKLIN D. JONES, M.D., F.A.P.A.*

*Colonel (ret), Medical Corps, U.S. Army; Clinical Professor, Uniformed Services University of the Health Sciences, Bethesda, Maryland; Past President and Secretary and currently Honorary President of the Military Section, World Psychiatric Association; formerly Psychiatry and Neurology Consultant, Office of The Surgeon General, U.S. Army

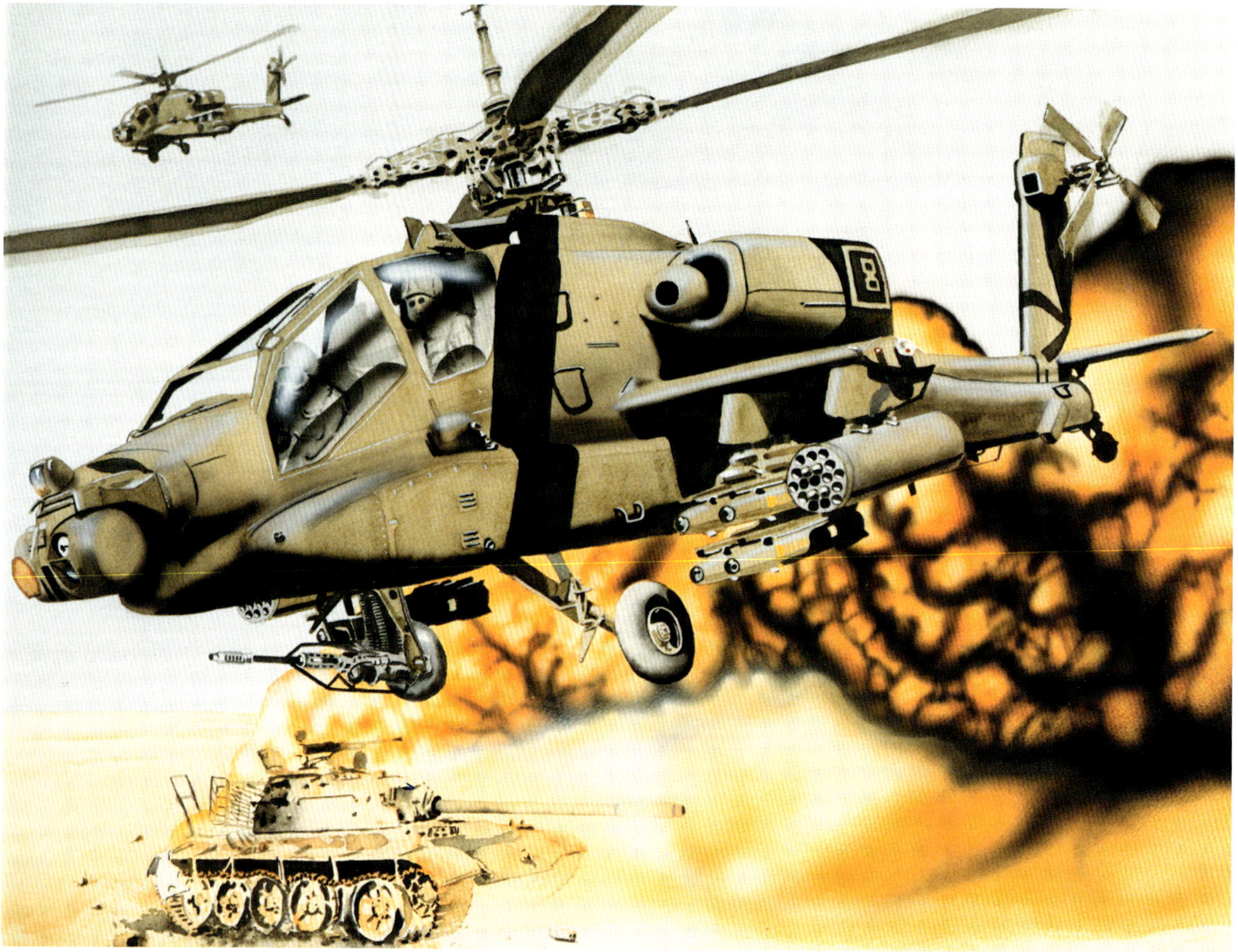

Mario H. Acevedo *The Attack* 1991

Mario H. Acevedo, a U.S. Army Combat Artist deployed to the Persian Gulf, depicts the aerial intensity of American gunships attacking Iraqi armor in the desert. Future warfare may occur in a variety of settings and intensity, ranging from the massive troop and materiel deployments of the Persian Gulf War to small peacekeeping missions. Such rapid and intense combat necessitates flexibility and innovation in the treatment and restoration of combat stress casualties.

Art: Courtesy of US Center of Military History, Washington, DC.

INTRODUCTION

Historical reviews of psychiatric interventions in past wars allow the exploration of the implications of a range of future combat scenarios.[1–5] A spectrum of combat intensities is possible, ranging from intermittent light-infantry combat (low-intensity conflict) to continuous, highly-mechanized battle (high-intensity conflict), possibly with nuclear, biological, and chemical (NBC) weapons. Whatever the combat intensity, the underlying stresses of dislocation from loved ones and home, the fear of the unknown, and the stresses of an unfamiliar environment will produce disorders of frustration and loneliness. Thus, higher-intensity conflict stresses will be superimposed on stresses associated with low-intensity conflicts.

While the holistic or psychosomatic approach emphasizes the unity of an organism's response to stress, it is convenient to separate factors producing stress and breakdown in battle into physical (or physiological) and psychological (or sociopsychological) categories.

The psychological factors, because they are potentially the ones more amenable to psychiatric interventions, have been emphasized the most in studies of breakdown in battle. Because of the nature of high-intensity, high-technology, and continuous combat, the physiological variables may still play a major role in breakdown in modern wars.

Psychological and physiological variables interact to prevent or promote illness. This can be seen, for example, in frostbite, the first combat psychiatric disorder described in the British literature during World War I.[6] More recently, Sampson[7] has described this interaction between the physiological responses to anxiety, particularly vasoconstriction, and to cold, also a vasoconstriction, when the soldier is immobile, stressed, and lacking in protective clothing. Similarly, the disorganized, immobilized soldier is less likely to attend to proper protective measures such as changing stockings frequently. This interaction of physiological responses to cold and behavioral and physiological responses to anxiety produces a cumulative effect of heat loss in peripheral tissues and thus of frostbite.

A large body of literature has documented the clinical relevance of stress not only to traditional psychiatric disorders but also to such apparently "physical" conditions as infections, cardiovascular diseases, and cancer.[8–10] Many of these deleterious effects of stress seem to be mediated by the neurotransmitter/neurohumoral and immune systems.

Although no one knows precisely what forms future warfare will take, the following possible forms of future warfare and available experimental studies related to combat performance are offered for consideration.

CHARACTERISTICS OF FUTURE WARFARE

From a historical perspective there appear to be two main groupings of combat stress casualties, which are to an extent dependent on the nature of the soldier's experiences. At one extreme are the disorders of frustration and loneliness (nostalgic casualties) that appear among troops engaged in intermittent, low-intensity combat, and in rear-echelon duties. These soldiers share the problems of anyone who leaves home to an inhospitable environment; they present with symptoms such as alcohol and drug abuse, disciplinary infractions, and venereal disease. Pre-Vietnam drafted soldiers in garrison settings manifested many of these behaviors, and U.S. soldiers in Europe and Korea continue to exhibit them. Terrorist and guerrilla tactics are deliberately calculated to maximize ambiguity and frustration. This provokes misconduct, including excessive brutality and atrocities which will alienate the local population, the home front, and world opinion. For the United States, the Vietnam conflict was the epitome of this type of conflict. Although it could be argued that they were not appropriately utilized, the traditional principles of treatment (proximity, immediacy, expectancy; reassure, rest, replenish, restore confidence) appear to have been less effective with these casualties in Vietnam.

At the other extreme is the high-intensity, high-lethality, continuous combat fought in some battles of World War I, World War II, and early in the Korean conflict, but best seen in the 1973 Yom Kippur War. Such casualties present with symptoms related to anxiety and physical and emotional exhaustion. The traditional principles of treatment, if the vicissitudes of battle allowed them to be used, worked best with these soldiers in the past; however, the severe stress of future warfare may exert psychological trauma of such severity as to lessen the effectiveness of these principles even if battlefield conditions allow their use.

Being unable to know what type of war the United States will be expected to win in the future, the armed forces must prepare for conflicts ranging from worst-case low-intensity operations other than war to very high-intensity wars. These two polarities will be addressed at this time in terms of psychiatric approaches. If psychiatric casualties can be appropriately treated in these extremes, those of a medium range of intensity should present no insurmountable or unforeseen problems. While future military missions may extend beyond combat, it is reasonable to expect that the combat intensity dimension will include the major varieties of future psychiatric problems.

Low-Intensity Future Warfare

A study of world conflicts since the Vietnam conflict would lead to the conclusion that the United States is likely to be involved in more low-intensity conflicts than high-intensity, 1973 Arab-Israeli-type wars. A chemical or biological low-intensity conflict would seem to be improbable, but chemicals have, in fact, most often been used against poorly equipped insurgents or dissidents, as by Spain and France against the Moroccans in the 1920s; by Italy against Ethiopia; by the Soviets or their clients in Yemen, Cambodia, Laos, and Afghanistan; and by Iraq against their Kurdish minority. U.S. forces, especially Special Operations Forces, could be on the receiving end of such weapons under circumstances which would be difficult to document.

In preparing for low-intensity combat stress casualties, there must be an attempt to strengthen ameliorating conditions. These include minimizing family stress, enforcing vigorous discipline in organized camp conditions, setting and enforcing strict but realistic rules of engagement, and promoting unit cohesion and pride in following the rules. At the same time, it will be necessary to eliminate or lessen the impact of aggravating conditions: prevent boredom, prepare for cultural differences, and strengthen social support from the unit, the family, and the community.

Fighting counterterrorist or counterinsurgency conflicts can result in successful outcomes. The British experienced such success in the Boer War in South Africa (1899–1902) and in a war in Malaysia (1948–1960), and the United States successfully put down the Moro rebellion in the Philippines (1902). Critical to these efforts was the use of professional soldiers and the ability to isolate the insurgents from resupply and indigenous support.

In counterinsurgency conflict the forces being allied with must be seen as legitimate to govern by the indigenous population. The U.S. troops optimally will be professional soldiers (and often Special Operations Forces) fighting in cohesive units, thus relatively impervious to the ambiguities universally present in civil wars. However, less frequently trained combat-service-support units, some from the Reserves, may also be deployed. The troop leaders should regularly explain the goals of the fighting and those goals should be explicitly formulated by the Commander-in-Chief. The mental health personnel must have a "mental-hygiene approach," emphasizing productive use of leisure time, and perhaps assisting in building schools and public works projects. Vigorous approaches to eliminating substance abuse and in-country treatment of substance abusers is mandatory. Realistic information about the risks and prophylaxis of venereal diseases should regularly be given by the medical personnel to the troops. Bushard-type counseling,[11] emphasizing *commitment* to the mission and *concurrence* of one's fellow-soldiers, should be readily available to temporarily disaffected or demoralized soldiers. The emphasis must be on current issues and on optimistic appraisal of the soldier's ability to overcome these challenges. Often, the best results occur when a senior sergeant or an officer can take the disaffiliated soldier "under his wing" and offer encouragement and support during a difficult time, a surrogate parenting for an immature personality.

The devastating effects of drug abuse by soldiers in Vietnam is detailed in Chapter 3, Disorders of Frustration and Loneliness. In his novel *1984*, George Orwell[12] suggested that drugs might be utilized to weaken a nation's fabric and assist a foreign power. In 1986, a U.S. Army general reported that communist Cuba was supporting the smuggling of narcotics into the United States, presumably to that end.[13] One of the most alarming terrorism trends in Latin America is the alliance between insurgency groups and narcotics traffickers, particularly in Peru and Colombia.[14] Most of the evidence supports the view that in Vietnam, market factors led to drug trafficking rather than deliberate subversion. However, the potential for such insidious subversion exists.

The mental health implications of drug dependence are obvious, but only recently have government and industry begun large-scale actions to counter the drug-abuse threat that afflicts primarily the age group most likely to be conscripted in the event of major hostilities. As mentioned, U.S. soldiers were deployed to Colombia to support that government's attempt to disrupt drug trafficking. The military has also assisted the Coast Guard and Immigration and Naturalization Service in guarding the borders against drug importation. Additionally, the U.S. government has used drug screening of personnel. Some industries have also begun such screening.

The senior U.S. Army leadership is aware of the potential stress issues in operations other than war, and is actively collecting data and developing policies and doctrine to control them. This doctrine includes the early deployment of mental health/combat stress control (clinical) teams and human dimensions (research) teams.[15-17] The focus of this chapter, therefore, will be on high-intensity combat, which presents formidable obstacles to traditional treatment delivery. While low-intensity conflicts and operations other than war are more likely than a high-intensity conflict, U.S. forces must be prepared for the high-intensity conflict (ie, a worst-case scenario such as NBC warfare). Even in the absence of NBC warfare, future combat may be sustained, highly intense, highly mobile, and highly technical.

High-Intensity Future Warfare

U.S. military forces must prepare for combat of unprecedented ferocity, lethality, and destructiveness. For example, modern combat offensive doctrine calls for continuous operations including conventional, airmobile, and airborne assaults possibly coupled with coordinated chemical strikes (and perhaps nuclear strikes) throughout the depth of the enemy's deployment.[18] Mobile combat groups will attempt to penetrate enemy defenses up to 150 miles, into the defender's rear positions, disrupting command, communications, and logistic activities.[19] Through the use of night vision devices and superior numbers, the attacking forces will fight continuously while allowing adequate rest by rotating spent units. If outnumbered, the defending forces would be engaged continuously,[20] resulting in fatigue and sleep deprivation. If opportunities for sleep did occur, the extraordinarily high noise levels and ground-shaking artillery and bomb blasts might make sleep impossible until the soldier approached physical collapse. This will maximize mental and physical stress on defending personnel and increase combat breakdown. If this seems an implausible scenario for the future U.S. Force Projection military, imagine what it would have been like for the lead U.S. contingency force Army and Marine brigades and divisions if the Iraqi Army in September 1990 had been able to press forward with a full armor attack, supported by their heavy artillery firing chemical shells, while improved Scud missiles dropped chemical, biological, and perhaps, nuclear warheads on the Arabian (and Israeli) ports, airfields, and cities (Exhibit 5-1).

A future regional power (perhaps even one of the current major powers under different leadership turned aggressively militaristic) could be tempted to pull a "high-tech" surprise, counting on an inadequate political and/or military response from the United States. It is conceivable that this could come after a period of economic hardship when the downsized U.S. military services were feeling the effects of decreased funding for maintenance, training, soldier and family benefits, and perhaps shortfalls in weapons research, procurement, and strategic lift capability. All these factors could have resulted in lowered

EXHIBIT 5-1

CHARACTERISTICS OF HIGH-INTENSITY WARFARE

High lethality with mass casualties
- "Disaster-fatigue" casualties

Continuous combat
- Sleep deprivation
- Increased fatigue

High mobility
- Radar localization
- Proportionally fewer forces

Dispersal of forces
- Nuclear/biological/chemical threat
- Infrared/radar "signature"
- Result of high mobility

Absence of air superiority
- Limited helicopter medical evacuation

Absence of rear battle-free area
- Limited traditional medical treatment

Adapted from Jones FD. Psychiatric lessons of low-intensity wars. Presented at Army Medical Department Division and Combat Psychiatry Conference, 1984; Fort Bragg, NC.

morale and retention of highly-skilled personnel, and lowered quality of new recruits, putting further strains on leadership and unit cohesion.

Strategically, the attacker in such a major regional conflict will focus on command, control, communications, and intelligence organs. The continuous assault will attempt to disrupt the small combat unit of 3 to 40 persons. Modern military planners are fully aware of the psychological factors in combat. A surprise attack with apparently overwhelming forces could lead to panic and collapse even when the opposing forces are about equivalent in strength. This occurred, for example, during the German blitzkrieg of French forces in 1940; the Israeli surprise attack on Egypt in 1967[21]; and the coalition attack, led by U.S. Forces, on Iraq in 1991. It almost occurred with the Arab surprise attack on Israel in 1973.

Surprise maximizes the psychological effect of an attack. A conventional rolling artillery barrage, finished by a salvo of rockets, need not kill the defenders. It will produce a state of "battlefield paralysis"—the temporary inability to use one's weapon—lasting from 30 seconds to 4 to 5 minutes depending upon the complexity of the weapon.[22] This would allow first-echelon attacking forces to advance immediately behind the rolling barrage with smoke and flame throwers. Their aim would be to pass through or bypass defending units rather than to engage them. First-echelon forces would then proceed rapidly to the rear to disrupt command, control, communication, and intelligence functions; to capture airfields, petroleum depots, and fire-support systems; and to link with airmobile and airborne forces. Second-echelon forces would then neutralize the remaining forward defending units to produce a swift and sudden collapse. NBC weapons, and even long-range improved conventional weapons, enable senior, rear-echelon military and political figures to influence directly the outcome of the battle.[23] Such weapons used against enemy command, control, communication, and intelligence, and nuclear means could paralyze a defending force. The response to such a scenario requires highly-mobile, dispersed forces.

CHALLENGES TO THE PRINCIPLES OF FORWARD TREATMENT

As discussed in Chapter 2, Traditional Warfare Combat Stress Casualties, the appropriate use of the traditional principles of forward treatment has resulted in the return of about one half to two thirds (or in optimal circumstances up to nine tenths) of combat stress casualties back to combat duty within days. Forward treatment consists of immediate, brief, simple interventions such as rest and nutrition in a safe place as near the battle lines as possible, with an explicit statement to the soldier that he will soon be rejoining his comrades. This approach to treatment also calls for soldiers evacuated rearward to be screened at a central collecting point from which they may still be returned to duty if further rearward movement is inappropriate.

In practice, this approach has required four essential elements:

1. A relatively safe and stationary place near the battle area (refuge);
2. A treating person (therapist) or team;
3. Time and resources for restoration of physiological needs (rest); and
4. A method for returning to one's unit (return).

Each element is critical to the process; and, as will be seen, each is jeopardized by modern, high-intensity warfare. High-intensity future warfare, therefore, challenges the application of the traditional principles of forward treatment (Exhibit 5-2). There may be no safe and stationary forward treatment area, because high technology has resulted in weapons and surveillance systems capable of discovering aggregations of personnel through the infrared "signatures" given off by heat radiation from groups of persons and their supporting machinery (eg, trucks, generators). Furthermore, rear areas may be preferentially attacked because they may be more vulnerable than front-line forces, which will be dispersed, camouflaged, and mobile.

Even if methods are found to shield and protect rear-area installations, the time needed to restore physiological and emotional needs, plus transportation limitations, will make it difficult or impossible to return the soldier to his own unit. This is because combat units must remain dispersed and highly mobile to avoid being targeted by their "signatures." However, studies from World War II and Korea make it clear that the returning combat stress casualty must rejoin his own unit or risk becoming a casualty again. Furthermore, the possible absence of local air superiority by U.S. forces will aggravate the difficulty of evacuation and return of casualties arising from dispersion and mobility of forces.

EXHIBIT 5-2

NEGATION OF PRINCIPLES OF FORWARD TREATMENT

No refuge:
- Absence of rear battle-free area

No therapists:
- Dispersal of forces
- Mass casualty situation (triage)

No rest:
- Absence of rear battle-free area
- High mobility
- Lack of time to treat

No return:
- Dispersal of forces
- High mobility

Adapted from Jones FD. Psychiatric lessons of low-intensity wars. Presented at Army Medical Department Division and Combat Psychiatry Conference, 1984; Fort Bragg, NC.

The psychological stresses of high-intensity combat will also be magnified due to the lethality and mass casualty nature of modern warfare. There is usually a direct relationship between wounded in action (WIA) and psychiatric casualties. The U.S. Army medical planning field manuals[24,25] give a conservative estimate of 1 psychiatric to 5 wounded-in-action casualties, but point out that some units in World War II fought battles in which the ratio reached 1:2. Being on defense increases stress casualties relative to wounded. However, being mobile tends to protect. Recent official casualty rate predictions have reduced the average division's daily wounded in action during the heaviest weeks of fighting from about 150 to 50. The U.S. Army does not expect to fight in massed formations with second-rate weapons, suffering mass casualties. However, war is not fought on the average day, and the enemy will not fight every division equally every day. The engaged brigade of an engaged division could easily suffer several hundred wounded out of a total of about 6,000 troops over 1 or 2 high-casualty days. This would result in more than 100 stress casualties arriving at the forward support medical company in the brigade support area over a few days. At least as many stressed soldiers would require special consideration without necessarily being held for restoration in medical units. Considering that rates were as high as one psychiatric to one wounded-in-action casualty in some Israeli and Egyptian units in the first high-intensity, sustained engagement of the 1973 Yom Kippur War, this stress casualty estimate may be too conservative.

Surgical casualties and combat stress casualties in a high-intensity scenario are projected to occur in such numbers that medical resources must utilize the triage principles developed for mass-casualty situations. Triage emphasizes treating first those who have the best chance of survival while postponing treatment of those seriously wounded or lightly wounded. In current civilian triage situations, surgical casualties have priority over psychiatric casualties in the allocation of medical personnel. Combat stress casualties, as the most likely to become effective with minimal intervention, will receive attention from division mental health and combat stress control unit teams. These assets will continue into the future force structure, but that alone is not enough to assure success. They must also be at the critical places on the fluid battlefield. They must be highly trained in peacetime to function in such a high-stress setting in a come-as-you-are war. Will the military be successful in recruiting and retaining psychiatrists, psychologists, and social workers who will enjoy the challenge of being true consultants and members of line units if the job involves this risk? Might it be necessary to train physician assistants for combat psychiatry positions? The plans for far-forward combat stress control in U.S. Army Force XXI are reviewed in Chapter 7, U.S. Army Combat Psychiatry.

If there were a threat of NBC warfare, the rate of stress casualties would rise. Stress casualties which mimic the symptoms of chemical, biological, or radiation injury may exceed the cases of actual injury by 2 or 3 to 1, based on World War I experience. The chemical protective suit and mask (mission-oriented protective posture or MOPP gear) would create heat buildup even in cool climates with excessive sweating and loss of salt and water. Furthermore, to minimize the need to urinate, soldiers in MOPP gear often do not drink fluids. In experiments conducted by Walter Reed Army Institute of Research (WRAIR) personnel,[26] soldiers in MOPP gear were observed to fail to eat and drink in order to minimize excretory functions leading to some degree of urine concentration. Even without MOPP gear, soldiers often do not eat or drink in the early days of combat. During the 1982 invasion of

Grenada by U.S. forces, casualties from dehydration occurred, indicating that U.S. forces need to be alert to this problem. The Israelis have made water drills a standard part of a combat commander's responsibilities, with failure in this area leading to punishment.

While overt heat prostration presents an unambiguous syndrome, the effects of mild dehydration are not so obvious. S.L.A. Marshall,[27] a man exposed to battle during World War I, World War II, and Korea, described the following incident during the strenuous invasion of a Japanese-held Pacific island during World War II:

Case Study: SLAM Finds Salt

The sniper fire had intensified.... When their officers got this company going again, I followed along for about a hundred yards into the bush. There, after just a few stumbling steps, I fell apart. My senses reeled. I was hit by such weakness that I dropped my carbine and could not unbuckle my belt, but that was not the worst of it. Within seconds my nerve had gone completely and I shook all over from fear.

I lay flat under a pandanus tree, telling myself: "It's combat fatigue. You've been kidding yourself. You are too old for the wars." Being unable to walk and scarcely able to think, I decided to stay where I was, wait for a stretcher-bearer to come along and get me back to the *Calvert* [ship], where I would stay. For possibly ten minutes I waited.

Before any aid man came my way, a rifleman stopped and stared at me. Then he took a bottle of pills from his jacket pocket and downed a couple of them.

I asked weakly, "What you got?"

"Salt."

"Gimme some. Nothing can make me feel worse than I do."

He gave me the bottle, saying he had another. I washed down eleven salt tablets with the lukewarm water from my canteen as fast as I could swallow. Within the next ten minutes my nerve and strength were fully restored, and I was never again troubled; yet that lesson had to be learned the hard way. No one had ever told me that one consequence of dehydration is cowardice in its most abject form.[27(p68)]

Comment: This vignette clearly demonstrates combat fatigue as a *psychophysiological disorder.*

RESEARCH STUDIES OF COMBAT STRESS

Psychological Factors

Combat does not lend itself to experimental studies because most of the variables cannot be controlled; consequently, few studies have been conducted during actual fighting. Perhaps the most extensive study of the stress of combat was done by Stouffer, DeVinney, Star, and Williams[28] during World War II. That study addressed primarily psychological factors and showed that cohesive, well-led units had fewer psychiatric casualties.

During the Vietnam conflict, Bourne, Rose, and Mason[29] obtained, over a 3-month period that included intermittent combat, behavioral data and urine samples from a 12-man Special Forces "A" team assigned in an enemy-controlled area. They found that the 2 officers experienced substantially higher levels of stress than the 10 enlisted men as measured by steroid excretion. It was also noted that on the day of an anticipated attack, an officer and his radio operator (command and communications positions) showed a modest rise in steroid excretion (increased stress) while the other subjects, all enlisted men, showed a drop. These findings (along with clinical observations and theoretical studies by Gal and Jones as discussed in Chapter 6, A Psychological Model of Combat Stress) suggest that assigned role in a group plays a major part in determining stress.

Bourne, Rose, and Mason[30] had also studied steroid excretion and obtained behavioral data on seven helicopter ambulance medics in combat in Vietnam. A surprising finding of the study was that comparison soldiers in basic combat training camps in the United States, as measured by steroid excretion, experienced greater stress than these soldiers engaged in highly dangerous combat operations (such ambulance crews averaged more medals for heroism than combat arms soldiers). They found that these combat soldiers utilized a variety of mental mechanisms to defend themselves from the stress of potential death and mutilation. These mental activities were highly individualized. One man was quite religious, believing that God would protect him. Another soldier, who tended to intellectualize, would make involved mathematical computations as to the probability of his being wounded or killed, would come up with figures indicating a low probability, and would dismiss such a low probability as being insignificant.

Similarly, in the Special Forces team Bourne[29] also found defensive mental operations but in this case the primary mechanism was an overwhelming emphasis on self-reliance, often to the point of om-

nipotence. In an unpublished study of explosive ordnance disposal (EOD) teams, often called "bomb squads," the author found similar mental operations used to protect the individual from the stress of potential death and maiming. In EOD personnel the primary defense was a belief that if one followed established procedures in a careful manner, there would be little danger. A sense of omnipotence and of fatalism ("I won't die until it's my time") were also frequent coping mechanisms.

Combat Role and Sleep Deprivation

In a simulated combat exercise the importance of leadership and cohesiveness was demonstrated in sustained operations when a good commander prevented soldiers suffering from cold exposure from disrupting his unit while another commander was not so effective.[31] During this same exercise Belenky[32] reported on the importance of physiological degradation of performance, particularly that caused by lack of sleep. He reported that a majority of soldiers deprived of sleep for 72 hours would experience visual hallucinations and illusions. However, the same study revealed that 3 or 4 hours of sleep in a 24-hour period would prevent most of the degradation of cognitive processes.

Johnson and Naitoh[33] have concluded from a comprehensive review of the literature that cognitive processes suffer earlier and more severely than muscular tasks during sleep deprivation. Experimenters at the U.S. Army Research Institute of Environmental Medicine[34,35] have explored the effects of sustained operations on artillery teams in simulated sustained combat. Their findings confirm earlier reports that cognitive tasks requiring abstract judgment, preplanning, and vigilance are degraded early and seriously from sleep loss and cumulative fatigue, while the ability to perform well-practiced, urgent tasks involving motor activity was preserved best.

Disrupted Circadian Rhythms

Experimenters at the Naval Health Research Center[36-38] have shown that performance is also related to circadian rhythms that, of course, are particularly susceptible to disruption from travel across several time zones, as would occur in any distant deployment of U.S. forces in an easterly or westerly direction. Abstract tasks such as reading comprehension have been shown to be best performed in the afternoon and evening, while performance speed was high in the morning and steadily fell during the day and evening.[37] In studies of nuclear submariners subjected to an 18-hour work-rest cycle, Naitoh and coworkers[38] found desynchronization of normal circadian rhythms, which could have implications for stress and health.

The situation is even more complicated in that circadian rhythms seem to be regulated by a "deep oscillator," which changes very little despite external changes in sleep cycle, and a "labile oscillator," which is more responsive to environmental changes.[39] The "deep oscillator," which may be reflected in persistent body temperature patterns, is more significant for tasks involving manual dexterity skills, while the "labile oscillator" is more significant for cognitive tasks.

A comprehensive review of the shift-work and jet-lag literature has drawn conclusions on reducing negative effects in the event of overseas deployment of U.S. forces.[40] They note that manipulation of the carbohydrate and protein components of the soldier's diet producing relative increases of serotonin or catecholamine precursors in the brain can result in a drowsy soldier when sleep is appropriate or an alert soldier when this state is appropriate. They have devised schedules not only in terms of optimal work-rest cycles but even appropriate diets of soldiers for sedating or alerting effects. They have suggested, for instance, that a high carbohydrate meal about 1 or 2 hours before sleep is desired will facilitate sleep through the insulin effect, which increases L-tryptophan transport through the blood-brain barrier. This precursor amino acid of serotonin increases serotonergic influence and thus sleepiness. There is increasing evidence that bright light exposure to the retinae can reset the circadian cycle. This can be accomplished by having the individual exposed to bright light in the new morning and decreased exposure at the new night, perhaps by wearing dark sunglasses.

Implications for Future Combat

Future commanders must maximize their soldiers' fighting ability and resistance to breakdown by insuring that the physiological needs of their soldiers are met. This involves a sensible doctrine of rest and sleep (at least 4 h sleep in a 24-h span), prevention of cumulative fatigue (by rotation from combat, preferably as a unit to maintain cohesion), adequate nutrition (especially fluids and salt), and frequent changes of socks to prevent frostbite in cold weather and fungal infections in hot weather. When initiating combat, U.S. commanders should seek to attack at a time when their sol-

diers' normal circadian rhythms are at a peak. For example, soldiers flown from the East Coast of the United States to fight in the Middle East could take advantage of the time zone dislocation by napping on the overseas flight and attacking at 0300 hours Persian Gulf time, physiologically early evening time for U.S. forces; and, for alertness, the lowest ebb of the biological tide for enemy soldiers accustomed to rhythms appropriate for the Persian Gulf region.

Future combat will also require close attention to psychosocial factors and revision of the principles of combat psychiatry. Because stress casualties have typically peaked among troops initially exposed to combat, prevention of these casualties will be critical to the outcome of a war of short duration. In addition to leadership and cohesion factors discussed previously, there is a need for ongoing educational efforts to minimize the effects of expected surprise attacks by the enemy. As mentioned in the Desert Rock studies discussed in Chapter 4, Neuropsychiatric Casualties of Nuclear, Biological, and Chemical Warfare, those soldiers most knowledgeable about nuclear explosions were least frightened. This need to educate soldiers should not only include the usual battle and NBC scenarios but also the possibility of atypical scenarios. By being familiar with such scenarios, the psychiatrist will be able to educate commanders concerning expected psychological reactions and potential interventions.

PRINCIPLES OF COMBAT PSYCHIATRY FOR FUTURE WARFARE

Because high-intensity warfare may make implementation of the traditional principles of combat psychiatry unworkable, new principles of treatment must be developed (Exhibit 5-3). It is obvious that preventing these casualties from occurring in the first place is the preferred course of action; however, this may be difficult given the intensity of warfare. Studies[41–44] have repeatedly shown that stress casualties occur in direct proportion to combat intensity and certain physical and morale factors. Factors tending to prevent such breakdown include the absence of fatigue, presence of good leadership and its consequence, unit cohesion, confidence of the soldiers in their weapons and in themselves, and an advancing or retreating military posture. Conversely, the negatives of these factors would promote psychiatric breakdown. Continuous, high-intensity warfare may prevent sleep and rest, thus producing fatigue and promoting breakdown. Dispersion will interfere with the ability of commanders to lead and may prevent the aggregation of comrades, impeding cohesion.

In the 1973 Yom Kippur War, an exemplar of a conventional high-intensity war, some of these factors were not appreciated. The hastily assembled (therefore less cohesive) Israeli forces were exposed to conditions of continuous, high-lethality warfare. Estimates[45] of Israeli acute psychiatric casualties were reported as between 30% and 50% of total casualties in some units. According to Egyptian military psychiatrists, the Egyptian psychiatric casualties at least equaled the "surgical";[46,47] that is, they were at least 50% of the total.

After the 1973 Yom Kippur War there was a concerted attempt by the Israelis to prevent future stress casualties; however, in the 1982 Lebanon War, which was not of as high intensity as the 1973 war, the percentage of acute psychiatric casualties is reported as 23%, mostly occurring during 2 weeks of active combat.[48] (A larger number of delayed and chronic post-traumatic stress disorder cases have

EXHIBIT 5-3

PRINCIPLES OF COMBAT PSYCHIATRY IN HIGH-INTENSITY WARFARE

Prevention:
- Unit cohesion
- Realistic training
- Doctrine of rest and nutrition

Battlefield treatment:
- Limited evacuation of psychiatric casualties
- Treatment in the midst of battle
- Emphasis on buddy care: Reassurance, Expectancy

Use of drugs:
- Nonsedating antianxiety drugs
- Nondepleting stimulants to reduce fatigue
- Reversible sleep and alerting agents

Adapted from Jones FD. Psychiatric lessons of low-intensity wars. Presented at Army Medical Department Division and Combat Psychiatry Conference, 1984; Fort Bragg, NC.

surfaced subsequently.[49]) It appears likely, then, that the United States must be prepared either to treat significant numbers of acute stress casualties in the event of a future war or to develop more effective methods of prevention. The most cost-effective approach would emphasize prevention.

Prevention

The chronology of combat stress breakdown was clearly described by Swank and Marchand.[50] It appeared that there are two groups of soldiers prone to become psychiatric casualties: those never before exposed to combat and those exposed to combat for a prolonged period of time. Swank and Marchand depicted this finding in a chronological chart of combat efficiency. Initial exposure finds low efficiency and high casualties. Efficiency improves after a few weeks with fewer casualties but again declines after 6 to 8 weeks of combat with increased casualties.

During the Korean and Vietnam conflicts the main preventive measure for prolonged exposure casualties, based on World War II experience, consisted of limiting the period of exposure to combat to prevent cumulative stress. Thus, the combat tour in Korea was 9 months and in Vietnam it was 1 year. In the absence of a lengthy war and with the probability of brief, intense future combat, the military has more recently focused on preventing the initial or "green troop" casualties. To do this the U.S. Army has initiated a number of programs to strengthen unit cohesion. This approach in recent years resulted in keeping commanders with the same unit for 18 months or more and in the COHORT (cohesion, operational readiness, training) Program of keeping groups of soldiers together from the time of basic training through assignment overseas. However, this program has largely been abandoned because of the administrative difficulties it creates. Confidence in weapons and selves is being achieved through an emphasis on physical fitness and realistic weapons training. This training is accomplished in part through use of laser "hits" in simulated combat, live-fire exercises, and realistic simulated combat exercises at the Combat Training Centers. A more exotic approach to prevention might consist of the use of performance-enhancing and anxiety-blocking pharmaceuticals, which the author will discuss later.

Battlefield Treatment in High-Intensity Warfare

In view of the problems posed by high-intensity combat for traditional treatment procedures, the original World War I principles of combat psychiatry must be revitalized (see Exhibit 5-3). The original concept for the care and evacuation of "nervous" and "mental cases" at the division level was stated in September 1918 as follows:

> 1. Each division in the area has a division psychiatrist who will be stationed at the triage [ie, the ambulance transfer point] when his division is engaged. There he will sort all nervous cases, returning directly to their organizations those who should not be permitted to go to the rear and resting, warming, feeding, and treating others, particularly exhausted cases, if there is opportunity to do so.
>
> . . . .
>
> 2. The advantages of these provisions for dealing with war neuroses and allied conditions in the divisions are:
>   (a) Control over the evacuation of cases presenting no psychoneurotic symptoms.
>   (b) Speedy restoration and return to their organizations of those in whom exhaustion is the chief or only factor.
>   (c) Cure of mild psychoneurotic cases by persuasion, rest, and treatment of special symptoms at a time when heightened suggestibility may be employed to advantage instead of being permitted to operate disadvantageously.
>
> . . . .
>
>   (f) Creating in the minds of troops generally the impression that the disorders grouped under the term "shell shock" are relatively simple and recoverable rather than complex and dangerous, as the indiscriminate evacuation of all nervous cases [suggests].[51(p309)]

Prevention and treatment must merge in a modern approach to managing stress casualties. Evacuation of stress casualties must be strictly limited. Becoming a stress casualty would, therefore, not result in an "evacuation syndrome."[31] Many stress cases, however, would still exist. The primary treating persons must be the soldier's fellow soldier ("buddy"), medic, squad, and platoon leader. If soldiers are too ineffective to remain in their squad or team, the next option is to rest them for a night or two in their battalion's headquarters and headquarters company (the "field trains" from which the maneuver companies receive their nightly resupply of ammunition, fuel, water, and food). Treatment would consist of reassurance, replenishment, expectancy, and possibly administration of a nonsedating antianxiety pharmaceutical.[52] This

would be monitored by the unit medic, physician assistant, or circuit-riding mental health officer and NCO. These mental health/combat stress control teams are already called for in current doctrine[25] provided by the division mental health section or the supporting combat stress control detachment.

In the future, the team might have a HMMWV (high mobility multipurpose wheeled vehicle) ambulance or armored personnel carrier in which they could provide mobile evaluation and restoration. For the soldier who appeared fatigued or depressed, nondepleting stimulants might be given. (A nondepleting stimulant is one that does not deplete the neurons of their neurotransmitters. Such depletion, which occurs, for example, with amphetamines, eventually results in rebound fatigue and depression as well as the dangers of heart arrhythmias and psychosis. Currently the amino acids L-tyrosine and L-phenylalanine come closest to being nondepleting stimulants. These can be defined as a "nutritional supplement," not drugs.) Only the small number of most impaired or diagnostically complex cases would be held for observation and restoration treatment by the combat stress control team's psychiatrist (or psychiatric physician assistant) at the forward support medical company, usually several kilometers from the battalion's headquarters companies. Because of the requirement for extreme mobility, this restoration might be provided in suitable vehicles, with built-in physiologic monitoring, biofeedback, and audio-video relaxation equipment. Such vehicles could be used for the prophylactic maintenance and enhancement of combat performance, as well as for restoration of soldiers who had already become stress casualties. Finally, there is growing evidence that the judicious use of pharmaceuticals may enhance combat performance and possibly prevent some forms of combat breakdown; therefore, the issues of the sanctioned use of drugs in combat will be discussed.

Ethical and Practical Issues Concerning Pharmaceuticals

The use of pharmaceuticals to sustain or enhance performance in combat is controversial. It raises important ethical and practical considerations. The U.S. government declared a war on drug abuse in the 1980s. As part of that effort, the U.S. armed forces have been assigned missions of drug interdiction overseas and on United States' borders to reduce the production and importation of illegal drugs.

The abused drugs include stimulants (cocaine, amphetamines) which are addictive because they produce (in high doses) feelings of intense well-being, power, alertness, endurance, and aggressiveness (as well as other less common but major psychiatric disorders). The abused drugs also include "depressants" (alcohol, barbiturates, benzodiazepine tranquilizers) which calm anxiety and produce feelings of well-being or promote sleep, as well as producing a drunken euphoria, dependence, addiction, and other negative effects. The narcotic painkiller drugs are abused because they produce a blissful euphoric state. Anabolic steroids are abused by body-builders and athletes because they increase muscle mass, strength, and endurance. They are banned in competitive athletics because they unquestionably increase speed, strength, power, and endurance, although at a potential (rare) cost of medical and psychiatric complications including violent attack behaviors ("'roid rages"). If the United States has declared war on drugs, how can it possibly justify prescribing similar drugs to American soldiers for use in combat?

The obvious answer in favor is that war is not a competitive sport. It is bound by the International Laws of War, but not by Olympic committee rules. Battles are fought by the nation's soldiers, at risk of death, to win the nation's military, and ultimately political, objectives. In such an environment it is necessary to give American soldiers every safe, feasible, and competitive advantage.

But are such drugs safe, especially in the highly unpredictable and unstable physical, logistical, and emotional context of combat? That question requires an empirical, not a philosophical, answer. All drugs are potentially double-edged swords. All will have side effects and overdose effects. Some may produce additional effects upon withdrawal or elimination of the drug. Some interact dangerously with environmental factors, diet, other drugs, or specific diseases. All drugs may have idiosyncratic effects on some individuals. It is unwise to dispense any drug lightly, without first evaluating the recipients and briefing them (and their support group) on what to expect and what to be alert for. It is then wise and ethical to follow them up periodically. For these reasons, any use of pharmacologic agents should be kept under appropriate medical supervision if not necessarily medical control.

After analysis of the risks, some drugs may be judged safe enough for "over the counter," self-administered use. Other drugs may be judged safe for routine prescription use with periodic follow-

up. Other drugs still may be so risky that they should be prescribed only in urgent, carefully defined situations. Like some medications used in treating highly lethal diseases, it may be reasonable to accept even a high risk of injury from the drug if there is little chance that the "patient" can live past the next week without it. Such situations can arise in war as well as in the emergency room.

Of course, if such a drug is administered as a calculated risk and if the soldiers do survive, the uniformed services owe it to them to provide long-term follow-up, and treatment or compensation for any complications of the therapy that may arise.

But will the parents and spouses of America tolerate soldiers being given drugs to induce them to risk their lives and possibly die? It is no longer doctrine to intimidate an enemy into surrender by the sheer bravery of American fighting forces. Rather, the intention is to "fight smart," using superior weapons and information technology on the future "digitized battlefield" to attack the enemy when he is much less capable of striking back.

The effective use of those sophisticated weapons systems requires keeping the operators' brains and bodies in fine tune. The continuous operation doctrine of the U.S. military demands initiative, agility, synchronization, depth, and versatility. Those battlefield imperatives task precisely the higher mental functions in all soldiers, from general officer to private, which are most susceptible to deterioration from sleep-loss, dehydration, fear, sensory overload, or sensory deprivation. If synchronization fails, American "high-tech" weapons kill other Americans or innocent noncombatants. If pharmacologic agents (or other technical solutions such as sensory stimulation, relaxation, or biofeedback) can help more than harm, should they not be used?

It is desirable to develop in U.S. soldiers such high levels of unit cohesion and patriotism that they will be willing, if necessary, to risk sacrificing themselves to save their buddies and accomplish the mission. However, it is not desirable to have anyone in the various weapons systems "high," "spaced out," or indifferent to his own safety. If a drug can help them sustain unit cohesion, good training, and good sense in the face of otherwise overwhelming fatigue or arousal, with an acceptable risk of other harmful effects, is it ethical to withhold it? The overriding question is whether the drug can be taken with an acceptable level of risk both for the mission and the soldier. That will require research, which will not be easy to accomplish.

Use of Pharmaceuticals in Combat

Undoubtedly alcohol was the first drug to be utilized to enhance combat performance. When Holland became a major source of gin, the widespread use of this alcoholic beverage by soldiers led to the expression "Dutch courage" to express the desired effect. The ancient Assyrians, Egyptians, and Greeks reportedly utilized opiates before and during battles to sustain or enhance bravery and courage.[53] Other drugs studied or used to enhance combat performance include ergot alkaloids, cannabis, amphetamine and other stimulants; Dramamine and other antihistamines; benzodiazepines; and L-tryptophan. It is the author's contention that the most extensive modern use of performance-enhancing drugs occurred among Soviet personnel during World War II shortly after amphetamine was synthesized. Amphetamine was useful not only to stave off fatigue and drowsiness but also to improve memory and concentration, particularly among Soviet pilots.

During the Vietnam conflict, methylphenidate (Ritalin) and sometimes dextroamphetamine (Dexedrine) were standard issue drugs carried by long-range reconnaissance patrol (LRRP) soldiers. The LRRPs found the most efficacious use to be upon completion of a mission when fatigue had developed and rapid return to the base camp was desirable. Other than mild rebound depression and fatigue after the drug was discontinued, no adverse effects were reported. Other investigators[54,55] studying the drug abuse problem later in the Vietnam conflict reported problems with abuse of these stimulants. Although there was no documented abuse of the morphine Syrettes, commanders suggested such abuse might be occurring,[56] causing them to be withdrawn from the soldiers.

Sedatives have also been studied as a method to improve performance in anxiety-producing situations such as paratroopers making low-altitude jumps or for reducing the emotional tension of young soldiers during the firing of guns.[57] Reports of improved target accuracy through use of the ß-adrenergic blocker, propranolol, and the anxiolytic, diazepam (Valium), have resulted in a U.S. Army ban on use of these drugs by soldiers engaged in marksmanship competition because they would confer an unfair advantage.

In the Vietnam conflict, neuroleptics (antipsychotic or major tranquilizer drugs) were widely utilized for psychotropic effects but benzodiazepines were also used. In the 1982 Falkland Islands

War, temazepam (Restoril) and triazolam (Halcion) were prescribed by the Royal Air Force (RAF) psychiatrist to British pilots on Ascension Island to ensure adequate sleep between the very long, multiple refueling flights to the Falklands and back.[58,59] Triazolam (Halcion) has been studied in U.S. Army field trials.[60] Recent benzodiazepine receptor research suggests ways that these drugs could be used carefully in combat settings not only to alleviate fear and anxiety but also as hypnotic and alerting agents.

Benzodiazepine Receptor Studies

Four functions mediated by benzodiazepines have been discriminated:[61,62] (1) antianxiety (anxiolytic), (2) anticonvulsant, (3) muscle-relaxant, and (4) sedative-hypnotic functions. A fifth possible effect, blocking panic, is relatively weak. Of drugs available on the U.S. market, a number of primarily antidepressant medications (eg, tricyclics and monoamine oxidase inhibitors) appear to have greater antipanic effects.[63,64] It is believed that these exert their effects by potentiating the inhibitory effects of γ-aminobutyric acid (GABA), which in turn is the neurotransmitter of 30% of the inhibitory synapses of the brain.[65] A careful modification of the molecular structures involved has resulted in the synthesis of experimental drugs that can act as agonists or antagonists of all four of the functions mediated by benzodiazepines. This selectivity suggests numerous clinical and military applications including both the prevention and treatment of combat stress disorders and enhancement of performance in certain circumstances.

As mentioned in Chapter 2, Traditional Warfare Combat Stress Casualties, the most consistent symptom of combat stress, whether occurring early in exposure to combat or after cumulative exposure, is anxiety. Such anxiety may be manifested by fear, hysterical conversion or dissociation, tremors, and similar symptoms. In the past, these conditions have been treated with sedatives ranging from chloral hydrate and bromides in World War I to barbiturates in World War II and even self-prescribed alcohol, cannabis, and heroin in Vietnam. These drugs often not only produced unwanted sedation but also decreased the probability of return to combat due to the fixation of a sickness role suggested by taking medication. Based on their experience in 1973, the Israelis promoted a policy prohibiting forward use of medications and even hypnosis.[66]

A drug, however, which would selectively reduce anxiety without diminishing mental or physical alertness and efficiency would go a long way toward "curing" the usual battle fatigue syndrome. To some extent this occurred in the Vietnam conflict when physicians treated psychophysiological symptoms of fear and anxiety with neuroleptics and antianxiety agents.[67] In Johnson's 1-month, mid-1967 survey, physicians' prescribing experience, when generalized to the entire troop population, gave an estimated prescribing rate of 12.5% per year of the assigned U.S. Army troops. Compazine, a major tranquilizer, accounted for 45% of prescriptions made by nonpsychiatrists, mainly used to treat gastroenteritis. Most of the 56 cases of battle fatigue reported in Johnson's study were treated with major tranquilizers (64%), particularly chlorpromazine (Thorazine). The neuromuscular, autonomic nervous system, and cognitive impairments produced by this drug make it a particularly questionable choice on the battlefield.

Future Sanctioned Pharmaceutical Use

The following discussion is offered to stimulate consideration of the potential uses of pharmacologic agents in combat. It does not reflect current official policies.

The ideal drug to treat combat stress breakdown would be an easily administered, stable compound that would reduce anxiety without significant neuromuscular or cognitive impairments, would be nonaddictive, and would permit an appropriate response to danger. Such a drug is not currently available in the U.S. market, but drugs selectively preventing severe anxiety without sedation are being studied, and they raise the possibility of developing a combat-appropriate drug.

Other drugs for selected purposes may also be developed. A drug with a short duration of effect reversible by an antagonist could prove to be a most useful battlefield hypnotic. Such antagonist drugs, primarily affecting the benzodiazepine receptor, are already in the experimental stage[61,62] and one, the benzodiazepine antagonist flumazenil (Romazicon) is commercially available. This drug, currently used in surgical procedures, could be given to a soldier who had received a short-acting benzodiazepine, to bring him awake quickly (within minutes to an hour) if it were necessary for him to resume critical duties.

Studies indicate that buspirone (BuSpar) relieves anxiety without producing cognitive impairment both in acute and chronic use and even in the presence of alcohol.[68,69] In fact, buspirone actually appeared to improve psychomotor skills in alcohol users.

Buspirone is now available in the United States. It has the advantage of causing no psychomotor impairment and no muscle relaxant or sedation effects greater than placebo. Vigilance tasks are improved by a slight alerting effect. Addiction potential seems low because there is no euphoriant effect, and a single large dose (40 mg or above) produces dysphoria. Patients have been given daily doses of over 2 g. One possible drawback is that, as part of its antianxiety effect, it also decreases anger and hostility, but it is arguable that cool professionalism is better than rage when operating modern weapons systems. A more important drawback is a latency or delayed-action period of about 10 days before the anxiolytic effect develops. The latency of anxiolytic effect also seems to occur with the benzodiazepines; however, their immediate sedative effects mask this latency effect.[70] The latency of effect need not limit buspirone to a prophylactic use in soldiers with preexisting anxiety disorders or undergoing reconditioning treatment for return to combat after being evacuated for battle fatigue. Key individuals or whole units could, hypothetically, be placed on buspirone 10 days prior to starting their rapid deployment standby mission cycles, and taken off at the end of the cycle. Buspirone has no adverse withdrawal syndrome.

Because certain individuals are vulnerable to panic attacks during episodes of heightened arousal such as combat, the use of antipanic agents might be appropriate in such individuals. Estimates of the incidence of panic disorder (repetitive, spontaneous panic attacks) range from 1%[71] to 6%.[63] At least two million Americans are thought to be afflicted. Because 25% of first-degree relatives of those with panic disorders are also afflicted in lifetime incidence and there is high concordance in monozygotic twins, a hereditary vulnerability has been postulated. In over two thirds of such patients, the attack can be brought on by infusing 10 mL/kg of 0.5 molar sodium lactate solution in a 20-minute time period. A simpler method of provoking panic in a vulnerable person is to have him or her hyperventilate. In periods of constrained manpower availability, those thought to be suffering from panic disorder who are otherwise fit for combat might be treated with antidepressants that block panic attacks. Antidepressants with minimal sedative side effects would have to be selected. The original monoamine oxidase inhibitors which are most effective as antipanic drugs are excluded because of the dietary restrictions against foods containing tyramine which trigger hypertensive crisis. A new class of monoamine oxidase inhibitors, RIMAs (reversible inhibitors of monoamine oxidase-A) do not have this problem. Imipramine (a tricyclic antidepressant) has too many anticholinergic side effects to be safe in most combat environments. The selective serotonin reuptake inhibitors have fewer side effects and may be demonstrated effective for panic disorder.

In summary, for millennia soldiers have utilized alcohol and other drugs to relieve the stresses of war. The time may now be opportune for the use of specifically tailored pharmaceuticals for these purposes without risking the dangers or decrements experienced in the past.

Thus, the revitalized principles of combat stress treatment involve maximizing preventive efforts and treating in the combat unit. This treatment approach eliminates stress reactions as methods to escape combat (evacuation syndromes), would obviate the need for large numbers of medical resources to treat such casualties (thus allowing them to treat surgical cases), and reduces the problems of returning soldiers to their own units.

The costs of this approach will be increased numbers of "psychosomatic" cases, inappropriate treatment of some misdiagnosed cases, and, perhaps, increased death rates among treated cases. As described above, this scenario is developed around one extreme of future combat, the high-intensity, possibly NBC, war. Lesser-intensity wars will call for varying degrees of traditional interventions depending on intensity.

SUMMARY AND CONCLUSION

This historical review of psychiatric interventions in past wars has explored the implications of a range of future combat scenarios. The spectrum of combat intensities ranges from intermittent light-infantry combat to continuous, highly-mechanized battle, possibly with nuclear, biological, and chemical weapons. Being unable to predict what type of war the United States will fight in the future, the armed forces must be prepared for both extremes. If psychiatric casualties can be appropriately treated in these extremes, those of a medium-range of intensity should present no insurmountable or unforeseen problems. Likewise, the military will be prepared for those future military missions that

extend beyond combat into areas of peacekeeping or humanitarian relief. However, even in these scenarios it is reasonable to expect that the combat intensity dimension will include the major varieties of future psychiatric problems.

In preparing for the extreme of low-intensity combat and the stress casualties associated with it, there must be an attempt to strengthen ameliorating conditions by minimizing family stress, enforcing vigorous discipline in organized camp conditions, setting and enforcing strict but realistic rules of engagement, and promoting unit cohesion and pride in following the rules. At the same time, it will be necessary to eliminate or lessen the impact of aggravating conditions: prevent boredom, prepare for cultural differences, and strengthen social support from the unit, the family, and the community.

High-intensity future warfare, in particular, challenges the application of the traditional principles of forward treatment because there may be no safe and stationary forward treatment area due to new weapons and surveillance systems capable of discovering aggregations of personnel. Also, rear areas may be easier to target because they are less dispersed, camouflaged, or mobile than front-line forces. Whatever the combat intensity in the future, the well-known stresses of dislocation from loved ones and home, the fear of the unknown, and the stresses of an unfamiliar environment will produce disorders of frustration and loneliness. Thus, the promotion or prevention of psychiatric morbidity will have significant implications for training and operational procedures in future warfare. Particular attention should be given to the interplay of physical and psychological variables in the prevention of combat stress reaction. Obviously, water and sleep drills should become standard in training scenarios. Perhaps not as obvious is the fact that, if feasible, planning sessions for combat should be held at the optimum time in the circadian cycle for highly complex and abstract cognitive tasks. For the soldier who is not experiencing a time zone dislocation, this would probably be in the afternoon and evening rather than in the early morning. Optimal times might also be considered in attacking the enemy. Troops who have rested during a transatlantic flight with proper planning could arrive at a battle at an optimum circadian period for themselves and at the least optimal period for an enemy. The enemy, of course, might not be so accommodating in allowing U.S. forces to prosecute the war on a favorable timetable.

It must be remembered that men have definite physical and emotional limits. A future war will produce levels of stress that unless prepared for in advance, will easily exceed these limits. Through thorough preparation and a sensible doctrine of human physical and emotional limits, a country can hope to deter war but, nonetheless, it must be prepared to fight and win if necessary. It is not enough that the medical community be aware of the limits of human mental and physical endurance in combat; the line commanders must be equally aware and be prepared to shape doctrine to conform to these human needs.

REFERENCES

1. Rosen G. Nostalgia: A "forgotten" psychological disorder. *Psychol Med.* 1975;5:340–354.

2. Jones FD. Lessons of war for psychiatry. In: Pichot P, Berner P, Wolf R, Thau K, eds. *Psychiatry: The State of the Art.* Vol 6. New York: Plenum; 1985: 515–519.

3. Salmon TW. The care and treatment of mental diseases and war neurosis ("shell shock") in the British Army. In: Bailey P, Williams FE, Komora PA, Salmon TW, Fenton N, eds. *Neuropsychiatry.* Vol 10. In: *The Medical Department of the United States Army in the World War.* Washington, DC: Office of The Surgeon General, US Army; 1929: Appendix; 497–523.

4. Hanson FR. The factor of fatigue in the neuroses of combat. Combat psychiatry. *Bull US Army Med Dept.* 1949;9:147–150.

5. Drayer CS, Glass AJ. Introduction. In: Glass AJ, ed. *Overseas Theaters.* Vol 2. In: *Neuropsychiatry in World War II.* Washington, DC: Office of The Surgeon General, US Army; 1973: 1–23.

6. Fearnsides EG, Culpin M. Frost-bite. *Br Med J.* 1915;1:84.

7. Sampson JB. Anxiety as a factor in the incidence of combat cold injury: A review. *Milit Med.* 1984;149:89–91.

8. Lipowski ZJ. Consultation-liaison psychiatry: An overview. *Am J Psychiatry.* 1974;131:623–630.

9. Brownell A, Shumaker S. Social support: New perspectives in theory, research and intervention. Part 1: Theory and research. *J Soc Issues.* 1984;40:1–144.

10. Brownell A, Shumaker S. Social support: New perspectives on theory, research and intervention. Part 2: Interventions and policy. *J Soc Issues.* 1985;41:1–171.

11. Bushard B. The U.S. Army's mental hygiene consultation service. *Symposium on Preventive and Social Psychiatry.* Washington DC: GPO; 1957: 431–443.

12. Orwell G. *1984.* New York: The New American Library of World Literature; 1950: 142.

13. Wilson GC. Raids said to cut Bolivian cocaine output: General reports of success of US-assisted helicopter operation. *The Washington Post,* 15 August 1986:A12.

14. McEwen MT. Psychological operations against terrorism: The unused weapon. *Milit Rev.* 1986;66(1): 59–67.

15. Martin JA. Combat psychiatry: Lessons from the war in Southwest Asia. *J US Army Med Dept.* 1991;PB8-92-1/2:40–44.

16. Dasey CF. US Army Medical Research and Development Command in support of Desert Shield/Storm. *J US Army Med Dept.* 1991;PB8-92-3/4:13–15.

17. Gifford RK, Marlowe DH, Wright KM, Bartone PT, Martin JA. Unit cohesion in Operations Desert Shield/Desert Storm. *J US Army Med Dept.* 1991;PB8-92-11/12:11–13.

18. Belenky GL, Newhouse P, Jones FD. Prevention and treatment of psychiatric casualties in the event of a war in Europe. *Int Rev Army Navy Air Force Med Serv (Paris).* 1982;55:303–307.

19. Hanne WG. AirLand battle: Doctrine, not dogma. *Milit Rev.* 1983;63(6):11–25.

20. Gans D. "Fight outnumbered and win"...against what odds?: Part 1. *Milit Rev.* 1980;60(12):31–46.

21. Cline WR, Rath FH. The concept of an army as a psychiatric casualty. *J R Army Med Corps.* 1982;128:79–88.

22. Donnelly C. The Soviet attitude to stress in battle. *J R Army Med Corps.* 1982;128(2):72–78.

23. Scott HF, Scott WF. *The Armed Forces of the USSR.* Boulder, Colo: Westview Press; 1979.

24. US Department of the Army. *Planning for Health Service Support.* Washington, DC: DA; 9 September 1994. Field Manual 8-55.

25. US Department of the Army. *Combat Stress Control in a Theater of Operations.* Washington, DC: DA; 29 September 1994. Field Manual 8-51.

26. Kant GJ, Smith R, Landman-Roberts L, Cardenales-Ortiz L, Mougey EH. The effect of sustained field operations on urinary electrolytes and cortisol. *Milit Med.* 1985;150:666–669.

27. Marshall, SLA. *Bringing up the Rear: A Memoir.* San Rafael, Calif: Presidio Press; 1979: 68.

28. Stouffer SA, DeVinney LC, Star SA, Williams RM. *The American Soldier.* Vol 2. Princeton, NJ: Princeton University Press; 1949.

29. Bourne PG, Rose RM, Mason JW. 17-OHCS levels in combat: Special Forces "A" team under threat of attack. *Arch Gen Psychiatry*. 1968;19:135–140.

30. Bourne PG, Rose RM, Mason JW. Urinary 17-OHCS levels: Data on seven helicopter ambulance medics in combat. *Arch Gen Psychiatry*. 1967;17:104–110.

31. Belenky GL, Jones FD. Evacuation syndromes in military exercises: A model of the psychiatric casualties of combat. In: Mangelsdorff AD, Furukawa PT, eds. *Proceedings, User's Workshop on Combat Stress*. Fort Sam Houston, Tex: Academy of Health Sciences; 1981: 140–142.

32. Belenky GL. Unusual visual experiences reported by subjects in the British Army study of sustained operations, Exercise Early Call. *Milit Med*. 1979;144:695–696.

33. Johnson LC, Naitoh P. *The Operational Consequences of Sleep Deprivation and Sleep Deficit*. London, England: Harford House; 1974. Sponsored by NATO Advisory Group for Aero-Space Research and Development (AGARD). AGARD-AG-193.

34. Banderet LE, Stokes JW, Francesconi R. Artillery teams in simulated sustained combat: Performance and other measures. In: Johnson LC, Tepas DI, Colquhoun WP, eds. *Biological Rhythms, Sleep and Shift Work*; New York: Spectrum; 1981: 459–479.

35. Francesconi RP, Stokes JW, Banderet LE, Kowal DM. Sustained operations and sleep deprivation: Effects on indices of stress. *Aviat Space Environ Med*. 1978;49:1271–1274.

36. Englund CE. The diurnal function of reading rate, comprehension and efficiency. In: *Proceedings, XIV International Conference of the International Society for Chronobiology*. Hanover, Germany: July 1979.

37. Englund CE. Human chronopsychology: An introduction and report of an autorhythmometric study of circadian periodicity in learning, mood and task performance. Presented at American Psychological Association Annual Meeting; 1981.

38. Naitoh P, Beare AN, Biersner RJ, Englund CE. *Altered Circadian Periodicities in Oral Temperature and Mood in Men on an 18-Hour Work-Rest Cycle During a Nuclear Submarine Patrol*. [Report Number 81-8], Naval Health Research Center, San Diego, Calif: 1981.

39. Monk TH. Sleep and circadian rhythms. *Gerontology*. 1991;26(2–3):233–243.

40. Hegge FW, Tyner CF. Deployment Threats to Rapid Deployment Forces. Presented to Division of Neuropsychiatry, Walter Reed Army Institute of Research; 1982; Washington, DC.

41. Appel JW, Beebe GW. Preventive psychiatry. *JAMA*. 1946;131(18):182–189.

42. Glass AJ. Psychotherapy in the combat zone. *Am J Psychiatry*. 1954;110:725–731.

43. Glass AJ. Observations upon the epidemiology of mental illness in troops during warfare. Presented at the Symposium on Social Psychiatry; April 1957; Walter Reed Army Institute of Research, Washington, DC: 185–198.

44. Glass AJ. Lessons learned. In: Glass AJ, ed. *Overseas Theaters*. Vol 2. In: *Neuropsychiatry in World War II*. Washington, DC: Office of The Surgeon General, US Army; 1973: 989–1027.

45. Noy S. Personal Communication, 1982.

46. Mansour F. Manifestations of maladjustment to military service in Egypt after prolonged stress. *Int Rev Army Navy Air Force Med Serv*. 1982;55:291–294.

47. El Sudany El Rayes M. Personal Communication, 1982.

48. Belenky GL, Tyner CF, Sodetz FJ. *Israeli Battle Shock Casualties: 1973 and 1982.* Washington, DC: Walter Reed Army Institute of Research; 1983. [WRAIR Report NP-83-4].

49. Belenky GL. Varieties of reactions and adaptation to combat experience. In: Menninger WW, ed. *Military Psychiatry: Learning from Experience.* Topeka, Kan: The Menninger Foundation; 1987: 64–79.

50. Swank RL, Marchand F. Combat neuroses: Development of combat exhaustion. *Arch Neurol Psychiatry* [superseded in part by *Arch Neurol* and *Arch Gen Psychiatry*]. 1946;55:236.

51. Zabriskie EG, Rhein JH, Strecker EA, Leopold S, Raynor MW, Steckel HA. Division, corps and army neuropsychiatric consultants. In: Bailey P, Williams FE, Komora PA, Salmon TW, Fenton N, eds. *Neuropsychiatry.* Vol 10. In: *The Medical Department of the United States Army in the World War.* Washington, DC: Office of The Surgeon General, US Army; 1929: 303–324.

52. Jones FD. Sanctioned use of drugs in combat. In: Pichot P, Berner P, Wolf R, Thau K, eds. *Psychiatry: The State of the Art.* Vol 6. New York: Plenum; 1985: 489–494.

53. Goldsmith M. *The Trail of Opium (The Eleventh Plague).* London, England: Robert Hale; 1939.

54. Holloway HC. Epidemiology of heroin dependency among soldiers in Vietnam. *Milit Med.* 1974;139: 108–113.

55. Robins LN. *A Follow-up of Vietnam Drug Users.* Washington, DC: US GPO; 1973. Special Action Office Monograph, Series A., No. 1.

56. Holloway HC. Thoughts about modern war. Presented at Army Medical Department Combat and Division Psychiatry Course; April 1984; San Antonio, Tex.

57. Roberts L. *Anxiety State and Battlefield Performance: A Negative Correlation.* [AST-266OR-031-83]. May 1983.

58. Pincus W. British got crucial data in Falklands, diary says. *Washington Post.* 23 December 1984: A1, A20.

59. Russell G. Falkland Islands: Explosions and breakthroughs. *Time.* 7 June 1982: 30–36.

60. Penetar D, Redmond D, Belenky G. Effects of triazolam on sleep and memory during long range deployments by air. *Aviat Space Environ Med.* 1980;60:594–598.

61. Skolnick P, Paul SM. Benzodiazepine receptors in the central nervous system. *Int Rev Neurobiol.* 1981;23:102–140.

62. Skolnick P, Paul S, Crawley J, et al. 3-hydroxymethyl-beta-carboline antagonizes some pharmacologic actions of diazepam. *Eur J Pharmacol.* 1981;69:525–527.

63. Shader RI, Goodman M, Gever J. Panic disorders: Current perspectives. *J Clin Psychopharmacol.* 1982;(6):2S–10S.

64. Muskin PR, Fyer AJ. Treatment of panic disorder. *J Clin Psychopharmacol.* 1981;1(2):81–90.

65. Paul SM. Interactions of antidepressants and anxiolytics with neurotransmitter receptors: Clinical implications. Presented at Army Medical Department Military Psychiatry Conference, Uniformed Services University of the Health Sciences; May 1982; Bethesda, Md.

66. Noy S. Combat psychiatry series. Presented to Division of Neuropsychiatry, Walter Reed Army Institute of Research; 1981; Washington, DC.

67. Datel WE, Johnson AW Jr. Psychotropic prescription medication in Vietnam. Available from Defense Technical Information Center, Alexandria, Va. [No. ADA 097610]. 1978.

68. Mattila MJ, Aranko K, Seppala T. Acute effects of buspirone and alcohol on psychomotor skills. *J Clin Psychiatry.* 1982;43(12):56–61.

69. Moskowitz H, Smiley A. Effects of chronically administered buspirone and diazepam on driving-related skills performance. *J Clin Psychiatry.* 1982;43(12):45–55.

70. Newton RE. Personal Communication, 1983.

71. Gorman JM, Liebowitz MR, Klein DF. *Panic Disorder and Agoraphobia: Current Concepts.* Kalamazoo, Mich: The Upjohn Company; 1984.

Chapter 6

A PSYCHOLOGICAL MODEL OF COMBAT STRESS

REUVEN GAL, Ph.D.* AND FRANKLIN D. JONES, M.D., F.A.P.A.†

*Colonel (res), Former Chief Psychologist, Israeli Defence Forces; Current Director, The Israeli Institute for Military Studies, 5 Kadesh St, Zikhron Ya'akov 30900 Israel

†Colonel (ret), Medical Corps, U.S. Army; Clinical Professor, Uniformed Services University of the Health Sciences, Bethesda, Maryland; Past President and Secretary and current Honorary President of the Military Section, World Psychiatric Association; formerly Psychiatry and Neurology Consultant, Office of The Surgeon General, U.S. Army

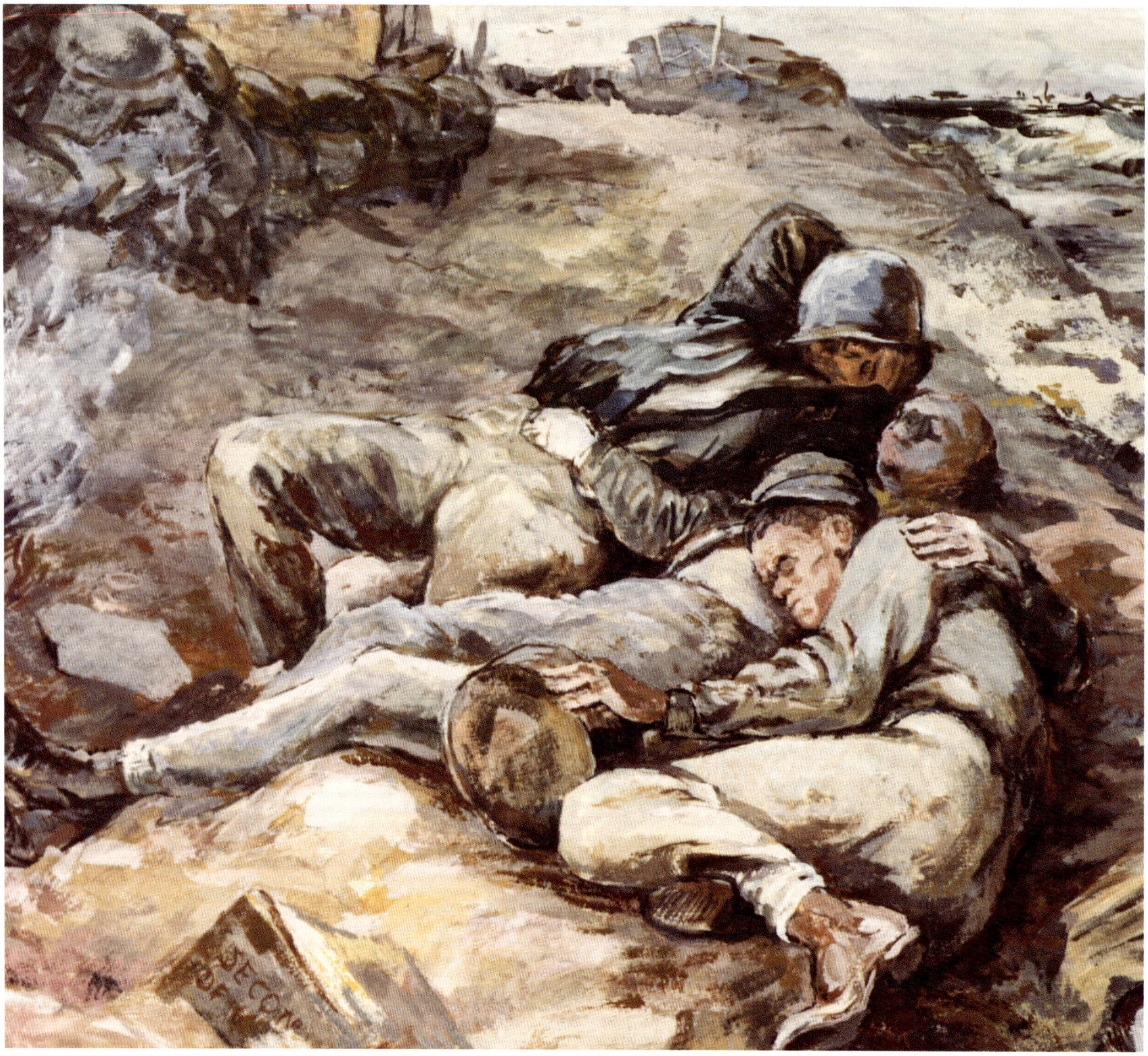

Manuel Bromberg *Soldiers Resting on Omaha Beach, Normandy* 1945

Manuel Bromberg was a member of the War Artist Unit for England and Ireland during World War II and was present during the invasion of Normandy. He does an exceptional job of visualizing the variables of combat stress (the individual, the unit, and the battlefield) in this watercolor of three exhausted soldiers from World War II trying to rest amidst the destruction about them.

Art: Courtesy of US Center of Military History, Washington, DC.

INTRODUCTION

The model presented in this chapter is a blend of theory and practice. The theoretical approach stems primarily from the cognitive theories of stress and coping, which emphasize the role of cognitive appraisal and active coping in the individual's response to stressful conditions.[1–4] The practical ideas are derived from the combat experiences of the senior author and those of his colleagues in the Israeli Defence Forces (IDF) and the junior author's combat experiences in Vietnam. These ideas were subsequently discussed and elaborated with well-seasoned IDF field commanders. The model has been used in lectures given at various senior command courses in the Israeli military and has been a useful tool for approaching the complexity of human behavior in groups under stress.

BACKGROUND TO THE MODEL

A number of studies related to World War II,[5,6] to the Korean and Vietnam conflicts,[7–9] and to the Arab-Israeli wars[10–12] have delineated variables that prevent or promote the individual's ability to cope with combat stress. These studies and the salient coping variables have been summarized by several authors.[10,13,14] Although these variables do not lack face validity, a coherent scheme of their interactions and their impact on subsequent combat stress reactions has been lacking. There have been attempts at a dynamic interpretation of the simple relation between nature, nurture, and combat stress, beginning as early as Salmon[15] and extending as recently as Shaw[16] and Milgram.[17] Yet the complexity of the combat situation calls for a multi-variable and rather complex, interactive model to account for the multitude of factors involved in the generation of, and consequent coping with, the stress of combat.

The proposed model is interactional in that it posits a number of antecedent variables acting through mediating variables to affect the individual's appraisal of the combat situation and subsequently result in the combatant's modes of response and coping with the realities of combat (Figure 6-1). Furthermore, the model is also dynamic wherein the individual's preferred coping behavior in turn affects his reappraisal of the situation and thus may further alter his combat responses.

The *antecedent variables* pertain to the individual, group, and environmental aspects and may conveniently be categorized as follows:

- Individual factors—personality, nonmilitary stress (family, etc), prior combat exposure, role in combat.
- Unit factors—cohesion and morale, training, leadership, and commitment.
- Battlefield factors—type of battle, surprise and uncertainty, environmental factors (weather, terrain, etc).

These antecedent variables, according to the proposed model, do not directly determine the soldier's appraisal of the combat situation; rather, they are mediated by other variables—the *mediating variables*—in an interactive manner. Of paramount importance in the soldier's expectation or interpretation of the immediate situation is the role his commanders (or persons in leadership positions) play in providing the information concerning the impending military operation. Thus, the way in which he is briefed and the way in which orders are given, interacting with the antecedent variables, will strongly color his evaluation (ie, appraisal) of both the nature of the stress and his ability to handle it. The role of the commander, then, becomes that of a *lens*, that is, either magnifying or minimizing the impact of the (objective) antecedent variables on the soldier's (subjective) cognitive appraisal.

The *appraisal process*, which is the central notion in this model, may vary along a wide range of alternatives: the exact situation may be assessed by different individuals or at different moments as a terrifying, benign, or challenging situation—depending upon the interactive consequences of the given antecedent and mediating factors. The individual's initial modes of response to and coping with a combat situation will reflect his own process of cognitive appraisal. *Response patterns* may be divided into the traditional categories of physical, emotional, cognitive, and social. These immediate, somewhat universal patterns of response will in

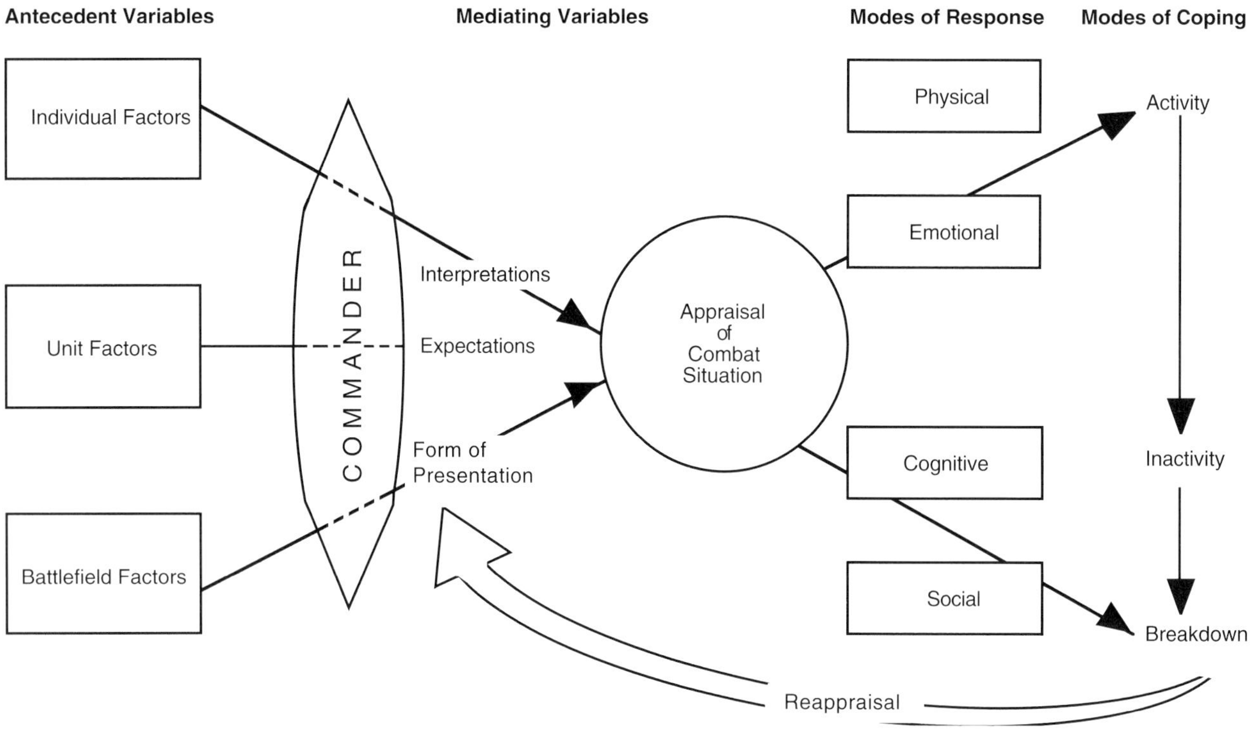

Fig. 6-1. A model of soldier behavior in combat stress conditions. This model is interactional in that it posits a number of antecedent variables acting through mediating variables to affect the individual's appraisal of the combat situation and subsequently result in the combatant's modes of response and coping with the realities of combat. The model is dynamic in that the individual's preferred coping behavior in turn affects his reappraisal of the situation and thus may further alter his combat responses. The role of the commander becomes that of a lens, magnifying or minimizing the impact of the (objective) antecedent variables on the soldier's (subjective) cognitive appraisal.

turn produce individual *modes of coping* ranging from an optimal mode (normally involving a high, goal-oriented level of activity) to limited coping (frequently characterized by passivity) to grossly disturbed coping (breakdown).

The modes of coping actually utilized will influence, in a feedback manner, the individual's *reappraisal* of the newly perceived situation and of his already tested capabilities to cope with it. Thus, the cognitive appraisal processes are in a state of dynamic flux, originally affected by the antecedent factors but consequently reflecting also the initial reactions made by the individual. The new appraisal will then lead to different modes of response leading to different modes of coping and a further new and different appraisal.

The following sections will further detail each of the components of the proposed model and will attempt to empirically substantiate the proposed relationships between them. This analysis will involve direct combat experience as well as relevant research.

ANTECEDENT VARIABLES

Two main groups of variables, antecedent and mediating, lead to the initial appraisal of the stress situation. The antecedent variables comprise those factors that are in the background of the combat situation; they may be categorized as individual factors, unit factors, and battlefield factors.

Individual Factors

Among the individual factors that any combatant brings along with him to the battlefield are his personality dispositions and his general well-being. These, together with his previous combat experience and his role in combat, determine the first category of the antecedent variables.

Personality Dispositions

Notwithstanding the almost obvious expectation that behavior in the face of battle should be somehow linked to the warrior's personality, very little empirical evidence has been found linking individual personality factors and combat behavior, either in terms of outstanding performance or breakdown.[18] One extensive study,[19] however, did find several characteristics that distinguish "fighters" (soldiers who had received, or had been recommended for, a decoration for valor in combat or were evaluated by peers as high performers) from "nonfighters" (soldiers who were evaluated by peers as poor performers, or admitted themselves as such). Among the differences revealed in that study, the "fighters" tended to be more intelligent, "masculine," and socially mature; and showed greater emotional stability and stronger leadership potential.

Indeed, military organizations tend to consider personality variables in selecting personnel for combat roles, particularly leadership roles and special operations. This preselection procedure may, in fact, by virtue of restricting the range for study, account for the difficulties in establishing empirical correlations between personality dispositions and combat performance. Gal,[20] for example, in a study of soldiers awarded medals for bravery in the 1973 Yom Kippur War found only a few differences in personality characteristics between the decorated soldiers and a matched sample of combat soldiers not so recognized. These personality characteristics were part of the officer selection process that many of the soldiers awarded medals had gone through. Medal recipients, as compared with their peers, showed higher scores in leadership, devotion to duty, decisiveness, and perseverance under stress. Sociability, social intelligence, and emotional stability did not distinguish the two groups.

With regard to psychiatric breakdown among members of combat units, Noy[21] found that while personality characteristics did not predict such breakdown, they were significant in recovery after breakdown. Men with massive repression of hostility or anxiety, particularly if coupled with situational stress at home, had a poorer prognosis. It is quite evident, then, as concluded by Glass in his summary of the "lessons learned" from World War II, that "the frequency of psychiatric disorders [in combat] seemed to be more related to the characteristics of the group than to the character traits of the involved individuals."[13(p995)]

Individual's Well-Being

While personality dispositions refer to longstanding traits of the individual himself, well-being refers to relationships between the individual and his environment.[22] Such relationships may directly affect combat behavior as shown in the Israeli experience of the 1973 Yom Kippur War.[21] In a group of 40 Israeli soldiers who suffered battle shock, 80% had prior or ongoing civilian stresses. About one half had pregnant wives or were new fathers during the year preceding the war and about one fourth of them had experienced a recent death in the immediate family. Other relevant civil stresses consisted of being newly married or separated and economic or family problems.

A World War II study[23] reported that 20% of psychiatric cases complained of "homesickness" as a significant stress. An even more striking difference between those who became psychiatric casualties and a nonafflicted comparison group was found when variables such as family, school, work, and social, recreational, and community adjustments were examined. Soldiers with impairments in these areas were found to have about a two to four times greater likelihood of breaking down.[23]

More recent studies have shown high levels of self-reported well-being to be a distinct characteristic of elite combat units.[24] Whether operating as a causal factor in facilitating volunteering to elite units, or emerging as a concomitant of belonging to such units, personal sense of well-being is evidently an important antecedent factor for any combatant facing the impending stress of combat.

Previous Combat Experience

The effect of previous experience on fear reactions was demonstrated in studies conducted with combat-like performance. Epstein[25] and his colleague[26] have demonstrated that experienced parachutists showed different patterns of subjective fear and physiological reactions as compared to novice jumpers.

Actual combat experience obviously has an even stronger effect. Indeed it has been recognized, at least since World War II, that initial exposure to combat on the one hand and cumulative combat stress on the other hand result in higher rates of psychiatric breakdown. Units with high percentages of "green" soldiers tended to have higher numbers of psychiatric casualties.[27] Clearly the soldier with prior combat experience has less chance of breakdown in subsequent exposure, until the point (about 30 combat days, defined as days in which a company suffered at least one wounded in action [WIA] or killed in action [KIA]) that cumulative stress begins to produce combat inefficiency.[28]

Apparently even the soldier who has broken down, if properly treated with "forward treatment,"[15] has no greater chance of breakdown again than his combat peers. Looking at Israeli soldiers who had become psychiatric casualties in 1973 and who subsequently served in the 1982 Lebanon War, Solomon, Oppenheimer, and Noy[29] found no significant increased recurrence of psychiatric breakdown among those with prior breakdown if they had been found fit for combat. It should be recognized, however, that a significantly smaller percentage of soldiers who had had psychiatric breakdowns were found fit for combat compared to those who had not (40% versus 75% in nonpsychiatric controls) but this may have been a result of lack of "forward treatment" in 1973.

It might be summarized, then, that previous combat experience may have an enhancing or an inhibiting effect on the soldier's reactions to subsequent exposure to combat—depending on whether the previous experience had been a traumatic or a nontraumatic one.

Role in Combat

One's role in combat, whether formally assigned or assumed during the vicissitudes of combat, plays a crucial role in his appraisal of the situation and thus in his method of coping. In general, engaging in an assigned role that involves some form of mission-oriented tasks will create a sense of mastery and control as well as distract the soldier from his impending danger.[4]

The leadership role in a combat situation is particularly important for coping behavior. Bourne, Rose, and Mason,[30] for example, in studies conducted during the Vietnam conflict, have shown significantly different patterns of hormonal responses (normally associated with stress) between officers and enlisted men of a 12-man group who were anticipating engagement in combat. The chronic levels of steroid excretion of officers were higher than those of their enlisted men and rose even higher on the day of anticipated attack. The senior radio operator's steroid excretion also rose; indeed, his role was closer to that of the officers, and reflected again the importance of his role assignment in combat.

Unlike Bourne and his colleagues, who equate steroid excretion with levels of psychological stress in combat, the authors believe that the level of steroid excretion reflects physiological arousal and that the leadership role may actually be less psychologically stressful because the leaders are better prepared for combat and have more control over combat situations. Support for this hypothesis may be seen in the work of Miller,[31] and Miller and colleagues,[32] with pilots and their radar intercept officers during stressful aircraft landing procedures. They found that while the radar intercept officers had lower levels of steroid excretion, the pilots, who had active control over the flights, reported fewer somatic complaints and significantly lower levels of anxiety than the radar intercept officers.

In support of these studies there are numerous personal observations that show that the leadership role supports superior combat performance and protects the leader from disabling psychological stress. The senior author both personally observed and had many communications from Israeli field commanders describing the mastery, confidence, and even daring they have derived, under fire, from the awareness of their leadership role and the expectations of their men.

During the 1973 Yom Kippur War, Israeli commanders were under the greatest combat danger, being in the forefront of the engagement. This danger is reflected in the fact that a commander had four times the chance of being killed compared with his men.[33] Despite the presumed increased risk of battle stress, Levav and others[34] showed that the rate of psychiatric breakdown among officers was one fifth that of enlisted men. On the other pole of battlefield performance, that of bravery in battle, the number of Israeli combat officers awarded medals for extraordinary acts of bravery was much higher (64% of the total) than their proportion in the line units.[20] When noncommissioned officers are included with commissioned officers, the percentage of medals for bravery rises to 88% awarded to persons in leadership roles, thus inverting the ratio of leaders-to-led.[35]

In conclusion, under battlefield conditions, perceived role is a critical factor in both combat effectiveness and resistance to breakdown. Perceived role serves adaptive coping purposes through the interplay of three psychosocial mechanisms: (1) the expectations attached to the role (especially the leadership role), (2) the sense of mastery and control associated with the role, and (3) concentration on the tasks required by the role distracts attention from the realistic dangers of combat.

To summarize, one can see that while there are only limited data to show that personality dispositions predict combat behavior, there is good evidence for the importance of background conditions such as the individual's well-being, his previous combat experience, and his perceived role in combat.

Unit Factors

In most cases the individual will not operate alone but will be part of a group in combat. The group's size (significant for the individual combatant) may vary from three or four (as in a fire team or tank crew) to larger formations such as companies or even battalions. These group characteristics, similar to individual characteristics, have important implications for combat behavior. Since the 1973 Yom Kippur War, the IDF has deployed field psychologists to all of its line brigades to survey morale factors at various organizational levels and report back to unit commanders. Systematic analysis[36] of these surveys revealed four general factors important in determining unit climate. These consisted of unit cohesion and morale; confidence in commanders; confidence in weapons and in oneself as a combatant; and ideology, values, and commitment.

Unit Cohesion and Morale

Unit cohesion and morale have repeatedly been found important in supporting individual coping behavior and unit performance both in wartime[5] and in peacetime.[37,38] Among other variables, they were found to affect critically the rates of psychiatric breakdown in combat.[13] In the words of Glass:

> Repeated observations indicated that the absence or inadequacy of such sustaining influences [which he termed "group identification," "group cohesiveness," "the buddy system," and "leadership"] or their disruption during combat was mainly responsible for psychiatric breakdown in battle. These group or relationship phenomena explained marked differences in the psychiatric casualty rates of various units who were exposed to a similar intensity of battle stress.[13(p995)]

In recent studies based on Israeli experiences during the 1973 Yom Kippur War, the relationship between unit cohesion and morale and coping behavior was reconfirmed. In a retrospective examination of 40 IDF soldiers who suffered psychiatric breakdown in that war, Noy[21] found that 40% of these casualties reported minimal group affiliation in contrast to only 10% in a control group of noncasualties. Similarly, Steiner and Neumann[39] found the following characteristics in 74 reserve soldiers presenting with acute or late onset of posttraumatic combat reactions after the 1973 Yom Kippur War: low morale, with little or no identification with their unit or team; lack of trust in leadership; frequent transfer or rotation; feelings of loneliness and not belonging to their units; and low self-esteem concerning their military performance.

Thus, a low level of morale and weak bonds with comrades and leaders may elevate the perceived stress of combat and ultimately result in severe combat reactions. This indeed happened in units with low cohesion and low morale. At the other end of the spectrum, elite units, famous for their high degree of cohesion and morale, have consistently had low psychiatric casualty rates despite frequent exposure to high-intensity battle stress.

Confidence in Commanders

The paramount importance of the role of leadership in combat has been recognized since antiquity. The history of battle has always been the history of leaders building their subordinates' confidence to achieve victories. Whether the fighting unit is a small band of warriors with spears or a vast army with laser-aimed rifles and bombs, their confidence in the leader is essential.

Contemporary studies[40–42] confirm the crucial role of unit commanders in preparing troops for combat, enhancing troop morale, and leading them courageously in battle. The soldier's confidence in the commander is also critical in protecting him from overwhelming battle stress. In Israeli studies during the 1982 Lebanon War, Kalay[43] found three elements that inspired confidence in the commander: (1) belief in the professional competence of the commander, (2) belief in his credibility, and (3) the perception that he cares about his troops. While in garrison all three components are equally important; in combat, trust in the commander's professional competence becomes primary.

In reviews of Israeli morale surveys during both the 1973 Yom Kippur War and the 1982 Lebanon War, the senior author[12] compared the levels of confidence soldiers had in commanders at various command levels, from platoon to division. While assessments before combat showed an almost linear increase in the confidence of troops in their commanders with increasing levels of command (ie, lowest at the platoon leader and highest at the division commander levels), after combat the trend was generally reversed with the highest levels of confidence shown in the more immediate commanders (platoon, company, battalion) and relatively lower confidence at the more remote levels of command (brigade, division). This difference may be accounted for on the basis that prior to battle the soldier perceives his welfare and success as being dependent on higher command plans and decisions; but, in actual combat, he finds that his very survival depends mainly on the actions of his more immediate leaders.

It is apparent, then, that despite marked changes in the configuration and technology of the battlefield, the confidence troops have in their commanders at all levels is a critical ingredient in the soldiers' process of coping with the stresses of battle.

Confidence as a Soldier

As described earlier, "green troops" suffer higher rates of psychiatric casualties than battle-experienced troops. This may well reflect the importance of increased confidence of the soldier in his own battle skills.

Confidence in one's weapons and in one's proficiency as a combatant has been shown to be important for the soldier's morale. In a morale survey among Israeli soldiers anticipating combat, Gal[36] reported high correlations between their personal level of morale and both confidence in themselves as combatants and confidence in the unit's weapons system.

Furthermore, Steiner and Neumann,[39] studying the combat experiences of Israeli veterans of the 1973 Yom Kippur War, examined among other variables the relationship between self-confidence in military performance and the development of posttraumatic stress disorders. They found that 46% of 74 soldiers suffering traumatic reactions evaluated their military performance and knowledge as poor. In contrast, only 3% of 100 soldiers in a nonafflicted control group reported such lack of self-confidence.

Another source of the soldier's confidence is his familiarity with his mission, with the operational terrain, and with the exact location of friendly and enemy forces.[36] Because one of the well-established sources of anxiety is fear of the unknown and the unfamiliar, introducing the soldier to the details of his mission, the terrain, and the deployment of forces will ultimately reduce his anxiety level.

These aspects of a soldier's self-confidence—trust in one's own combat skills, in weapons systems, and familiarity with missions and terrain—are all created within the unit framework during training periods. Knowledge of missions and terrain is not learned during training in the United States as it is in Israel because of the wider range of scenarios. The more realistic the training, the better prepared the soldier will be. However, the growing sophistication (and expense) of modern weaponry has resulted in the increasing use of training by simulation devices, which may act against the accomplishment of such realistic training. Simulation training, while usually accurate in its technical aspects, is quite dissimilar from the arduous and horrifying conditions of combat.[44] Military training, therefore, must aim not only at producing technical proficiency with one's weapon but also at developing soldierly skills and proficiency to serve the soldier as a psychological defense mechanism against the strenuous conditions of the battlefield.

Ideology, Values, and Commitment

It is commonly believed that a strong ideological conviction plays a significant role in combat motivation. Obviously, when a soldier believes that he is defending his homeland, he may derive additional strength to face the horrors of battle. However, while it is evident that such ideological convictions foster the joining of a military organization, there is little empirical data supporting the position that such feelings enhance performance or prevent breakdown in the midst of a combat situation. In fact, observations by acknowledged military experts have deemphasized the importance of ideology when survival on the battlefield is at stake. For example, S.L.A. Marshall, after visiting Israel and discovering the importance of nationalist feelings to its citizens, gave his own judgment:

> But for my own part, I reject finally the idea that the extraordinary elan of that Army in combat comes from self-identification of the individual with the goals of his nation in the hour when his life is in danger. That is not the nature of man under battle; his thoughts are as local as is his view of the nearest ground cover, and unless he feels a solidarity with the people immediately around him and is carried forward by their momentum, neither thoughts about the ideals of his country nor reflections on his love for his wife will keep him from diving toward the nearest protection.[45(p304)]

In a similar vein, Field Marshall Montgomery, in referring to patriotic feelings and historical roots of combat motivation, deliberately downplayed these factors: "[I]n the crisis of battle the majority of men will not derive encouragement from the glories of the past but will seek aid from their leaders and comrades of the present."[46(p21)]

Despite this discounting of idealistic feelings as a factor in actual combat, there is evidence that a soldier's perception of the legitimacy of his side's participation in war is important for his morale. A morale survey conducted among IDF troops prior to the Israeli incursion into Lebanon found a positive correlation between the soldiers' morale level and their belief that invading Lebanon was justified.[36]

A similar relationship between morale and perceived legitimacy of one's side in a war probably could have been found in Vietnam. Renner[47] and Gabriel and Savage[48] have argued that after 1968, soldiers' perceptions that the U.S. presence was not legitimate led to unit disintegration as evidenced by "fragging" (assassination of one's leaders), desertion, drug abuse during combat, and combat refusals.

It was reported[49] that Soviet soldiers stationed in Afghanistan during the mid-1980s invasion suffered low morale and engaged in widespread drug abuse and some fragging similar to U.S. soldiers in the late phases of the Vietnam conflict. Defecting soldiers in Afghanistan related this to loss of belief in the legitimacy of the war: "It's a stupid war, not useful to anyone."[49]

Ideological concerns thus seem most important when legitimacy is questionable, or in wars of low intensity with intermittent combat, and in the anticipation before battles or during lulls between battles. In the heat of battle, however, ideological motivation is replaced by other unit factors such as leadership, unit cohesion, and combat skillfulness.

Battlefield Factors

The third group of antecedent variables, battlefield factors, may play a decisive role in promoting combat stress because they include the nature of the threat and the environment of the battlefield. Most battlefields have unique features that generate different levels of stress. The World War II U.S. battles on Okinawa and Normandy, for example, both beginning as amphibious invasions, had vastly different characteristics and quite different rates of psychiatric casualties: very high in Okinawa and overall relatively low in Normandy. The Israeli 1967 Six-Day War and 1973 Yom Kippur War were both brief and of high intensity but differed markedly in the impact on troop morale and psychiatric casualties: almost none in the former and relatively high in the latter.

The main components in this last category of antecedent variables are the type of battle, its length and intensity, the uncertain elements of battle, and the physical characteristics of the battlefield.

Type of Battle

Offensive and defensive operations differ in generating stress reactions. In defensive operations, especially with impending danger but without active engagement to break the tension, the soldier is subjected to an enforced passivity and experiences a feeling of helplessness. By contrast, in offensive operations, even though the risk may be greater, the soldier is active, has a vicarious sense of control over the situation, and is distracted from personal concerns.[4] Similarly, during static situations such as being pinned down for long periods, perhaps by artillery fire or similar situations of immobility, stress casualties are higher than in mobile situations such as advancing or even retreating.[50]

Day vs night operations may also generate different stress reactions in synergy with other situations. For example, at nighttime the soldier in a defensive posture may have his feelings of isolation accentuated by darkness. On the other hand, daytime operations with active engagement of the enemy may allow the soldier to see his wounded and dead comrades, adding to his battle stress. Unfortunately, no clear data indicating increased pathogenicity for either situation exist.

Length and Intensity of Combat

Length of exposure to combat has been correlated with cumulative stress[28,51] while intensity of combat is more related to acute stress.[50] In furthering this distinction, some authors refer to the consequences of cumulative stress as "combat exhaustion" or "fatigue" and of acute stress as "battle shock."

Several authors have attempted a predictive model of breakdown based on duration of combat exposure[28,51] or intensity of combat.[52–54] Swank and Marchand[28] found that most psychiatric casualties occurred after 30 to 45 days of exposure to combat.

Beebe and Appel, on the other hand, predicted that "the breaking point of the average rifleman seems to have been reached at about 88 days of company combat [days in which a company casualty occurred]."[51(p163)]

A number of authors[10,13,50,52–55] have observed the relationship between combat intensity, as indicated by wounded and killed in action (WIA and KIA), and combat breakdown. Normally, the rate of psychiatric casualties will fluctuate in proportion to the WIA. In prior wars this ratio has ranged from 1:3 to 1:1; however, in low-intensity, intermittent combat, psychiatric casualties are less directly related to combat and take different forms.[47,56,57]

To summarize what is known about the relationship between duration of exposure to combat and the likelihood of combat stress breakdown, it appears that some minimum amount of exposure to combat is necessary to enhance soldiers' confidence and decrease their vulnerability to breakdown. Beyond that exposure threshold, increased exposure to combat eventually weakens the soldiers' defenses against breakdown.

Battle Anticipation, Uncertainty, and Surprise

As alluded to earlier, the anticipation of battle may be more stressful than actual battle.[4] A well-known syndrome described by World War II physicians as the "precombat syndrome"[58] consisted of vague complaints without identifiable physical findings among those scheduled for combat, for example, air crews awaiting a bombing run. Furthermore, Jones[59] noted that there were numerous psychiatric complaints in the 25th U.S. Army Division in the several months when deployment to Vietnam was uncertain, but fewer when it became definite.

Generally, troops prefer to avoid impending threats of combat; however, long periods of anticipation may result in paradoxical positive feelings concerning impending combat. The first author has monitored the feelings of combat anticipation of a group of infantrymen stationed in a combat zone for 3 weeks. He found an inverted U-shaped curve peaking at 10 days measuring strong anticipation of actual engagement with the enemy. This response pattern reflects the mounting anticipation during the ascending limb and a growing desire to relieve the anticipatory anxiety with action. The descending limb may reflect a desire to avoid combat altogether because relief was becoming imminent.

Breznitz,[60] among others, has discussed this reaction pattern in his study of "incubation of threat." According to Breznitz, two conflicting tendencies may operate simultaneously in an anticipatory period. On the one hand, the person gradually relaxes after the initial introduction of the threat. On the other hand, there is increasing excitation as actual occurrence of the threatening event approaches. In cases where a U-shaped curve is exhibited by stress reactions, this curve may be the net result of these two processes.

Uncertainty can take two forms: temporal uncertainty in which the time when an event will occur is unknown and event uncertainty in which the time is known but the nature of an event is unknown. Situations involving both types of uncertainty are common in combat. In general, the greater the uncertainty, the greater the stress.[61,62]

Although anticipation and uncertainty create high levels of stress, a surprise aversive event is even more stressful. The initial phase of a surprise attack may maximize panic and psychiatric breakdown. According to senior Egyptian Army psychiatrists, this was reflected in high psychiatric casualties among Egyptian soldiers in the early period following the 1967 surprise attack by Israel.[63] Likewise numerous psychiatric casualties among Israeli troops occurred in the first hours and days following the surprise attack by Arab forces in the 1973 Yom Kippur War.[11]

Environmental Conditions

Some of the antecedent factors are not necessarily born in combat, but they affect combat performance. For example, when combatants are rapidly transported to a new and unfamiliar environment, they must first adjust or acclimate before performing at their optimum.[64] Furthermore, harsh environments such as arctic or tropical climates, wet, or other inclement weather increase combat stress casualties, probably through the increased physiological stresses added to the psychological stresses of combat. Numerous authors have commented on the deleterious effects of adverse environmental conditions on morale[5] (ie, strange terrain such as that found in the desert, the jungle, the steppes—lacking usual landmarks) and on the soldier's ability to cope in combat.[65]

Masked psychiatric conditions ranging from frostbite or immersion foot in cold or wet climates to dehydration in hot or dry climates exemplify the relationship between combat breakdown and adverse environments.[66]

MEDIATING VARIABLES

While antecedent variables are important in the soldier's appraisal of the combat situation, their impact on the individual's response and coping behavior is determined by mediating variables. These variables are, in the first place, cognitive in their nature, involving cognitive interpretations of the antecedents, a logical evaluation of the situation, and a buildup of expectations both of one's behavior and of the consequences of the entire situation.

A second characteristic of these mediating variables is that they are largely controlled by the commander who may give them a positive or negative connotation. For example, a determined, confident commander, who conveys to his troops his optimistic view, will actually increase the chances of success, assuming that the optimism is realistic. On the other hand, an unenthusiastic, subdued, or frightened presentation will create uncertainty or fear and result in less resolute, more pessimistic appraisals, increasing the possibility of failure.

The commander plays a central role in creating the individual's appraisal of the situation by acting as a lens (see Figure 6-1) that focuses the antecedent variables into a unified interpretation of the situation. Like in a telescope, this "lens" works (with regard to the stress of combat) to amplify the perceived threat or to reduce it, make it closer or more remote, better focused or more blurred. Though it may not be possible to modify many of the antecedent variables, the commander can be trained to present and interpret information regarding these antecedents in an optimal manner and hence create an expectation of success.

A third characteristic of the mediating variables is their dynamic quality. While the antecedent factors may change or remain the same, the interpretation given to them may vary as new information becomes available or as behavior changes as a consequence of the appraisal. A heroic or cowardly act by oneself or a comrade, for example, will change the initial interpretation of the situation and lead to changed responses.

It must be realized that there are not clear-cut distinctions between the antecedent and mediating variables. Interpretations and expectations may stem directly from the individual's predispositions or be part of a unit characteristic. These antecedent and mediating variables are schematically presented separately in the model for purposes of clarity only.

THE APPRAISAL PROCESS

The appraisal is the bridge between the external conditions and the soldier's response. It is the combination of the soldier's perception and evaluation of both the situation and his own capability to cope with it. The same situation may result in a whole spectrum of appraisals by various individuals or by the same individual at different times. Thus, a given combat situation may appear lethal, hazardous, adventurous, or auspicious, while the individual reaction to it may range from being terrified or threatened to challenged or excited.

The appraisal process further determines the course of action that an individual might take when faced with a stressful situation. This is reflected directly, for example, in the work of Grinker and Spiegel on combat stress in World War II. As these authors noted, "appraisal of the situation requires mental activity involving judgment, discrimination and choice of activity."[6(p122)]

Lazarus and his colleagues[3,67] have empirically demonstrated the dominance of the cognitive appraisal process in determining the emotional and behavioral responses of groups and individuals to stress. In a series of studies[3] in which audiences viewed highly distressing films, the responses of the audience were clearly determined by a narrative voice that interpreted the ordeal as ranging from traumatic to neutral, intellectualized, or benign (through denial-like processes). Though the subjects all saw exactly the same film, their reactions were drastically different as a function of the sound track the introduction provided before the film. Using the neutral group as a reference, the trauma group showed marked elevation of physiological and psychological distress while the intellectual and denial groups showed reduction in distress. Subsequent experiments using the same paradigm revealed different stress reactions as a function of the conditions (ie, length of anticipatory time, level of uncertainty) on which the appraisal process depended, the type of cognitive activities (ie, detachment or involvement) required from the subjects, and as a function of individual differences.

Thus, the same situation may generate different responses depending on the type of interpretation or expectation suggested prior to or during the situation. Likewise, an individual or group reaction to battlefield conditions can be determined by the mediating variables (interpretations, expectations, form of presentation), which are primarily controlled by the commander. From these different appraisals will result the different modes of response or coping.

MODES OF RESPONSE

The modes of response to stressful combat situations may be categorized as follows:

- *Physical:* includes autonomic changes (tachycardia, vasoconstriction, sweating, increased gastrointestinal motility), musculoskeletal changes (increased tonicity and perfusion of blood to muscle), and glandular changes (release of medullary and cortical hormones from the adrenal glands producing many of the foregoing effects).
- *Emotional:* includes a variety of affective reactions varying from enthusiastic excitement to apprehensive fear, anxiety, or depression.
- *Cognitive:* includes distortion of perception with narrowing of attention span, hyperalertness to certain stimuli, and increased utilization of automatic or overlearned responses.
- *Social:* includes increased dependency on leadership and need of affiliation, sometimes expressed by seeking reassurance and physical clustering. Negative aspects may be an increased tendency to make demands and irritability.

These reactions are universal. Alerting the soldier to their anticipated appearance under stress by reassuring him that they are normal and are preparing the body for combat will serve a preventive and therapeutic purpose. The appraisal plays a lesser role in eliciting or controlling these responses than it does with the coping responses, which will be discussed next.

While the modes of response (in this model) are relatively involuntary or automatic, immediate, and brief, the individual's modes of coping are more flexible, voluntary, and may be delayed and prolonged. The former may only to some extent be conditioned through training; the latter are highly influenced by training and strongly determined by the instant conditions of combat.

MODES OF COPING

The individual's appraisal of the situation and the variety of modes of response are incorporated into an integrated or holistic mode of coping, ranging from various levels of activity through passivity to actual breakdown. The active mode of coping may take various forms. During combat anticipation (almost always present on the battlefield), activity may take the form of preparation—checking gear, plans, or last minute details. Activity may not necessarily be directly related to the threat, and can include card playing, book reading, letter writing, and so forth. These activities, nonetheless, serve as successful coping behavior because they distract the individual from considering the death or wounding that may await him in battle, and sustain and promote cohesion and resolve. This behavior, particularly when it takes the form of combat preparations, also gives the soldier a sense of mastery over the situation, diminishing anxiety.[4]

During combat, the active-coping mode is seen in controlled aggression by the combat soldier: seeking shelter, firing weaponry, scanning or scouting the terrain, etc. Similarly, the combat-support soldier will stay active in his respective duties. The consequences of this active mode are usually greater initiative, innovation, bravery, and successful accomplishment of the mission. Rarely, this activity is not mission-oriented and results in inefficiency in combat.

Relative inactivity or even passivity in the combat situation is manifested by decreased movements, relative apathy to the surroundings and mission, and lack of initiative. The observation during World War II and the Korean conflict that only a small percentage of soldiers fired their weapons[68] probably applies to this group of combatants. A consequence of this unsuccessful coping mode is not only a failure to perform effectively but also a beginning of a psychological collapse, exhibited by increasing fatigue, mounting anxiety, and a sense of burnout. The ultimate result of a passive mode of coping may be a complete breakdown, whether labeled combat fatigue, battle shock, or war neurosis. This breakdown occurs when the soldier's preoccupation with his own anxieties leads to removal from battle, shutdown, immobility, and erratic behavior.

Whatever mode of coping is utilized by the individual, it is not only an outcome of the combat appraisal and modes of response but also serves as an input into the ongoing reappraisal of the situation. Based on his own mode of coping, the soldier may now reinterpret the combat situation. This in turn may generate new modes of response and coping that further modify the appraisal. Typically, if a successful active-coping mode took place, the reappraisal process tends to be in the direction of optimism. Conversely, passive coping usually will lead to a pessimistic appraisal, resultant less-effective modes of response and coping, and increasingly negative appraisals. Thus, the behavior of the soldier in combat is an ongoing process of appraisals and reappraisals (largely unconscious appraisal and reappraisal) that are affected by his perception of the situation on one hand and his initial responses and coping on the other hand. The leader can optimize his own coping by good training, keeping himself functioning, and taking care of junior leaders, and by intervening at key times and places with his troops.

SUMMARY AND CONCLUSION

This model of combat stress is complex in that there are multiple interacting variables in its application and, furthermore, the variables interact in an ongoing, circular fashion. Despite its complexity, the model is operationally applicable. A combat leader who is aware of the multiple variables mediating stress in battle can understand and anticipate both the behavior of troops and of himself, and take preventive measures to diminish the stress. Understanding the ongoing, circular nature of these variables, he can intervene to reduce the stresses, the anxiety, and ultimately the potential for breakdown.

This model can be taught in varied types of leadership training. For example, in the Israeli Defence Forces Staff and Command School, officers who were combat veterans were presented with the model and encouraged to test it against their personal experiences. Almost unanimously, these officers gave positive evaluations of the validity of the model for combat. The best didactic approach seemed to be through an initial presentation of the model followed by small-group interaction in which instructors guided the discussion. The small-group participants explored the applicability of the model to their own experiences.

Students of war and combat agree that the most precious commodity in battle is not armaments but people. The understanding and application of this model may conserve and increase the efficiency of the vital human resource.

REFERENCES

1. Lazarus RS. *Stress and the Coping Process*. New York: McGraw-Hill; 1966.
2. Arnold MB. *Emotion and Personality*. New York: Columbia University Press; 1960.
3. Lazarus RS, Folkman S. *Stress, Appraisal, and Coping*. New York: Springer; 1984.
4. Gal R, Lazarus RS. The role of activity in anticipating and confronting stressful situations. *J Human Stress* [now *Behav Med*]. 1975;1(4):4–20.
5. Stouffer SA, DeVinney LC, Star SA, Williams RM. *Studies in Social Psychology in World War II*: Vol 2. *The American Soldier: Combat and its Aftermath*. Princeton, NJ: Princeton University Press; 1949.
6. Grinker RR, Spiegel JP. *Men Under Stress*. New York: McGraw-Hill; 1945.
7. Davis SW. Stress in combat. *Sci Am*. 1956;194:31–35.

8. Bourne PG, ed. *The Psychology and Physiology of Stress: With Reference to Special Studies of the Vietnam War*. New York: Academic Press; 1969.

9. Jones FD, Johnson AW. Medical and psychiatric treatment policy and practice in Vietnam. *J Soc Issues*. 1975;31(4):49–65.

10. Solomon Z. *Combat Stress Reactions: The Enduring Toll of War*. New York: Plenum Publishing; 1993.

11. Belenky G, Noy S, Solomon Z. Battle stress, morale, cohesion, combat effectiveness, heroism, and psychiatric casualties: The Israeli experience. In: Belenky G, ed. *Contemporary Studies in Combat Psychiatry*. Westport, Conn: Greenwood Press; 1987: 11–20.

12. Gal R. *A Portrait of the Israeli Soldier*. Westport, Conn: Greenwood Press; 1986.

13. Glass AJ. Lessons learned. In: Glass AJ, ed. *Overseas Theaters*. Vol 2. In: *Neuropsychiatry in World War II*. Washington, DC: Office of The Surgeon General, US Army; 1973: 989–1027.

14. Jones FD. Combat stress: Tripartite model. *Int Rev Army Navy Air Force Med Serv (France)*. 1981;55:303–307.

15. Salmon TW. The care and treatment of mental diseases and war neurosis ("shell shock") in the British Army. In: Bailey P, Williams FE, Komora PA, Salmon TW, Fenton N, eds. *Neuropsychiatry*. Vol 10. In: *The Medical Department of the United States Army in the World War*. Washington, DC: Office of The Surgeon General, US Army; 1929: Appendix; 497–523.

16. Shaw JA. Comments on the individual psychology of combat exhaustion. *Milit Med*. 1983;148(3):223–225, 229–231.

17. Milgram NA. Personality factors in military psychology. In: Gal R, Mangelsdorff AD, eds. *Handbook of Military Psychology*. West Sussex, England: John Wiley & Sons; 1991: 559–572.

18. Gal R. Personality and intelligence in the military: The case of war heroes. In: Saklofske D, Zeidner M, eds. *International Handbook of Personality and Intelligence*. New York: Plenum Publishing; in press.

19. Egbert RL, Meeland R, Cline VB, Forgy EW, Spickter MW, Brown C. *Fighter 1: An Analysis of Combat Fighters and Non-fighters*. Monterey, Calif: US Army Leadership Human Research Unit; 1957. HumRRO Technical Report #44.

20. Gal R. Courage under stress. In: Breznitz S, ed. *Stress in Israel*. New York: Van Nostrand Reinhold Company; 1983: 65–91.

21. Noy S. Stress and personality as factors in the causation and prognosis of combat reaction. In: Belenky G, ed. *Contemporary Studies in Combat Psychiatry*. Westport, Conn: Greenwood Press; 1987: 21–29.

22. Campbell A. *The Sense of Well-being in America*. New York: McGraw Hill; 1981.

23. Brill NQ, Beebe GW. *A Follow-up Study of War Neuroses*. Washington, DC: US GPO; 22 January 1958.

24. Manning FJ, Fullerton TD. Health and well-being in highly cohesive units of the US Army. *J Appl Soc Psychol*. 1988;18(6):503–519.

25. Epstein S. Toward a unified theory of anxiety. In: Maher BA, ed. *Progress in Experimental Personality Research*. Vol 4. New York: Academic Press; 1967.

26. Epstein S, Fenz WD. Steepness of approach and avoidance gradients in humans as a function of experience: Theory and experiment. *J Exp Psychol*. 1965;70(1):1–12.

27. Drayer CS, Glass AJ. Introduction. In: Glass AJ, ed. *Overseas Theaters*. Vol 2. In: *Neuropsychiatry in World War II*. Washington, DC: Office of The Surgeon General, US Army; 1973: 1–23.

28. Swank RL, Marchand WE. Combat neuroses: Development of combat exhaustion. *Arch Neurol Psychiatry* [superseded in part by *Arch Neurol* and *Arch Gen Psychiatry*]. 1946;55:236–247.

29. Solomon Z, Oppenheimer B, Noy S. Subsequent military adjustment of combat stress reaction casualties: A nine year follow-up study. *Milit Med.* 1986;151(1):8–11.

30. Bourne PG, Rose RM, Mason JW. 17-OHCS levels in combat: Special Forces "A" Team under threat of attack. *Arch Gen Psychiatry.* 1968;19:135.

31. Miller RG. Secretion of 17-OHCS in military aviators as an index of responses to stress: A review. *Aerosp Med* [now *Aviat Space Environ Med*]. 1968;39:498.

32. Miller RG, Rubin RT, Clark BR, Crawford WR, Arthur RJ. The stress of aircraft carrier landings: I. Corticosteroid responses in naval aviators. *Psychosom Med.* 1970;32:581–588.

33. Gabriel RA, Gal R. The IDF officer: Linchpin in unit cohesion. *Army.* 1984;34(1):42–49.

34. Levav I, Greenfeld H, Baruch E. Psychiatric combat reactions during the Yom Kippur War. *Am J Psychiatry.* 1979;136(5):637–641.

35. Gal R. Combat stress as an opportunity: The case of heroism. In: Belenky G, ed. *Contemporary Studies in Combat Psychiatry.* Westport, Conn: Greenwood Press; 1987: 31–45.

36. Gal R. Unit morale: From a theoretical puzzle to an empirical illustration—an Israeli example. *J Appl Soc Psychol.* 1986;16(6):549–564.

37. Manning FJ, Ingraham, LH. An investigation into the value of unit cohesion in peacetime. In: Belenky G, ed. *Contemporary Studies in Combat Psychiatry.* Westport, Conn: Greenwood Press; 1987: 47–67.

38. Shirom A. On some correlates of combat performance. *Admin Combat Q.* 1976;21:419–432.

39. Steiner M, Neumann M. Traumatic neurosis and social support in the Yom Kippur War. *Milit Med.* 1978;143(12):866–868.

40. Bartone PT, Kirkland FR. Optimal leadership in small army units. In: Gal R, Mangelsdorff AD, eds. *Handbook of Military Psychology.* West Sussex, England: John Wiley & Sons; 1991: 393–409.

41. Hunt JG, Phillips RL. Leadership in battle and garrison: A framework for understanding the differences and preparing for both. In: Gal R, Mangelsdorff AD, eds. *Handbook of Military Psychology.* West Sussex, England: John Wiley & Sons; 1991: 411–429.

42. Donohue KS, Wong L, Jones SM. Leadership. In: Dupuy TN, ed. *International Military and Defense Encyclopedia.* McLean, Va: Brasseys; 1993.

43. Kalay E. The commander in stress situation in IDF combat units during the "Peace for Galilee" campaign. Presented at the *Third International Conference on Psychological Stress and Adjustment in Time of War and Peace*; 1983; Tel Aviv, Israel.

44. Driskell JE, Salas E. Overcoming the effects of stress on military performance: Human factors, training, and selection strategies. In: Gal R, Mangelsdorff AD, eds. *Handbook of Military Psychology.* West Sussex, England: John Wiley & Sons; 1991: 183–193.

45. Marshall SLA. Combat leadership. In: *Symposium on Preventive and Social Psychiatry.* Washington, DC: US GPO; 1957: 303–307.

46. Montgomery B. *Morale in Battle: Analysis.* Germany: British Army of the Rhine; 1946.

47. Renner JA. The changing patterns of psychiatric problems in Vietnam. *Compr Psychiatry.* 1973;14(2):165–181.

48. Gabriel RA, Savage PL. *Crisis in Command.* New York: Hill & Wang; 1978.

49. Klose K. Defectors say morale is low in Afghan war. *Washington Post.* 2 Aug 1984: A1, A28.

50. Glass AJ. Observations upon the epidemiology of mental illness in troops during warfare. In: *Symposium on Preventive and Social Psychiatry.* Washington, DC:US GPO; 1957:185–198.

51. Beebe GW, Appel JW. *Variation in Psychological Tolerance to Ground Combat in World War II.* Washington, DC: National Academy of Sciences; 1958.

52. Glass AJ, Ryan FJ, Lubin A, Ramona CV, Tucker AC. Psychiatric prediction and military effectiveness, Part 1. *US Armed Forces Med J.* 1956;7(10):1427–1443.

53. Glass AJ, Ryan FJ, Lubin A, Ramona CV, Tucker AC. Psychiatric prediction and military effectiveness, Part 2. *US Armed Forces Med J.* 1956;7(11):1575–1588.

54. Glass AJ, Ryan FJ, Lubin A, Ramona CV, Tucker AC. Psychiatric prediction and military effectiveness, Part 3. *US Armed Forces Med J.* 1957;8(3):346–357.

55. Beebe GW, De Bakey ME. Incidence of Hits and Wounds. In: *Battle Casualties: Incidents, Mortality and Logistic Considerations.* Springfield, Ill: Charles C Thomas; 1952: 16–73.

56. Crocq L, Crocq MA, Barrois C, Belenky GL, Jones FD. Low-intensity combat psychiatric casualties. In: Pichot P, Berner P, Wolf R, Thau K, eds. *Psychiatry: The State of the Art.* Vol 6. New York: Plenum Publishing; 1985: 545–550.

57. Jones FD. Psychiatric lessons of low-intensity warfare. *Ann Med Milit Fenn* [Finland]. 1985;60(4):128–134.

58. Johnson AW. Combat psychiatry, Part 2: The US Army in Vietnam. *Med Bull US Army Europe.* 1969;25(11):335–339.

59. Jones FD. Experiences of a division psychiatrist in Vietnam. *Milit Med.* 1967;132(12):1003–1008.

60. Breznitz S. Incubation of threat: Duration of anticipation and false alarm as determinants of the fear reaction to an unavoidable frightening event. *J Exp Res Pers* [now *J Res Pers*]. 1967;2:173–179.

61. Epstein S, Roupenian A. Heart rate and skin conductance during experimentally induced anxiety: The effect of uncertainty about receiving a noxious stimulus. *J Pers Soc Psychol.* 1970;16:20–28.

62. Folkins CH. Temporal factors and the cognitive mediators of stress reaction. *J Pers Soc Psychol.* 1970;14:173–184.

63. Salama A, Mansour F, El Sudany El Rayes M. Personal Communication, 1983.

64. Krueger GP. Sustained military performance in continuous operations: Combatant fatigue, rest and sleep needs. In: Gal R, Mangelsdorff AD, eds. *Handbook of Military Psychology.* West Sussex, England: John Wiley & Sons; 1991: 255–277.

65. Lewis NDC, Engle B. *Wartime Psychiatry: A Compendium of the International Literature.* New York: Oxford University Press; 1954.

66. Chermol BH. Psychiatric casualties in combat. *Milit Rev.* 1983;58:26–32.

67. Lazarus RS, Averill JR, Opton EM. The psychology of coping: Issues of research and assessment. In: Coelho GV, Adams JE, Hamburg DA, eds. *Coping and Adaptation.* New York: Basic Books; 1974.

68. Marshall SLA. *Men Against Fire.* New York: William Morrow Company; 1950: 54–58.

Chapter 7

U.S. ARMY COMBAT PSYCHIATRY

NICHOLAS L. ROCK, M.D., F.A.P.A.[*]; JAMES W. STOKES, M.D.[†]; RONALD J. KOSHES, M.D.[‡]; JOE FAGAN, M.D.[§]; WILLIAM R. CLINE, M.D.[¥]; AND FRANKLIN D. JONES, M.D., F.A.P.A.[¶]

*Colonel (ret), Medical Corps, U.S. Army; Formerly Chief, Department Psychiatry, Walter Reed Army Medical Center, Washington, D.C.; Formerly Neuropsychiatric Consultant and Chief Drug/Alcohol Abuse, and Psychiatry and Neurology Consultant, Office of The Surgeon General, U.S. Army

†Colonel, Medical Corps, U.S. Army; Chief, Combat Stress Actions Office, Department of Preventive Health Services, Academy of Health Sciences, Army Medical Department Center and School, Fort Sam Houston, Texas 78234-6133

‡Colonel, Medical Corps, U.S. Army; Chief, Combat Stress Actions Office, Department of Preventive Health Services, Academy of Health Sciences, Army Medical Department Center and School, Fort Sam Houston, Texas 78234-6133

§Colonel, Medical Corps, U.S. Army, Special Assistant to the Deputy Director for Program Operations, Office of the Civilian Health (CHAMPUS), Aurora, Colorado 80045-6900; Formerly Psychiatry and Neurology Consultant, Office of The Surgeon General, U.S. Army

¥Colonel, Medical Corps, U.S. Army, Walter Reed Army Medical Center, Washington, D.C.; formerly Neuropsychiatry Consultant, U.S. Army Europe (USAREUR) and 7th Medical Command (MEDCOM)

¶Colonel (ret), Medical Corps, U.S. Army; Clinical Professor, Uniformed Services University of the Health Sciences, Bethesda, Maryland; Past President and Secretary and current Honorary President of the Military Section, World Psychiatric Association; Formerly Psychiatry and Neurology Consultant, Office of The Surgeon General, U.S. Army

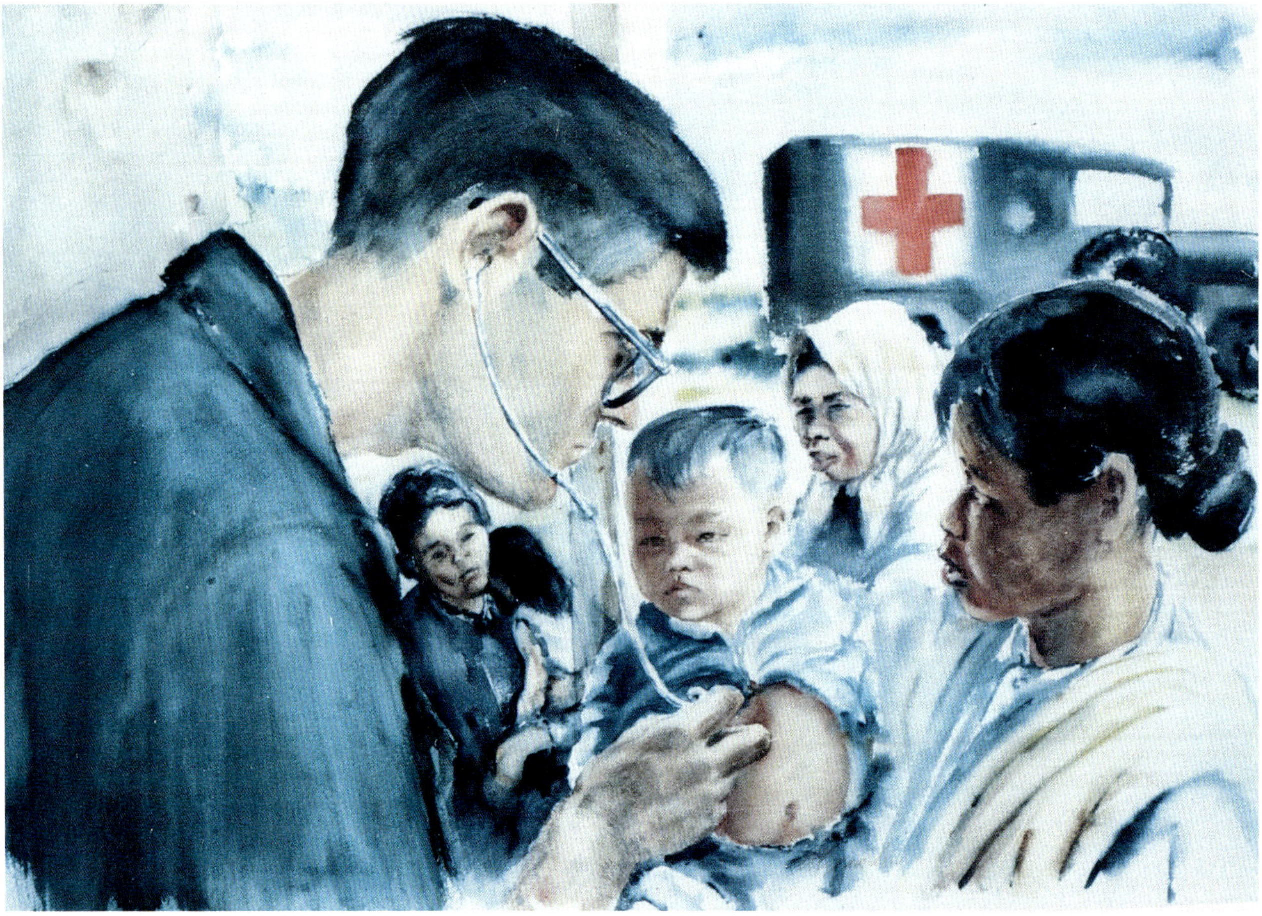

Samuel E. Alexander *American Doctor II—Field Force Doctor Examines Vietnamese Child* 1968

Samuel E. Alexander was a member of the U.S. Army Artist Program and was in Vietnam in 1967. His painting depicts the other functions of U.S. Army Psychiatry in the theater of operations. When not evaluating and treating combat stress casualties, or providing consultation services to commanders, psychiatrists and other physicians routinely provide medical care to the local civilian population under the MILPHAP (Military Public Health Action Program) which was unofficially known as the MEDCAP (Medical Civilian Action Program).

Art: Courtesy of US Center of Military History, Washington, DC.

INTRODUCTION

The Mission of the U.S. Army

The mission of the U.S. Army is to deter potential enemies from using force against the interests and security of the United States and its allies. If deterrence fails, the U.S. Army's mission is to fight and win the nation's land wars, whether they be waged with conventional weapons or weapons of mass destruction. Throughout its history, and increasingly since the end of the Cold War, the U.S. Army has also been tasked with numerous military operations other than war (MOOTW). These include humanitarian and civil assistance, infrastructure building, and disaster relief. Such missions can be within the United States (classified as "domestic support operations") or in foreign lands; they do not involve combat; and often involve medical personnel and medical units in lead roles.

Other military operations other than war are: peacekeeping; noncombatant evacuation operations; search and rescue; intelligence gathering; training missions to assist foreign countries with internal and external defense; demonstrations or shows of force; and the restoration of public order. In these missions, it is hoped that U.S. forces can avoid or deter combat, but must be prepared to defend themselves. Missions to restore order, training missions in countries that are resisting armed insurgencies, and the ambiguous category of "peace enforcement" can degenerate into sporadic low-intensity conflicts. The U.S. Army must wage and "win" these armed conflicts short of war, although in these the political objectives far outweigh the purely military ones. Conflicts short of war include counterterrorism, some counternarcotics operations, strikes and raids, support for insurgencies, and counterinsurgency (guerrilla) operations. Whatever the immediate mission, all U.S. Army personnel of all branches must be ready to perform their duties and defend themselves in the extreme stress of combat.

The Mission of the U.S. Army Medical Department

The mission of the U.S. Army Medical Department (AMEDD) is to "conserve the fighting strength" and to care for the sick and wounded. Patient care responsibility is primarily to the active duty service members, although the U.S. Army and the nation recognize the importance of assuring quality medical care to retirees and to U.S. Army family members as part of sustaining a combat-ready force. U.S. Army doctors, researchers, medical administrators, and workers of many specialties have led the way in preventive medicine. Contributions include sanitation and hygiene practices, the prevention and treatment of infectious diseases (from malaria and yellow fever to hepatitis and acquired immunodeficiency syndrome [AIDS]), and the identification of the hostility (anger) factor as the chief contributor to the risk of coronary artery disease in persons with "Type A" personalities.

U.S. Army experience has stimulated dramatic improvements in the acute stabilization, evacuation, and definitive treatment of severe physical trauma. Recently, the combat support mission of the U.S. Army Medical Department has been distilled into six battlefield roles. From the front-line medic to the continental United States (CONUS) hospital staff, all AMEDD personnel must be prepared for the personal stress of being in combat and for the stress of caring for wounded combat casualties.

The U.S. Army Mental Health/Combat Stress Control Mission

The primary mission of U.S. Army psychiatry and the mental health team is to conserve the fighting strength by assuring a sane, stress-tolerant, mission-effective force. This must be accomplished in considerable part by assisting the chain of command (officer commanders), the chain of support (noncommissioned officers), and the chain of concern (chaplains, other special staff, unit medical personnel, rear detachments, and family support groups) with professional advice, education, and assistance. It also involves screening out the mentally unsuitable and psychiatrically disabled. Direct care involves treating or counseling soldiers with temporarily distracting problems or disabling mental disorders to quickly restore them to effective duty. It also involves initiating the longer-term treatment of those who must be separated from the military.

The U.S. Army Mental Health/Combat Stress Control team in combat fulfills the AMEDD's six battlefield rules as delineated in Exhibit 7-1. In 1984, Combat Stress Control (CSC) was finally recognized as an autonomous AMEDD (and U.S. Army) battlefield functional area. This was the delayed culmination of an honorable history in which U.S.

EXHIBIT 7-1

HOW COMBAT STRESS CONTROL FULFILLS THE ARMY MEDICAL DEPARTMENT'S IMPERATIVE ROLES

Maintain presence with the soldier

The combat stress control concept places behavioral science experts forward on the battlefield and throughout the theater, where they provide immediate, on-site training, mentoring and assistance to leaders (especially at company grade), medical personnel and unit ministry teams, and the soldiers.

Maintain the health of the command

The actions of the combat stress control team prevent stress casualties, and enhance unit cohesion, soldier performance, and organizational capability under stress. They enhance mental health effectiveness of the command's Family Support Groups, through regular advice and liaison. By contributing directly to mission accomplishment, combat stress control also reduces other types of casualties.

Save lives

The combat stress control personnel save lives directly by identifying and stabilizing those neuropsychiatric or stress cases whose disturbed behavior endangers themselves or others. In a world of lethal weapons, suicidal, homicidal, or psychotic behavior can create mass casualties. Correctly diagnosing surgical and medical emergencies which have been mislabeled as psychiatric behavior also directly saves lives. The combat stress control personnel save lives indirectly by enhancing decision-making and mission execution through command consultation.

Clear the disabled from the battlefield

The combat stress control team contributes to clearing the battlefield by identifying and stabilizing for transportation those psychiatric cases who need rapid evacuation, while screening out and treating the much larger number of stress cases who can quickly return to duty far forward. Without combat stress control, these cases overload the limited evacuation assets or interfere with operations.

Provide quality care

Combat stress control personnel assure appropriate quality of care at each echelon for battle fatigue and psychiatric cases. For battle fatigue cases, premature evacuation can cause permanent disability, and constitutes malpractice unless it is unavoidable under the tactical situation. Also, the American people clearly expect the Army to take all feasible measures to prevent misconduct stress behaviors and post-traumatic stress disorders in our soldiers. Through their top priority consultation-liaison mission, the multidisciplinary combat stress control team personnel train, mentor, and provide technical supervision throughout the Army medical, combat service support, and combat arms systems to assure quality stress and mental health care to all soldiers. Through their advice and liaison mission to unit leaders, family support groups, and the supporting medical systems in garrison and Reserve Component units, they extend this quality assurance to the Total Army family.

Return soldiers to duty

The combat stress control organization returns many soldiers to duty quickly. This reduces the burden on the evacuation system and returns trained, seasoned soldiers to their own units, instead of unknown, combat-inexperienced replacements who have to be flown into theater. It also benefits the casualties' future mental health.

Adapted from the Draft Concept Statement of the Combat Stress Control Panel, Medical Re-Engineering Initiative, AMEDD Center and School, Fort Sam Houston, Texas, April 1994.

Army neuropsychiatry and its allied mental health professions established doctrine, organization, and an operational concept that was truly distinct from the rest of U.S. Army medicine.

The American soldier of today is highly technically trained and not easily replaced in a short time. The prevention of stress casualties and the early return to duty of stress-disabled soldiers requires more focus in peacetime on neuropsychiatry and mental health programs in preparation for mobilization. The transition of mental health professionals from a civilian practice to military can take 6 months and may be too late to be effective at a time of national emergency. The mental health personnel must master military-specific clinical and organizational skills which have no civilian counterparts. Direct application of civilian mental health experience to combat stress cases or functioning military units can cause harm. Military stress control expertise must be acquired by military providers working in the military unit context, not in a garrison version of civilian direct-patient care. The operational planning and coordination of stress control in war and operations other than war requires that experienced mental health staff officers and noncommissioned officers (NCOs) be integral members of medical, U.S. Army, and joint services command headquarters.

History of U.S. Army Neuropsychiatry in Combat

The history of U.S. Army neuropsychiatry is covered in considerable detail in *Neuropsychiatry*,[1] the history of neuropsychiatry in World War I, and in *Neuropsychiatry in World War II*,[2,3] the two volume series. Chapter 1 of this volume, Psychiatric Lessons of War, also discusses the history of military psychiatry, especially in terms of the evolution of concepts. The following discussion highlights the important conceptual and historical developments in military psychiatry while emphasizing the structural components of the delivery of patient care. The materials presented draw heavily from those found in the official histories.[1-3]

The U.S. Army began as the Continental Army under the leadership of General George Washington. There was no subspecialty of psychiatry or other mental health professions at that time, although chaplains supported the spiritual and moral health of the troops. Dr. Benjamin Rush served as the prototype Surgeon General from 1776 to 1778. Rush advocated abstinence from alcohol. Later, as a civilian physician at the Pennsylvania Hospital, Rush preceded and paralleled the more famous French physician, Philippe Pinel, in championing the "moral treatment of the insane." He advocated asylums in the quiet countryside for the mentally ill—clean buildings with bathing facilities, where violent patients were kept separate from passive ones and all were treated with kindness, work, and diversion (occupational therapy). He wrote "We assume that insanity has its seat in the mind. And nevertheless we attempt with remarkable inconsistency to cure it by physical methods. The disease affects the body and mind alike and can be cured only by methods which reach both."[4(p28)]

In the Continental Army and the U.S. Army which it became, the importance of morale or "esprit de corps" was recognized. It was needed to keep soldiers steady in the line of battle and to prevent desertion in the long periods of inactivity under deprived conditions far from home, such as the winter at Valley Forge during the American Revolutionary War. Also recognized were many of the same mental health disorders seen today, although without the current more elaborated diagnostic understanding: alcohol abuse and alcoholism ("drunkenness"), homesickness and chronic situational depression ("nostalgia"), and more overt psychotic disorders ("insanity" and "melancholia"). Joseph Lovell, the Surgeon General from 1817 to 1828 and an advocate of temperance who eventually succeeded in abolishing the daily rum ration, attributed more than one half of the deaths in the U.S. Army over that period to alcohol.[5(p29)]

In 1852, Dorothea Dix persuaded Congress to fund the U.S. Government Hospital for the Insane (now St. Elizabeths Hospital). The Government Hospital was to receive the insane of the U.S. Army and U.S. Navy. However, during the Civil War, so many insane Union soldiers were discharged locally to find their own way home that complaints led to an 1864 War Department order requiring transfer to the Government Hospital until the soldiers' families could come for them.

Nostalgia cases in the Civil War numbered 5,547 (with 74 deaths). It is likely that the differentiation between nostalgia ("a species of melancholy or mild type of insanity caused by disappointment and longing for home") and physical diseases such as tuberculosis was not always made. Little treatment was attempted, and most cases were discharged home.[6]

"Functional heart disease" was described by DaCosta in 1862, who also termed it "the irritable heart of the soldier."[7] The condition usually originated in combat as a prompt and persistent tachycardia (120–130 bpm) on slight exertion. DaCosta reported that most cases improved with hospitalization and tincture of digitalis three times a day. On one occasion when 4,900 soldiers were discharged from the Union Army, 2,300 were diagnosed as heart disease, of which 1,200 were "functional." Today, a patient presenting with a psychophysiological manifestation of hyperarousal and conditioned anxiety might well be considered an "evacuation syndrome."[8]

The first formal training in psychiatry to Regular Army Medical Officers began at the U.S. Army Medical School, consisting of four clinical sessions at the Government Hospital. There were also lectures in military law and malingering. By 1915, the total training in mental illness had increased to 24 hours.

Perhaps the first organized military mental health unit was with the Russians in the Russo-Japanese War (1904–1906).[9] During this war the Russian Red Cross established mental health programs and recording of neuropsychiatric cases. In addition physicians, functioning as neuropsychiatrists, were put as close to the front as possible to perform special evaluations of nervous and mental cases. Eventually other countries developed such programs during World War I.

As World War I was waged in 1914 and 1915, newspaper and journal reports of "shell shock" ("le syndrome commotionnel") aroused interest among U.S. psychiatrists. Prominent American psychiatrists during World War I advocated to the U.S. Army Surgeon General (Major General Gorgas) the formation of a psychiatric organization. The plan included developing psychiatric units in general hospitals staffed by psychiatrists throughout the United States.

Dr. Thomas Salmon,[10] medical director of the National Committee for Mental Hygiene, offered the committee's services to the U.S. Army. He and others visited U.S. Army medical facilities supporting the operations against Pancho Villa in Mexico and Canadian hospitals with psychiatric evacuees from France. In 1917, Dr. Salmon visited England for several months. By then, the psychological nature of "war neurosis" and the value of forward, brief treatment had been well documented by the French and confirmed by the British. Dr. Salmon recommended to the U.S. Army Surgeon General that a similar echeloned system of prevention and treatment be adopted. When the United States entered the war, Salmon was commissioned a major. He was appointed Director of Psychiatry to the American Expeditionary Forces (AEF) in December 1917, and immediately implemented his plan.[1]

> The experience of the French and British medical services showed, within a very few months after the beginning of the war, that patients with war neuroses improved more rapidly when treated in permanent hospitals near the front than at the base, better at casualty clearing stations and postes de chirurgie d'urgence than even at advanced base hospitals, and better still when encouragement, rest, persuasion, and suggestion could be given at a combat organization itself. It was for the purpose of applying this well-established fact that plans were made to station a medical officer with special training in psychiatry and neurology in each combat division, since the division was to be the great combat unit of the American Army in France. It was deemed impractical to consider detailing a consultant in neuropsychiatry to a combat unit smaller than the division.[1(p303)]

By order of the chief surgeon of the AEF, the division psychiatrists were under the direction of the chief surgeons of the division, but were not members of the division headquarters staffs. Rather, they were attached to the "sanitary trains" (the equivalent of the current medical units that are organic to the division). Later, Salmon concluded that putting the psychiatrists in the headquarters under the chief surgeons worked better. The psychiatrist's specified duties included examining all cases of mental or nervous diseases (including malingering and self-inflicted wounds) and advising on their diagnosis, management, and disposition; forensic testimony when requested; giving "informal clinical talks" to medical officers and others on the nature, diagnosis, and management of the disorders; keeping careful records of all cases; and submitting regular reports to and advising the chief surgeon.

> The division psychiatrist was stationed at the advanced field hospital, or triage, and his range of activity extended forward to the ambulance dressing stations and beyond as far as he cared to go and backward as far as the rear field hospital, which was the unit treatment center [ie, still within the division]. The triage, or sorting station, was apt to be anywhere from 2 to 9 miles, or more, from the front line, and the treatment field hospital 4 to 7 miles further removed. The former was usually an abandoned strong barn; and the latter, generally under canvas, capable of caring for about 150 patients in five or six large tents. At the treatment field hospital the division psychiatrist was generally able to count on one enlisted man...to care for each 15 patients.... An assistant divisional specialist would have proven a valuable adjunct. It is true that even with an active combat division there were times when there was scarcely enough [patient care] work to keep the division psychiatrist occupied; yet these periods were succeeded by days or weeks of stress and strain...when the services of a trained assistant would have been invaluable. The small "pool" of neuropsychiatrists under the

> control of the corps or army [neuropsychiatry] consultant proved a useful means of meeting this need.[1(pp309–310)]

At the forward triage, the division psychiatrist sorted all nervous cases, returning directly to their combat units those who should not be permitted to go to the rear and resting, warming, feeding, and treating others, particularly exhaustion cases, if there was opportunity to do so.[1]

Salmon had learned from British experience the importance of not using dramatic or diagnostic labels for stress casualties, and adopted the British policy of using "N.Y.D.N." for "not yet diagnosed (nervous)." This avoided the suggestion of physical brain injury implied in the dramatic name "shell shock" or the implication of mysterious psychiatric illness implied by the official diagnosis, "war neurosis." Under optimal conditions, over 70% of the casualties held for treatment at the 150-cot field hospitals in the division rear returned to duty within 5 days. However, when the tactical situation forced the emptying of the field hospitals after only two days of treatment, the return-to-duty percentage dropped to 40%.[1(p333)]

The second echelon, only a few miles behind the divisions, was the three neurological hospitals. These were located in old French barracks buildings, staffed by general medical personnel and commanded and supervised by psychiatrists. The sole function of these 150-bed units was to provide additional brief rest and intensive rehabilitation for those NYDN cases who had had to be evacuated from the divisions. About 55% of these cases returned to duty after an average of two weeks.

The third echelon, further to the rear, was Base Hospital No. 117, whose sole purpose was to provide several weeks of even more intensive reconditioning treatment to the soldiers who had not returned to duty from the neurological hospitals or who had somehow slipped through the first two echelons and been evacuated to regular hospitals. Another base hospital, No. 116, was the neuropsychiatric specialty hospital dedicated to the "true" neuropsychiatric cases who were judged not suitable for return to duty. Base Hospital No. 117 also had a high rate of return to duty, although many were to noncombat jobs in the rear. The staff of Base Hospital No. 117 included psychiatrists, U.S. Army psychiatric nurses, on-the-job-trained enlisted medics, and civilian volunteer occupational therapists. The official history describes in detail the importance of the nursing staff in establishing and maintaining a positive, return-to-duty ward morale. The occupational therapists provided both shop work and outdoor work details; the official history emphasizes the importance of these tasks in restoring confidence. In the last weeks of the war, occupational therapists were sent forward to the neurological hospitals where they enabled some soldiers to return to duty who otherwise would have been evacuated to Base Hospital No. 117.

In the continental United States, the American Red Cross established a psychiatric social worker program to aid military patients. Clinical psychology programs were not recorded at that time.

It should be apparent from this brief history that the forbears of military psychiatry during World War I knew much of what is known today about combat stress casualties, and practiced prevention and treatment very well. It was recorded in the official history, but then forgotten.

From World War I to World War II hospital psychiatry functions continued, but unlike the assignment of medical and surgical consultants, there was no representation of the mental health specialties on The Surgeon General's staff. At the beginning of World War II Harry Stack Sullivan, psychiatric consultant to the Selective Service Commission, promoted policies that resulted in the rejection of young men being conscripted if they showed any taint of anxiety or neurotic tendencies, including so-called "neuropathic traits" such as nail biting, enuresis, or running away from home. These policies were also applied to soldiers after induction, resulting in what Ginsberg et al[11] labeled "lost divisions" of about 2.5 million men. Of 18 million screened, nearly 2 million were rejected because of an emotional or mental defect and another three quarters of a million were prematurely separated for the same reasons. The total ineffective group included approximately one out of every seven men called for service.[11]

Besides the absence of representation at the War Department or even the Department of the Army (DA) staff, the division psychiatric positions were abolished in 1939 as unnecessary. In August 1940, Lieutenant Colonel (later General) Patrick Madigan was assigned to the Professional Services Division, Surgeon General's Office, but his duties were purely routine and administrative. Not until February 1942, after the attack on Pearl Harbor, was he able to upgrade his position to a Neuropsychiatry Branch under the Professional Services Division. However, in 1941 troop clinics were established outside of the hospitals and psychiatrists were assigned. A training center at Fort Monmouth, New Jersey, developed a community clinic in early 1942 and had an enlisted social worker and later an enlisted psychologist to assist the psychiatrist. This program led to the establishment of the Mental Hygiene Consultation Service (MHCS) at all replacement training centers. Its purpose was to help the maladjusted trainee. This concept of MHCS continues to the present in the Community Mental Health Services in the Medical Activity of each post.[12]

World War I style forward treatment was relearned during two battles of the Tunisian Campaign in March and April 1943.[3] Captain Fred Hanson, who served with Canadian forces prior to U.S. entry into the war, was assigned with American forces in North Africa. Hanson may have been familiar with Salmon's principles because the British were using *The Medical Department of the United States Army in the World War, Volume 10, Neuropsychiatry* in their planning.[1] He avoided evacuation and returned more than 70% of 494 neuropsychiatric patients to combat after 48 hours of treatment, which basically consisted of resting the soldier and indicating to him that he would soon rejoin his unit. On April 26, 1943, in response to the recommendations of his surgeon, Colonel Perrin Long, and psychiatrists, Captain Hanson and Major Tureen, General Omar Bradley issued a directive that established a holding period of 7 days for psychiatric patients and further prescribed the term "exhaustion" as the initial diagnosis for all combat psychiatric cases. The word exhaustion was chosen because it conveyed the least implication of mental disturbance and came closest to describing how the patients really felt. Division psychiatrists were hastily reassigned. This move proved its worth in the Italian campaign.

The ineffective psychiatric criteria for screening at initial entry were also tightened to disqualify only the overtly psychotic or seriously mentally retarded. A later study demonstrated that the "neurotics" who would have been screened out by the earlier criteria were not significantly more likely to become stress casualties or less likely to be decorated for valor than the men who had passed that screening.

Colonel (later Brigadier General) William C. Menninger became The Surgeon General's Chief of the Neuropsychiatry Branch in December 1943, and the branch became a division, on an equal level with medicine and surgery, in January 1944. A School of Military Psychiatry, plus some civilian schools, addressed the serious shortage of psychiatrists. Initially, a 4-week course trained physicians who already had more than a year of psychiatric training. Later, a 12-week course was conducted to prepare physicians with no psychiatric training to function in psychiatric positions.

By late in the war, the Mediterranean and European theaters had psychiatrists assigned to each division, although some divisions received only inexperienced general medical officers. Many maneuver battalions had "rest centers" in their "kitchen trains," where exhausted soldiers were monitored by the nearby battalion surgeon. There were "exhaustion centers" in many regimental or combat command "trains" (equivalent to today's brigade support areas), run by the adjutant but monitored by the regimental surgeons. Combat exhaustion cases were rested here for several days. In some divisions, company commanders were even required to select some number of individual soldiers for rotation back to these centers for brief "R and R" (rest and recreation). It was the primary duty of the division psychiatrist to train the battalion and regimental surgeons in the principles and practice of combat psychiatry. Toward the end of the war a distinguished group of civilian psychiatrists were commissioned to evaluate U.S. military psychiatric treatment in Europe. They found that about half of the stress casualties were never recorded because of the success of forward treatment at the battalion and regimental aid stations and rest centers.[13]

During combat late in World War II, the division psychiatrists in Europe triaged and treated more severe combat exhaustion cases at the division clearing company in the division rear, holding them for 1 to 2 days. They then supervised their further rehabilitation for 3 to 5 days at the division's Training and Rehabilitation (T&R) Center. The T&R Center was controlled by the Adjutant, and staffed with combat veteran officers and NCOs, often ones who were on profile with minor wounds or injuries (including combat exhaustion!). The soldiers shared pup tents and were led through a program of calisthenics and realistic combat drills, often conducted in the ruins of nearby towns that had been recent battlefields. Return-to-duty rates from the T&R Centers ranged between 50% and 70%.[14]

Behind the divisions, there were U.S. Army-level Neuropsychiatry Centers. These were 250-bed holding companies with supervisory psychiatric staff. Like the World War I Neurological Hospitals, these received the cases that the division psychiatrist judged too disruptive for the division clearing company and T&R Center, plus those who failed to respond sufficiently to the 5- to 7-day treatment, and the overflow caused by tactical demands.

The Neuropsychiatry Centers continued the highly structured program of physical reconditioning, hot showers, good food and comfortable cots, and recreational and work activities. Some of these soldiers returned to their original units. Others were sent to nearby combat service support units for further useful "occupational therapy" and reclassification into support roles. The few who failed to respond were sent to base hospitals with psychiatric wards. Approximately 90% of the stress casualties who received specialized psychiatric care were returned to useful duty in the theater.

In addition to rediscovering the principles of treatment applied so effectively in World War I, and the ineffectiveness of large-scale screening, World War II psychiatrists learned about the epidemiology of combat stress casualties. They documented the direct relationship to intensity of combat, modified by physical and morale factors, and the importance of unit cohesion both in preventing breakdown and in enhancing combat effectiveness. During the war, prospective studies conducted by Stouffer et al[15] conclusively showed that units with good morale and leadership had fewer combat stress casualties than those without these attributes when variables such as combat intensity were comparable. Regarding combat intensity it was found that there was a direct relationship between combat intensity as measured by rates of wounded and killed in action and psychiatric casualties.[16]

Another finding during World War II was the chronology of breakdown in combat. It had long been recognized that "new" and "old" men in combat units were more prone to breakdown. "New" or inexperienced troops were more likely to become stress casualties, and have usually accounted for over three fourths of stress casualties; however, with increasing exposure to combat after 1 or 2 combat months, an increasing rate of casualty generation also occurs.[17] Beebe and Appel[18] analyzed the World War II combat attrition of a cohort of 1,000 soldiers from the European Theater of Operations (ETO) and found that the breaking point of the average rifleman in the Mediterranean Theater of Operations (MTO) was 88 days of company combat, that is, days in which the company sustained at least one casualty. A company combat day averaged 7.8 calendar days in the MTO and 3.6 calendar days in the ETO. They found that due to varying causes of attrition including death, wounding, and transfers, by company combat day 50 in both theaters 9 out of 10 "original" soldiers had departed. In their projections Beebe and Appel found that if only psychiatric casualties occurred, there would be a 95% depletion by company combat day 260; however, due to other causes of attrition (transfer, death, wounding, illness), the unit would be virtually depleted by company combat day 80 or 90, approximately the breaking point of the median man.[18]

From studies of cumulative stress such as these as well as observations of the efficacy of a "point system" (so many points of credit toward rotation from combat per unit of time in combat or so many combat missions of aircrews) used during World War II, the value of periodic rest from combat and of rotation came to be understood and applied in the Korean and Vietnam conflicts with fixed combat tours. The fixed tours did, however, result in the "short-timer's syndrome," an anxious, tense state not uncommon in combat participants during the final weeks of the stipulated tour of combat duty.[19,20]

The final and perhaps most important lesson of World War II was the importance of group cohesion not only in preventing breakdown, but also in producing effectiveness in combat.[19] Cohesion is so important in both prevention and treatment of psychiatric casualties that Matthew D. Parrish, an eminent psychiatrist who served in combat aircrews during World War II and as U.S. Army Neuropsychiatry Consultant in Vietnam, has suggested it as another principle of forward treatment that might be termed "membership."[21]

After World War II key commands kept neuropsychiatric consultants, particularly in Europe and at the Department of the Army. The specialty of social work officer was established along with the conversion of the enlisted psychologist from the Sanitation Corps to an officer in the Medical Service Corps.

The experience of World War II was documented in the two-volume official history, *Neuropsychiatry in World War II*.[2,3] This included the plan for the way that special neuropsychiatric teams would support the division mental health capabilities and provide backup and mobile consultative support in the corps. However, the U.S. Army was substantially deactivated in the late 1940s, and the invasion of South Korea by North Korea caught the United States unprepared. Task Force Smith, hastily mobilized from garrison troops in the Pacific area and reinforced by reactivated World War II veterans from the United States, suffered heavy losses in killed, wounded, and captured during the retreat to the Pusan perimeter. Although the veterans remembered that combat exhaustion cases ought to be treated in the combat zone close behind their units, most were unavoidably evacuated to Japan. There, proper treatment at the hospitals salvaged many for combat service support duties, but very few returned to combat duty.

After the first months of the Korean conflict, Colonel Donald Peterson, the Neuropsychiatry Consultant, assigned Lieutenant Colonel Albert Glass as the Neuropsychiatry Theater Consultant for the forces in Korea. Glass[22] immediately established a comprehensive mental health program. He had served in World War II and was able, based on his experiences, to quickly organize an effective, forward program that has remained the basis for current military mental health programs. The division mental health sections were trained to provide active training to the regimental and battalion surgeons. In addition, the Table of Organization and Equipment (TO&E) was developed for a mobile psychiatric detachment. This new unit was designated a "KO Team." "KO" was not an acronym. Rather, it was only one in a series of "K" teams, with "K" arbitrarily indicating that these were hospital augmentation detachments. The first KO teams were deployed to Korea, where they reinforced the division mental health sections at times of heavy fighting, and could enhance the use of a divisional clearing company as a temporary exhaustion center. They also provided mobile consultation throughout the corps and U.S. Army areas, like the fictitious psychiatrist, Major Sidney Greenfield, did on the television series "MASH."

In April 1952, a third-echelon treatment facility (equivalent to Base Hospital No. 117 in World War I) was established near Seoul by adding a psychiatric detachment to a 300-cot medical holding company. This facility had an average census of 45 soldiers with an average duration of stay of 7.4 days. It returned 76% to duty.[23]

A comparison of treatment efficacy data near the end of World War II and the 1953 Korean conflict reveals the following: World War II—60% of psychiatric casualties were returned to duty within their own division, while in Korea it was 88%; World War II—90% were returned to duty somewhere in the combat theater compared to 97% in Korea.[23] In 1957, the first version of Army Regulation 40-216, *Neuropsychiatry and Mental Health*, codified the roles and responsibilities of division psychiatry in wartime and peacetime.

The first U.S. Army psychiatrist to be assigned in Vietnam, Major Estes G. Copen[24] provided support to approximately 8,000 American advisors. He noted the prevalence of misconduct and psychosomatic complaints among the service support troops, in contrast to those in combat units, that was to become the hallmark and curse of the Vietnam conflict. With the buildup beginning in July 1965, divisions deployed to Vietnam, each with their one division psychiatrist, and social work officer, plus two enlisted specialists with their medical company supporting each brigade. The enlisted specialists were often college or graduate level draftees with behavioral science training. They staffed mental health consultation services at the division base area and went forward when appropriate to the brigade and battalion fire bases. The theater neuropsychiatrist consultant established his office at Headquarters, U.S. Army Vietnam in November 1965.

The first KO team to deploy was activated at Valley Forge General Hospital in Pennsylvania in October 1965, deployed by ship 29 November 1965, and was operational by January 1966. It consisted of three psychiatrists, one neurologist, two social workers, one clinical psychologist, one psychiatric nurse, and 12 to 15 enlisted social work, psychology, and neuropsychiatric specialists. Its mission was to establish a "Psychiatry and Neurology Treatment and Evacuation Center" in Vietnam. (The adoption of this title at that time is interesting in that it emphasizes the two functions that current doctrine, as practiced in the Persian Gulf War, would deemphasize. The more "doctrinally correct" translation might be the "Psychiatry and Neurology Evaluation and Return to Duty Center.") The center provided psychiatric and neurological evaluation and treatment for up to 30 days as inpatients, if necessary, prior to evacuation to the continental United States or return to duty. The detachment was assigned to an evacuation hospital 20 miles northeast of Saigon, where it occupied its own Quonset buildings. It quickly also established an active MHCS for the many units in the vicinity that lacked organic mental health services.

Despite its title, the Psychiatry and Neurology Treatment and Evacuation Center aggressively applied the time-proven principles of combat psychiatry and returned about 90% of its inpatients to duty. It maintained a military-, not patient-, care milieu with strong expectation of return to duty. Although distant from most of the tactical units, the center maintained a psychological proximity and unit identity by requesting the parent unit to make regular visits to its soldier, bring his mail, and give him his pay on the ward. The ubiquitous helicopters made this possible, and most line commanders cooperated fully with the visitation program.

Less than 5% of the caseload presented with well-defined psychiatric illnesses. The majority of soldiers referred to the KO team had behavioral difficulties or somatic complaints. The latter were either physiologic manifestations of stress (headache, back pain, gastrointestinal symptoms, syncope and vertigo), conversion-type symptoms affecting vision, hearing, speech, pseudoseizures, "narcolepsy," or somnambulism, and amnesias. The KO team also provided extensive consultation to medicine and surgery regarding stress and somatic symptoms in soldiers recovering from physical wounds.

As the buildup in Vietnam continued, eventually two KO teams were assigned in Vietnam. The incidence of traditional "combat exhaustion" remained very low (below 2%). This was attributed to the rotation policy (365-day tours), scheduled R and R, the sporadic nature of combat in most of the heavy artillery, armor, and air weapons support of U.S. forces, the effectiveness of helicopter evacuation of the wounded, and the prevention (by division mental health and the KO teams) of a "psychiatric" evacuation syndrome. Another factor in the low utilization of the "combat exhaustion" label was the criterion that the soldier had to show "fatigue, whether produced by physical causes such as exertion, heat, dehydration diarrhea and loss of sleep...[or] anxiety and insomnia." This effectively excluded most of the anxious, depressed, conversion and dissociative subtypes who would now be counted under the umbrella of "battle fatigue," as they would have in World War II.

As noted elsewhere in this volume, the division mental health teams and KO teams were less successful in recognizing the contributing causes of misconduct stress behaviors and in helping the chain of command to prevent them. Measures such as the individual 365-day tour, while protecting against battle fatigue or combat exhaustion, fragmented unit cohesion. Liberal availability of alcohol, with frequent excess use, did not set a good example for the prevention of marijuana, heroin, and other illegal drug abuse, which became epidemic by 1970. Those factors, plus an unwise short rotation policy for junior officers and the unpopularity of the war, led to epidemic indiscipline, including the threatening and "fragging" of leaders. Failure to instill understanding and respect for the Vietnamese (both South and North, friend, neutral, and foe), the frustrating and ambiguous rules of engagement, and the nature of terrorist guerrilla war, led to numerous small and some major acts of brutality and outright atrocity. The turmoil in the U.S. Army only reflected that of the nation, where violent political dissension, substance abuse, and racial animosity and overt antimilitary demonstrations were rampant.[25]

Following the withdrawal of all U.S. combat forces from Vietnam after the cease-fire signed by the United States, North Vietnam, and South Vietnam in Paris (1973), the U.S. Army entered the period of the "hollow army." While undergoing a major reduction in force and maintaining supposedly "fully manned" units to deter Soviet aggression in Europe, the U.S. Army continued to be plagued by drug abuse, indiscipline, low morale, and reduced readiness. The division mental health sections (now also including clinical psychologists) were too preoccupied with the daily referrals of disturbed, problem soldiers for most to train with their units much in the field. While the mental health team was valued for their ability to process problem soldiers for administrative or "chapter" discharges, they were also to some extent sullied by association with their workload clients.

The KO team TO&E was redesigned about 1973 into the "OM Team." ("OM" is also not an acronym. The "O" signifies that it is one of a series of medical teams that provide area support.) This designation more properly defined the units' mission than had the "K" (hospital augmentation detachments). However, the issue was confounded by taking inpatient services out of all the combat zone deployable hospitals and adding it to the OM team. The OM team had a small headquarters with a psychiatrist commander, clinical psychologist, field medical assistant (officer) and several enlisted. It had three mobile consultation teams, each with a psychiatrist, social worker, six behavioral science specialists (91G), and two vehicles. The treatment section had a psychiatrist, two psychiatric nurses, eleven psychiatric specialists (91F), and a 91G. Apparently, the plan was for OM detachments to augment one or two evacuation hospitals in a theater (reinforcing the evacuation hospital's one psychiatrist, one psychiatric nurse, and two psychiatric specialists) to provide 25-cot psychiatric wards. Other OM detachments might reinforce a general hospital or two in the communications zone. In fact, only one active component OM detachment was authorized, and it had no personnel assigned. Six OM detachments were established in the U.S. Army Reserves, but no doctrine was written regarding their expected employment. Not until 1984 did the OM teams begin to take part in realistic annual field training exercises.

Belated recognition of the Soviet offensive NBC (nuclear, biological, and chemical) threat to the North Atlantic Treaty Organization (NATO), made vivid by the intense fighting in the 1973 Yom Kippur War and the Israeli experience of stress casualties, led to renewed awareness of combat stress by the senior U.S. Army leadership. Army Regulation 40-216, *Neuropsychiatry and Mental Health,*[26] was updated in 1984, its first revision in 30 years. Staff studies at the Academy of Health Sciences at Fort Sam Houston, Texas, in the late 1970s and early 1980s, led to recognition of combat stress control as an autonomous AMEDD functions area in 1984. This finally put the combat mental health doctrine organization and employment on a par with preventive medicine, combat dentistry and veterinary medicine, if still less prestigious than hospitalization and evacuation.

In an intensive revision of all U.S. Army field medical support to meet the Soviet threat and support AirLand Battle (later called Medical Force 2000 or MF2K), the AMEDD was held to a strict personnel ceiling. However, within this ceiling, the newly proposed combat stress control (CSC) "companies" and "detachments" were authorized a 400% increase in active duty slots and a 280% increase in U.S. Army Reserve slots over those already available for modification from the old OM teams.

The TO&Es for the 85-person medical company CSC, and the 23-person medical detachment CSC were developed between 1986 and June 1989 and forwarded for Department of Army approval. These units have a modular design that packages a psychiatrist, social worker, and two enlisted, with vehicle, into a CSC preventive team that can reinforce a division mental health NCO and officer at the maneuver brigade level. A clinical psychologist, a psychiatric nurse (clinical nurse specialist) and an occupational therapist, with two each of their enlisted assistant and two more enlisted, are combined into an 11-person CSC restoration team. This team can staff a program of 1- to 3-day restoration treatment in the division rear, as well as sending two to three person teams to provide consultation in the vicinity or to reinforce the CSC preventive teams forward on short notice.

The CSC preventive and restoration teams' personnel can also be task organized in any combination to provide reconstitution support to units that have been pulled back after suffering heavy attrition. The task-organized elements can also conduct 1- to 2-week reconditioning programs in the corps area for slow-improving stress casualties. For more description of CSC doctrine and units, see Chapter 10, Joint Operations.

In the area of CSC doctrine, paragraphs and chapters were added to other medical field manuals starting in 1991.[27,28] Field manuals specific to the combat stress control functional area were written and staffed through multiple revisions starting in 1989, finally to be printed in September 1994.[29,30]

Meanwhile, however, events were calling for CSC support to U.S. Army combat operations. In December 1989 through January 1990, Operation Just Cause, the U.S. invasion of Panama, involved a night air assault by U.S. Army Ranger battalions; followed by an 82d Airborne Division brigade; the air-landing of 7th Light Infantry Division forces; reinforcing elements of those divisions; the 5th Mechanized Infantry Division; a separate brigade; and many other units already in Panama. There were several days of intense, but brief and local fighting, that included a number of psychologically traumatic incidents.

No division mental health assets were deployed to theater, although both the 82d and 7th sections were ready to go. The garrison and hospital psychiatric/mental health assets already in Panama were not readily adaptable or sufficient to the task of postcombat preventive activities. Subsequent problems with post-traumatic stress disorder (PTSD) and less obvious attrition or misconduct in a number of units confirmed the importance of such activities, preferably in the theater of operations, even after brief, successful contingency operations in which American and local civilian losses are sustained.

When Iraq invaded Kuwait in August 1990, the new CSC TO&Es were still in queue awaiting their Department of the Army staffing. The new field manuals were circulating in preliminary draft form. The mobilization for Operation Desert Shield (the multinational show of force to deter further Iraqi aggression and encourage withdrawal from Kuwait) first deployed the division mental health sections with their units, although some personnel had had little or no prior field training. Each of the Psychiatry Consultants was given copies of the drafts of the first five chapters of this volume for distribution. Fortunately they had some time in theater to prepare themselves.

In September, the one active component OM team was mobilized at Fort Benning, bringing together its Professional Officer Filler System (PROFIS) officers, levied enlisted complement and second-hand equipment for the first time. Anticipating the new CSC detachment TO&E,

it incorporated an occupational therapist officer and NCO in the place of other, unfilled specialties. The unit deployed in late October, set up a restoration program at the one combat support hospital then in Saudi Arabia, and immediately began sending out mobile consultation teams. Within days it had reversed the tendency to evacuate all "psychiatric cases" out of theater. As the one preventive psychiatric unit for 18th Airborne Corps, it quickly established a high degree of credibility.

Two of the six U.S. Army Reserve OM Detachments were activated just after Thanksgiving and deployed to Saudi Arabia the first week in December. One became the CSC asset for 7th Corps, that was then arriving from Germany. The second was assigned to the echelon above corps at Riyadh, and collocated with a general hospital. The neuropsychiatry consultant for U.S. Army Central Command (ARCENT) also reached Saudi Arabia in December. As planning for the expulsion of Iraqi forces from Kuwait proceeded, the ARCENT psychiatrist and command surgeon concluded that the OM team assets needed to be divided into their mobile teams and sent forward as close behind the combat maneuver brigades as the tactical situation allowed. Projected estimates for U.S. wounded and chemical injuries were high, if the veteran Iraqi soldiers were able to put up a stubborn defense and use their chemical arsenal and long-range artillery despite the planned U.S.-led air campaign. Stress casualties in such a scenario could equal one per three or even two wounded, and one or two per chemical injury.

Accordingly, ARCENT directed the two OM detachments, which were allocated one to each corps, to send their teams to join the "medical task forces" that would go forward into Iraq behind each division. It was judged that they did not yet have the logistical capability and field experience to try to accompany the maneuver brigades medical companies, as the draft field manuals advocated. As the air campaign progressed, the third OM detachment at Riyadh split into four teams. One team remained in Riyadh, two were sent to reinforce the OM teams supporting the corps, and the fourth team established a second-echelon restoration/reconditioning center at one of the major hospital complexes.[31]

During the short, fast-moving ground campaign, the stress control teams from the OM detachments moved forward with the surgical teams, holding cots, and preventive medicine teams that collectively comprised the medical task forces. Most of these were directly behind the maneuver brigades, leaving the main support medical companies of the division support commands far to the rear. Some stress control teams in 18th Corps reached the Euphrates valley. Few stress casualties were seen during the successful offensive, as prior experience predicts.

In the conferences that the AMEDD assembled to formalize lessons learned, the ARCENT surgeon stated that combat stress control had been one of the success stories of the Persian Gulf campaign in preventing unnecessary evacuations and returning soldiers to duty. However, it was recognized that there had been too few assets to simultaneously support the combat divisions and the rear areas that were subject to Scud missile attacks, as well as stressful environmental conditions. The medical leaders of 18th Corps, in particular, strongly encouraged the rapid fielding of the new CSC units, doctrine, and training. This advocacy assisted the expeditious fielding of these new CSC units, despite the downsizing of the U.S. Army following the breakup of the Soviet threat.

Equally important was that the active duty detachments were authorized most of their officers and all of their enlisted personnel full time (not as PROFIS fillers with full-time duties in the hospitals). This enables them to train with the units they support, to provide preventive stress control services to those units in garrison, and to deploy rapidly in war or operations other than war. In fact, the first CSC detachment activated on schedule on 16 December 1991 and one half of its personnel deployed to Somalia for Operation Restore Hope on 5 January 1993. It maintained teams in Somalia until February 1994.

Combat stress control detachment teams deployed to Haiti in September 1994, early in Operation Restore Democracy, and continued to rotate there after the mission was turned over to the United Nations. Another team deployed to Saudi Arabia in October 1994, supporting a show of force and training exercise in Kuwait in response to threatening Iraqi troop movements. In December 1994, part of a CSC company, most of a CSC detachment, and the neuropsychiatric ward of a combat support hospital deployed to Guantanamo, Cuba, to provide inpatient and outpatient treatment to Cuban refugees, as well as stress control support to the U.S. troops running the camps. These missions demonstrated the versatility and value of CSC units in military situations other than war, as well as war.

U.S. ARMY COMBAT ENVIRONMENTS

To be effective combat stress control consultants and treaters, the psychiatrist and other mental health officers and NCOs must have an exceptional degree of military credibility and knowledge of the supported units. They must understand and be conversant in the unit's missions, equipment, internal organization, special language and acronyms, and typical stressors and stress profiles. In this regard, CSC personnel are analogous to flight surgeons (see Chapter 8, U.S. Air Force Combat Psychiatry). They can only achieve the necessary expertise and credibility by "flying" some hours and days with similar units in realistic field training and operations. This textbook can only provide a brief overview and introduction to a few of the major branches of the U.S. Army.

Within each branch, specific types of units (and specific officer areas of concentration and enlisted military operational specialties) have their own mission profiles and typical physical and psychological stressors. To advise a commander on how to sustain and enhance his unit's performance, or to assure him that one of his soldiers is again ready for duty, requires more than a second-hand knowledge of what that performance and duty involves.

Combat Troops

Infantry

Infantrymen (there are as yet no infantrywomen) are men who engage the enemy in close combat, sometimes hand-to-hand, standing on their feet, lying on the ground, or dispersed in holes which they have found or dug in the dirt. In battle, and sometimes between battles, they must carry everything they need to fight and survive on their persons. Infantry can be categorized by how much they must rely on their own physical strength and endurance, separated from mechanical support. Special Operations Forces (the "Green Berets") and Rangers are all airborne (parachute) qualified, but may undertake prolonged and grueling missions, with only rare, air-dropped supplies. Airborne infantry are delivered by parachute or airlanding, but are reinforced by heavier units within a few days and continue to fight as light infantry. Light infantry and air assault infantry also must travel very light on the ground, but usually have helicopters and a few light trucks for rapid redeployment and resupply.

The mechanized infantry normally work as integral members of the "combined arms team" with armor. They travel in infantry fighting vehicles (IFVs) or armored personnel carriers (APCs) that enable them to keep up with the tanks. IFVs provide some ability to fire while on the move, but most of the squad dismounts to fight on the ground when assaulting or defending a position or clearing an area. Mechanized infantry therefore share many of the stressors discussed below for armor while having more logistical support (and logistical requirements) than other infantry.

Infantry make up the most numerous component of most combat forces. Because of their relative numbers and the degree of unprotected exposure to enemy weapons and the elements, they usually suffer the highest number of casualties and make up a large percentage of the battle fatigue cases. However, the percentage of battle fatigue casualties to killed and wounded among well-trained infantry units is typically lower than in armor, artillery, or combat services support units. An average rate for conventional combat is one battle fatigue casualty per five wounded, with at least an equal number treated and returned immediately to duty. Rates of 1:3 to 1:2 are seen in very prolonged and especially static combat.

In the elite special forces, ranger, and airborne units, the ratio has been strikingly low (less than 1:10 or 1:20) even in mass casualty battles. This is attributed to the benefits of tough training, close contact with trusted leaders and comrades ("vertical and horizontal unit cohesion"), and a sense (most of the time) of having some personal control over one's fate. The ground is the infantryman's protection, allowing dispersion and shelter if wisely used. To quote a Bill Maudlin World War II cartoon, Joe is looking at a tank and says to Willie, "I'd rather dig. A moving foxhole attrac's the eye." Mines, booby traps, and chemical contamination of the ground (requiring wearing of the protective ensemble) make the ground no longer a reliable friend, and are therefore especially stressful.

Infantry soldiers are especially prone to combat exhaustion as they are deployed rapidly and are subject to extreme physical work, sleep loss, and limits on available food, water, and hygiene. They can often feel unprotected or unsupported in the field of operations. Communication can get very difficult, especially at night or in restrictive terrain when visual contact with the rest of the unit may be nearly impossible. Often moving quickly through difficult terrain or behind enemy lines, the special operations forces (SOF), light infantry, or mechanized infantry soldiers can become separated and anxious about being wounded and left on the battlefield. While this may heighten the soldiers' sense of unit cohesion, the effect of a lost or wounded member on the whole unit can be devastating.

It is in the field of battle that unit bonds are often tested and an entire unit can be immobilized or destroyed because of the one weak link in communication or trust. Prior to mobilization the unit members must get to know each other and especially to be confident in each of their abilities to fight together as a team. No unit should be deployed without the commander's having the opportunity to portray himself as a thoughtful and knowledgeable leader; a unit without confidence in its leader can fail, generating a large percentage of both emotional and physical casualties.

Because of the newer weapons technologies and the rapidly moving forward edge of the battlefield, fragmentation among infantry units can often occur. Devastation of life by enemy or friendly fire may be great, and the exposure to dead and wounded comrades as well as enemy is magnified. In this setting, human soldiers must often charge ahead and their sense of "neglecting" their buddies is intense. Sensory overload under these conditions can only be countered by the unit cohesiveness and bonding developed long before the mission is begun.

Ongoing development and testing for the "digital battlefield" of the "Information Age" of the 21st century proposes to give each infantry fire team leader, and perhaps each infantryman, a global positioning device that gives precise coordinates for his location on the terrain and short-range voice communication with other team members. There may even be a "heads-up" display inside the visor to his helmet that advises him of the locations of all other friendly forces and identified enemies in the vicinity, as well as much other information. Assuring that this technology increases combat effectiveness rather than creating distraction and dependency, especially in tired, fearful soldiers, will be an urgent topic for combat stress control in future field trials, training, and combat operations.

Armor

The armor branch soldier fights inside a tank—a heavily-armored, tracked vehicle capable of rapid cross-country movement on suitable terrain. The tank has a heavy gun for destroying other tanks and hard targets by direct (line-of-sight) fire, and machine guns for destroying exposed infantry and other "soft" targets. Tanks are most effective in the offensive in open country where, in combination with mechanized infantry and supporting artillery and air attacks, they can break through enemy defenses and spread havoc in the rear.

Much of the time, however, armor works in the offense or defense on more restrictive terrain, moving from position to position in coordinated movements with each tank much like an individual infantryman. Unlike the infantryman, however, the tank protects against bullets and artillery fragments, giving a relative sense of invulnerability. Modern tanks also have collective protection against chemical agents. Tanks are disabled (and less often destroyed) by other tank's guns, by direct artillery hits, by mines, and by a variety of infantry- or vehicle-carried antitank rockets, many of them now precision-guided.

Speed in firing first or in taking protective countermeasures (measured in seconds, if not split-seconds) can be crucial to survival. When the crew compartment of a tank is breached or the tank burns or explodes, escape may also be a matter of seconds, and death can be especially gruesome. Battle fatigue rates are therefore high among the survivors or witnesses of the deaths of fellow crew, relative to the number of wounded who get out alive. Battle fatigue to wounded ratios of 1:2 and 1:1 have been reported when armored units were caught at a disadvantage or unexpectedly found themselves outclassed by superior tanks or infantry antitank weapons.

Tanks, while giving the soldier a sense of confidence, can be sources of problems. Highly technical in today's U.S. Army, these weapons are at best finicky, subject to heavy vibration and jolting in operation, require continuous maintenance, and demand specialized skills to operate. Armor crews tend to be closely knit units, where deviance, defiance, and "specialness" are not readily tolerated. Individuals working in tank crews have to rely on the skills of their comrades, live for weeks to months together in very close proximity, and often get to know each other on an intensely personal level. The operation of the tank is dependent on each person's doing his job; the tank does not operate fully if one member of the crew is incapacitated. Maintenance units that take care of the machinery have to be reliable and known by the operators; "slacking off" is not tolerated.

Tankers rarely see their human victims close up. The mission of armor units is to neutralize other similar or smaller-sized enemy weapons. Because of this, tankers are prone to periods of heightened enthusiasm and letdowns after the mission is accomplished. Debriefing is especially important and the tendency to focus on the mechanical details of the mission, create distance from the destruction, or overpersonalize the killing, may be compelling dynamics with these crews that must be dealt with constructively.

Modern tanks have night vision and infrared sights and laser rangefinders that can make true combat sensorially much like a complex team computer-simulation task or arcade game. Individual crews now train at their tasks in "high-tech" simulators, "moving" over virtual-reality terrain and engaging virtual-reality targets that, although still substantially abstracted, are not that different from what would actually be seen. Multiple simulators can be linked together so that three to five tanks in a platoon can be maneuvering together on each other's scopes.

The combined arms team can even train together in virtual reality, with attack helicopter crews and mounted mechanized infantry all in their own simulators (perhaps even located on distant posts) working in concert on the same computer-generated terrain, supported by field artillery fire direction centers who respond to calls for artillery fire that the computer faithfully represents in real time. Research and development for the "digital battlefield" is equipping each tank with global positioning devices linked by computers and computer-generated displays in each tank and at its higher headquarters.

The successful integration of information technology into armored formations may be technically easier than with dismounted infantry, but it will still require extensive human factors evaluation and training. It must be remembered that ground war, more than air, sea, or space war, is fought under very "dirty" physical and emotional conditions. Continuous and even sustained operations are often required. Strict limits on the size and weight of equipment demand compromises: air conditioning may be necessary for the computers, but little has traditionally been invested to provide comfort for the crew members. If the "high-tech" systems break down under the strain of field operations, the crew must be capable of fixing them or carrying on without them. Fear, grief, rage, guilt, or simple sleep loss must not be allowed to impair the crucial human components of the system.

Field Artillery

The mission of field artillery is to lob projectiles of high explosives or other munitions to places relatively far away and out of sight on the battlefield. Artillery crews are usually eight to ten people, working in sections of three to four crews. Two sections comprise a battery, the equivalent of an infantry or tank company.

The towed, tube artillery are wheeled guns (technically "howitzers") that can be air-transported to support light infantry and are towed behind their "prime movers" (relatively light-weight trucks). They provide minimal protection for their crews. Firing the large shells at a rapid rate is heavy physical work. Self-propelled tube artillery are large howitzers mounted on tracked vehicles, less armored than tanks, but providing some crew protection. They are supported by other tracked vehicles carrying additional ammunition. The latest versions provide more mechanization for moving and loading the heavy shells. Missile artillery such as the Multiple Launch Rocket System (MLRS) are also tracked vehicles with considerable mechanization, but still require substantial heavy work.

Field artillery batteries and sections may be stationary at "fire bases" in some low-intensity or static combat scenarios. In "high-tech" combat, they must be highly mobile, whether to keep close behind the moving armor or to avoid the enemy's own "counter-battery fire." Modern radars can locate the source of artillery fire quickly, perhaps even before the shells ("rounds") have landed. The addition of global positioning devices and on-board, interactive computers to the most modern howitzers or rocket launchers greatly increases their ability to "shoot and scoot"—to stop, fire rapidly at a mathematically determined location, and move elsewhere. Without this enhancement, emplacing the battery is a very deliberate and precise process.

Like tank crews, soldiers in the field artillery are highly specialized technicians, especially the NCOs and officers. The potential for destruction by enemy action, while less than for infantry or armor, may be catastrophic when it occurs. The potential for error injuring one's own crew or distant friendly units is also great. Artillery units avoid direct combat with enemy ground forces, but must defend themselves against harassment and, rarely, by direct fire against infantry or armor attack (which they are likely to lose). When casualties are suffered, the ratio of battle fatigue casualties to wounded is likely to be higher than in the infantry.

Certain psychological defenses must be encouraged and supported during these soldiers' missions. Artillery soldiers have to closely rely on each other for both support and technical expertise. Training constitutes a large portion of these soldiers' days. The artillerymen have specific team drills with built-in double checks to process technical and mathematical data without error. As long as these drills are followed, tired and stressed teams are able to function accurately, if perhaps less rapidly. When stress or overconfidence leads to taking short cuts, disasters can occur, as shown in this case known to the second author.

Case Study 1: Live Fire Error

On a U.S. Army post, one artillery shell killed several infantrymen far from the allowable "impact area" on post. Investigation revealed that an artillery battery had fired that round with all seven bags of gunpowder instead of the appropriate four bags. The battery was in the last hour of a 3-day continuous operations field exercise and was firing all of the remainder of its ammunition in a sustained barrage. The enlisted soldier whose job in the drill was to take three bags out and drop them on the ground had simply failed to do so. The second soldier whose task was to count the bags and throw them into a common pit had fallen behind in his task. Bags had accumulated on the ground, so that double-checking was not simple. While the battery had had a sleep plan, both junior soldiers had stayed awake during their last "down time," helping out. The defense lawyer called the second author for advice on who was at fault.

Comment: This is the type of error of omission that is most likely with sleep loss. The muscular work of rapidly loading artillery rounds can have an almost hypnotic rhythm, punctuated by the highly reinforcing "ritual" firing and recoil of the howitzer. The final "crescendo" before going home would have produced a euphoric "adrenalin high" in the sleep-deprived brain. The ultimate responsibility has to fall on the crew chief (with some for the section chief), first for failing to assure that every double-check in the team drill was being faithfully performed and second, for not having enforced the sleep plan. Predictably, the officer and senior NCOs had not enforced the sleep plan for themselves, and were substantially more sleep-deprived than any of their enlisted soldiers.

The coordination and computation of the firing data are calculated for the entire battery by a Fire Direction Center (FDC) team. These teams are equipped with computers and radios, but can also perform manual (chart) calculations. The following case illustrates the potential effects of fatigue on these and other types of Tactical Operations Center (TOC) team performance.

Case Study 2: Fire Direction Control Research Study

Fire direction teams of one officer and four enlisted from an elite unit conducted sustained operations for up to 42 hours in a realistic mockup of an FDC tent. The scenario provided a detailed sequence of events in a combined arms operation across a map that provided comparable measures of speed, accuracy, and preplanning every 6 hours. The teams' tasks (as in combat before the fielding of special field artillery digital computers) was to manually plot the location of targets called in over the radio, and to derive range, bearing, angle of gun elevation, and charge. Some targets were called in with requests for immediate fire ("fire missions") while others were called in to be plotted for firing "on-call" or at a future scheduled time ("preplanned targets"). The FDC was also expected to update its situation map based on messages from the simulated units and to establish that targets were not at the locations of friendly units, in no fire areas, or otherwise requiring clearance from higher headquarters under the rules of engagement. Ammunition requisition and other self-initiated preplanning was expected.

Throughout the sustained operations, the teams' ability to perform their highly practiced and precise team plotting tasks, even under urgent time pressure, was unimpaired. However, after about 24 hours, they fell behind in updating their situation maps and precalculating the positions and firing data for the preplanned target lists. They lost their grasp of their place in the operation. They no longer knew where they were relative to friendly and enemy units. They no longer checked what they were firing at. When called upon to fire at several urgent targets concurrently that involved preplanned targets (which they had accomplished well early in the exercise) long delays and random serious errors occurred. Some of those errors involved their fire falling on friendly locations.

Comment: Similar and even worse problems of preplanning and internal and external communications can be expected in the headquarters staffs and tactical operations centers of infantry, armor, and higher echelon commands whose tasks do not provide the highly practiced and double-checked drills of the FDC. The development of automated data processing (computers) will reduce the need to depend on memory or make mathematical calculations. However, they may compound the problems in communication, decision making, and preplanning by lulling the staff into a false sense of security and concealing signs of system error until they are irreversible. Sleep plans are essential for all command, control, communications, and intelligence (C^3I) staffs.[32]

Artillerymen can feel more important than the average soldier because of the killing power of their weapons, the supposed "smarts" required, and the relative "luxury" of being able to transport comfort items. Conflicts can arise because of this. Artillerymen may also feel guilt (or defend against feeling disgust or guilt) at a killing process that, in most situations, keeps them relatively secure and comfortable. Mental health professionals must pay attention to the possibility that anger and depression may be present in these soldiers as they alternately feel important and useless in the overall mission on the battlefield. Another risk for artillerymen is that of fatigue.

It should be remembered that forward observer teams of artillery officers and NCOs deploy forward as integral members of infantry and armor formations. They share all of their hosts' environmental risks and stressors, with the additional stressor of being responsible for calling down devastation out of the sky, sometimes dangerously close to themselves or other friendly units.

Air Defense Artillery

This branch is responsible for the defense against enemy aircraft and ballistic missiles. Small teams with shoulder-held anti-air missiles are attached to infantry, armor, and field artillery units and share most of their hosts' stress environments. Teams with "high-tech," mobile missiles and ultra-rapid-fire guns, supported by mobile radar teams, are deployed to protect key targets such as the brigade and division support areas and corps base defense clusters. Larger missiles such as the Patriot are used to protect key air bases and ports throughout the theater of operations against ballistic missiles and long-range aircraft.

Unlike the field artillery, which are rarely totally idle, most air defense artillery in recent wars have had to sustain vigilance with little or no opportunity to fire; the exception was the Patriot missile units in the Persian Gulf War, deployed both in Saudi Arabia and Israel. There, the political impact of their presence far outweighed their actual (subsequently determined) performance, and placed upon them a heavy burden of responsibility. Fatigue and stress became a significant factor for those crews. The deployment of Patriot batteries to South Korea in 1993 as a show of resolve suggests that the responsibility will continue, and become even heavier if a potential opponent is known to have chemical, biological, or nuclear warheads.

Army Aviation

U.S. Army Aviation is currently restricted to rotary (helicopter) aircraft. Because of their ability to hover, fly "nap of the earth," and land on many kinds of terrain, helicopters are especially suited to the close support of land battles. Attack helicopters are well armored and very heavily armed, with "high-tech" target acquisition and navigation equipment. Scout helicopters are lightly armed and armored, and often work in teams with the attack helicopters. Cargo helicopters are used to ferry combat troops, ammunition and supplies, sometimes into "hot" landing zones. They have minimal armor, and may mount machine guns for self-defense. Medevac helicopters are unarmed, in accordance with the Geneva conventions. All helicopters are vulnerable, to a greater or lesser degree, to small arms fire and especially to missiles from the ground, as well as to other attack helicopters and jet fighters.

A special pride is felt by soldiers who fly aircraft. Perhaps the most technically trained and responsible soldiers, these men are proud of their contribution to the Persian Gulf War, and believe that their "machines" are the best, the most sophisticated, and the most expensive. Fliers also rarely see their victims close up. The thrill of hitting the target in a gunship raid, sneaking through enemy lines to guide troops and spot aggressors may be counterbalanced by unconscious guilt at the mass destruction caused, yet unseen. Aviators have to train as a group, but when any group of young, highly trained professionals converges, competition can become quite intense.

Pilots tend to be highly aggressive and individualistic, as noted in Chapter 9, U.S. Air Force Combat Psychiatry. Many of the author's observations about U.S. Air Force pilots also apply to U.S. Army pilots. These soldiers must be subtly reminded that they are part of a larger organization that they need as much as it needs them. Fliers can be demanding, privileged individuals who have to rely on the cooperation of air support troops, those who service the craft and provide all logistical support. Like U.S. Air Force aircrews, U.S. Army aircrews have a unit flight surgeon to monitor their physiologic and mental status and ground them if they have become unsafe. However, the U.S. Army environment is more dirty, dispersed, mobile, and spartan, perhaps leading to more fatigue and physiologic stress than in the U.S. Air Force.

Mental health professionals may have to take a humble and reassuring stance when interacting with pilots and others in the aviation corps to allow for adequate ventilation of frustrations and anxieties. Pilots are very concerned about being taken off flight status if they admit to emotional problems

(especially suicidal thoughts). They will not open up to a mental health officer they do not know and trust, as was also noted in Chapter 8.

Combat Support/Combat Service Support Troops

There is a poorly defined distinction between the "combat arms" (who actively try to kill the enemy, as attack helicopters do), and the combat support and combat service support branches. Combat support, in theory, refers to those who actively facilitate the battle (such as the Signal Corps, Military Intelligence, Engineers, Military Police, and the Special Operations Forces' Psychological Operations and Civil Affairs units) while combat service support (CSS) refers to those who sustain the ability of the combat arms to fight by transporting the ammunition, fuel, food and water, servicing and repairing the equipment, providing health care, sorting the mail and providing other personnel and administrative services.

The distinctions between "combat" and "support" are often arbitrary and inconsistent across soldiers within a branch or corps. The combat engineers are a macho "combat arm" who share and often exceed the risks of the infantry and armor as they precede them into battle to clear minefields and bridges or blow up obstacles. They rely on sophisticated armored vehicles or brute strength, and defend themselves or attack enemy positions with personal and heavy weapons. The civil engineers use military versions of civilian equipment to build roads, buildings, and other infrastructure in the rear. The combat signalman crouches alongside the infantry platoon leader under fire, while signal battalions set up and operate the mobile subscriber telephone nodes, satellite uplinks, and other communications throughout the theater of operation. The military police may be far forward or far to the rear, maintaining route security, securing and guarding enemy prisoners of war, or enforcing the Uniform Code of Military Justice (UCMJ) on U.S. service members who misbehave.

Mechanics can be found in contact teams operating recovery vehicles on the battlefield, in maintenance companies in the brigade and division support areas, and in large depots in the corps rear. Truck drivers in infantry battalions drive forward in convoys at night to deliver supplies at a rendezvous with the maneuver companies' first sergeants, scant kilometers from the enemy. Truck drivers of division and corps transportation or petroleum distribution companies may drive cross-country through minefields at night, trying to keep the advancing armored formations supplied, or may drive only along well-secured main supply routes in the rear with military police escort.

Even the personnel clerks, supply clerks, and cooks may be assigned in an infantry battalion headquarters company, performing guard duty at night for the brigade support area. Alternatively, they may be in a corps headquarters or quartermaster ordnance or personnel administration unit, in a "safe" rear area with only periodic charge-of-quarters (CQ) or staff duty at night. The cooks everywhere work extra-long hours. Of course, on the modern battlefield, no place is totally safe. Even the U.S. Army stevedores unloading ships at the port of embarkation may be subject to ballistic missile or terrorist attack.

Because most CSS troops are further from direct contact with the enemy and further from enemy artillery than the combat arms, fewer CSS troops are killed and wounded in action. However, when they do suffer attack, their ratio of battle fatigue casualties to battle casualties is typically higher than in the "combat hardened" combat arms.

It can be hypothesized (but should never be presumed) that the combat support/service support soldiers who are *integral* to forward combat units will take on some of the typical psychological characteristics and stress profiles of their assigned units. Those who are only *habitually* attached may be a little less so inclined. Soldiers or teams who are only *temporarily* attached or recently arrived far forward will be in transition and under the highest stress. Personnel who are in familiar units of their own kind in areas with very low probability of attack may come closest to fitting the stereotype of the rear area soldier (the "REMF," or Rear Echelon Mother F—er, as the combat soldiers in Vietnam labeled them).

The stereotypic REMFs are managers, not leaders. At his worst, the REMF is the petty (or senior) bureaucrat who enjoys exercising arbitrary power over others and uses the rules and regulations to do so. The REMFs take advantage of their positions to acquire even more benefits and comforts than their rear-area positions naturally provide them, often at the expense of the combat soldiers for whom those comforts (supplies, equipment, R and R facilities) were intended. Low-ranking REMFs who have no power (and even some higher-ranking REMFs who do) are prone to the disorders of frustration and loneliness, as discussed in Chapter 3.

The rear-area soldiers (whether REMF or "regular Joe or Jane") may feel not part of the battle, unappreciated, and left out of both the excitement and tragedy of war. Some secretly wish to participate in the battle and can feel inadequate, cheated, and inauthentic as soldiers. They may take dangerous risks or violate regulations to gain macho souvenirs such as enemy weapons. They may have too much boring time without meaningful duties, and too much access to the temptations of substance abuse, unsafe sex, or other misconduct. These misbehaviors need the special intervention of mental health workers because they are contagious, and because without supplies and other logistical support, the combat troops cannot fight.

Some features of the Persian Gulf War worked to counteract many of the traditional causes of the REMF syndrome. The strict prohibitions on alcohol, substance abuse, and nonmarital sex of the host nation, and the deliberate segregation of most U.S. units from the local population in Saudi Arabia were protective, but will not occur in all future deployments. The U.S. Army does have a strict drug abuse prevention policy and may adopt a "no alcohol-in-theater" or "only 2 beers at unit functions" policy, very different from the active pushing of alcohol in Vietnam.

The priority of deploying combat forces to deter further aggression during Operation Desert Shield (the mobilization phase of the Persian Gulf War) meant that there was a very low proportion of combat service support troops, who accordingly worked extremely long, hard hours. Living conditions were initially as austere for the CSS units as for the combat arms, and the senior U.S. Army leadership deliberately kept it that way. They did not build up a comfortable supporting base. In part that was to reassure the host nation that there was no intention to stay. The logistical system was also too tasked with bringing in war materials to bring in luxuries. The senior leaders also remembered, however, how much they and their troops had resented the REMFs when they were junior officers and NCOs in Vietnam. They deliberately lived spartanly themselves, and required austerity of all their subordinate CSS units. Some leaders required their rear area CSS soldiers in safe areas to wear helmets and even flak jackets when there was no threat, as a symbol of solidarity with the combat soldiers.

Finally, when the Scud missile attacks began, and later when the ground offensive proceeded with relatively few U.S. casualties, whatever guilt or sense of unimportance many CSS personnel may have felt was absolved. The senior leadership did praise the logisticians' part in winning the war. However, many CSS units did miss out on the victory parades and felt unappreciated by civilian society when they returned home late after staying to clear up the battlefield and store or ship the equipment.

It should also be remembered that a large percentage of CSS units are in the reserves, and so face the additional stressors of seriously disrupted occupational, financial, and family affairs. The importance of building high unit cohesion and strong family support groups in reserve units is obvious, but is not easily accomplished except in units from small towns with strong roots in the civilian community.

The following disguised case history illustrates inadequacies of leadership and questionable conduct in a CSS unit, as revealed in a delayed end-of-tour debriefing following the Persian Gulf War.

Case Study 3: Leadership Problems in a CSS Unit

A reserve transportation battalion was deployed to the theater shortly before combat began. As expected, its companies and teams were widely dispersed, attached to other units for logistic and administrative support while performing heavy, sometimes dangerous, duties. The dispersed elements felt that their headquarters did not keep track of them or assure their support. The commander was perceived as having several favorite officers (all white males), while devaluing minority and female officers and all NCOs. Rules were applied unfairly; for example, even married enlisted couples in the unit were denied conjugal privileges while it is alleged that the favorite officers slept with whomever they could "persuade." The battalion chaplain was perceived as the commander's spy, since retribution seemed to follow soon after any complaints were shared with him.

All awards and decorations after the war went to the white male favorites. The unit cooks who had been levied to drive trucks in a heroic night convoy to take supplies through minefields (illuminated only with blackout lights and following in the tread marks of the tanks that had gone before) did not even receive certificates of appreciation because "they were just doing their jobs." The company commander who had organized the convoy but stayed behind at headquarters received the decoration for valor.

The unit was late in redeploying home, missing all the victory parades. The soldiers rejoined unsympathetic employers, families, and creditors who said they'd "only been support troops, not in combat." The commander and favorite officers immediately left the unit, taking their awards with them, and leaving the previously devalued NCOs plus new officers in charge. Within a year, many unit members were reporting symptoms of fatigue, trouble concentrating, hair loss, joint pains, and other complaints. They attributed their symptoms to exposure to antimissile radar emissions (from an installation near their headquarters in the theater) or chemicals.

Comment: The question of whether the symptoms were caused by some exposure or exposures deserved, and received, intensive medical evaluation. What was unquestionable during the debriefings that these units participated in over a year after their return was the open anger and sense of betrayal expressed by the junior NCOs and enlisted. The senior NCOs retained their professionalism during the debriefings, but confirmed the enlisteds' memories of the events in private conversation. The role of a sense of betrayal and injustice in the etiology of PTSD has been emphasized by Shay.[33] It was unfair to accuse the chaplain of violating confidentiality—the commander could have simply been good at guessing, or indiscriminately punished every suspect when the chaplain advised him of low morale and the reasons for it. However, had the unit's elements been visited routinely by mental health/CSC (MH/CSC) teams while in theater, the original poor leadership and questionable conduct could have been corrected.

Evolving U.S. Army doctrine and organization[30] calls for the area support medical battalion mental health section, reinforced by teams from the CSC Company, to visit every company-sized unit every few weeks to conduct unit survey interviews with the troops. These structured interviews serve both a data gathering and a ventilating function. The MH/CSC teams' command consultations might have inspired the commander to improve his ways or, that failing, have advised his senior commander.

The unit should also have had an end-of-tour debriefing and scheduled homecoming debriefings before redeploying home. The family support groups should have been involved in posthomecoming activities that validated the spouses', and their own, honorable service under hardship and (for some) real danger. Those measures would have decompressed the anger and facilitated constructive action a year sooner.

One group of CSS troops deserves special attention from the MH/CSC organization and others. These are the formal Mortuary Affairs units (previously called Graves Registration). Those who must recover, process, and transport the bodies of the dead and their personal effects are at very high risk of developing post-traumatic stress disorder. This is often of the delayed type because of the tough emotional shell they form to perform their gruesome duties day after day. There are also many other soldiers in all other branches and military specialties who are temporarily detailed to body recovery and disposition duties, or who are exposed to human remains. These include the tank turret mechanics or ordnance specialists who cannot repair the tank until they have washed out the remaining blood and pieces of tank's crew, who had been lying under the sun for several days. Chapter 10, Combat Stress Control in Joint Operations, provides a summary (information card) on measures these people should take to enable them to perform their very important morale-sustaining duties and return home feeling proud about what they have done without being haunted by the dreams and memories they may have for the rest of their lives.

The Medical Combat Health Support Troops

Combat medics share all of the stressors of the combat arms units they support. Battalion aid stations (Level I care) follow close behind. Medical companies maintain clearing stations and treatment teams in the brigade support and division support areas close to the front and at base defense clusters in corps. These companies can move themselves rapidly, tearing down and setting up within hours. Although technically privileged against attack by the Geneva Convention, they are often forbidden by the tactical commanders from showing the red cross on white background emblem.

Forward surgical teams (replacing the current Mobile Army Surgical Hospitals) can reinforce the medical companies as far forward as the brigades. Dental teams set up to support troop concentrations. Preventive medicine and veterinary teams routinely visit units to inspect sanitation, disease vectors, and food supplies. Ground and air ambulances are prepositioned or deploy forward to bring casualties quickly back to the clearing station (Level II) and hospital (Level III) care.

The hospitals use Deployable Medical Systems (DEPMEDS) expandable shelters, TEMPER (tent, extendible, modular, personnel) tents, and prepacked sets to assemble a climate-controlled complex of wards, operating rooms, laboratory and x-ray radiographic facilities, pharmacy, administrative, and admission and disposition areas. The hospital staff are usually quartered in general purpose (GP) large tents without climate control. Hospitals take days to set up and break down, and many trucks from nonmedical sources to move. They also require extensive logistical support to operate. They are therefore normally located in the corps, although some may be close to the divisions. Hospitals normally do show the red cross, indicating privileged status.

Casualties with medical diseases and nonbattle injuries may reach the aid stations, clearing stations, and hospitals at a fairly steady rate, barring some epidemic illness or mass casualty accident. The war-wound surgical caseload, like battles, are likely to come in surges separated by lulls. It is the role of the medical regulating officer at the medical group headquarters to spread the casualties somewhat evenly, and to direct patients who need specialty team care to the hospitals that have those specialty teams. In major battles, all hospitals may experience mass casualty conditions. Sick or wounded enemy prisoners of war are also brought to U.S. hospitals. The Geneva Convention[34] requires that they be treated the same as U.S. casualties, according to the same triage categories.

What are some of the stressors unique to medical units? The AMEDD professionals and specialty technicians often do not train frequently under field conditions, and so are unfamiliar with the sets, kits, and outfits. They may not appreciate why they do not have their familiar, latest drugs, sutures, and diagnostic equipment, in field-portable form. They may have difficulty acclimatizing to the dirt, discomfort and primitive hygiene facilities, as well as to the separation from home and the potential of personal danger. Many are PROFIS or IRR (Individual Ready Reserve) individuals who are joining unfamiliar units that may or may not already have a unit cohesion that incorporates them. The highly specialized professionals and technicians are often very concerned if they are unable to practice their specialized procedures, lest they lose their skills and their credentials.

Treating seriously wounded casualties is stressful, but justifies to the medical personnel why they themselves are there. It quickly builds and sustains unit cohesion unless something disrupts the patient care. However, the casualties can arouse several distressing ethical issues. How do different individuals deal with the moral dilemma of placing patients in the "expectant" triage category, especially the patients they know they could save if they only had fewer patients, more supplies, or the "high-tech" equipment back in their stateside hospital? How do they face the moral dilemma of saving the grossly, pitifully disabled patient when they *do* have the resources to do so, especially if the patient begs to be given "grace" (euthanasia)? How do they face the moral dilemma of returning soldiers to duty, perhaps to be wounded again or killed, when they themselves do not have to risk direct combat? May they become overwhelmed or depressed by their inability to relieve the suffering or save the lives of so many young Americans with whom they identify? How do they deal with their anger, hatred, and perhaps guilt, when treating the injured enemy prisoner who may have been the one who wounded those not-quite-so-urgently triaged American soldiers next to him? May they be upset at being forbidden to treat local foreign civilians in need who are not the U.S. Army's responsibility? May they be horrified at receiving the victims of atrocity, including women and small children, who *are* their responsibility to treat, as when the Iraqi Shiite victims of Republican Guard massacres in southern Iraq were air evacuated to U.S. hospitals in theater after the Gulf War?

Medical personnel often tend to deny stress in themselves, and may have to be approached diplomatically or indirectly by mental health/CSC consultants. Special attention should be given to those personnel who are not normally direct patient care providers. Those persons usually have less "stress inoculation." They include the food service, maintenance, administrative, and laboratory personnel. These are the ones most likely to be detailed to be litter bearers for the severely injured, attendants for the expectant patients, or handlers for the bodies in the morgue.

Hospitals are nominally staffed for two 12-hour shifts a day, but mass casualties can require continuous or sustained operations for periods of several days to weeks. Fatigue impacts heavily on patient care as well as on morale and stress tolerance. Medical personnel can become battle fatigue casualties, and require treatment according to PIES (**p**roximity, **i**mmediacy, **e**xpectancy, and **s**implicity), with the five Rs, as discussed in Chapter 10. Stress and fatigue can also disrupt interpersonal communication and cooperation, impairing unit efficiency in subtle ways. Misconduct stress behaviors can occur. These include "self-medication" with alcohol and with the drugs that are available (by pilfering or "skimming") in medical facilities. Seeking solace in sexual relationships is a natural reaction to loneliness and "living on the edge." However, fraternization (heterosexual as well as homosexual) and adultery are criminal violations of the UCMJ. Consensual heterosexual misconduct has rarely been punished, but its occurrence in medical units adversely impacts upon unit morale, especially when unit leaders are involved. The rumors and aftermath of "deployment affairs" can also have harmful effects on families back home.

Monitoring these many stress issues and intervening when indicated is a command and leadership responsibility.[29] The hospital or battalion chaplain can often be helpful. Responsibility is also given, by doctrine,[30] to the neuropsychiatric ward and consultation service in the hospitals and to the medical combat stress control company or detachment that is providing area support in the vicinity. Interventions are reviewed elsewhere in this textbook.

MEDICAL/PSYCHIATRIC ORGANIZATION AND THE COMBAT STRESS COMPANY

The neuropsychiatric and mental health team consists of neurologists, psychiatrists, clinical psychologists, social workers, psychiatric and mental health nurses, occupational therapists, and the various enlisted technicians in those specialties. Mental health professionals in the Army Medical Department (AMEDD) are those commissioned officers and enlisted personnel specialists trained and credentialed to provide the various mental health functions. In addition to those previously mentioned, other professionals can be qualified for these specialized services such as physician assistants (PA), counselors, and chaplains. Para-professionals or technicians are the behavioral science specialists (91G), psychiatric specialists (91F), and occupational therapy specialists (91L).

The Mental Health Program

The mental health program of the military is somewhat different in peacetime from that during mobilization. The U.S. Army regulation that is the basis for both is *Neuropsychiatry and Mental Health*.[26] The regulation prescribes and refines policies and concepts regarding neuropsychiatry (NP) principles for mental health staff and facilities. This directs the neuropsychiatry/mental health staff to advise and assist command to conserve and maintain manpower at maximum efficiency. While the emphasis is on mobilization, it is important during peacetime to prepare by employing common neuropsychiatry and mental health principles. Neuropsychiatric and mental health personnel must be ready and responsive for mobilization and other missions as required.

Basic Principles

Based on experiences gained during World War I and World War II, the Korean conflict, and the Vietnam conflict, the following principles have evolved for the prevention, treatment, and administrative management of neuropsychiatric and stress disorders. Major emphasis is placed on *preventive* psychiatry and mental health programs that lead to early recognition and preventive treatment of potential mental health problems. This is similar to preventive medicine concepts. Neuropsychiatric personnel make a primary contribution to this program by fulfilling the appropriate responsibilities outlined in the U.S. Army mission.

While neurology and psychiatry functions are generally separate during peacetime, in mobilization the neuropsychiatric emphasis collocating neurology with psychiatry is used. Both battle and nonbattle injuries and illnesses are thus coded in those categories. In addition, the "neuropsychiatric" term clearly includes the organic (physical) as well as the functional (mental) types of disorder. This is particularly important in trauma, and nuclear, biological and chemical (NBC) scenarios. In Medical Force 2000, the only neurologist is in the general hospital. In the proposed Force 21 AMEDD, neurologists may not be included in the TO&E of deployed hospitals or CSC units, but will be available to provide consultation via telemedicine.

In combat, treatment of battle fatigue and other types of neuropsychiatric casualties will be *instituted early*, as near the unit of origin as practicable. Proper psychiatric treatment of neuropsychiatric casualties requires a military environment rather than a traditional hospital atmosphere. Mild "duty" cases should be treated and returned to duty immediately from the battalion aid station, brigade, or division or area support medical company medical treatment section or hospital admissions and dispositions section, or in nonmedical units whenever the tactical situation permits.

Early return to duty is the therapeutic objective. This can be accomplished only if the medical officer accepts full responsibility to make often difficult diagnostic or disposition decisions objectively and without delay. Neuropsychiatric referrals from supporting or noncombat troops should be made to the nearest mental health personnel who are often stationed forward of the combat service support unit. Moderate "rest" cases who cannot return to their units immediately but who do not need medical or mental health observation and treatment or both should be sent to rest for 1 to 2 days.

Patients suffering from severe battle fatigue (hold or refer), or other neuropsychiatric patients who cannot be returned to duty at the forward facilities, are to be channeled to the division medical support unit(s) having mental health/CSC capability. These teams must have a capability of providing rest and restorative therapy for up to 72 hours prior to return to duty. Those casualties who prove to need longer treatment will be evacuated to a 7- to 14-day reconditioning program at CSC facilities in direct or general support of the unit. After that period, the individual will be returned to duty or evacuated to the communications zone or CONUS Level-IV reconditioning program.

In noncombat situations the evaluation, treatment, and disposition of nonpsychotic psychiatric patients, except in unusual cases, will be on an *outpatient basis.* Their retention on duty status facilitates therapy and reduces ineffectiveness. In both combat and noncombat situations, *direct communication and liaison* among neuropsychiatry (MH and CSC) staff (for example, between division psychiatrists and the theater neuropsychiatry consultant) through technical channels as approved by appropriate command surgeons, are indispensable to monitoring evacuation and issuing policy. Such communication must be actively encouraged.

The *rapid communication* of technical information, especially in combat, is essential to an effective mental health program. It should be recognized that the greater the combat pressure, the more difficult it becomes to maintain necessary communication. Therefore, maximum use of direct forwarding of technical reports must be done, consistent with good judgment and propriety.

The overall effectiveness of any neuropsychiatry program is dependent on the proper *numbers, distribution, and assignment* of qualified mental health personnel. It is essential that the staff promote training and make accurate evaluations of mental health personnel to assure their appropriate assignment. Neuropsychiatry personnel should ensure that all medical personnel have some familiarity with basic combat psychiatric principles.

All mental health combat stress control personnel should be cross-trained in specialized topics and techniques to include:

- Briefing on CSC unit status, functions and capabilities.
- Educating leaders, chaplains, and medical personnel on stress casualty identification, management and disposition; substance abuse; suicide prevention; family violence prevention.
- Teaching stress management, relaxation techniques, coping skills, grief and anger management, conflict resolution, parenting.
- Facilitating small team after-action debriefings by unit leaders.
- Leading critical event debriefings of functioning military teams.
- Conducting individual and small group debriefing of stress casualties.
- Assessing interviews, basic mental status, and recognition of signs requiring additional mental or physical status workup by specialists.

Each of the five MH/CSC disciplines also brings areas of special expertise, which may be partially cross-trained to the others. The psychiatrist, as working physician, practices psychiatry in the triage, diagnosis, brief intervention treatment, and disposition of soldiers and patients. The psychiatrist assists with triage and acute trauma life support during mass casualties, and assists with routine sick call and care of the ill, wounded and injured, especially those with return-to-duty potential. The psychiatrist should be ATLS- (Advanced Trauma Life Support) qualified by the Combat Casualty Care Course, and have completed the NBC casualty care course.

The occupational therapist (OT), assisted by the NCO and enlisted specialist, increases the capability to evaluate physical and mental functional capacity related to combat duty performance; prescribes and supervises therapeutic work and recreational activities for recovery battle fatigue cases in support of the host medical facility; and assesses alternative duty assignments for soldiers who cannot return-to-duty in their original specialty. The OTs also advise unit commanders regarding work schedule organization and time management, constructive structuring of rest and tension-relieving activities, and use of work assignments in preventing battle fatigue and misconduct stress behaviors and in restoring recovered cases to full duty. The OTs provide rehabilitative care for minor orthopedic injuries, especially of the upper extremity.

The psychiatric nurse (66C)/clinical nurse specialist (66C7T), assisted by the 91Fs, greatly increases the capability to stabilize and hold potentially disruptive cases at forward locations for further evaluation. Some cases can be returned to duty at this echelon, if they improve in 24 to 36 hours with sleep and a structured military milieu, instead of having to be evacuated immediately to a hospital in the corps area. If the position is filled by a clinical nurse specialist, as authorized by the TO&E, this nurse may be credentialed to prescribe selected psychotherapeutic drugs. The psychiatric nurses are especially suited for consultation and preventive interventions with other medical and nursing staffs in medical facilities. Psychiatric nurses in the corps hospitals provide further stabilization for either transfer to CSC reconditioning programs or for air evacuation out of theater.

The social work officer, assisted by the 91Gs, applies the principles, knowledge and skills of social work to the psychosocial systems of U.S. Army units and their Family Support Groups. They are prepared to coordinate with other Department of the Army, Department of Defense, and civilian support agencies. The social worker provides mental health assessment and treatment, coordinates support for division soldiers and families, and has expertise in prevention/intervention for family violence and substance abuse control.

The clinical psychologist, assisted by 91Gs, provides diagnostic assessment, and can administer and interpret psychological and neuropsychological tests to diagnose problem cases and assess potential for recovery. The psychologist's treatment and consultation skills include the behavior therapies and focused applications of learning theory. Doctoral-level psychology training in research methods and statistics contributes in unit surveys and the analysis of trends.

THE FUTURE

The U.S. Army's battlefield tenets of initiative, agility, synchronization, and depth are designed to surprise and overstress enemy forces.[35] They make the enemy incapable of cohesive action. Those same tenets demand high-level mental skills from leaders and soldiers at every echelon. It is these mental skills that are most vulnerable to degradation by stress. The enemy seeks to impose stress on U.S. troops, and U.S. Army planners, in turn, accept stress as a calculated risk in the U.S. Army's plan to impose greater stress on the enemy.

Control of stress is the commander's responsibility. Before, during, and after operations, the commander is aided in this responsibility by specialized AMEDD CSC/Mental Health personnel. These personnel work in concert with the NCO chain of support, the chaplains, unit medical personnel, and principal and special staff. Commanders and their other supporting personnel must give priority to their primary missions. Stress control is so important to mission accomplishment that AMEDD mental health personnel have been assigned in every war since World War I with combat stress control as their primary duty.

Evolving doctrine calls for the United States to use technological superiority to win decisively on the digitized battlefield. These weapons systems call for an extremely high level of knowledge, skill, and sustained mental acuity on the part of every soldier. Human error due to stress can lead to devastating failures in "high-tech" systems, such as that seen on the U.S. Navy guided missile cruiser, the *Vincennes*. Combat stress control—the continual monitoring of stress levels and prompt intervention when indicated—takes on increased importance in the "high-tech" environment.

The combination of highly lethal, mobile, and interspersed weapons systems from different branches, services, and allies, with interpretation of enemy doctrine and movements, creates an intrinsic risk of friendly fire casualties. This risk must be calculated and the stress consequences, which extend far beyond the involved units, must be assessed and controlled. The combat stress control system assists this process.

Advanced communications technologies so vital on the battlefield also make modern warfare a very public enterprise. News, video, and private telephone can take the battle to the homefront almost instantaneously, complicating operations security and bringing battlefield stressors into living rooms across the country and around the world. Telephones and media can also bring homefront stressors to the soldier overseas. The interaction between unit leaders and their units' families is vitally important to mission readiness. Active Family Support Groups have been effective in decreasing the historically large percentage of battlefield stress related to issues back home.

The U.S. Army will continue to leverage existing and emerging technological capabilities to enhance support operations across the full range of military operations. Application of technologies to enhance and assure communications is vital to the CSC concept.

SUMMARY AND CONCLUSION

The basic concept in management of neuropsychiatric casualties is increasingly higher, multitiered echelons of care. Mental health personnel and programs must be flexible and mobile. Assessment and triage at clearing stations by trained specialists and professionals is essential. Exercise in peacetime of all elements of the program is important. Communication nets are critical if coordination is to be effective. Successful capability of the various elements to hold and carry transient casualties needs planning and practice. Developing a personnel program to return soldiers to duty will require staff action at various headquarters. Ability to provide rest and restorative care (sleep space, food, and so forth) in a protected but accessible area must be planned early. Personnel needs above the standard TO&E requirement must be anticipated if sufficient augmentation is to be made possible. Training in basic stress management for neuropsychiatric problems and cross-training in life saving techniques is essential. Education of all health professionals in basic neuropsychiatric concepts is important.

REFERENCES

1. Bailey P, Williams FE, Komora PA, Salmon TW, Fenton N, eds. *Neuropsychiatry.* Vol 10. In: *The Medical Department of the United States Army in the World War.* Washington, DC: Office of The Surgeon General, US Army; 1929.

2. Glass AJ, Bernucci R, eds. *Zone of Interior.* Vol 1. In: *Neuropsychiatry in World War II.* Washington, DC: Office of The Surgeon General, US Army; 1966.

3. Glass AJ, ed. *Overseas Theaters.* Vol 2. In: *Neuropsychiatry in World War II.* Washington, DC: Office of The Surgeon General, US Army; 1973.

4. Rush B. Cited by: Shafer HB. *The American Medical Profession, 1783–1850.* New York: Columbia University Press; 1936: 27–31.

5. Lovell J. Cited by: Shafer HB. *The American Medical Profession, 1783–1850.* New York: Columbia University Press; 1936: 27–31.

6. Rosen G. Nostalgia: A "forgotten" psychological disorder. *Psychol Med.* 1975;5:340–354.

7. DaCosta. Cited by: Deutsch A. Military psychiatry: The Civil War, 1861–1865. In: Hall JK, Zilboorg G, Bunker HA, eds. *One Hundred Years of American Psychiatry: 1844–1944.* New York: Columbia University Press; 1944: 367–384.

8. Jones FD, Johnson AW. Medical and psychiatric treatment policy and practice in Vietnam. *J Soc Issues.* 1975;31(4):49–65.

9. Richards RL. Mental and nervous disorders in the Russo-Japanese War. *Milit Surg* [now *Milit Med*]. 1910;26(2): 177–193.

10. Salmon TW. The care and treatment of mental diseases and war neurosis ("shell shock") in the British Army. In: Bailey P, Williams FE, Komora PA, Salmon TW, Fenton N, eds. *Neuropsychiatry.* Vol 10. In: *The Medical Department of the United States Army in the World War.* Washington, DC: Office of The Surgeon General, US Army; 1929: Appendix; 497–523.

11. Ginsberg E, Anderson JK, Ginsberg SW, Herma JL. *The Ineffective Soldier: Patterns of Performance.* New York: Columbia University Press; 1959: 11.

12. Cohen RR: Mental hygiene for the trainee. *Am J Psychiatry.* 1943;100: 62–71.

13. Bartemeier LH, Kubie LS, Menninger KA, Romano J, Whitehorn JC. Combat exhaustion. *J Nervous and Mental Disease.* 1946;104:358–389.

14. Glass AJ, Drayer CS. Italian campaign (1 March 1944–2 May 1945), Psychiatry established at division level. In: Glass AJ, ed. *Overseas Theaters.* Vol 2. In: *Neuropsychiatry in World War II.* Washington, DC: Office of The Surgeon General, US Army; 1973; 47–109.

15. Stouffer SA, DeVinney LC, Star SA, Williams RM. *The American Soldier.* Vol 2. Princeton, NJ: Princeton University Press; 1949.

16. Beebe GW, De Bakey ME. *Battle Casualties: Incidence, Mortality, and Logistic Considerations*. Springfield, Ill: Charles C Thomas; 1952.

17. Swank RL, Marchand F. Combat neuroses: Development of combat exhaustion. *Arch Neurol Psychiatry* [superseded in part by *Arch Neurol* and *Arch Gen Psychiatry*]. 1946;55:236–247.

18. Beebe GW, Appel JW. *Variation in Psychological Tolerance to Ground Combat in World War II, Final Report*. Washington, DC: National Academy of Sciences; 1958.

19. Glass AJ. Lessons learned. In Glass AJ, ed. *Overseas Theaters*. Vol 2. In: *Neuropsychiatry in World War II*. Washington, DC: Office of The Surgeon General, US Army; 1973: 989–1027.

20. Jones FD. Experiences of division psychiatrist in Vietnam. *Milit Med*. 1967;132(12):1003–1008.

21. Parrish MD. Personal Communication, 27 July 1991.

22. Glass AJ. Observations upon the epidemiology of mental illness in troops during warfare. Presented at the Symposium on Social Psychiatry; April 1957; Walter Reed Army Institute of Research, Washington, DC. 185–198.

23. Reister FA. *Battle Casualties and Medical Statistics: US Army Experience in the Korean War*. Washington, DC: Office of The Surgeon General, US Department of the Army; 1986: 58–59.

24. Copen EG. Discussed in: Jones FD, Johnson AW. Medical and psychiatric treatment policy and practice in Vietnam. *J Soc Issues*. 1975;31(4):49–65.

25. Camp NM. The Vietnam war and the ethics of combat psychiatry. *Am J Psychiatry*. 1993;150:1000–1010.

26. US Department of the Army. *Neuropsychiatry and Mental Health*. Washington, DC: US Government Printing Office; 1 September 1984. Army Regulation 40-216.

27. US Department of the Army. *Health Service Support in the Theater of Operations*. Washington, DC: DA; 1 March 1991. Field Manual 8-10.

28. US Department of the Army. *Brigade and Division Surgeon Handbook*. Washington, DC: DA; 1991. Field Manual 8-10-15.

29. US Department of the Army. *Leaders' Manual for Combat Stress Control*. Washington, DC: DA; 29 September 1994. Field Manual 22-51.

30. US Department of the Army. *Combat Stress Control in a Theater of Operations*. Washington, DC: DA; 29 September 1994. Field Manual 8-51.

31. Johnson LB, Cline DW, Marcum JM, Intress JL, Effectiveness of a stress recovery unit during the Persian Gulf War. *Hosp Community Psychiatry*. 1992;43(8):829–833.

32. Banderet LE, Stokes JW, Francesconi R. Artillery teams in simulated sustained combat: Performance and other measures. In: Johnson LC, Tepas DI, Colquhoun WP, eds. *Biological Rhythms, Sleep and Shift Work*. New York: Spectrum; 1981: 459–479.

33. Shay J. *Achilles in Vietnam: Combat Trauma and the Undoing of Character*. New York: Athenium; 1994.

34. *Geneva Convention for the Amelioration of the Condition of the Wounded and Sick in Armed Forces in the Field. 21 April–12 August 1949*. Geneva, Switzerland: Geneva Convention; 1949: D-1.

35. US Department of the Army. *Force XXI Combat Health Support Operations* [draft concept], Annex I, Combat Stress Control. Fort Sam Houston, Tex: US Army Medical Department Center and School; May 1995.

Chapter 8

U.S. AIR FORCE COMBAT PSYCHIATRY

DAVID R. JONES, M.D., M.P.H.*

*Colonel (ret), Medical Corps, U.S. Air Force; Chief Flight Surgeon, Aeropsych Associates, 4204 Gardendale, Suite 203, San Antonio, Texas 78229-3132; Clinical Professor of Psychiatry, Uniformed Services University of the Health Sciences, Bethesda, Maryland; Clinical Professor of Psychiatry, University of Texas Health Science Center at San Antonio, Texas

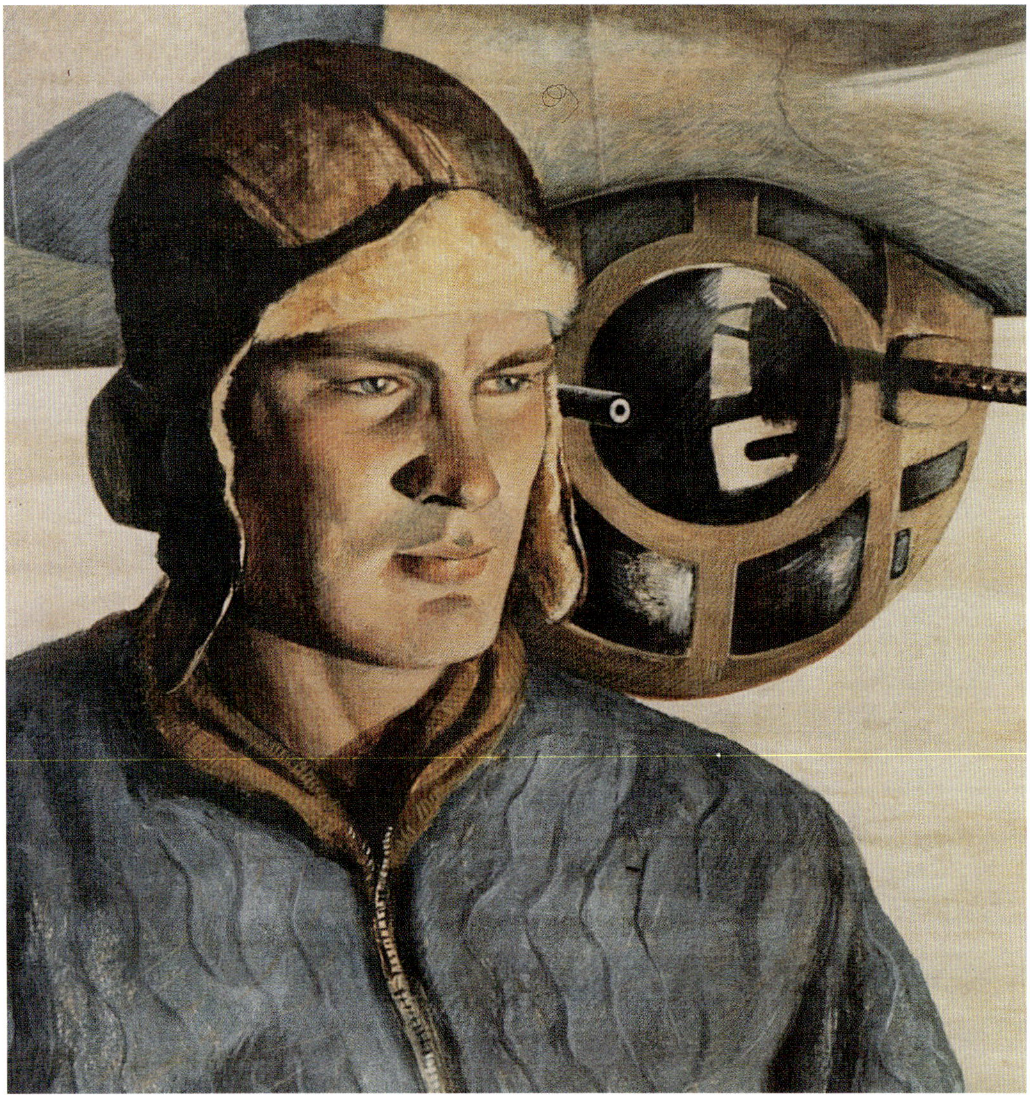

Peter Hurd — *Aerial Gunner, England* — 1944

Peter Hurd was a Life Magazine artist during World War II, assigned to cover the action on Ascension Island and also in England. His painting depicts a gunner standing in front of his turret on the belly of a bomber. For sheer terror, few jobs in the U.S. Army Air Forces in World War II could compare to his—relying on his own composure, wits, and agility to shoot down enemy aircraft, while totally exposed to return fire

Art: Courtesy of US Center of Military History, Washington, DC.

INTRODUCTION

The U.S. Air Force mission and its possible combat scenarios differ considerably from those of other services. Traditionally, the people at risk in the U.S. Air Force have been the fliers—the pilots, navigators, weapons systems operators (WSOs), electronics countermeasure operators, radio operators, gunners, loadmasters, flying crew chiefs, and other highly skilled and carefully selected personnel. These fliers have been the tip of the arrow, supported by the rest of the U.S. Air Force. Thus, at a 3,000-person airbase, only the 300 or so fliers might be exposed to combat. Security police armed with light weapons provide perimeter security against small attacks, but most of the personnel on base are usually not even issued personal weapons. The U.S. Air Force has no tradition of arms, little training in the use of rifles and pistols, and essentially no tactical field training in self-defense. In case of ground attack, most personnel are expected to take cover and wait while some other military service or the base's own aircraft and security police fight off the attacking enemy. Leadership training of U.S. Air Force officers and noncommissioned officers (NCOs) does not address handling troops in deadly peril, and the average service member knows little about how to behave under attack. Few role models are available, either through tradition or in real life.

Thus, two differences come immediately into focus when comparing the U.S. Air Force role to the roles of the other services[1]:

1. In the past, the brunt of battle has been borne by a select, highly trained small group of U.S. Air Force fliers, with whom the mass of troops may not be able to identify personally.
2. In the event of enemy attack, most U.S. Air Force members will have to take cover and wait while others decide their fate. This passive role carries with it a particular vulnerability to combat reactions. [This is further discussed in Chapter 6, A Psychological Model of Combat Stress.—Ed.]

The combat stresses borne by the fliers and by those nonflying members who may have to suffer through a ground attack on the base will be considered separately, drawing examples from wars of the past in order to develop and discuss future preventive and therapeutic measures to preserve the fighting strength.

SUPPORT OF FLIERS IN COMBAT

The nature of war dictates that, certainly in the beginning phases and perhaps for several weeks, fatigue is the order of the day. Operation Desert Storm, the combat phase of the Persian Gulf War, followed that rule, and so, no doubt, will the next conflict. As usual, all did not go according to plans. The uncertainty of the length of deployment contributed to general tension. Combat air patrols up to 8 hours long could be followed by alert scrambles of equal length. Tanker schedules sometimes consisted of 12 hours flying, 12 hours rest, and 12 hours of alert. Some crews flew 36-hour crew days. Sleep was interrupted by aircraft noise and Scud missile alerts. Some line commanders seemed not to understand the effects of stress and chronic fatigue. Some flight surgeons felt that aircrews were pushed to the limits of their endurance, to the point where flying safety suffered. Fatigue was a consideration in at least two noncombat fatal accidents. Other problems included missed meals because of scheduling conflicts, crowded billeting of crews flying different schedules when all fliers were brought on base for security reasons, and environmental stressors such as heat and isolation. The pace of the war was so rapid that there seemed to be no time to deal with emotional reactions to the deaths of squadron mates.[2] In brief, the emotional aspects of war have not changed much in the last 50 years.

Most of the literature concerning the effects of combat stress on fliers derives from World War II; little was written on this subject during the Korean conflict, and there is essentially no psychiatric literature on the U.S. Air Force experience in Southeast Asia during the Vietnam conflict. No significant publications on this topic have emerged from recent U.S. Air Force operations in Libya, Grenada, Panama, or Kuwait and Iraq. This is a regrettable lack, for several demographic factors have changed during this period.

Fliers today differ considerably from their predecessors. The fliers in World War II were wartime volunteers, high school graduates or college students commissioned through the Aviation Cadet Program, trained in a specific aircraft, and sent into combat with perhaps 200 flying hours altogether. Most of these fliers separated from the service after the war, having no intention of a career in military aviation. Some joined the reserves, probably thinking that they would be recalled to active duty only in the unlikely event of a national emergency.

The call came sooner than anyone expected. Many of the reservists were reactivated in 1950 for the Korean conflict. This "police action" did not generate the sense of national unity that World War I and World War II had, and many reservists were quite bitter about having their lives and careers interrupted to fight in a war not linked to a clear threat to the nation. (Their feelings were expressed in the sardonic song, "Here's to the Regular Air Force, they have such a wonderful plan: They call up the Goddam Reservists, whenever the shit hits the fan!") Somewhat older, not as committed, and with considerably less motivation to fly, those recalled fliers became a problem because of their increased incidence of refusal to fly combat missions due to "fear of flying."[3–5] Harking back to lessons learned during World War II, flight surgeons would check such fliers to assure that they had no psychopathology, and then clear them medically for flying duties. Any further refusal to fly was handled administratively rather than medically.

The demographic characteristics of U.S. Air Force fliers have continued to change since the mid-1950s. All fliers (indeed, all officers) must have a college degree, and most obtain their commissions either through the U.S. Air Force Academy or through Reserve Officers' Training Corps programs. Many go on to obtain master's degrees after entry on active duty. Except for the few older officers commissioned through the old Aviation Cadet Program or Officer Candidate School, this was the complexion of the force in Southeast Asia. These young, bright, well-educated fliers had thus spent at least 5 years (4 in college, 1 in flight training) directed toward the goal of becoming a U.S. Air Force officer and flier. Many were seriously considering 20-year careers, and most of those who were not were hoping for careers as airline pilots. Thus they went to war older and better educated, and with a longer career view than their predecessors. Many were fairly "high-time" fliers when they arrived in Southeast Asia, although the younger ones might arrive with only 200 to 300 flying hours. The professional fighter pilots were a subgroup of the U.S. Air Force, a tactical cadre that rotated between Southeast Asia, the Tactical Air Command in the United States, and tactical fighter wings in the U.S. Air Force, Europe (USAFE). Some of these men served two, three, or four tours in Southeast Asia. These fliers differed from the U.S. Army helicopter pilots, who were younger, less educated, and more like the World War II volunteers.

The U.S. Air Force today has continued its policy of producing highly selected, educated, and trained pilots. The increasing complexity of aircraft (frequently called "weapons systems" to underline this complexity) requires continued high-grade training. Many frontline pilots, navigators, weapons systems operators, and electronic warfare operators are in their 30s, and some are in their 40s. They are, as stated earlier, considerably different from their predecessors in World War II, and more like those who flew in Southeast Asia. Yet there are almost no specific data about combat reactions of fliers in action in Southeast Asia, the Libya raid, the invasions of Grenada and Panama, or the Persian Gulf War, or about the types of support most effective in maintaining their morale and fighting spirit. Thus, any ideas or plans for furnishing such support in a future conflict must be based on the reports of U.S. experiences in World War II and Korea, along with anecdotal data and reminiscences from Southeast Asia, data obtained from the performance and support of fliers from the U.S. and other nations in the more recent conflicts, and projections of all of this information onto present U.S. Air Force fliers. Added to these changes will be the effects of the drawdown of the U.S. Air Force since the collapse of the Soviet Union, the increase in the proportion of women and their new roles, and the outcome of the present debate about homosexuals and lesbians in the service. Still, one may reasonably assume that principles of support to morale and flying efficiency that have been effective in a variety of past conflicts are probably basic enough to prove useful when flexibly and thoughtfully adapted to the particular circumstances of future conflicts.

U.S. Air Force fliers may fill a number of roles in a combat situation. Some tactical fighters will fly air-to-air combat missions to establish air superiority over the battlefield by attacks on enemy aircraft. Others will fly tactical air-to-ground missions, attacking enemy troop concentrations, armor, artillery, supplies, and equipment. These aircraft may be single-seat (pilot only), or may be crewed by a pilot and a weapons system officer. Forward air controllers will coordinate some strikes and will identify targets. Reconnaissance pilots will take photographs before and after air strikes to use in planning missions and to assess damage. Tactical helicopter pilots may fly special missions, inserting or extracting troops, rescuing downed fliers, and carrying patients to the rear. Tactical transport crews will airlift supplies, delivering them from the air by parachute or by special low-altitude extraction systems, or by landing to off-load in the conventional way.

These and other tactical aircrew will be exposed to specific dangers: ground-based small-arms fire, surface-to-air missiles, conventional antiaircraft fire, and attack by enemy aircraft. The threat of chemical or biological warfare at base or just prior to takeoff may act as a stress multiplier. Tactical missions tend to be fairly short, lasting from 1 to 4 hours, and thus the aircrew may fly two, three, or even four missions in a day. Israeli fighter pilots in the 1967 war, expected to fly an average of three or four sorties a day, flew an average of seven a day; some pilots flew as many as 10.[6] The dangers of such missions may vary considerably; some are the proverbial "piece of cake" while others may be extremely lethal. At times the danger—or lack of danger—will be familiar to the fliers. Other missions or target areas will be known as unpredictable, thus adding the considerable stress of uncertainty to all the other stresses of combat.

For the tactical fighter pilot, the success both of air-to-air and air-to-ground missions depends on personal skills. Dual-crewed aircraft such as the F-15E integrate the weapons system officer into the equation, but the skill of the pilot is still paramount. Whether a pilot lives or dies in such combat depends upon personal prowess to a degree that may be unique in modern warfare.

Such a pilot must have supreme confidence in personal skills and a strong narcissistic component recognized when he is selected for training. This narcissism, an almost magical sense of personal invulnerability, is nourished by the U.S. Air Force's system of training. It displays itself in the "typical fighter pilot personality" that is immediately apparent to the most casual observer of human nature. This pilot's effectiveness in battle depends on boldness, self-sufficiency, situational awareness, and an internal locus of control. Such pilots may depend to some extent upon a wingman and a squadron for support, but deep in their hearts, each knows that one can ultimately depend only upon oneself. Maintenance of this narcissism in the face of mounting losses to the enemy of friends—fliers who were known to be skillful and brave—requires a healthy initial motivation to fly, a strong ego, and well-developed denial skills to defend against personal fear and sense of mortality. Magical thinking and superstition may also be observed. Deaths are briefly acknowledged and then consciously suppressed in order to continue the squadron mission.

Support of tactical fliers in the combat arena has been similar during each of America's last four wars. Airfields have been reasonably free from enemy attack in most cases, and fliers have lived in a base environment in which a great deal of effort has been devoted to their personal comfort and support. Nourishing meals available 24 hours a day, specified crew-rest periods with exceptions granted only by higher headquarters, personal health care and welfare overseen by a squadron flight surgeon and his staff, quiet quarters that are air-conditioned or heated—all these amenities and more are provided by regulation, if not always in fact.

Transport crews will be affected by some but not all of these considerations, with added stresses deriving from their particular mission profiles. Tactical transport aircraft, particularly the C-130s and the cargo helicopters, may be used for resupply under fire of troops and bases, or of besieged civilians receiving humanitarian aid. The resupply of the besieged Khe Sanh defenders during the Vietnam conflict is an example of such an endeavor. Not only the pilots' skills count here, but also those of other aircrew members and even the ground crew who must help off-load the aircraft under fire. The stress of flying in such a large, unarmored, defenseless "sitting duck" target during the approach, landing, taxiing, off-loading, takeoff, and departure under fire is enormous, especially because each of these activities must take place in a location known in advance to enemy gunners, whose weapons may already be ranged and sighted in. Transport crews may be called upon to make a half-dozen or more landings during a day's missions, and their vulnerability to ground fire leads to a constant state of arousal; there are only limited options to counter such fire when it occurs. Flying such missions when attack by enemy aircraft is possible will add to the strain. This was exemplified by the slaughter in April 1943 when American fighters caught about 100 JU-52 transports carrying troops to reinforce the German Army in Tunisia, shooting down 52 of them over the Mediterranean Sea.[7]

Strategic bomber crews may face different perils. Penetration of enemy defenses depends upon surprise, electronics countermeasures, such technological advances as the cruise missile, and whatever escort aircraft may be used. The venerable B-52s are neither fast nor maneuverable when compared with air-defense aircraft or with surface-to-air missiles. Presumably, their airfields will be far enough from the conflict on the ground to be safe from attack with conventional arms and will be vulnerable only to long-range missiles, to enemy strategic attacks, or to saboteurs.

Strategic bomber crews had the highest proportion of combat losses among fliers in 1944, 7.7 per 1,000 hours flown, compared to light bombers (3.4) and fighters (1.1).[8(p10)] The B-52 experience in Vietnam shows the difference in attacking targets with and without air defense. Between June 1965 and August 1973, the Strategic Air Command flew more than 124,000 B-52 sorties against targets in Southeast Asia, losing 29 B-52s altogether. All of the 17 B-52s lost to hostile fire were shot down over North Vietnam; none were lost to hostile fire over the lightly-defended South. (The other 12 were lost through accidents or midair collisions.)[9]

Fifteen of these 17 were shot down during the 11 days of Operation Linebacker II, when some 740 sorties were flown against targets in Hanoi and Haiphong in December 1972.[9] These B-52s were based on Guam and in Thailand, secure from enemy attack, but the cumulative and rapid losses caused considerable concern among the fliers involved. According to their flight surgeon, this concern manifested itself as a rapid and forceful statement up the chain of command of the need to change tactics over the target, a statement that quickly led to the needed changes.[10]

In addition to the operational factors already mentioned, three other matters distinguish the support of U.S. Air Force fliers in combat. One is the similarity between the "fear of flying" syndrome, which may occur in peace as well as in wartime, and the signs and symptoms usually associated with combat fatigue.[11] The second is the use of *rest* as a primary preventive and therapeutic measure. The third is the specific relationship between the fliers and the flight surgeon who is directly responsible for furnishing their preventive health measures and medical support. These three factors will be considered separately.

"Fear of Flying" and Combat Fatigue

"Fear of flying" has been called a symptom without a disease.[12] Recognized early in the history of powered flight, it was the subject of two of the nine chapters in one of the first textbooks of aviation medicine.[13] Through the years, it has had about as many synonyms as has combat fatigue itself: aeroneurosis, chronic fatigue, staleness, aviator's neurasthenia, flying phobia, and others.[14] The crux of the problem appears to be that humans have an instinctive fear of falling, which is overcome to some extent during the early years of muscular development as children learn to control their environments by their own efforts. Some youngsters conceive of flying as the ultimate mastery and power ("Put out my hand, and touched the face of God") and thus present themselves for flying training saying, "I've wanted to fly as long as I can remember" (ie, since age 5 or so).

> The central unifying force through the Air Corps is the intangible yet powerful devotion to aircraft felt in different degrees by all its members....Planes receive an almost libidinal investment of interest...the aircraft became anthropomorphized ....This devotion and enthusiasm for aircraft is of such a compelling force that it to some extent supercedes military discipline.[1(p99–101)]

Other fliers may be motivated less by such a long-lived desire than by their perception of flying as a way to enhance a career in the U.S. Air Force. In other words, motivation to fly may be largely emotional, or it may be largely cognitive.[11] Most fliers are probably motivated by some mixture of the two, and fliers at either end of the motivational spectrum may serve complete careers in the cockpit, honorably and well. Yet the underlying instinct to avoid heights persists. Many pilots joke about being mildly afraid of heights in the ordinary sense, but show no carryover of this fear to flying in their aircraft. Through their desire to fly, they deny, suppress, or repress their primitive anxiety about heights. "You can get killed just crossing the street" is their common response to questions about their view of the dangers of flying.

Still, the dangers are real and, with continued exposure to the world of flying, a military flier's ability to deny them is slowly eroded. "There are old pilots, and there are bold pilots," goes the old saw, "but there are no old, bold pilots." Youthful enthusiasm is tempered by maturity and the lessons of experience. "Flying is 99% boredom and 1% pure terror." The jokes and sayings reflect the realities. As youthful fliers begin to comprehend the realities, the strength of their motivation is tested. When it is flawed, it fails early.

A few fliers are driven by psychologically overdetermined factors—an anxiety-driven need to "prove" something to someone (usually father) may be seen in some. When success is near, the primitive symbolism of succeeding (defeating father) arouses basic anxieties that interfere with successful flying, and the flier either quits, fails through "lack of adaptation," or presents with disabling medical or psychiatric symptoms.

Others fail in less spectacular ways, with symptoms that are similar to the effects of combat on infantry. They may be restless and irritable, with nerves on edge. They may have insomnia, and whatever sleep comes is light or fitful, disturbed by unpleasant dreams or actual nightmares. They may report profound dread or apprehension about flying, with tremors, sweating, and palpitations. They may have difficulty with concentration, begin to experience airsickness, or report that they are so preoccupied with their fears that they must concentrate on not activating the ejection seat in normal flight. Symptoms may be of disabling and phobic proportions, or they may be mild and only slightly distressing. At times, symptoms may have begun with a specific and clearly recognized traumatic event, such as a personal close call or the crash of a friend. Other cases may begin as the accumulation of stresses which gradually and finally overcome a strong motivation to fly and the flier comes to the reluctant realization that the joy is gone from flying.[11]

Some fearful fliers, having no conscious recognition of their underlying anxiety, may also present with psychophysiologic disorders. Headaches, vasovagal syncope, obscure visual problems, gastrointestinal upsets, and many other systemic complaints may be presented for diagnosis. The astute clinician may note that the chief complaint is presented in a framework of "I'd like to fly, but ... " which indicates that the flier has linked the symptoms with a hoped-for result of *not* flying. This attitude distinguishes this particular flier from the other fliers who complain about possibly being grounded, or conceal their symptoms, fearing that they will lose their flying status.[11]

All this and more occurs in military flying in times of peace. U.S. Air Force doctrine[15] calls for evaluation to determine whether medical or psychiatric disease is present. If so, medical grounding and treatment are in order. If no physical or mental disease is present, the flier is returned to his or her commander as medically cleared to fly. Further refusal to fly is handled administratively and may result in simple reassignment to ground duties (especially if the precipitating event is acknowledged to be catastrophic and the resultant fear understandable to all), or may involve adverse administrative action.

Estimates of the incidence of such cases of fear of flying (the U.S. Air Force term for this symptom in the absence of psychiatric disease) are difficult because they are not routinely tabulated through medical channels, but the best guess was about seven cases per year during the period from 1975 to 1984.[16] Thus, fear of flying may be regarded as a peacetime paradigm for combat fatigue, admittedly on a much smaller scale. Such cases are difficult to handle in the local fishbowl environment of the squadron.

The author, in his past capacity as a psychiatrist at the U.S. Air Force School of Aerospace Medicine, has worked with flight surgeons in the field who were wrestling with the problem of a flier—and friend—who developed some manifestations of fear of flying. Such fliers were not mentally ill, in which case they would be medically grounded; they had simply lost their motivation to fly and presented themselves as no longer safe. Every instinct cries out against requiring someone to fly who no longer wants to do so; such a flier will clearly be unsafe, and requiring one either to fly against his will, or to face possible adverse administrative action seems the height of folly. How much more difficult, then, will it be for a flight surgeon to take similar action to require a flier to fly into combat? Yet this is exactly the kind of judgment required, to extract from each flier every possible combat mission before allowing him to step down to nonflying duties or to return to noncombat flying. Thus the role of the flight surgeon in maintaining the operational strength of the squadron must be considered.

The Use of Rest for Prevention and Treatment

As *fatigue* is a primary underlying pathologic process, *rest* is a prime restorative. Rest may be used in several ways that may be stated as "rules," if those responsible understand the need for exceptions in individual cases.

Crew Rest

The major problem with research in this area derives from the lack of any agreed-upon objective measure of fatigue. Many biochemical and behavioral factors have been studied in this regard, and recently such manifestations as characteristics of eye blinks, voice stress analysis, and rate of mistakes in flight simulators have been studied to see if they could be quantified. However, the final "gold standard" is the flier's subjective appraisal of his condition. Further adding to the complexity are the numerous combinations of work-rest-sleep cycles available.

Hartman[17] reviewed some of the current literature and discussed some of the differences between various kinds of missions: *tactical, strategic, airlift, and ground-based control centers.* Briefly, his opinions are:

- *Tactical missions* involve brief multiple sorties in one day. The special stresses include high workload environments, highly hazardous missions, acute fatigue effects (the physical results of pulling high-G loading, for instance), and rapidly cumulative chronic fatigue. Circadian factors are also involved in all-weather aircraft.
- *Strategic missions* (bombers, AWACS [Airborne Warning and Control System aircraft], tankers) may involve longer missions, in some cases extending beyond 24 hours. In-flight work/rest cycles become a factor, as do reasonable in-flight rest facilities, nutrition, and the different jobs performed by flight crew and mission crew in AWACS and command post aircraft.
- *Airlift missions* may involve multiple short sorties (tactical) or long-range missions crossing many time zones (strategic). There is more scientific information on such flights and also on the use of multiple crews for one aircraft. One particular problem involves "ramp-pounding," a pernicious and frustrating form of nonwork experienced while waiting for an aircraft to be loaded, repairs to be made, passengers to be rounded up, or during any of the many other occurrences that may delay an aircraft for minutes, hours, or days. Circadian stresses cause a small but appreciable decrement in performance, but may be magnified by other stresses. The conventional wisdom of the many studies in this area is reflected in U.S. Air Force crew-rest regulations.
- *Ground-based centers* (command posts, towers, radar sites, and the like) may have unique stresses based on workload, the facility itself, its location, its dangers, and other unforeseen factors.

Rayman[18] reported on a heavy flying schedule for C-130 crews during a 2-month emergency airlift. The crews flew almost 180 hours per month (the usual limit is 125 h), involving three or four shuttles per day. He defined "fatigue" as cumulative effects that were not relieved by a single day's rest and "tiredness" as the acute effects that were. His practical conclusions, listed below, are applicable to all flying circumstances, regardless of their complexities, because they derive from the subjective effect of daily stress, yet allow for a reasonably objective aeromedical judgment.

- Understand that crew duty limitations are due to variables and must be established by experience and precedent, as well as by local needs. Be flexible.
- With good motivation and good support, aircrew members can exceed normal crew-rest requirements for at least 2 months.
- Routine aeromedical surveillance suffices for the first month. Extra surveillance (defined as the flight surgeon's meeting each aircrew member before each takeoff and after each landing) is necessary after that.
- Assess fatigue frequently. One may do this by daily contact; occasional anonymous questionnaires; aircrew briefings on fatigue factors; assuring the best available crew-rest quarters, food, and in-flight provisions; and establishing rapport with aircrew and supervisors.
- The decision to restrict an aircrew member temporarily from flying because of fatigue should be made jointly by the flight surgeon, the operations officer, and the aircrew member. Remember that grounding one flier means more work for another.
- Aircrew members should be relieved of all additional duties, so as to direct all their energies to the flying mission.
- Bend every effort toward flying the schedule as scheduled; avoid needless changes, delays, and excessive ramp time. Quarters near the flight line (but not so near as to cause the crews to be kept awake by the noise) reduce wasted travel time.
- Incentive pay for extra effort is a strong motivating factor for paramilitary flying.

Each U.S. Air Force major air command has its own crew-rest regulations. Variables that contribute to these regulations include size of crews, type of aircraft, flying hours each day, hours of rest between flights, hours of nonflying duty, and hours flown each month. All of these factors may be waived if the exigencies of the situation demand it, but the wise commander will consult with the flight surgeon before doing so, and the wise flight surgeon will look at the fliers on an individual basis before giving advice on the subject. The difference between granting a crew-rest waiver for a single-seat fighter mission and a similar waiver for a transport mission where one pilot may take a nap in a bunk during the mission is immediately apparent, even in principle.

The literature is specific, however, that one must consider more than the hours of crew rest available. Sleep disturbances are a consistent early symptom of cumulative combat stress in fliers, and thus the flight surgeon must discuss the quality of their sleep with individual fliers. If sleep is disturbed by nightmares or insomnia to the point that the flier remains as tired upon awakening as when going to bed, the cumulative fatigue after 2 or 3 days may well render him or her ineffective at best and unsafe at worst.

The social role of alcohol in the ambiance of combat fliers deserves brief consideration. The drinking habits of aircrew are the stuff of legends. The stories, the songs, the customs, the superstitions, the very social fabric of the squadrons of old are celebrated and, in the opinion of this author, reasonably accurately presented in plays, movies, books, television, and folklore. For more than 30 years to which the author can attest, flight surgeons in training have been urged to go to the bar with "their" fliers in order to meet them socially, to learn what's really going on, to find out what makes them tick. From the 1940s through the 1970s, at least, the Officers Club bar was a center of aviation society.

These habits are changing as American society changes, as the realities of working spouses and modern family dynamics have affected the social structures of flying squadrons, and as the incredible demands of modern military aviation have demonstrated that "you cannot hoot with the owls if you want to fly with the eagles." Still, the tendency of many fliers to treat their fatigue symptoms with alcohol has been well-observed in the past, and will probably continue in the future. Many books attest to this. Gene Basel's *Pak Six*[19] contains repeated references to bar conversations, and the personal experiences of the author's generation of flight surgeons in Southeast Asia corroborate Basel's writings. One does not need a postgraduate education to understand that alcohol abuse is dangerous in such circumstances. It is not necessary to belabor the point beyond observing that drinking serves several purposes: as a self-administered and socially acceptable psychotropic medication, as a social lubricant to allow personal conversation among somewhat emotionally distant people, and as a sedative.

There is one specific observation, based on the author's experiences as a flight surgeon, that may not be quite as intuitive as "Alcohol abuse is bad for flying safety," or "Alcoholics should be identified, grounded, and treated." That observation stems from the use of alcohol as a sedative. If a flier takes a couple of drinks late in the evening to help get to sleep, that amount of alcohol may be seen as benign and insignificant. The flier may, however, go to sleep easily, dream extravagantly, and awaken feeling refreshed and invigorated. Glancing at the clock, the flier notes that it's only 0130; 2 hours of sleep have passed, not a whole night, and there's plenty of time left to sleep after all. But now the flier can't go back to sleep, or sleeps only fitfully, with many awakenings, and much punching of the pillow. Finally, perhaps about 0430, the flier does fall hard asleep for an hour, only to be awakened at 0530 to prepare for the day's flying. A couple of cups of coffee help, although the flier may feel a bit dulled all day.

This is not really a big deal, once. But repeat that drinking pattern for a week or two, and the flier's edge is definitely dulled. Fatigued, he continues to take a couple of late evening drinks as a sedative, not getting drunk, but interfering with the normal sleep cycles on a chronic basis.

The giveaway is the extravagant dreaming early in the night's sleep. Alcohol may produce a self-sustaining dysregulation of the normal sleep cycle. Its effects are complex, but the end result is a diminution of concentration and memory, and an increase in fatigue, anxiety, and irritability. These changes can persist even after the drug is no longer present.[20,21]

It is this author's opinion that aircrew should be taught this signal: if they dream and awaken early in the night, they've had too much to drink and should change their pattern. Again, it's no big deal once in a while, but common sense indicates that interfering with the normal sleep cycle on a recurrent basis is not good for the flier who must be sharp and prepared for anything that combat flying (or, for that matter, ordinary flying) should bring along.

What should the flight surgeon do to help aircrew sleep? Should hypnotic agents be allowed? The general rule is that one should not use hypnotic agents unless, using mature and informed judgment, one decides that it is less dangerous to use them than it is not to use them. The British used 20 mg of temazepam (Restoril) as a hypnotic for fliers during the South Atlantic (Falkland Islands) campaign. Group Captain Michael Fisher commented:

> We were particularly impressed by a short-acting drug for ensuring our aircrews adequate sleep before flights. Very often they were having to get their sleep at unusual hours of the day under very noisy, cramped conditions. [Temazepam] is rapidly excreted, though it's rapid in its effect. People were able to sleep and wake up and go flying without any sort of hangover effect. Aircrew eventually were permitted to fly within only six hours of taking the drug.[22(p10)]

The decision to use temazepam during the South Atlantic campaign was based upon British recognition of demanding operational workloads, the need for extension of permissible flying hours, and the potential for these conditions to continue for several weeks. Their experience included transport crews logging up to 150 hours in 24 days, with single bomber missions lasting up to 28 hours. Even without the use of test doses, they encountered no problems with this medication.[23]

Temazepam is a short-acting benzodiazepine most active 20 to 40 minutes after oral administration, with peak effect in 2 to 3 hours, and a biphasic half-life with a 30-minute short peak and a 10-hour terminal half-life. Temazepam does not affect rapid eye movement (REM) sleep and somewhat decreases slow wave sleep. Exigencies of combat may dictate its use, or the use of a similar short-acting benzodiazepine, but *only* after ground testing by administration to the individual flier on a night prior to a nonflying day, in order to detect any unusual or idiosyncratic effects on the ground rather than in flight. A new, nonbenzodiazepine hypnotic, zolpidem tartrate (Ambien), may offer some advantages over benzodiazepines(BDZs). It is important to remember that many BDZs induce a retrograde amnesia that could interfere with last minute instruction before sleep.[24]

Amphetamines have been used by pilots during deployments and on prolonged combat missions for several decades. Most recently fighter pilots deploying from the United States to Saudi Arabia were permitted their use, and 5 mg dextroamphetamine tablets were made available to tactical pilots for combat air patrol missions. Of 464 fighter pilots surveyed by the Tactical Air Command after the Persian Gulf War, 65% said they used amphetamines during Operation Desert Shield (the mobilization phase of the war), and 57% during Operation Desert Storm (the combat phase of the war). The U.S. Air Force subsequently decided to reevaluate this policy, and authorization for their use was withdrawn effective 13 March 1992. No untoward occurrences or reactions were reported, but a decision was made "to make sure that what we were doing was correct."[25(p3)]

Lyons and French et al[26] published an aero-medically-oriented review of modafinil, a nonamphetamine stimulant developed in France. Unlike the amphetamines, it apparently has a low abuse potential. It also has minimal peripheral side effects at therapeutic doses. The authors concluded that this medication might be an ideal replacement for amphetamines in short-term operations in which fatigue might be a limiting factor. They recommend further study of modafinil, or a similar alpha 1 receptor agonist.

In the opinion of this author, sedative and stimulant medications should only be used when, in the best judgment of the most operationally experienced line and medical authorities available, it is more dangerous not to use them than it is to use them. Further, they should be used only by fliers who have been previously ground-tested, and who (*a*) have had no untoward effects, (*b*) are familiar with their primary effects, and (*c*) wish to use them.

Also in the author's opinion, tactical pilots—especially those who fly single-seat aircraft—should be ground-tested regardless of the current policy allowing or not allowing their use in flight, because such policies can change quickly, and the circumstances mandating the change may not allow time for proper ground-testing.

Ground-testing is carried out in the following manner. Information about the medications to be used is gathered by the flight surgeon from the most up-to-date sources available. A questionnaire is developed that inquires specifically after primary effects, secondary ("side") effects, and any significant idiosyncratic reactions. Open-ended and nondirective questions are added for anything else the flier may have noticed, desirable or undesirable.

On a Friday when the flier will dependably not be flying until the following Monday, he (alone, or in a group briefing) is informed about the ground-test and its purposes. Alcohol is specifically forbidden during the test, and, needless to say, the flier should take no other medications during the test.

At the agreed-upon hour (say, 2200), the flier takes the sedative medication and retires 1 hour later. Upon awakening the next morning, the flier notes the quality and quantity of sleep, and fills out the questionnaire regarding medication effects.

If all is well, the flier then takes the first dose of stimulant (at, say, 0800). Four hours later, the flier notes any reactions on the questionnaire. If all is well, the flier then takes the second dose. Four hours subsequent to that, the flier notes any further observations. He uses no further medications, and no alcohol, that Saturday evening.

Sunday, no medications are taken.

Early Monday, the flier sees the flight surgeon (or vice versa), individually goes over his questionnaire, and confirms its information. The flight surgeon asks any follow-up questions indicated.

The flier and the flight surgeon both sign the questionnaire, which is placed in the flier's medical records. The bottom line (literally) is that the flier is signed off as ground-tested and approved for the supervised use of the two medications tested while flying, or the flier is not approved for their use.

Two points should be stressed. First, *not* being approved for their use does not disqualify the flier for anything—any mission, any flight, any profile. Second, even if approved for their use, the actual choice to use medications is always left up to the flier. The flight surgeon may only offer to make them available for certain missions. No one—commander, flight surgeon, or anyone else—may order the flier to take them. The flier is now familiar with the medications, and may make up his own mind about their use.

The Interval Between Missions

World War II flight surgeon reports generally agreed that missions should not be flown on more than 3 consecutive days.[27,28] All involved were aware that standing alert was as wearing as flying an actual mission, if not more so, in that there was no release of anxiety through action. Further, flight surgeons reported that the period between learning about a mission and flying the mission was the most stressful. Weather holds, slipped takeoff times, and scrubbed missions were extremely nerve-wracking and, at least from the point of view of generating combat fatigue, should be counted as a mission day.[28]

A day off must be *off*, with no duty requirements whatsoever. Further, the flier should know about it ahead of time, so that its relaxation may be anticipated as a short-term goal. Specific recommendations for time off in the Eighth Air Force area were 10 to 15 hours of operational flying per week, 24 hours of leave per week, 48 hours of leave every 2 weeks, and 7 days of leave per 6 weeks.[29] Grinker and Spiegel commented on the strength of the group identification among fliers, that there was little relaxation available to a flier on the ground if his friends—or especially his crew—were flying.[1] Thus, if possible, a wing stand down will provide much more release of anxiety for fliers than will an individual day off. Exigencies of combat, however, rarely allow such a policy.

The author's conversations with Southeast Asia combat fliers have underscored the value of trusting the flier's own judgment in determining when one should not fly a given mission because of fatigue. A flier in a well-run squadron may be allowed to take his name off the flying schedule every now and then without question if that flier feels not fit to fly that day. Clearly, any flier whose overuse of such a privilege points to an unwillingness to do his share should be evaluated by the operations officer or flight surgeon. Giving the fliers a bit more control, balanced by the self-policing action of a well-integrated squadron, may enhance morale and delay combat fatigue.

Rest and Recreation

A prolonged combat tour should be split by a 1-week rest-and-recreation ("R and R") break. Realistic flight surgeons recognized during World War II, and again 20 years later in Southeast Asia , that fliers do not necessarily rest on R and R. It is wise not to schedule them to fly for 1 day after they return from R and R, but to use this period to accomplish ground training or administrative duties.[29] Some fliers will object to time off, wishing to hurry through their tour and get home. If the rest causes more stress than it relieves, such a schedule may be modified a bit. In general, though, its beneficial effects will be obvious throughout the squadron.

Tour Length

The length of a combat tour is a decision that should be made by line commanders at the highest level. It is discussed here because of its immense importance to fliers' morale and its epidemiologic role in shaping the patterns of susceptibility to combat fatigue.

In World War II, the tour length for heavy and medium bomber crews depended upon the number of missions flown, with the "magic number" being predicated on giving each aircrew member a better-than-even chance of surviving the tour. The Twelfth Air Force determined "the maximum effort of the average flier," essentially based upon attrition rates, to be based on a 60% to 80% chance of completing a tour, if the military situation permitted.[8] Attaining the desired number of missions or flying hours became a valued short-term goal for fliers, and the demoralizing effects of shifting the magic number, always upward, furnished one of the themes for the novel *Catch-22*.[30] The uncertainties of when personnel deployed for the Persian Gulf War would return, and the effects of those uncertainties on morale, recapitulated this theme.

The knowledge that the combat tour has a finite duration becomes more important in maintaining tolerance of the growing anxiety, and

> [E]xperience...repeatedly demonstrated that this factor has been responsible for many individuals achieving the expected level of operational missions. Without this certainty of relief, the ego in many instances would have succumbed much sooner, and an appreciable decrease in the number of combat missions flown by available personnel would have resulted.[31(p9)]

How long should such a tour be? The answer depends on many factors: (*a*) the type and severity of the flying operation, (*b*) losses to combat and accidents, (*c*) the physical conditions of the bases, and (*d*) the realities of the combat needs. However, once a tour is announced, it should be changed only for absolutely critical reasons, and such a change should be accompanied by a responsible explanation to the fliers of the exigencies leading to the decision.

From a pragmatic point of view, a combat tour, usually measured in number of missions, should allow each flier *at least* a better-than-50% chance of going home in one piece. In the author's opinion, odds less than 50% should apply only in last-ditch efforts, such as in the Philippines in 1942.

Completing a combat tour in prior wars was not without a striking psychological and psychosomatic cost to the fliers. The prolonged tension led to progressive loss of normal personality features. Aircrew became quieter, more serious and cautious, sometimes seclusive and depressed, with loss of interest in other pursuits, loss of spontaneity, and a decreased love of flying. Sleep disturbances included insomnia and nightmares, with battle scenes a frequent theme. Fliers would have little appetite for food, but their intake of coffee, cigarettes, and alcohol would increase. Their increased tension would also be manifested as irritability, jumpiness, and tremors. Fantasies of omnipotence and invulnerability would be replaced by obsessive fantasies of death and ruminations about lost friends. Physical fatigue in periods of prolonged or intense flying would accelerate this process and might lead to a clearly visible decline in a flier's ability to fly and to fight, which the whole squadron would recognize. At this point, if not removed from operational flying, the flier would either experience such severe symptoms as to develop full-blown combat fatigue, or might become so ineffective as to be at special risk in combat.

The Role of the Flight Surgeon

As this discussion has demonstrated, fliers are different from other combat troops. This difference extends to their medical support, which is provided on a highly personal and individualized basis by the squadron flight surgeon. Thus, morale support and first-echelon mental health care may well be furnished by the flight surgeon rather than by enlisted medical technicians or by "buddy care" from peers. The flight surgeon is an intrinsic part of the squadron's internal support system and should be present on a day-to-day basis to furnish primary medical care and to advise the squadron commander on matters of preventive medicine, including matters of morale.

Flight surgeons have only a few tools with which to slow the inevitable progress of combat fatigue in fliers, but these are powerful therapeutic agents if properly used. Above all, flight surgeons must understand that combat fatigue is a normal reaction of a normal group of people to a dreadfully abnormal situation. As a normal reaction, combat fatigue cannot be prevented or avoided, but may be delayed. The frame of reference must not be "Does anyone in my squadron have combat fatigue?" but rather, "I must understand how each of my fliers is dealing with this stress and watch for defenses that are crumbling." With this attitude, the flight surgeon is ready to support the flying mission by helping each flier to fly as long and as effectively as possible.

Combat Flying for Flight Surgeons

The flight surgeon must fly combat missions, if at all possible. This sets in motion a complex set of tried-and-true interpersonal dynamics that pay off with several specific benefits.[27(p81)]

Understanding the Mission. Flying the mission will enable flight surgeons to understand the stresses of combat at a visceral level. By thoughtful reflections upon their own reactions, a level of understanding develops that would not otherwise be possible. Good flight surgeons identify strongly with "my" squadrons and "my" fliers. The use of the possessive pronoun is universal among the best flight surgeons, who are much like fliers in their own personalities. Yet they must recognize that they are *not* pilots, navigators, electronic warfare operators, or gunners. Overidentification can lead to prostitution of medical ethics and to fuzzy professional thinking. It can also lead flight surgeons to think that flying, rather than caring for the fliers, is their own mission. How much should a flight surgeon fly? That depends on the aircraft, the mission profiles, and the press of other duties. In general, based on the author's experience in Vietnam, a flight surgeon should log not less than one nor more than two missions per week during duty hours, except in support of aeromedical evacuation. After-hours flights should be negotiable with the squadron or wing commanders, depending upon the flight surgeon's being able to sleep normally and to be fully functional in all medical duties.

Credibility. By flying the squadron mission, the flight surgeon establishes credibility. The fliers know that the flight surgeon flies and the flight surgeon can "speak the language" without being awkward or pretentious. More importantly, the flight surgeon can discuss his own personal fears, anxieties, and reactions in such a way as to give these strong (and often unacknowledged) feelings a legitimacy of expression. Such modeling of openness is quite healthy. A flier who is terrified, and who is also ashamed of that terror, may experience considerable relief in laughing with the flight surgeon who says "I thought I was going to wet my pants on *that* one!" Other fliers may have had precisely the same feeling but were unwilling to admit it, each feeling like the only coward in a group of heroes.

Acceptance. The flight surgeon, by flying and by being accepted by the fliers as "one of us," assumes a symbolic importance within the squadron, perhaps second only to that of its command echelon. Such a flight surgeon is a person whose judgment is trusted, a confidant of the commander and the operations officer. Understanding, tolerant, noncritical, realistic, yet firmly committed to the squadron goals, the flight surgeon develops an image as an important person, one whose good opinion the flier values. Giving sympathy, affection, and protection to the fliers, still the flight surgeon expects of them dedication, perseverance, and a willingness to continue the mission. The excellent flight surgeon does not overidentify with the squadron, does not fear their rejection (a healthy personal sense of self-esteem comes from within), and deals adaptively with personal internal conflicts between protective drives and the need to keep the fliers flying even if some die. This requires a well-integrated personality structure, buttressed by professional skill, and a strong personal value system.[31]

Intercession. The flight surgeon who flies combat missions can see firsthand the reactions of the troops to real-life combat stress, can observe their discipline, sees the fliers *in vivo*, as it were, and can then use the information to keep the commander informed about morale. These words may look a bit cynical in print, but the matter is quite practical. As a flight surgeon with an Air Commando wing in Vietnam, the author flew with enough different crews to appreciate how the fliers behaved in routine flight and in combat. He carefully avoided any actions that smacked of "informing" on specific fliers, but was able to keep the wing commander up to date on how well his fliers followed crew rest procedures, in-flight safety measures, and general flight discipline. Being known and trusted both by the commander and the fliers, the author was able to explain and interpret each to the other, informally and nonthreateningly. He represented a way by which petty gripes and problems could be taken outside the chain of command to the one who could fix things, in matters that might have led to hard feelings if official action had been necessary. The credible flight surgeon thus may become a sort of ombudsman within the squadron and the wing, able to get things done that need to be done, and to interpret—and occasionally to soften—policies imposed from above. Such an outlet, serving also as a safety valve, may contribute considerably to the fliers' morale.

Ventilation, Observation, and Early Intervention

In common with combat troops in other situations, some psychological relief may be afforded aircrew by allowing them to ventilate after missions and by participating in group activities. These functions are served to some extent by the intelligence debriefing that takes place after combat missions for fighter and bomber crews and by the natural tendency of crews to gather at the bar at the end of a day's flying. Again, excessive drinking is a danger to be guarded against, but such activities in moderation have a cathartic and mutually supportive role for the squadron and are of real value in the world of the flier. If conditions allow, an intramural sports program (softball, volleyball) has a similar value, as well as serving as a physical outlet. Such activities must be voluntary, however. Some troops can lose themselves in reading, and a library or other source of books and magazines is a useful asset. Informal reports from the Persian Gulf War also indicate the value of hand-held computer games. The value of mail from home cannot be overstated.

The flight surgeon may also keep in touch with the reactions of individual fliers to the combat situation. Any group of fliers reflects the strain of combat, and the flight surgeon will have to become acquainted with the ways that fliers show the strain. Most of the literature on combat fatigue speaks of the effects of war on infantrymen who are exposed to death for days, weeks, or months at a time, without letup. The flier goes on a mission, faces death, sees comrades die at a distance (or, rarely, on the same aircraft), and returns to a generally safe environment.

The ego of the flier uses various strategies to cope with the stress of combat. These strategies are familiar from the peacetime environment, but are generally discussed only in the context of psychopathology, rather than as useful adaptive mechanisms. During the prolonged combat tours of World War II, flight surgeons became familiar with a pattern of coping mechanisms in fliers progressing through their tours. Ignorance or denial of the realities of combat protected the fliers' egos against fear at first, because their perceptions of dangers were only intellectual and theoretical. This attitude would disappear after a few flights, as the realities intruded. Fliers might feel some anxiety, but the continued flying, the acquisition of combat survival skills, and the reassurance of peers and of the flight surgeon would generally suffice to keep the anxiety tolerable. Successful aggressive action against the enemy served as a powerful way to discharge anxiety and helped the flier maintain some sense of control over the flying environment.

The individual aircrew member would identify strongly with a unit or with his crew (a small group of men to whom he might ascribe almost magical powers) or even with a single flier. Similarly, some would identify strongly with an aircraft as a powerful and deadly champion. It was but a short step to superstitions about flying as magical defenses: "lucky" items, rituals, and so forth.[32(p16)] (The recent movie *Memphis Belle* showed several examples of such superstitions, rituals, and amulets.) Freedom from anxiety in flight depended upon the fantasy of the aircraft as safe and upon a flier's identification with its strength and invulnerability. Fliers also identified with leaders and with particularly skillful comrades. Such identification might be badly shaken if an accident or combat loss claimed these magical objects, because the identification was now with a wounded or dead person, rather than with an invincible, potent one. Some magical feeling of immunity and omnipotence would also help carry the flier along, strengthening ego defenses against reality, because many elements in aerial warfare are truly beyond anyone's ability to control.[1] Denial of these realities ("They'll never get *me!*") would bolster such magical fantasies for a while, but the accumulation of combat experience would gradually erode this fantasied invulnerability and the ego would begin to lose its power to protect itself against crippling anxiety.

> Not one man in a hundred looked forward to an operation with relish, although most of them derived considerable satisfaction from doing an operation well and returning safely...all that most aircrew wanted after furnishing their reports was breakfast and bed and sleep. They did not remember vividly every detail of all their operations, but they were conscious of no urgent desire to forget them....Their attitude to losses and the death of friends was particularly striking; it was one of supreme realism, of matter-of-fact acceptance of what everyone knew perfectly well was inevitable. They did not plunge into outspoken expression of their feelings, nor did they display any compromise with conventional reticence about violent death. They said "Too bad...sorry about so-and-so...rotten luck." Their regret was deep and sincere, but not much displayed or long endured. They were apt and able to talk of dead and missing friends, before mentioning their fate, just as they talked of anyone else or of themselves. It took the loss of particular friends or leaders, flight commanders or squadron commanders to produce a marked reaction among a squadron. Then they might feel collectively distressed, have a few drinks because of that, go on a party and feel better.[32(p15)]

These words were written about British night bomber crews in World War II, but they apply just as well to the Air Commandos (now Special Operations) and tactical fighter pilots with whom the author worked in Vietnam. The men had seen friends die in aircraft accidents before the war, and combat losses were regarded in much the same light. There was some corporate acknowledgment of those who were killed, but relatively little grief was expressed. Spontaneous expressions of anger or acute grief at the loss were heard as the news was delivered, and then the old mechanisms of denial, intellectualization, rationalization, altruism, humor, and magical thinking reasserted themselves and the loss was thenceforth discussed more coolly. Toasts might be drunk in the bar; a few (but by no means all) of the squadron would attend a memorial service; and the war went on. Symonds[33] speaks of the mental state ("confidence") that carries a flier through such experiences, ascribing it to a blend of resolution, bravery, and frankness. As frankness ebbs (as reality intrudes), bravery and resolution to see the job through keep the flier going.

Still, fliers did, and will, break down in combat. A number of authors in World War II and Korea commented on a pattern that most likely will be seen in future prolonged aerial conflicts.[1,3,28,32,33] There will be a few fliers who suffer disabling symptoms of anxiety early in their combat flying (Group A). A few of these fliers may be returned to flying, but most seem not to have the capacity to tolerate combat flying and may need to be relieved from duty. These fliers may represent the U.S. Air Force equivalent of the U.S. Army's early breakdowns among men with immature, dependent, or other maladaptive personality structures[34] as discussed in Chapter 1, Psychiatric Lessons of War, and Chapter 2, Traditional Warfare Combat Stress Casualties. Other cases of combat fatigue tend to occur in two clusters: toward mid-tour (Group B), and as the tour nears its end (Group C). Finally, there will be a scattering of fliers who undergo extremely stressful events, who then break down in consequence (Group D). Such events may be scattered throughout the tour. Stafford-Clark[32] and Symonds[33] concur that the prognosis is poor for Groups A and D, and better for Groups B and C.

Some of the fliers in Group A are described in terms that today would place them among those having antisocial personality traits: lack of allegiance to others than themselves and little regard for the social conventions or expectations of the squadrons. One would hope that most potential fliers with such personalities have been detected and eliminated by the preselection interview with the flight surgeon, the Adaptability Rating for Military Aviation (ARMA).[35] If not, such fliers may show their true colors during the extensive flying training and combat crew training process or by their behavior in squadron operations during peacetime. Failing that, there is no way to treat such an ingrown personality pattern, and these fliers must be administratively eliminated from flying status if they are detected.

It is axiomatic that it is impossible to predict who will do well in combat and who will not, until they are actually exposed to enemy fire. Some fliers will be unambiguous in their refusal to fly combat missions. Because they are not psychologically conflicted about their determination not to fly into danger, they do not become symptomatic. (Symptoms arise from unresolved internal conflicts.) They may even express their surprise that no one understands their feelings and excuses them. Appeals to duty, to squadron or personal loyalty, or to pride will have no effect. Such aircrew must be grounded in disgrace by their commanders. The wise flight surgeon will counsel administrative authorities that, if these fliers are not punished, they should at least not be rewarded by being administratively grounded and given a job seen as desirable by squadron members.

Whether combat fatigue occurs early in the tour or toward its midpoint, the first contact of the anxious flier will be with the flight surgeon, who certainly does not need to be a psychiatrist to deal with most such cases. The flier may come in of his or her own accord, or the flight surgeon may have noted the classic early symptoms: gradual withdrawal from social contact, loss of sense of humor, lack of spontaneity, passivity leading to moroseness, the onset of multiple complaints of vague symptoms that would hitherto have been ignored or even hidden from the flight surgeon to avoid grounding, and diminished energy and appetite. Later symptoms will almost certainly include irritability; increased use of cigarettes, coffee, and alcohol (which obviously make things worse); digestive disturbances; weight loss; insomnia; and the disturbance of sleep by bad dreams or nightmares. The flier may develop tics, frank tremors, or an increased startle reaction. Further symptoms of anxiety, depression, and psychophysiological reactions will be superimposed on these symptoms if matters are not corrected.

The best early intervention is to talk things over privately with the troubled flier. Whether the interview is initiated by the flier, flight surgeon, or squadron commander, the flight surgeon should take the role of a sympathetic and concerned counselor who wishes to help the flier regain composure and return to the cockpit, once more fully effective. Thus the flight surgeon supports that part of the conflicted flier that wants to return to effective duty. How long has the flier felt below par? Was it due to a particular event, or to an accumulation of things?

If an accident or a particular mission is on his mind, allow him to ventilate. What was he doing? Where? When? Then what happened? How did he react? How did others react? How does he think he *should* have reacted? What is he telling himself now about the whole thing?

If it were cumulative stress, how has it affected him? What is he afraid of? How does he see others reacting to the situation? How do they react to him? How much does he feel a part of the group and how much ego support does he derive from them and from the leaders? At times one may encounter marked misperceptions about how others feel, how they handle things, and how "I have let them down."

In each case, the flight surgeon can reflect the reality of the situations involved, correcting misapprehensions, clarifying the flier's status in the squadron, and helping to strengthen the ways in which the flier has dealt with the stress so far. An understanding, noncritical, tolerant acceptance and explanation of the flier's anxieties (unrealistic) and fears (realistic) is essential, so that the flight surgeon then assumes a warm but firm parental role that allows for sympathy, affection, and protection while expecting and demanding the utmost dedication to the mission, to the point of possible self-sacrifice.

By allowing the flier to talk about his anxiety, especially if it is manifested through psychophysiological mechanisms, the flight surgeon may help clarify that which the flier really fears: injury or death. Verbalizing this fear allows the flier to examine it directly, rather than dealing through a smoke screen of symptoms and vague apprehensions. It also allows the flier to deal realistically with anxiety about being seen as afraid, which may be perceived as a strong taboo within a "macho" squadron: "Better to die than to look bad."

When the flight surgeon accepts and defines this fear as natural and universal, the flier's tendency to view it as an unnatural, exaggerated personal failing may be corrected. Thus he reassures himself that he is normal and that if his squadron mates are dealing with similar feelings and yet can continue to function, so can he. Reassurance, accepting support, and firm encouragement to return to duty will strengthen his ego and help him deal with the doubts, self-criticisms, and guilt with which his superego may be taxing him about his not being the perfect flier. Remembering that the flier *is* conflicted (or else he would have quit long ago!) will help the flight surgeon deal with personal uncertainties about such a therapeutic approach.

Gratification of the need for the flight surgeon's approval may do much to relieve anxiety, particularly in the more passive or dependent members of the squadron. The amount of positive feedback needed obviously varies from person to person.[31,36]

At a deeper level, an individualized psychotherapeutic technique must be used. This may be performed by some particularly adept flight surgeons, or may require the services of more skilled psychotherapists. Uncovering therapy will help aircrew members express their honest fears; they frequently lack insight into their own apprehensions. The insight gained may be only intellectual; but, even expressing it verbally gives the emotion legitimacy. Furthermore, the flier may be relieved by no longer being afraid and unwilling to acknowledge emotions he regards as unworthy. The more that the anxiety is expressed verbally, the less the need to express it physiologically or psychosomatically; thus, the flier is relieved of the added fear of bodily disease.

> The ego, weakened and shaken by anxiety, needs strong and repeated doses of reassurance, support and encouragement....Many men despise and often condemn fear as unmanly and cowardly, and therefore suppress or repress their own, out of guilt or the hurt to self-esteem. These superego tensions must be relieved by appropriate explanations.[31(p82)]

If fears are already conscious, uncovering is not necessary; ventilation and reassurance may suffice.

Should such fliers be unwilling to tolerate their fears or somatic concerns, they may respond to an appeal to pride and conscience by pointing out the obvious secondary gains. For example, being grounded would remove them from danger, but would transfer the risk to comrades. Use the transference relationship with the flight surgeon and squadron for leverage: "We will think better of you if you fly in spite of your feelings." This may be tempered by simultaneously gratifying dependency needs through allowing extra time with the flight surgeon, or a special system of appointments after missions.

In the case of fliers who attempt to compensate for these needs by denying them and rejecting proffered help, an especially sensitive and tactful approach may be necessary. The therapist may encounter displaced hostility, especially if morale in the squadron is low. This symptom may need to be interpreted to the flier: "I know things are bad in the squadron, and I know you're unhappy with them. Still, we've got a mission, and you're not really sick and don't need to be grounded. I know you can fly and I'll be willing to check you over after every flight to be sure nothing else is going wrong with you. This tension gets to everybody, but I know you can gut it out for a while longer."

Levy,[31] whose approach has been paraphrased, noted that no one had good statistics on what went on within the squadrons. He felt that about 40% of medical/operational failures were primarily psychological and that about half of these failures occurred in the first 10 missions. He went on to point out, as do all authorities, that all fliers would finally break down if not eventually relieved from duty.

Captain Robert Rehm[27] carried his interest in the progression of responses to combat stress beyond that of most flight surgeons. After a year as a flight surgeon in Italy, he felt that he had merely scratched the surface in dealing with his fliers' psychological problems; therefore, he began flying regularly with the crews to better understand their experiences. Although he does not specify, he was probably assigned to a B-24 heavy bomber squadron. He reports various common psychological factors occurring in three segments (the first 10 missions, the subsequent 30, and the final 10) during his 50-mission experience. He expresses the certainty that anxiety was the greatest during the initial missions over the target, especially when the new flier is confronted with serious occurrences such as flak wounds, aircraft damage, or witnessing the loss of another aircraft.[27(p5)] Such a "mild catastrophic event" [!] will shake the resolve of unaggressive aviators. Captain Rehm states that he found it necessary to take a firm attitude and *not* to leave the decision to continue flying up to the flier, but to explain—repeatedly, if need be—that he had no medical reason to ground the flier, who must continue to fly. Such a firm stance was usually effective.

During his own "tour," Captain Rehm describes mostly short and rather easy missions at first, with some exhilaration at actually being in combat and taking some flak hits. However, a near crash on takeoff laid the basis for a later phobia—he preferred to sit where he could not see the ground on takeoffs. One such episode was not sufficient to keep him anxious, but an accumulation of similar phobias could become disabling.

After his first 10 missions, he found that the excitement was subsiding as familiarity increased. The many novel experiences were now accepted as routine, given that no truly catastrophic event occurred. He felt less alone in the aircraft and more homogeneous with the other aircrew members. The war was no longer a personal matter between him and the enemy, but the cooperative effort of a force of which he was a part. He also felt a growing blind faith in his pilot, something quite common in his squadron. "All the dangers which have been safely encountered and surmounted are epitomized in that particular pilot. He stands as a tribute to experience and a symbol of their safety."[27(p7)]- This statement clearly delineates the identification with the pilot and the magical powers attributed to him by an ego defending itself against reality.

As the second period progressed, Captain Rehm describes his emotional plateau as being able to relax over friendly territory and more nervous in the briefing for a bad target (Ploesti, for example) than during the actual mission. After seeing one of their planes shot down, he became somewhat anxious and was insomniac for a few nights. However, his assurance reasserted itself when all went well on subsequent flights.

He comments here on the importance of keeping men flying regularly, "regardless of unusual or catastrophic episodes ... [I] returned a man to duty as soon as physically able, following any injuries which he has sustained. The longer he has to think about his injuries and how they occurred, the more the mental 'gremlins' play on his emotional stability."[27(p8)] He experienced the effects of a long stand down after his 35th mission, just after seeing a plane crash and burn on takeoff, when bad weather grounded the squadron for 10 days. This exacerbated his growing fear of takeoffs, which was relieved only when a trusted pilot had him sit on the flight deck during takeoff and explained how little danger they were in once takeoff speed was attained. (This explanation is, of course, somewhat irrational when one considers that Captain Rehm had, in 35 rides, seen two planes crash and burn on takeoff. One sees how the weight of reassurance from a valued authority transcends logic.) The flight surgeon must understand that a flier who is conflicted about continuing to fly is just that, *conflicted*. That part of him that wants to fly will seize on any information from a valued figure, such as the flight surgeon, as an excuse to return to what he knows he should be doing anyway. Flight surgeons must never underestimate their power in such instances, even though they understand the irrationality involved.

At about this point in a combat tour, Captain Rehm comments upon the "benign hypochondria" in many fliers who develop vague somatic symptoms, some real, such as head colds, some not. Wise flight surgeons will not overemphasize the importance of such symptoms by initiating "junior medical student" workups for minor complaints, sometimes thereby attempting to exorcise their own anxieties. In others, Captain Rehm observed overuse of alcohol and tobacco, irritability, insomnia, nervousness, and temper outbursts. As he began his last 10 missions, he summarized his own situation:

> I realized how all important the factor of physical fatigue was. I became nervous and irritable and I had a great deal of trouble controlling my emotions. I had little zest for the squadron activities.

> My appetite decreased materially and I noted that during the past two and one-half months my weight had dropped from 178 to 156 pounds. I found that I was smoking two packs of cigarettes daily instead of one. The most noticeable factor was my inability to sleep, especially before each mission. This was most marked on the event of my fiftieth mission. Missions to (various targets) were met and completed with much trepidation. The easier missions...gave much relief but seemed much more hazardous than formerly. However, throughout this entire period, the interest and encouragement of the men in the squadron and group spurred me on to greater efforts than before.[27(p10)]

If a flier must be grounded for combat fatigue, and local treatment is not sufficient, that flier must be evacuated to a treatment facility where specialized psychiatric care is available. The author's experience in Vietnam was that the few fliers who were evacuated for psychiatric care to the hospital at Cam Ranh Bay 25 miles away were returned in a week or two and were able to return to flying duties without further difficulty. The author has heard anecdotal reports from multiple sources about several fliers who were grounded for similar symptoms during the Persian Gulf War, and who were evacuated to the United States for treatment. Upon their hospital discharge, no administrative route was available to return them to duty with their squadrons; thus, they were returned to their Stateside bases. There they and their spouses were shunned by other fliers' families, and when their squadrons returned from overseas, they were not accepted back. In essence, their careers are ruined. While these stories cannot be confirmed, their consistency among the sources rings true. If so, they furnish a stark example of the loss of competent fliers because of aeromedical evacuation beyond the point of return to duty. This provides another reason to give treatment as far forward as possible. Medical authorities should also plan to provide an administrative mechanism for return of such fliers to their overseas squadrons.

As combat flying draws to a close, several changes may be noted. Jones[37] speaks of the "short-timer's syndrome" in soldiers, a mixture of mild anxiety and phobic symptoms near the end of a fixed 1-year tour. Some commanders kept men off tough patrols and assignments during their last month, which unfortunately tended to move the onset of the symptoms to the 11th month rather than the 12th. Thus, the division psychiatrist discouraged this policy, in order to maintain consistency in all units and to avoid premature onset of symptoms.

The author saw two sorts of reactions in fliers near the ends of their combat tours. The first was a tendency to "beat up the sky" on the last mission, a tendency that resulted in some unnecessary losses from enemy fire or from crashes. One squadron adopted the policy of suddenly announcing to a flier, "That was your last mission—turn in your gear," about 10 days before the end of the tour.

The second reaction was to become progressively cautious and super-safe, which at times resulted in mission ineffectiveness. This reaction may represent the flying equivalent of "short-timer's syndrome." If so, this author agrees with Jones' approach, which is to advise the commander not to make special allowances for a flier near the end of the tour, in order to avoid adding a secondary gain to the natural tendency to let down right at the end.

Any person, flier or nonflier, needs a chance to debrief and "decompress" at the end of a combat experience. This process should be led in a sympathetic setting by a knowledgeable practitioner. Ideally, the squadron could undergo the process together, giving all a chance to achieve closure on matters of self-esteem, of group validation of individuals' performances, and of an agreed-upon remembrance of how things were. This process should be formalized by such elements as a memorial service for lost comrades and a military parade, with awards and decorations, and a casing of the colors. Ratification of the worthiness of one's service by a valued authority is a powerful antidote for a stressful experience that may be used to balance the doubts and emotional reactions yet to come.

Summary

Plans for dealing with combat fatigue in fliers must be based on experiences of flight surgeons and psychiatrists in past wars with the clear caveat that conditions in future wars may be quite different. Flight surgeons must understand the basic principles underlying the prevention, or at least the delay, of combat fatigue; and they must use their two major therapeutic modalities wisely: (1) the judicious prescription of rest as a palliative and restorative and (2) their own influence in sympathetic yet authoritative roles that offer understanding while expecting faithful service.

Psychiatrists to whom flight surgeons refer fliers must also understand these principles and must take care not to preempt the role of the flight surgeon, nor to belittle or ignore the need for coordination between the two disciplines in decisions regarding flying status.

SUPPORT OF NONFLYING PERSONNEL IN COMBAT

U.S. Air Force doctrine currently calls for four echelons of medical care in combat situations. The first echelon (1-E) consists of care given before a physician becomes involved: preventive measures, first aid, buddy care, and the attention given by enlisted medical personnel. The second echelon (2-E) is the first care given by a physician's assistant, nurse practitioner, or physician, perhaps in a base medical facility or in one located just off-base. Third echelon (3-E) care is given in a larger medical facility (250 to 300 beds) located well off-base, either in a presited hospital or in a transportable hospital brought in by air or by truck. The fourth echelon (4-E) facilities are larger still, and are located well away from the primary battle zone. From these hospitals, patients requiring long-term care will be evacuated back to the United States.

By the nature of these facilities, psychiatric care at the 3-E and 4-E level will be given by specialists. Information in this chapter is primarily intended for nonspecialists, and thus it will deal almost exclusively with the 1-E and 2-E care.

As mentioned in the Introduction, there is little historical information on the effects of combat upon the support troops who make up the majority of any U.S. Air Force base population. In contrast to the classical estimates of psychological casualties as comprising about a one fourth to one half of all battle-induced casualties in combat, during the Persian Gulf War psychiatric diagnoses among U.S. Air Force troops averaged about 3/1,000/wk, about 5% of the total morbidity. This may be compared to the reported average for respiratory diseases of 21/1,000/wk, or the nonbattle injuries rate of 12.3/1,000/wk. Psychiatric diagnosis peaked at about 5.8/1,000/wk during the third week of the air combat campaign.[38(p30)]

These relatively low numbers would have undoubtedly been higher had the bases been under concerted attack, and one might reasonably assume that the particular vulnerability to stress found in U.S. Army support troops under fire would apply here also. Sir Winston Churchill once said, "Nothing in life is so exhilarating as to be shot at without result," but the more common experience seems to be, "Few things in life are as stressful as being shot at and not being able to shoot back."

Consider the situation of an overseas U.S. Air Force base under conditions of impending combat on which troops might come under attack by enemy air and land forces or by missiles that might bear nerve gas or mustard. There is little precedent in today's U.S. Air Force for a line chief to tell his armament troops, "You have to upload that F-16 right now! I know there's persistent nerve gas around, but all of you have your chemical assemblages on. We fixed up the rips the best we could with plastic tape. If any of you get gas symptoms, try to get back here. The rest of you will have to keep uploading the plane, so don't stop to help each other. We have to get that plane off before they hit us again!" Grinker and Spiegel[1] describe similar stress on ground maintenance troops in North Africa who came under attack by German fighters.

> Especially in the early days of the Tunisian campaign, although the forward airfields were constantly patrolled by the fighter aircraft, these were no match for enemy aircraft coming in considerable numbers. The planes appear from nowhere, announcing their presence by the spatter of machine gun bullets and the thump of explosive cannon shells. They appear mysteriously, almost magically, flying out of the sun in the early morning, or diving from behind a cloud to lay a string of bombs throughout the dispersal area. One minute all is peaceful, a scene of quiet, busy activity. There may be a roar of motors in the air, but that is the normal state over an airfield. The next minute enemy fighter planes are buzzing the field, bullets kick up dirt all about, and the tremendous crump [*sic*] of exploding bombs deafens the ears. There is no time to look for shelter, hardly time to put on a helmet—nothing to do but lie flat on the ground and hope for the best. The ack-ack batteries contribute to the general noise and confusion—ineffectively in most instances, because the planes usually come in too low and too fast for effective anti-aircraft fire. In no time at all, the enemy planes are gone, leaving behind them a few twisted, burning planes, a few injuries and deaths, and a number of incipient anxiety states.
>
> Because in this kind of attack the ego has actually no time for defensive activity, its helplessness is real and actual. There is nothing in the environment which can be used to anticipate the approach of danger. Under such circumstances, any stimuli, any loud noise, even the roar of aircraft motors, may actually mean the beginning of an attack. Inhibition of anxiety becomes increasingly difficult. When enemy attacks become incessant, almost everyone on the field develops some degree of free-floating anxiety. The development of the symptoms of neurosis, aside from those of anxiety, in this situation, is directly dependent on the capacity of the individual ego to tolerate free anxiety.[1(pp103,104)]

Marquez reports a similar scene 25 years later, during the Tet attacks on Bien Hoa Air Base in South Vietnam, 0200, 29 January 1968.

> People were running around trying to find shelter anywhere....The 120-mm rocket was an especially frightening weapon because, in addition to doing damage as a fragmentation weapon, it made a lot of noise....Great fires were started, and the firefighters were unable to put them out. People were standing around staring and were too frightened to act...Through it all, there was rampant confusion and no one knew if another attack was imminent....It's hard, but important, to keep busy in the aftermath of one of these things. Some were scared; some were totally out of their minds; others were enjoying it![39(p22)]

Marquez goes on to describe that someone issued weapons to the U.S. Air Force troops on the base, and suddenly there were

> 500 armed aircraft mechanics running around with weapons, no enemy to shoot at, and no one in charge....They were just firing at noises. It took me four hours to retrieve those guns....My reasons were clear—I was afraid my troops would kill each other before dawn....Fear drives people to do very irrational things ... It takes a lot of discipline to get people back together and working productively.[39(p22)]

What can be done today to prepare for such stresses tomorrow? What should be done as the war begins? General preparation should include attention to education, training, group cohesion, morale, and sleep discipline, as well as to other elements leading to improved or prolonged combat effectiveness. These preventive measures will be considered individually. They serve as prophylaxis and, in a sense, as early treatment measures at the 1-E level of medical care.

First-Echelon Measures

Education and Training

The medical officer on base who is most knowledgeable in such matters must be sure that all officers and senior NCOs understand the basic message of this chapter, that they will have to deal with acute stress reactions from the announcement of deployment through the first few days of combat, and that more chronic combat fatigue will inevitably build as time goes on. They must understand that they should take preventive measures before and during the conflict. Briefings should be given by mental health professionals if possible, and, if not, by the senior flight surgeon.

This information must be transmitted down through the ranks to the working level. Leaders should tell their troops ahead of time as much about the combat conditions as possible. They may want to say that it is almost certain that everyone, themselves included, will be afraid, and that it is normal to experience the physical manifestations of that fear. They must expect dry mouths, sweaty palms, palpitations, rapid heartbeats, breathlessness, stomach flutters, and perhaps even nausea and vomiting, urinary frequency, or diarrhea. They will surely be tremulous. All these symptoms are to be expected, as is a realization of their fear about what is about to happen.

Leaders must also make it clear that they expect all of their troops to do their jobs in spite of their fears and to help each other out. In a phrase, "It is all right to be afraid, and your body may let you know that it feels the fear, but you must not let that fear keep you from doing your duty." This may be compared to an athletic contest in which the players know they are nervous and yet go into the game to do the best they can, knowing that they will lose much of the tension as soon as the first contact is made. At that point, they will revert to the skills that they have worked so long to acquire.

By discussing their feelings ahead of time, each individual will know that he or she is not the only one who is aware of being afraid, not the only coward in a band of heroes. Each will know that it is all right to feel fear, as long as each performs assigned duties when the time comes for action. A poll of infantry veterans has shown that, prior to battle, 69% were aware of a racing, pounding pulse; 45% had sweaty palms; 15% had cold sweats; and a lesser percentage felt faint, were nauseated or vomited, or had strong urinary or defecation urges.[40(p11)] *Most of these men were aware of the physical symptoms of fear before they were aware of the emotion which caused them!*[40(p24)]

This poll also emphasized the importance of the control of behavior in action. Of the infantrymen surveyed, 94% said that seeing others act calmly under fire helped them to feel better and act better themselves. Many found that concentrating on their own duties helped, as did cracking jokes about the situation. Some 97% said that knowing morale was high in their unit made them better soldiers.[40(p47)]

All troops must understand the importance of the unit mission and must know how their own work helps the unit achieve its goals. They must understand how they fit into the big picture and why that picture is important, or they will certainly not risk their lives to do what must be done. More concretely, they must understand exactly what they are to do under attack, whether by land or air, by conventional, chemical, or other means. Warnings and all-clears must be crystal clear, to avoid unnecessary or panicky decisions. All concerned should understand that people tend to regress in their behavior when under acute stress, and a simple rote performance of duty may see them through until they become more accustomed to combat conditions. Actions to be taken under attack should be rehearsed so as to be well-nigh automatic. As noted, knowing that training is excellent and that readiness is high is a powerful antidote to fear in combat and will help prevent acute combat stress reactions.

In a study of British unexploded ordnance disposal personnel, Rachman noted qualities of underlying resilience which he described as present in a great many military individuals. When combined with "adequate training, good and reliable equipment, high group morale and cohesion," he found that a sense of calmness, awareness of physical fitness, and general psychological health nearly completed the picture. The single factor that, he felt, distinguished the "courageous" (decorated) individuals was a singular lack of any hypochondriacal features at all. Most had "*no* bodily or mental complaints whatsoever."[41(p102)]

If one regards the desired outcome of a battle or an attack as the transformation of a disciplined and effective enemy military force into a disorganized and powerless rabble ["Inside every army is a crowd struggling to get out,"[42(p175)] then this issue of performance of duty under attack becomes the proper focus of all military training. People on air bases under attack must understand that failure to do their work under the conditions of noise, smoke, confusion, death, and destruction that have accompanied warfare since the invention of gunpowder, will result in defeat. As different as battles and warfare have become from those of the past, what they retain is the human element:

> the behavior of men struggling to reconcile their instinct for self-preservation, their sense of honour and the achievement of some aim over which other men are ready to kill them. The study of battle is therefore always a study of fear and usually of courage; always of leadership, usually of obedience; always of compulsion, sometimes of insubordination; always of anxiety, sometimes of elation or catharsis; always of uncertainty and doubt, misinformation and misapprehension, usually also of faith and sometimes of vision; always of violence, sometimes also of cruelty, self-sacrifice, compassion; above all, it is always a study of solidarity and usually also of disintegration—for it is toward disintegration of human groups that battle is directed.[42(p303)]

Understanding these elements of battle, the wise physician, who has the commander's ear, will assure that everyone within the command understands them also. It is a message seldom heard in the peacetime U.S. Air Force, and then heard only faintly. Much in battle is sociologic and psychologic, and those who understand these factors and can communicate them to the troops in a manner that is understandable and memorable may have much to do with winning.

With this background, the junior officers and senior NCOs should get into the habit of having small "how-goes-it" sessions to assure that everyone gets "the word" at the working level. Hocking[43] comments that an excellent indicator of good morale among troops is the liberty felt by their officers to tell the truth in times of difficulty or failure. Tempering the truth is a sign of distrust of the troops and an attempt to manipulate morale from the outside. As such, it is immediately suspect. Morale is a state of faith between the leaders and the troops and must not be abused. If one does not know what the situation is, one should say so and do everything possible to discover what it is, rather than lying about it. Faith, once betrayed, is almost impossible to reestablish. Troops who know the truth, and know that they know it, are much better prepared to deal with it than those from whom it has been concealed.

Group Cohesion and Morale

At the lowest unit level, a buddy system (the British call it "battle friends") should be established whereby pairs of troops are specifically instructed to look after each other. This system should reflect natural friendships whenever possible, rather than being imposed from above. Thus, each person is aware that there is another person who will be specifically looking out for his welfare when things get rough, that no one will be forgotten or unaccounted for. As a corollary, each unit should maintain small group integrity so that individual bonds and loyalties are not arbitrarily disrupted. Such small groups should be together off-duty as well as on in order to foster their interdependence. Working groups should live together in barracks or shelters, rather than being split up as sometimes occurs in peacetime living.

This point was emphasized by Manning and Ingraham,[44] who surveyed U.S. Army units to establish some of the underpinnings of unit cohesion. One element, usually missing but of inestimable value when present, was the presence of commanders or senior NCOs in after-duty, informal settings *if* they felt socially at ease doing so. By doing so, they shared experiences other than those of the workplace. "The more people interact, the more varied the settings, and the more time the group maintains stable membership, the more the members have in common and the higher the resultant cohesion."[44(p65)]

Skillful Leadership

The small unit leader must be familiar enough with the troops to recognize when an individual's stress symptoms are getting out of hand. The leader should be willing to give a little extra rest and time off to those whose fears are beginning to get the best of them. In his book *Fighting Spirit*, Major General F.W. Richardson, a retired British Army physician, discusses the here-and-now treatment of acute combat stress reactions.[45] Two hundred yards behind the battle line he had established

> a sheltered rest station ... at the bottom of the hill ... (S)omeone had given this place the name of 'Tranquility House.' Once its value had been clearly recognized and the...medical officers instructed about the early handling of cases of threatened breakdown, it was enough for them to mark men's field medical cards 'T.H.' After 12 to 24 hours of rest and hot meals at this post, many men, who might otherwise have had to be sent to hospital, were able to rejoin their units...without loss of face.[45(p106)]

Such an arrangement may or may not involve a medical professional, but the circumstances described certainly should not involve a formal admission in the medical sense, which would reinforce the "sick" role. The message should be "You're not sick and you're certainly not a coward; you're just worn out and need a bit of rest before you go back to duty."

Obviously, medical advisors should assure that officers and NCOs understand the early symptoms of combat fatigue, those at the mild end of the spectrum that might otherwise be ignored: insomnia, nightmares, restlessness, decreased appetite, irritability, increased startle reflex, decreased efficiency, increased smoking or drinking, loss of sense of humor, and changes in normal temperament beyond those that are taking place in the unit as a whole. Troops showing these symptoms should, if possible, be given a little extra time off, or at least the opportunity for a good night's sleep ("three hots and a cot"). A little consideration in these matters may go a long way in prolonging the efficiency of the unit, as well as its individual members' ability to function well.

Richardson went on to report that hundreds of British soldiers were sent out of battle in World War II by their officers because they were showing physical signs of fear. This practice not only was a waste of manpower, but had the potential for a snowball reaction among the troops not yet affected, to whom the secondary gain for the symptoms was all too clear. He points out the clear necessity for commanders to learn to

> distinguish between men who are simply afraid and those who are beginning to find fear uncontrollable. To distinguish between a man who needs to be encouraged to carry on and one who should quietly be got rid of, for the time being, lest his fear become infectious, can test experienced leaders. During the trial by court martial of a soldier for cowardice in Korea, a civilian counsel for the accused was trying subtly to shift the blame onto the shoulders of the platoon commander who, he claimed, should have seen that the man was on the verge of a breakdown. 'Could you not see,' he demanded aggressively, 'that Fusilier L... was trembling involuntarily?' The young officer's splendid reply was 'We were ALL trembling involuntarily.'[45(p111)]

In the same vein, the leader should provide the best amenities possible under the circumstances, including food, shelter, and cleanliness. The troops who know that their leaders are living up to this valuable and venerable military tradition will understand the implicit message that underlies it: "As I show that your physical comforts are important to me, you can see that I consider each one of you valuable, and you know that I will not waste your lives needlessly in battle." Loyalty in battle is, after all, a two-way process.

Leaders should also be alert to undue confusion or agitation in their troops while under fire, and should set a firm, calm example. The timely joke is of inestimable value in this respect. The leader should help turn their minds outward, away from their own troubles and toward their comrades, reinforcing each other's efforts, doing the job at hand, and supporting the base fighting mission. The emphasis should be on teamwork and accomplishment ("We're all counting on you") to appeal to that part of each person's ego that wants to perform honorably under fire, to be thought well of by comrades, and to be part of the best unit in the winning force. By setting a calm example, not minimizing the occasion but instead helping the troops rise to its demands through pride and loyalty, by making them part of something bigger than themselves, the U.S. Air Force leader is following the example of the great leaders of history. Morale, in this context, becomes a matter of concentration of purpose, competence, honesty, selfless generosity, dignity, and exemplary behavior.[43]

Sleep Discipline

Medical personnel must impress on commanders the importance of making sure that their troops get adequate sleep, to the extent that the situation allows. Studies have shown that 4 hours of uninterrupted sleep, especially if it includes the 3 hours between 2 AM and 5 AM, are necessary to maintain the efficiency of the troops over the long haul. In these studies, the 4 hours of sleep consisted of the total amount of Stage 4 sleep and of REM sleep that the troops would have gotten under more normal conditions; that is, their sleep became more condensed and efficient in refreshing them in the field conditions of relative sleep deprivation. Less than 4 hours of sleep led to progressive fatigue and inefficiency.[46]

This doctrine may be hardest to apply to the commanders themselves, who may believe that they are indefatigable. The military writings of Wellington, of Napoleon (whose ability to nap was legendary), and of Montgomery (in contrast with Rommel, who exhausted himself) all bear witness that "the high commander who, under the strain of a prolonged campaign, can preserve an undisturbed sleep pattern is the right man in the right place!"[45(pp76,77)] This may be contrasted with the old saw that "the military regard sleep as monks do sex: the really competent ones get along without it!"[45]

Other Factors

Commanders should be aware that there are some specific factors that may increase their troops' susceptibility to fear: being alone, darkness, rumors, lack of plans, and insidious silence punctuated by loud or unexplained sounds. Knowing ahead of time that such things increase apprehension may help to reduce their effects, and the troops should be warned about them. At best, the men may recognize their own fears and joke about them. At least, they will not be surprised that they feel afraid. They will understand that there is no disgrace in feeling fear, only in giving way to it.

Commanders must also be aware of the insidious effects of prolonged inactivity or unstructured time on morale, especially if accompanied by an undertone of anxiety about what might happen. Several traditional antidotes are available, tailored to the specific circumstances.

A good sports program is worth its weight in gold. The one drawback is a tendency to cause injuries, so be careful about activities involving physical contact, and provide referees to keep things in hand. Educational offerings will attract some: lessons in the local language, history, and customs, or even a formal course program if available. An enlightened leave program may be possible, with tourist-type day or overnight trips to local attractions. For prolonged campaigns, consider an R and R policy.

Pay attention to work-alert-rest schedules. Avoid switching personnel on and off night duty; it may be possible to have reasonably stable day and night sections, to avoid undue circadian disturbances. Rotate tasks. Provide military training and upgrade. Cross-train if it is reasonable; this will also benefit the organization in case of losses through combat or illness.

As Hoffman[47] points out, these factors, combined with a sense of good leadership, fairness, competence, and caring, will demonstrate to the troops that their commanders are looking out for their welfare. Attention to details, alertness to signs of stress in self and buddies, and open lines of communication up and down the chain of command during lulls will help assure good performance when things get rugged.

Medical personnel must assure that line officers and NCOs understand that the best way to counter the demoralizing and fearful effects of combat is to foster good morale. The wise leader knows that there are clear indicators of poor morale available, such as an increase in abuse of alcohol and drugs, venereal disease, fights, AWOLs (absent without leave), and similar Article 15 offenses. One may also see an increase in a constellation of medical conditions, the prevention of which is a function of personal discipline: sunburn, frostbite, immersion foot, malaria (the troops are not using insect repellent, taking their prophylactic medications, or sleeping under their mosquito netting), food-borne diseases (improper hygiene), and other such maladies.

Further, a unit that is well-led, and knows it, will identify itself with its leader and will begin to use his way of speaking, habits of behavior, and even personal mannerisms.[48] This magical identification with a leader who is perceived as wise and powerful is a notable indicator that morale is high. Although a unit with good morale may not display its discipline in the "snappy salute" sense, it will take good care of itself. It will practice the essentials necessary to preserve its own health and its operational readiness, and the troops will reinforce each other in following the formal and informal rules that maintain and increase their collective effectiveness.

Second-Echelon Measures

Almost all of the literature concerning the initial care of combat fatigue victims has been written by U.S. Army psychiatrists. One of the clearest descriptions of this care was given by W.C. Menninger[49] in his classic monograph, *Psychiatry in a Troubled World,* in which he discussed the treatment regimen developed by the psychiatrists in the Mediterranean Theater in World War II.

> By their plan the battalion aid station surgeons were indoctrinated with "first aid" psychiatry. It was they who had to decide whether a man should be returned to duty, given a brief respite, or evacuated to the clearing station. It was fully appreciated that many soldiers, if returned to the battalion kitchen area and permitted a night of sound sleep with the aid of a mild sedative and some warm food, would be ready in 24 hours to return to combat. No record was ever kept of the men so handled, but it is known to be a sizable percentage of the men seen at the battalion aid station.
>
> The seriously upset soldiers were sent 2 to 5 miles farther back to the division clearing station where the division psychiatrist had his headquarters and treatment center. This sometimes was in a tent or in a commandeered building such as a schoolhouse, factory, or whatever might be available. The soldier arrived here from his foxhole within 1 to 3 hours. Each one was seen initially by the psychiatrist and interviewed briefly. If he was recognized to be too sick to benefit from brief rest and such psychotherapeutic help as could be given in a short time, he was immediately evacuated farther back. The largest percentage of the soldiers who came to the clearing station remained there for 48 hours. These men were given sufficient sedation to insure a good 12 to 24 hours of sleep, only interrupted when awakened for food. On the second day, they had an opportunity to shave and bathe. Approximately 40 per cent could return to combat on the third day. Follow-up studies suggest that many of these men carried on indefinitely. Perhaps 25 per cent of this group had recurrence of symptoms and became repeaters."[49(pp306–307)]

Menninger goes on to describe the treatment of those not handled at the clearing station (which, in U.S. Air Force terminology, would be an off-base 2-E facility). The worst casualties, or those not responding to brief intervention, were sent to "exhaustion centers" 16 to 24 km (10–15 mi) behind the lines. These were staffed by 12 officers and 99 enlisted and were equipped to take care of 200 to 500 psychiatric casualties. Patients remained there 5 to 8 days and were treated with rest, recreation, and narcosynthesis using sodium pentothal. These centers developed training platoons, directed by line officers, "which provided an additional 2 to 5 days of military activities at a graded tempo to prepare the men for return to combat. Of the combat casualties, 20 per cent were returned to combat from these centers."[49(p307)]

Menninger notes specifically that, besides adhering to the classic treatment principles of proximity-immediacy-expectancy, the entire program assumed that the chief preventive efforts were a function of commanders, not of the medical personnel, and that the active support of the line officers was required in order to assure its success.

Thus the elements of care at the 2-E level include the location of the unit, its staffing, its function, the treatment setting, the principles of management, the use of medications, and the options available for disposition of those treated there.

Location and Staffing

Plans for locating the U.S. Air Force 2-E mental health services change from time to time, but the doctrine, configuration, and location will probably not differ greatly from what will be described below, and will correspond in function, if not in location, to the system of which Menninger wrote. Medical personnel remaining on a base under continuing attack or threat of attack will probably consist of a few flight surgeons, perhaps a surgical specialist, some medical technicians and ambulance drivers, and a mental health team consisting of a psychiatrist, a psychologist, a clinical social worker, and some mental health technicians. The remainder of the local medical and mental health personnel, perhaps augmented by others brought in under mobilization plans, will work at one or more sites located 5 to 10 km (3–6 mi) off-base; each site will be independently capable of giving stabilizing medical care in support of approximately 4,000 troops. It should be noted that distances given are rather arbitrary. The important concept is "psychological distance": far enough from combat to be safe, near enough to return to one's own unit.

Although preliminary plans call for a psychiatrist, a psychologist or a clinical social worker, and two mental health technicians to augment some 2-E facilities as part of the 50-bed Air Transportable Hospital, current U.S. Air Force manning levels make it unlikely that more than one off-base 2-E facility per base will be so staffed. Thus, each local Director of Base Medical Services (DBMS) may well have to decide how best to use the available mental health staff, considering the on-base situation, the off-base situation, the adequacy of communication and transportation links, the combat/casualty situation, the nature of the threat, and other such variables. The disposition of local mental health resources may be changed as the situation dictates, and such local flexibility should not be hampered by excessive doctrinal rigidity. Common sense should prevail, and all concerned should be aware that their experience with the realities of the situation may quickly supersede set-piece planning.

Why be so insistent that early treatment be given at the on-base 2-E facility rather than off-base? In a lecture to U.S. Air Force mental health professionals in 1983, an Israeli psychologist pointed out the value of having mental health professionals use their knowledge and experience close to the fighting:

- They can use their professional stature to resist local unit commanders who want to evacuate troops with symptoms of combat fatigue. Less knowledgeable people might give way to such pressure.
- They can respond realistically to any troops who say "You don't know what it's like," because they live on the same base and under the same conditions. This corresponds to the principle that flight surgeons should fly in unit aircraft, both in peace and in war, to meet the flier on equal footing in terms of understanding the situation personally. Although some 2-E facilities off-base may also need a mental health capability, it is crucial that patients with only mild or early symptoms be kept on-base, along with a contingent of mental health personnel.[50]

To his two reasons, a third may be added. Few U.S. Air Force medical personnel today, officer or enlisted, have personal combat experience. To leave the triage decisions concerning patients with psychiatric symptoms in the hands of the flight surgeon or DBMS, neither of whom is likely to have either combat *or* psychiatric experience, is to put the troops doubly at risk of the wrong decisions being made. Mental health workers must be on-base, making every effort toward rapid, effective interventions: reassuring, explaining, exhorting, and above all, returning troops to their units as rapidly as possible.

What, then, might be the function of a 2-E site off-base? The author sees this as an overflow facility, used for patients who are truly mentally ill, or who have not been able to return to duty as expected and are awaiting evacuation. This facility may also receive patients when the on-base 2-E facility is overrun with troops. The realities of the situation faced by the DBMS and the mental health staff should quickly result in the available facilities being used in the most efficient manner possible, if the tried-and-true principles outlined here are intelligently applied.

Function of the Second-Echelon Facility

Clearly, the burden of the initial management of acute symptoms immediately after a base is first attacked will fall upon whatever medical personnel remain on that base, whether or not they have had formal mental health training. Another Israeli Defense Force psychologist has emphasized that such reactions may overwhelm unprepared medical personnel, especially if they themselves have also just experienced their first attack.[51] Human nature leads one to look to any perceived authority for help in crises, and the disaster literature leaves no doubt that anyone who is seen as having special knowledge or skills in such a case will quickly be sought out. When confronted with troops having combat shock reactions, medical personnel will certainly look to colleagues with mental health training—*any* mental health training—to handle the unwounded stress casualties.[51]

By now the reader must be aware that all military mental health authorities agree on the necessity *not* to overreact to such circumstances by evacuating troops to the rear—not even a little bit to the rear—because of the perceived secondary gain. *"If they ain't hurt, don't ship 'em out!"*

This inelegant slogan is easy to remember in a crisis, and may be used by medics and line personnel alike. If the mental health troops on a base overwhelmed with somatic casualties are pressed into triage, litter-bearing, or treatment teams, they may join in following the course of least resistance and shipping the unhurt but stunned and sobbing troops off-base to a less harassed 2-E facility. This impulse must be resisted, or there will be an intolerable loss of unwounded troops to off-base locations from which it may prove very difficult to reclaim them.

An on-base holding facility must be provided to the DBMS by a wing commander who understands the principles involved, explains them to the commanders of the various squadrons, and supports the DBMS in their application. Reflecting upon Richardson's Tranquility House described above,[45] this author recommends that such an on-base facility be established in a reasonably secure location, away from primary targets, and run by the available mental health personnel. Flexibility in assigning mental health nurses and occupational therapists to this facility may also prove useful.

In the personal communication previously noted,[51] Levy commented that the Israeli medical service organizes its combat stress casualties along military lines, with unit names rather than medical names. Under this model, each U.S. Air Force psychiatric technician might direct a "flight" of 10 or more casualties. Three or more flights would comprise a "squadron," with the squadron command element consisting of the psychiatric social worker, an NCO-in-charge (NCOIC), and, if available, an occupational or physical therapist. This latter function might even be filled by a knowledgeable physical training technician from the base gymnasium.

The structure of this local treatment team would thus emphasize the military aspects of the situation and minimize the medical aspects. At this level, treatment essentially consists of acknowledging a temporary inability to work, without falling into the medical model (taking a history, writing up a chart, making a formal diagnosis), that reinforces the patient role. Such troops—do *not* call them "patients"!—should not be formally admitted to the facility. "You're not a coward, you're not sick, you're just worn out, and you'll be all right in a day or two" must be the constant theme. A chance to rest, a hot meal (the U.S. Army's "3 hots and a cot"), a physical examination, however perfunctory, to reassure that there is no physical problem, and an appeal to honor, group loyalty, and the mission may be all that is necessary. In fact, at his first contact with the medics, all that a scared kid may need is for someone in authority to tell him that he's all right, and that he must get back to work, do his part, and not let his buddies down.

Principles of Treatment

The treatment of acute combat reactions or of combat fatigue on-base may be summarized in the acronym BICEPS (brevity, immediacy, centrality, expectancy, proximity, and simplicity). The author coined this acronym in 1980 for use in the U.S. Air Force Surgeon General's Medical Red Flag training program. The principles of proximity, immediacy, and expectancy, so named by Artiss, were articulated by Glass[52] in World War II and were derived from Salmon's forward treatment during World War I.[53] The principles of brevity, centrality, and simplicity were discussed by F. Jones, after the war in Southeast Asia.[37] Each principle might, of course, be discussed at length, but, in the total context of this discussion, they are identified as follows:

- ***Brevity.*** Treat briefly, from 12 to 72 hours, with the explicit goal being a rapid return to duty.
- ***Immediacy.*** Treat as soon as the person's behavior makes it clear that he or she can no longer function as a productive squadron member. Do not wait for full collapse of function, especially if squadron authorities or buddies indicate that this individual is becoming nonfunctional. Do not wait for an outside consultant, either. Begin treatment now.
- ***Centrality.*** Treat combat fatigue cases who are being considered for evacuation in a single location, separate from somatic casualties and "sick" patients, preferably administered by a single individual. At this single location skilled personnel may be able to prevent further evacuation.[34,37]
- ***Expectancy.*** Treatment should be aimed at getting the individual back to duty, and all concerned must expect this to be the inevitable and only outcome. The therapists should ally themselves with the patient's conscious will to remain and do the necessary duty, and should work together toward that goal so the fatigued person can return to friends, unit, and job. The therapeutic alliance must not allow any other goal to interfere with getting the person well, and the functional definition of "getting well" is a return to duty.
- ***Proximity.*** Treat close to the unit, so that cohesion continues. This will be most concretely demonstrated by having the person's friends and commander visit, thus proving

that they do not reject combat fatigue victims as cowardly or unworthy. Those who repudiate their stricken comrades may be unable to tolerate any such tendencies in themselves and thus reject those who symbolize their own fears. Such people will contribute to the problem by increasing the victim's guilt; and, if they are leaders themselves, may lose troops unnecessarily because of this attitude. Close liaison between therapists and the parent unit will not only help the troops in question, but will demystify the whole experience for the unit as well, and will show the lack of secondary gain: becoming symptomatic is not an automatic ticket out of combat. Here again, the value of keeping this 2-E function on-base rather than several kilometers away is obvious.

- ***Simplicity.*** Treat in the here-and-now, aimed at a return to duty. This is not the time for a full-scale psychiatric evaluation and formulation, or a treatment contract extending into the indefinite future.

Medications

Psychopharmacology, like other areas of drug therapy, is a dynamic and rapidly changing field. Each physician uses medications in a highly personal way, and psychiatrists are no exception. Some are chemical nihilists, while others write a prescription for almost every patient they see. Thus, the precedents for the use or nonuse of medications in combat situations are by no means applicable to all situations or to all therapists.

In World War II, psychiatrists frequently used sodium pentothal or Sodium Amytal[1(p52)] to help soldiers abreact their emotional turmoil. A review of the use of medications in the Vietnam War by some 40 U.S. psychiatrists revealed that a large proportion of them used anxiolytic and neuroleptic agents, even in early or mild cases of combat fatigue.[54] These therapists reported the use of recuperation, social therapy (the milieu of expectancy), and medications, in that order of frequency, in the 2-E environment.

They used anxiolytics in about 30% of their cases, mainly for early symptoms, including apprehension (especially the "short-timer's syndrome"), sleep disturbances, tremors, and increased startle reactions. They used neuroleptics in about 20% for threatened assaultive behavior, defects in judgment, or other behavioral changes which concerned or alarmed the unit. Neuroleptics were used with increasing frequency in patients with increasingly disturbed behavior, especially in those for whom recuperative facilities seemed to be of little use.[54]

More recent practices contradict these findings. The Israelis, as has been noted, are much more interested in behavioral treatment. One source cites the use of medications, and only tricyclic antidepressants at that, in only 8% of the 60 soldiers referred for 3-E and 4-E treatment out of the 600 soldiers who were evacuated as combat fatigue casualties in the 1982 Lebanon War. The treatment program for the majority consisted of "walking and talking," abreactive individual and group psychotherapy, individual and group sports activities, and combat-oriented military training.[55] By contrast, the British, in the Falkland Islands War, used short-acting benzodiazepines as a prophylaxis against excessive fatigue due to insomnia, evidently with good results.[23]

Two major cautions are offered against the early use of medications. First, their use tends to reinforce the sick role, because the giving of medications is one of the hallmarks of the physician-patient relationship in American society. Second, many psychotropic medications have a duration of action longer than the 72 hours that a combat fatigue victim may spend in a 2-E facility, especially if one takes into account the active metabolic products of some of the drugs. Sending a person back to combat duty still under the influence of psychoactive drugs may be dangerous. Even in peacetime, people in the many combat support positions covered by the Personnel Reliability Program would not be allowed to take such medications and continue to work in their sensitive, demanding jobs. The use of such medications under combat conditions must thus be thoughtfully weighed for the risk-to-benefit ratio, both for the individual and for the mission.

In the end, the decision to use or not to use psychotropic medications rests with the physician on the scene. There is much information on this subject elsewhere, and anyone potentially faced with this situation would do well to know as much as possible about a few psychotropic drugs before the combat situation occurs, when there will be no time to look them up. Use such drugs sparingly and for specific target symptoms, with full consideration of the two negative factors noted above.

Treatment Setting

Although one may find it impossible to imagine what a 2-E facility might look like, on- or off-base, perhaps Enoch's[56] description of such a function in the Israeli campaign in Lebanon will be useful, especially when compared and contrasted with Menninger's description of a similar function in World War II, cited above.

> Initially, (the) team would conduct an interview to establish where the soldier had been, what he had done, and what had happened to him. This interview was oriented objectively rather than toward thoughts and feelings. The team confirmed two of the observations made in previous wars. First, thoughts and feelings inevitably followed the description of the objective events. Second, just describing what had happened clarified events and reduced the emotional turmoil. The team would allocate the next 6 to 8 hours of treatment to physical replenishment (water, food, and rest). Then the soldier was given useful tasks to do and invited to join in supportive individual and group psychotherapy. Next, the team arranged for comrades from the soldier's unit and for the unit commander to visit the soldier. Then the soldier himself was taken to visit the unit. In these ways, mutual confidence between the soldier and his unit was restored. When the soldier had recovered enough to return to the unit, the team would arrange for comrades from his unit to pick him up. This team took advantage of its proximity to the front and the soldier's unit to maximize expectation that he would return and to reinforce the soldier's link to his comrades and commander. The team observed that units were happy to receive the soldier back, confirming the finding from other sources that under stress group members prefer someone they know to someone they do not know, regardless of presumed competence. With respect to themselves, the members of the psychiatric team noted that, because of their proximity to the front, they were all afraid. However, sharing the dangers of combat with the soldiers being treated reduced their reluctance to return a soldier to his unit. They noted that their fear was diminished to the degree that the (medical) commander was competent in ensuring their supplies of gasoline and other essentials. When this was not the case, they became more afraid, hoarded supplies, and saw their clinical effectiveness decline. The team observed their tendency to overidentify with the soldier they were treating; to want to be the "good father," and to protect their new-found "son" from harm. This difficulty was reduced through once-a-day staff meetings for the purpose of discussing cases, providing mutual support, and working through emotional conflicts.
>
> The Israelis observed that the psychiatric symptoms changed from the time the soldier broke down at the front to the time he arrived at the (medical station). At the front, soldiers suffering psychiatric breakdown complained of an inability to perform—termed by the Israelis "the ticket out" of combat, while upon reaching the (medical station) they complained of difficulties with thoughts and feelings—termed "the ticket in" to treatment. The Israelis concluded that severity of initial symptoms had little to do with prognosis for recovery; the most important indicator of a good prognosis was the soldier's labeling himself as healthy, taking initiative in his own care, helping others, and helping run the treatment team's area.[56(p14,15)]

With the applications of the BICEPS principles there is a deemphasis on medications and the "sick" role. Troops in this ambiance must not be treated as patients. They must spend the day in uniform, not in pajamas, unless they are specifically supposed to be in bed resting for the first 12 to 24 hours. Their days should be structured and should be used purposefully to maintain the identity of each as a functional military person. Daily roll call, announcement of the day's schedule, physical training, useful activities such as digging trenches or bunkers, filling sandbags, improving the local area, playing sports, and attending meetings should be the order of the day. The value of occupational and physical therapists in planning and carrying out such activities is clear.

In the 528th Medical Detachment, already mentioned, the role of occupational therapy personnel as "environmental managers" both in the consultation role and the therapeutic role proved extremely valuable during the Persian Gulf War. Presentation as "work therapy" furthers the sick role, so the presentation as "work assignment," "work detail" or "work activity," may be more appropriate to the "return to duty" ambiance of this modality. Ellsworth and colleagues[57] have presented a review of this subject, together with a model schedule for patient activities (Exhibit 8-1).

Group therapy sessions must be carefully monitored and one must be particularly careful not to let them turn into "my experience was worse than your experience" sessions. Such an ambiance may be perceived as rewarding symptoms, and troops may escalate each other into brief reactive psychoses if not restrained.[51] Thus, such sessions should be goal-directed, here-and-now, and oriented toward health rather than emphasizing symptoms and disability. Sports programs, which by their nature reward healthy behavior, are of particular value. Coaches urge one to perform in spite of symptoms.

The programs of Menninger[49] and the Israelis[56] were reflected in that of the U.S. Army in the Gulf War. "PSYCH-FORCE 90" was the self-designation of the 528th Medical Detachment, a psychiatric OM (combat stress prevention and treatment) organiza-

EXHIBIT 8-1

SECOND-ECHELON TREATMENT FACILITY: MODEL SCHEDULE FOR PATIENT ACTIVITIES

A typical day might include:

0545–0730	Wake up, clean up, formation, breakfast
0730–0800	Morning details
0800–0830	Morning physical training
0830–1200	Work assignments (after initial rest and hygiene)
1200–1300	Formation and Lunch
1300–1530	Classes (stress management, relaxation, assertiveness training (after initial rest and hygiene)
1530–1600	Change for afternoon physical training
1600–1700	Physical training, recreation
1700–1830	Formation and Dinner
1830–1930	Group discussion
1930–2200	Evening activity, personal time
2200	Lights out

Adapted with permission from Ellsworth PD, Sinnott MW, Laedtke ME, McPhee SD. Utilization of occupational therapy in combat stress control during the Persian Gulf War. *Milit Med*. 1993;58:383.

tion of 15 officers and 33 enlisted troops deployed to Saudi Arabia in October, 1990, to support the Persian Gulf War.[58] This unit operated three consultation teams that made proactive visits to U.S. Army units, and one base camp treatment team that furnished outpatient and inpatient therapy (20 beds). Between November 3, 1990 and January 10, 1991, the unit performed 600 unit consultations. Several thousand soldiers were seen altogether. The units performed 387 formal psychiatric evaluations, and held 123 soldiers for treatment. Fifteen percent were evacuated out of theater. (Of all the soldiers evacuated to Europe, less than 6% had psychiatric diagnoses.)[59] This effective use of psychiatric treatment teams involved two facets. First, in consultations with commanders, they actively sought to advise the field units about psychological stress, work-sleep cycles, heat stress, buddy-aid, critical event debriefings, and follow-up consultations when necessary (as with training accidents or firing weapons in anger).

Their second mission was to triage and treat dysfunctional soldiers. After one interview, they would make disposition: evacuate the truly mentally ill, hold a soldier for treatment if suicidal. Otherwise, they attempted simple ventilation, focusing on solutions in the here-and-now. Problems involving the family back home were referred to the chain of command. (Their experience, and that of the author 30 years earlier, was that evacuating troops from a combat zone for family reasons was folly, and would result in an epidemic of family problems within the unit.)

Soldiers held for duty were kept in a military environment—cots in tents. Therapeutic emphasis was on healthy functioning through an intensive work-therapy program, promoting adaptation through psychological educational classes and small group therapy. This involved only limited ventilation, restructuring problems into here-and-now resolvable issues, and acquiring adaptational skills. Command consultation was obtained when warranted.

A common factor associated with developing adjustment disorders was the soldier's assignment to a new unit within 90 days of deployment (ie, the soldier was not yet strongly bonded to the unit). Most soldiers presented for treatment within their first month in theater, pointing up the need for some stress training *prior* to deployment. Also, problems reflecting troubles at home indicated the usefulness of strong family support programs.

Other patient clusters centered around: (*a*) mothers leaving small children, losing their bonding; (*b*) Reserve or Guard troops taking psychoactive medications prescribed by their civilian physicians, being cut off these medications through lack of availability, or contraindicated because they lowered heat tolerance; (*c*) functional symptoms found to be due to organic conditions; and (*d*) veterans of prior wars undergoing exacerbations of traumatic stress reactions. This latter situation frequently involved medical troops, and was possibly associated with their easy access to psychiatric care.

After the OM team arrived in theater, the evacuation of personnel because of personality disorders fell by 50%; most evacuations after that were for major psychiatric disorders.[58] The success of this unit should light the way for U.S. Air Force mental health professionals.

Options for Disposition of Troops

Therapists working at on-base or off-base 2-E facilities will have a number of choices for disposition

EXHIBIT 8-2

OPTIONS FOR DISPOSITION OF TROOPS PRESENTING AT 2-E FACILITIES

1. Immediate return to duty.
2. Hold for a brief period, perhaps with a meal, rest, and return to duty without having been admitted.
3. Hold overnight, as in (2) without admission. Possible use of a single dose of short-acting benzodiazepine for sedation.
4. Relieve from duty (admit) and treat as indicated for 2–3 days. Use BICEPS principles. Return to duty.
5. Use of (4), with return to limited duty or to less hazardous or less demanding duty. This may be especially useful in the "old sergeant's syndrome."
6. Use of (4), with unsatisfactory results and with subsequent evacuation to a 3-E facility.
7. Treatments (1–5), with subsequent return to commander for administrative action, in instances where the problem is due to personality disorder rather than to medical or psychiatric problem.
8. Evaluation and immediate evacuation to the 3-E level when the diagnosis is a true and severe mental disease. This procedure should occur only rarely.
9. Evaluation leads to a diagnosis of probable somatic disorder and the patient is transferred to the appropriate treatment facility.

of troops who come under their care (Exhibit 8-2). Precedent, imagination, and experience suggest the outcomes delineated in the exhibit; others may be developed as the exigencies of the situation dictate.

In the section on care of fliers, the value of a formal ending to a unit's combat experience has been mentioned. Current literature also underscores the value of a stress debriefing of the entire unit. This is a formal process, and should be undertaken only by trained professionals, preferably not assigned to the unit. It is modeled on the Critical Incident Stress Debriefing,[60] used by many civilian fire and police departments, and similar organizations. This process has been termed the "After-Action Stress Debriefing."[61]

This process is too involved to be discussed here, but is discussed extensively in Chapter 11, Debriefing Following Combat. Authors who served in the Gulf War have attested to its value, and to the consequences of not having such a program available.[62,63] Medical personnel of many disciplines know of the concept, and the absence of a chance to process their combat experiences will be missed and commented upon.

Summary

Future wars may replicate past wars in which air crews carried out transportation, bombing, and fighting missions from a relatively safe support base. In this case, little change from prior practices in the care of nonflying personnel is required. In a large-scale engagement, however, modern tactics, reflecting technological advances, call for pressing the battle to support facilities, perhaps through long-range missile or air assaults. In such a situation (eg, the Persian Gulf War) nonflying U.S. Air Force personnel may become combat targets and thus combat stress casualties. Currently, little provision is made for such casualties; however, there is good reason to believe that the traditional principles of U.S. Army combat psychiatry, as described by the "BICEPS" acronym, can be effective in treating and returning to duty the majority of these casualties. Provision of this treatment will require education and training of all personnel and medical and mental health personnel assigned "forward" at first- and second-echelon support installations. As always, good leadership and cohesive units will minimize combat stress casualties.

CONCLUSION

The author has studied this topic, lectured on it, and discussed it with colleagues since 1979. He has also read historical and current military biographies, histories, aeromedical reports, and the literature of military medicine and psychiatry. In a most introspective way, he has reexamined his service as a flight surgeon with the Air Commandos in Vietnam, and would add the following remarks to this chapter.

To begin with, physicians and others thinking about combat must understand that they will have to deal with combat from three points of view. The first of these has already been thoroughly discussed—the care of others. The second of these is that they must also think about caring for themselves. The realities of combat will also reach those trying to ameliorate its effects, often in a most intrusive and distressing way. Those feelings will have to be dealt with. It is vital that mental health providers take care of themselves and their colleagues. And the third point of view is that they must care for their colleagues. This includes being alert for the abuse of alcohol as a solvent for pressures and emotions, and be aware that medics, too, need time off, especially those in the surgical arena, confronted daily with carnage beyond comprehension. Patients, self, and fellow medics: one must be aware of all three.

Commander Sandra Yerke's graphic description of the difficulties encountered in molding a group of strangers into a competent staff on a hospital ship during the Persian Gulf War[64] should be required reading for each medic on active duty. Anyone may deploy at any time, if the circumstances are right, and all must be prepared, always.

Wars tend to be come-as-you-are events, and there will be little time to read up on them once one starts. Field medical units usually do not include libraries, and thus mental health providers most often deploy with only the knowledge they carry in their baggage or in their heads. Base or post libraries usually have very good military sections and the author urges the reading of some books written by medical personnel about their experiences. The thoughtful perusal of a few such books, combined with constructive thinking about what the role of the mental health provider might be in such a situation, may help prepare such personnel in ways that would not otherwise occur to them or to those who train them.

In addition, medical officers and NCOs may well have to exercise command of troops in the combat ambiance, a fact that may never have occurred to them until now. The responsibility for giving orders that may result in the loss of life or limb by those carrying out the orders is not a subject taught in medical school or emphasized in unit training exercises. It is an awesome responsibility, and all medical personnel would do well to learn a bit more about combat leadership than the service usually teaches medics. Military medical officers are accustomed to maintaining currency in their medical literature. It is vital that they maintain currency in the military literature as well. Through long experience, line officers will tend to believe that a medic is a good medic unless proven wrong. They will also tend to believe that a medical officer is not a good officer until the medical officer proves that he is. Medics must be as good at their job as those on the line are at theirs.

Principles of conservation, training, planning, and execution of war plans apply to the medical commander as surely as they do to the line commander.

> (T)he physician-soldier must be able to make the hard decisions that are required ... with little time to reflect, depending instead on the education and training that has led him [or her] to a leadership position and the medical intelligence available....The troop commander must be prepared to make decisions that place the lives of those that he is responsible for at risk. So must the physician who commands others in war."[65(p375)]

Finally, and most personally, the author recalls the well-known words of General Robert E. Lee as he viewed the appalling battlefield at Fredericksburg after his victory over General Burnside: "It is well that war is so terrible, else we should become too fond of it." Having spent a year in Vietnam, and having been immersed in the medical literature of war since 1979, the author agrees. His wish and his prayer are that none who read these words may ever have to put into practice the principles of combat psychiatry.

REFERENCES

1. Grinker RR, Spiegel JP. *War Neuroses in North Africa.* New York: Josiah Macy Jr Foundation; 1943.

2. Consolidated Aerospace Medicine Desert Shield/Storm After Action Report. Department of the Air Force. HQ, SAC: Offutt AFB, Neb; 1992.

3. Lifton RJ. Psychotherapy with combat fliers. *US Armed Forces Med J.* 1953;4:525–532.

4. Schultze HA. Fear of flying. *USAF Med Svc Dig.* 1952;3:25,51.

5. Spiegel FS. Problems of the flight surgeon in Korea. *US Armed Forces Med J.* 1953;4:1321–1324.

6. Marshall SLA. *Swift Sword.* New York: American Heritage Publishing Co Inc; 1967.

7. Payne LGS. *Air Dates.* London, England: William Heinemann Ltd; 1967.

8. Link MM, Coleman HA. *Medical Support of the Army Air Forces in World War II.* Washington, DC: Office of The Surgeon General, US Air Force; 1955.

9. Berger C, ed. *The United States Air Force in Southeast Asia.* Washington, DC: Office of Air Force History; 1977.

10. Farmer RA. Personal Communication, 1984.

11. Jones DR. Flying and danger, joy and fear. *Aviat Space Environ Med.* 1986;57:131–136.

12. Bucove AD, Maioriello RD. Symptoms without illness: Fear of flying among fighter pilots. *Psychiatric Quart.* 1970;44:125–142.

13. Anderson HG, ed. *The Medical and Surgical Aspects of Aviation.* London, England: Oxford University Press; 1919:67–95, 96–135.

14. Armstrong HA. A special form of functional psychoneuroses appearing in airplane pilots. *JAMA.* 1936;106: 1347–1354.

15. US Department of the Air Force. *Medical Examinations and Standards.* Washington, DC: USAF; 15 November 1994. Air Force Instruction 48-123, Attachment 6.

16. Touhey JE. Personal Communication, 1984.

17. Hartman BO. Management of irregular rest and activity. In: *AGARD Lecture Series 105: Sleep, Wakefulness, and Circadian Rhythm.* London, England: AGARD;1979: 13-1–13-15.

18. Rayman RB. Cambodian airlift. *Aviat Space Environ Med.* 1977;48:460–464. (Reprinted 1993;64:319–323).

19. Basel GI. *Pak Six.* New York: Jove Press; 1992.

20. Mendelson WB. *Human Sleep: Research and Clinical Care.* New York: Plenum Medical Book Co; 1987.

21. Knowles JB, Laverty SG, Kuechler MA. Effects of alcohol on REM sleep. *Quarterly Journal of Studies on Alcohol.* 1968;25:342–349.

22. Fisher M. British physician reports on Falkland Islands campaign. *US Medicine.* 1983;February:3,10.

23. Nicholson AN. Long-range capability and the South Atlantic campaign. *Aviat Space Environ Med.* 1984;55:269–270.

24. Merlotti L, Roehrs T, Koshorek G, et al. The dose effects of zolpidem on the sleep of healthy normals. *J. Clin Psychopharmacol.* 1989;9:9–14.

25. Landry R. Cited in *The Air Force Times.* 27 April 1992:3,20.

26. Lyons TJ, French J. Modafinal: The unique properties of a new stimulant. *Aviat Space Environ Med.* 1991;62:432–435.

27. Rehm R. Fifty missions over Europe. In: Wright DG, ed. *Observations on Combat Flying Personnel.* New York: Josiah Macy Jr Foundation; 1945: 4–11.

28. Krosnick G. Anxiety reactions in fighter pilots. In: Wright DG, ed. *Observations on Combat Flying Personnel.* New York: Josiah Macy Jr Foundation; 1945: 53–64.

29. Hastings DW, Wright DG, Glueck BC. *Psychiatric Experiences of the Eighth Air Force.* New York: Josiah Macy Jr Foundation; 1944.

30. Heller J. *Catch-22.* New York: Dell; 1955.

31. Levy NA. *Personality Disturbances in Combat Fliers.* New York: Josiah Macy Jr Foundation; 1945.

32. Stafford-Clark D. Morale and flying experience: Results of a wartime study. *J Ment Sci.* 1949;95:10–50.

33. Symonds CP. Human response to flying stress. *Br Med J.* 1943;2:703–706,740–744.

34. Jones FD, Johnson AW. Medical and psychiatric treatment policy and practice in Vietnam. *J Soc Issues.* 1975;31(4):49–65.

35. Mills JG, Jones DR. The adaptability rating for military aeronautics: A historical perspective of a continuing problem. *Aviat Space Environ Med.* 1984;55:558–562.

36. Layden M. Experiences with anxiety states in combat flying personnel. In: Wright DG, ed. *Observations on Combat Flying Personnel.* New York: Josiah Macy Jr Foundation; 1945: 13–18.

37. Jones FD. Experiences of a division psychiatrist in Vietnam. *Milit Med.* 1967;132:1003–1008.

38. Butts DW, Potts D. HQ TAC/SG Operations Desert Shield/Storm Environmental Health and Bioenvironmental Engineering Post-Deployment Workshop Report, 2–3 May 1991. Cited in Ferguson R, Operations Desert Shield/Storm: Air Force Medical Plans and Operations. 25 November 1991: 28–32. Available from the Air University Library, Maxwell AFB, Ala (Document #M-U 44093).

39. Marquez L. A general's reflections: Stress and combat. *Air Force J of Logistics.* 1986;10:22,26.

40. Dollard J. *Fear in Battle.* Westport, Conn: Greenwood Press; 1977.

41. Rachman S. Fear and courage: Some military aspects. *J R Army Med Corps.* 1982;128:100–104.

42. Keegen, J. *The Face of Battle.* New York: Penguin Books; 1978.

43. Hocking WC. *Morale and Its Enemies.* New Haven, Conn: Yale University Press; 1918.

44. Manning FJ, Ingraham LH. An investigation into the value of unit cohesion in peacetime. In: Belenky GL, ed. *Contemporary Studies in Combat Psychiatry.* Westport, Conn: Greenwood Press; 1987: 47–67.

45. Richardson FW. *Fighting Spirit.* New York: Crane, Russak; 1978.

46. Haslam DR. The military performance of soldiers in sustained operations. *Aviat Space Environ Med.* 1984;55:216–221.

47. Hoffman K. Medical concerns of the desert soldier: Establishing a model for comprehensive care in a war zone. *J US Army Med Dept.* 1992;Nov–Dec:19–27.

48. Blumenson M, Stokesbury JL. *Masters of the Art of Command.* Boston: Houghton Mifflin; 1975.

49. Menninger WC. *Psychiatry in a Troubled World.* New York: Macmillan; 1948.

50. Hess A. Personal Communication, 1983.

51. R. Levy, Psychologist, Chief of Israeli Defence Forces Mental Health Department, Personal Communication, 1984.

52. Glass AJ. Lessons learned. In: Glass AJ, ed. *Overseas Theaters.* Vol 2. In: *Neuropsychiatry in World War II.* Washington, DC: Office of The Surgeon General, US Army; 1973: 989–1027.

53. Salmon TW, War neurosis ("shell shock"). *Milit Surg.* 1917;41:674–693.

54. Datel WE, Johnson AW Jr. Psychotropic prescription medication in Vietnam. Available from Defense Technical Information Center, Alexandria, Va. 1978. No. ADA 097610.

55. Belenky GL, Tyner CF, Sodetz FJ. *Israeli Battle Shock Casualties: 1973 and 1982.* Washington, DC: Walter Reed Army Institute of Research; 1983. Report NP-83-4.

56. Enoch D, et al. Cited by: Belenky GL, Tyner CF, Sodetz FJ. *Israeli Battle Shock Casualties: 1973 and 1982.*. Washington, DC: Walter Reed Army Institute of Research; 1983. Report NP-83-4.

57. Ellsworth PD, Sinnott MW, Laedtke ME, McPhee SD. Utilization of occupational therapy in combat stress control during the Persian Gulf War. *Milit Med.* 1993;58:381–385.

58. Holsenbeck LS. "PSYCH-FORCE 90": The OM (Combat Stress) team in the Gulf. *J US Army Med Dept.*1992;3/4 (Mar–Apr):32–36.

59. Sosa, I. The Journal interviews—LTG Frank F. Ledford, Jr., Surgeon General, United States Army. *J US Army Med Dept.* 1992;3/4 (Mar/Apr):unpaginated.

60. Mitchell JT. When disaster strikes: The critical incident stress debriefing process. *J Emerg Med Svcs.*1983;8:36–39.

61. Shalev A, Ursano, RJ. Group debriefings following exposure to traumatic stress. *Proceedings of the Wartime Medical Services, Second International Conference.* Stockholm, Sweden: IFS Institute for Hospital Planning; 1990: 192–207.

62. Martin JA. Health issues: Lessons from Operation Desert Shield/Storm. *Proceedings of Psychology in the Department of Defense.* Thirteenth Symposium, 15–17 April. Colorado Springs, Colo: US Air Force Academy Department of Behavioral Sciences and Leadership; 1992: 221–225.

63. Garland FN. Combat stress control in the post-war theater: Mental health consultation during the redeployment phase of Operation Desert Storm. *Mil Med.* 1993;158:334–338.

64. Yerkes SA. The "Un-Comfort-able": Making sense of adaptation in a war zone. *Milit Med.* 1993;158:421–423.

65. Carter BS. The military physician and conservation of force. *Milit Med* 1993;158:374–375.

Chapter 9

U.S. NAVAL COMBAT PSYCHIATRY

JOHN MATECZUN, M.D., M.P.H., J.D.*

*Captain, Medical Corps, U.S. Navy; Chief of Staff, DoD TRICARE Managed Care Program, Region 1 Staff Office, Washington, D.C.; formerly Force Surgeon and Assistant Chief of Staff, Health Services Support, Headquarters, U.S. Marine Corps Forces Pacific, Camp H.M. Smith, Hawaii

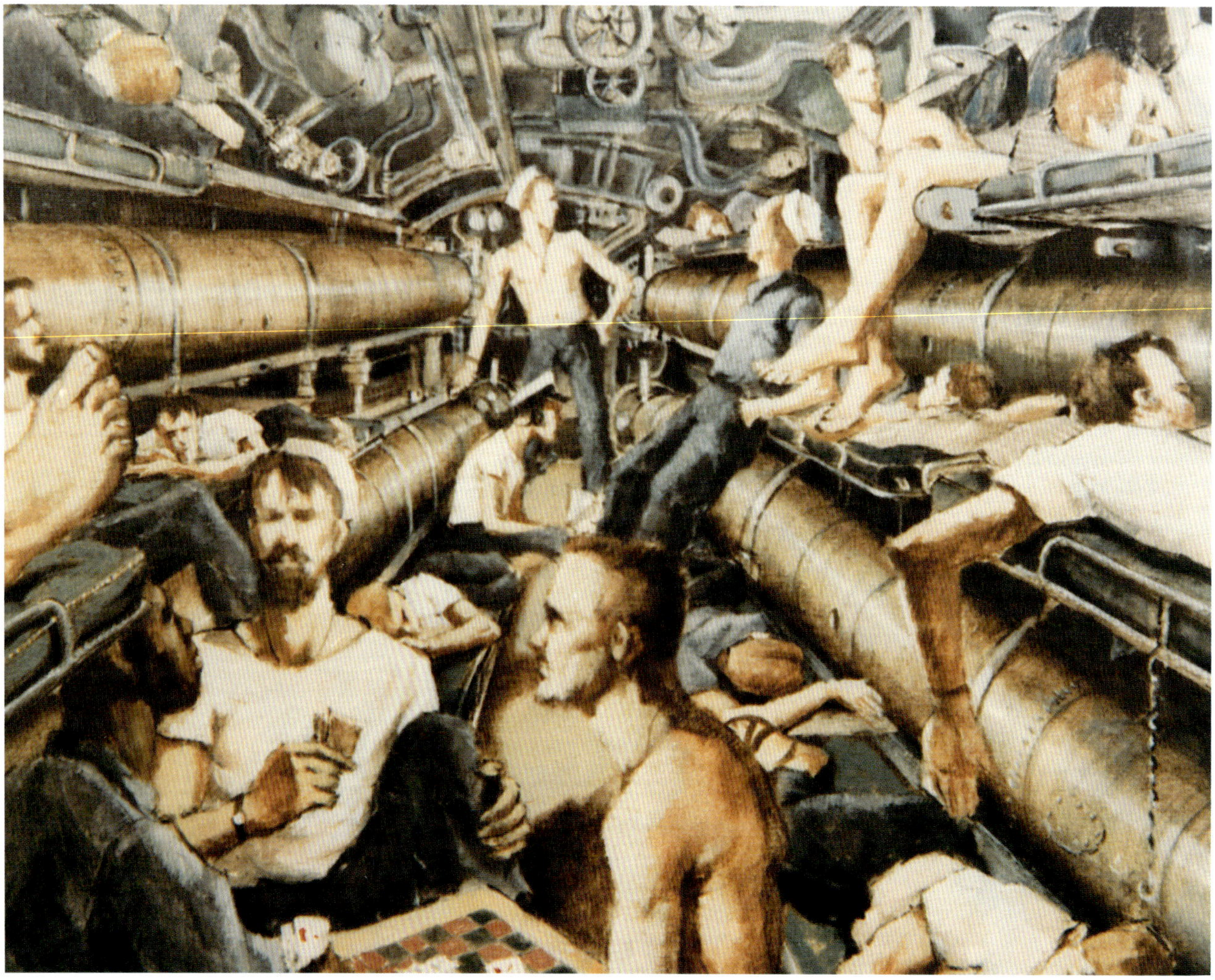

Paul Sample *Crew's Quarters Aboard U.S. Submarine, Pacific* 1943

Paul Sample was a war correspondent and artist for Life Magazine during World War II and spent time with a submarine crew on routine patrol in the Pacific. His painting depicts leisure time activity in the very cramped quarters of a submarine. Naval combat is extremely diversified due to the varying fighting components and missions of the U.S. Navy, however, all naval combat is similar in that most of it is characterized by periods of intense activity, followed by lulls, such as shown in this painting.

Art: Courtesy of US Center of Military History, Washington, DC.

INTRODUCTION

Naval Mission

Since its inception, the United States has been a typical maritime power looking to the oceans for trade, ideas, and culture; colonized from overseas; and threatened only by potential adversaries across the seas.

The United States reached the zenith of maritime power in the period immediately following World War II at which time it had the strongest armada of naval and merchant vessels ever assembled by any one nation. At that time, the U.S. Navy had complete superiority at sea with no opponent left capable of contesting use of the seas. Such sea control (the capability to assert one's own use of the seas and to deny that use to others) has been the fundamental role of the U.S. Navy.

During the period of the Cold War, the U.S. Navy's force structure and capabilities were oriented towards sea control and three other missions: (1) strategic deterrence, (2) naval presence, and (3) projection of power ashore. Deterrence was carried out by ballistic-missile submarines, a crucial part of the deterrent "triad" (Strategic Air Command [SAC] bombers and intercontinental ballistic missiles [ICBMs] were the other two). Presence was carried out by the use of naval forces below the level of hostility and ranged from informal ship visits to patrols just outside a nation's waters. The method for projecting power ashore was an outgrowth of U.S. expertise developed in the amphibious assaults of the island campaign in the Pacific during World War II and consisted of operations putting U.S. Marines on a beach or the use of naval air or surface forces to destroy targets ashore.

In September 1992 a new direction for U.S. Naval forces, called "... From the Sea," emerged. The national security strategy shifted from a focus on global threat to a focus on "regional" challenges. There was a concurrent emphasis on joint and combined operations. This resulted in a fundamental shift away from open-ocean war fighting *on* the sea towards joint operations conducted *from* the sea. The mission of the U.S. Navy during a regional conflict became controlling the ocean adjacent to the littoral battlefield, the ground from the shore to objectives, and the skies above both.

Naval Organization

Even before the United States had a Constitution, it had an organized navy. In 1775, the Continental Congress created a congressional oversight committee for the Continental Navy. On 10 November 1775, the Continental Marines were established. They celebrate their birthday annually on 10 November even though the present U.S. Marine Corps was established by an Act of Congress on 11 July 1798.

The Department of the Navy (DON) was formalized in 1798 and has been in evolution since that time. The Secretary of the Navy (SECNAV), a civilian, is in charge of DON. The Chief of Naval Operations (CNO) is the senior military officer of DON and commands the operating forces and shore establishments of the U.S. Navy. The Commandant of the Marine Corps (CMC) is responsible to SECNAV for Marine Corps matters. Both the CNO and the CMC are members of the Joint Chiefs of Staff. CMC is not part of the command structure of the CNO; there is, however, close cooperation between the two military heads who report to SECNAV. Both U.S. Navy officers and U.S. Marine Corps officers are considered U.S. *Naval* officers, although the two services have unique cultures and traditions.

The operating forces of the U.S. Navy are included in the fleets; Pacific Fleet includes the Third and Seventh Fleets, Atlantic Fleet the Second Fleet, and U.S. Naval Forces, Europe, the Sixth Fleet. The operating forces of the U.S. Marine Corps include the U.S. Marine Corps Forces Pacific which includes the I Marine Expeditionary Force (I MEF), and the III Marine Expeditionary Force (III MEF), and the U.S. Marine Corps Forces Atlantic, which includes the II Marine Expeditionary Force (II MEF).

There is a dual chain of command to the operating forces. There is an operational chain from the President through the Secretary of Defense to a Commander of a unified or specified command. In this chain of command the unified commanders pass orders to naval service component commanders such as the Commander in Chief, U.S. Pacific Fleet (CINCPACFLT) or the Commander in Chief, U.S. Atlantic Fleet (CINCLANTFLT). In August of 1992 Marine Corps service component commands were established and U.S. Marine Corps Forces Pacific (MARFORPAC) and U.S. Marine Corps Forces Atlantic (MARFORLANT) became Echelon II commands within their unified commands.

There is also an administrative chain of command through SECNAV and CNO or CMC to the operating forces. Within this dual chain the administrative chain of command is permanent while the operational chain of command is task oriented and can be restructured as necessary.

The U.S. Navy and U.S. Marine Corps together are responsible for developing and maintaining an effective amphibious warfare capability. This team is unique with mobility and versatility enabling it to fight multidimensionally on land and at sea as well as under the sea and in the air.

The naval environment is unique as well. Because of the historical isolation during long, harsh sea voyages command at sea has been filled with great responsibility. Perhaps in no other military organization is the effect of a commanding officer on morale so keenly felt.

> Naval medical officers noted variations in the incidence of neurosis in different ships in which they served. There was a great depth of meaning in the old naval term 'a happy ship,' implying a unit in which there was mutual trust and respect between officers and men, and dependent to a great extent on officers and senior raters who not only knew their jobs but who also had a sympathetic understanding of the men under them and could get the best out of them.[1(p647)]

Ships themselves are known to take on a personality and a life of their own to the crew.

> She was to become the ruler of my life, and the most beautiful and responsive creature I had ever known; a hard, exacting mistress, but loyal, generous, and courageous. All ships have souls, and all sailors know it, but it takes a while to learn to commune with one. It took me a long time for *Trigger* had to find her own soul too.[2(p11)]

Naval Medicine

Physician services for the Continental Navy were often contracted for by the ship's master and attached to the ship for a specific cruise. Most were surgeon's mates who had some medical training but who were relatively inexperienced. Some held medical degrees. In 1811 Congress established U.S. Navy hospitals and a U.S. Navy hospital fund. The fund was to be collected from U.S. Naval personnel, a small portion of whose pay would provide for the service. The first U.S. Naval hospital was built in Washington, D.C., about 1821. The oldest hospital building in service in the U.S. Navy is Building One at the Naval Hospital in Portsmouth, Virginia, which still houses the inpatient psychiatry services.

The Bureau of Medicine and Surgery (BUMED) was established in 1842. Dr. William P. Barton became the first Chief of the Bureau of Medicine and Surgery with a staff of four. In 1871 the Medical Corps was first mentioned in an Act of Congress which established it as a separate entity and as a staff corps of the U.S. Navy. U.S. Navy medical department personnel provide services to both the U.S. Navy and U.S. Marine Corps. The U.S. Marine Corps has no medical branch but does have U.S. Navy medical personnel assigned to U.S. Marine Corps units and under U.S. Marine Corps operational command.

Naval Psychiatry

There were few psychiatrists in the U.S. Navy, or for that matter in the country, until World War II. In 1940, the U.S. Navy had 10 Regular Navy psychiatrists doing clinical work and 7 in training; a total of about 25 medical officers performed neurology and psychiatry duties.

The neuropsychiatric branch at BUMED was established in 1942. Dr. Francis Braceland took charge of U.S. Navy Psychiatry in World War II, initially as a special assistant to the Surgeon General, and subsequently as the Head of the Neuropsychiatric Branch. The number of psychiatrists reached a maximum of 693 at the end of World War II. Out of the wartime training programs grew the current U.S. Navy psychiatry residency programs. By 1948 the number of psychiatrists on active duty had declined to 74 with 32 in training. That year the Surgeon General reported "personnel needs in Psychiatry are still critical and an active procurement program has been initiated."[3(p412)] (*"Ce plus le change...."*)

The Neuropsychiatry Branch at BUMED lasted some 35 years through several name and mission changes until 1977. A few years later a system of specialty advisors to the Surgeon General was put in place and the Specialty Advisor for Psychiatry (SAP) has been a focal point for U.S. Navy psychiatry since that time.

HISTORY OF MARITIME PSYCHIATRY

Ship differs from shore and the challenges of shipboard life make life different for sailors. Much of the following was adapted from the excellent review by Captain Rolf Steyn.[3]

The Vikings of the early middle ages were sea warriors who bequeathed the term 'berserk' for a peculiar battle frenzy by which they were seized (probably enhanced by mead—beer fermented from honey). In the early Renaissance, communities loaded their maladaptors, for a fee, on ships (the ship of fools) for transport to unknown destinations. Some modern parallels are occasionally carried out by judges who encourage maladaptors to go to sea instead of jail. "It is a popular delusion that the ne'er-do-well, the black sheep of the family, will be picked up and made a man of by the discipline of the military life."[4(p408)]

Sailors in the 16th through 19th centuries manned great fleets which conquered the world. Their crews are suspected of spreading syphilis that was a major cause of mental illness and other diseases which proved devastating to previously unexposed populations. Many showed the weakness, irritability, and depression associated with scurvy. Crews had general ill health so mental troubles alone did not stand out. The annual death rate in the British Navy was 1 in 8 in 1779.[3]

Sailors were known to consume large amounts of alcohol. Admiral Edward Vernon, known in the English fleet as "old grog" directed in 1770 the issue of a daily half-pint of rum mixed with a quart of water to sailors of the West Indies fleet. This was designed as a temperance measure to remedy abuses stemming from straight rum drinking. The mixture, which was also called "grog," won general acceptance in the British Navy as well as the American Navy which was patterned after it. Congress incorporated the rum ration in legislation in March of 1794. In 1806 whiskey was substituted as cheaper and more wholesome.[3]

In the 19th century about 80% of floggings in the U.S. Navy were administered for drunkenness and alcohol-related offenses. Flogging was abolished in 1850, possibly related to Dana's publication of *Two Years Before the Mast*. President Lincoln abolished the grog ration on 1 September 1862. In the 20th Century improvements in nutritional knowledge and food handling greatly improved the physical health of naval forces with concomitant mental health improvement.

During World War II psychiatric diagnoses in the U.S. Navy and U.S. Marine Corps were common with some 150,000 patients being admitted for psychiatric illness. Over 100,000 sailors and marines were separated for psychiatric disorders, constituting 34% of total medical separations. Not included in these numbers are 90,000 recruits who were discharged for mental reasons.[3]

Group therapy first became an accepted treatment modality during World War II, largely because of the large numbers of patients and paucity of therapists.

> Group therapy, born of necessity, was soon found to have other things to commend it. The individual undergoing treatment lost the feeling of uniqueness and of shame when he saw that other persons were suffering the same emotional distress as he himself was undergoing. There is no reason to believe that this type of therapy cannot be carried on in civilian life.[5]

Variability in diagnosis during World War II led to work towards a definite nosology with Captain George Raines contributing with Brigadier General William Menninger to a joint Armed Forces nomenclature and method of recording psychiatric conditions in 1949 which later led to the first American Psychiatric Association nomenclature, the Diagnostic and Statistical Manual (DSM).[6]

Literature on the subject of psychiatric casualties at sea is almost completely nonexistent. This is in part a problem with the collection of medical statistics in an environment where there may be few medical personnel, such as on a small ship. The loss of a ship may mean the loss of an entire crew so combat stress casualties cannot be ascertained. As a ship continues to function after a battle, it may be that many sailors who would otherwise have been identified as casualties are able to stay with their division until acute reactions have subsided. This may be particularly true if they were in close contact with shipmates and working within their division in which case only the most dysfunctional casualties would ever have been evacuated.

Ursano and Holloway[7] note that psychiatric combat casualties are a unique class of conditions defined by etiology (eg, combat), rather than by symptomatology and that the behavior and psychophysiological manifestations of the combat casualty are protean.

This author would argue that there is a "plasticity" in the presentation of psychiatric symptoms related to cultural or subcultural environments that exist in the military and the expectations that such cultures engender which determines a large part of the protean nature of such casualties. In the following sections some of the subcultures which make up the U.S. Naval culture will be explored.

NAVAL COMBAT ENVIRONMENTS

Submarine Warriors

History of Submariners

Submarines were born in 1620 when Cornelius van Drebbel, a Dutch physician, launched a wood vessel covered with greased leather in the River Thames. This ship was really little more than an oar-driven diving bell which was not capable of submersion and probably ran awash during its trip.

Although a submarine first saw action during the U.S. Civil War, submarine warfare came of age in World War I. The U-boat arm of the German Navy demonstrated what could be achieved in the interdiction of trade routes. They sank almost 6,000 ships, mostly defenseless, merchant vessels grossing a little over 11,000,000 tons and in so doing rendered it almost impossible for the Allies to continue the war. There were 13,333 noncombatant merchant seamen and passengers who died during these attacks.[8(p7)] U-boats also sank nine British and French battleships and 14 cruisers. A single German submarine U-9, in a brief engagement, destroyed three British cruisers, an event which had a profound effect on maritime strategy during the war.[8(p7)]

World War II saw submarine warfare continue in the same strategic role that had begun in the previous war. The tactical introduction of the wolf pack and the night surface attack decimated Allied convoys attempting to cross the North Atlantic. The Axis Powers sank almost 3,000 merchant ships with a tonnage approaching 15,000,000. German U-boats also sank two battleships, eight aircraft carriers and some 50 destroyers.[8(p228)] Only the development of the convoy system and depth charges allowed the United States to continue supporting the allies.

The Submarine Service of the U.S. Navy adopted U-boat tactics to the Pacific and sank more enemy warships than had the U-boats. They were also able to sink more than 1,100 Japanese merchant ships with a tonnage of almost 5,000,000.[8(p228)] The size of the Submarine Service was only 1.6% of the U.S. Navy's total strength yet they suffered a heavier proportion of casualties than any other branch of the U.S. Navy. In the Pacific theater, more than 3,500 submariners were killed[8(p154)] and there were many examples of extraordinary heroism. The trials of the submariner have been brought to popular attention through novelizations and motion pictures such as *Run Silent, Run Deep*[9] and *Das Boot*.[10]

Psychiatric Casualties

The hazards encountered by submariners can be seen as unique and extremely stressful.[11] During patrol allied submarines were "lone wolves" and subject to intense attack when sighted by enemy air and surface antisubmarine units. The depth charge was the primary antisubmarine weapon and the men could not help but wonder when the next bomb or depth charge would make a direct hit. All knew that submarines were being lost to enemy counterattacks.

While being hunted, they were unable to fight back and "ran silent" with all, except those necessary to control the ship, in their bunks. Those who were up and about removed their shoes. Talking and unnecessary noise was kept at a minimum for everyone. The interior became excessively hot and humid because of secured ventilation, air conditioning and refrigeration units. All of this resulted in enforced inactivity and helplessness during the trauma of exploding depth charges. Even when not being attacked there were the stressors of mines, shallow water operations, air-sea rescue operations, reconnaissance operations, and days of patrolling without enemy contacts.

During World War II there were no studies of U.S. psychiatric casualties occurring aboard submarines while on war patrols. A review after the war[11] noted that there were approximately 1,520 war patrols completed by U.S. submarines, of which 1,489 patrol reports were available for study. An attempt was made to extract from those reports instances of "psychiatric casualties." These were essentially those men who were unable to continue with their duties secondary to what was thought to be some psychiatric-related problem. The total number of cases so identified by the authors was 56. This would have been a rate of .00044 casualties per man-patrol. Estimating another way this would have equalled an "admission rate" of 2.2 per thousand men in the Submarine Service. These figures also suggest that the role of an evacuation syndrome was essentially unavailable in the submarine setting.

Case Study 1: Depth Psychiatry

That there were frequent stress reactions short of "breakdown" is illustrated in extracts from the reports. General manifestations of responses to the conditions were described as "excessive physical weariness with headaches, lethargy and sometimes heat exhaustion." Also noted were frequent somatic symptoms.[11(p608)]

For the first two hours we were in a mighty tough spot....The predicament of the ship was a fact fully recognized by the older and more experienced men. As the youngsters folded up, the others took over....The most startling effect was the apathy engendered by the combination of heat, pressure, physical effort and mental stress....

[W]ithin a period of 24 hours following the depth charge attack, several cases of mild gastric disturbance consisting of light nausea and cramp-like feeling developed; rapid recovery without treatment followed...[A]pproximately one-half the crew complained of headaches, slight diarrhea and acidosis for three or four days following the depth charge attack.[11(p608)]

Comment: The World War II casualty figures may be incomplete and underestimated but still present an enviable record. The authors believed the low casualty rate could be ascribed to factors of selection (every man was a volunteer), training, morale, pre- and post-patrol physical examinations to detect men in need of rest and rehabilitation, rest camps and rotation (after two consecutive patrols), and confidence in submarines, officers, and shipmates.

Behnke[12] relates the comments of a former sub commander on this unique environment:

> To operate a complicated mechanism like a submarine, each individual must be free to volunteer information, to discuss when discussion is profitable, to exercise initiative and discretion in carrying out his duties; yet in other situations he must obey instantly, without question and without thought as to his safety. The recognition of the subtle changes in a situation that determine where and when and in what circumstances these two widely different attitudes are demanded is what makes a good submarine man.[12(p724)]

The British Submarine Service during the war reported a 40/1,000/y rate of psychiatric casualties.[13(p343)] Disparities between countries in reported rates have been hypothesized to be a tendency of commanding officers of U.S. submarines to transfer or separate a crewman for other than psychiatric reasons.[14] Other labels such as chronic maladapter, upper respiratory disease, or environmentally unadaptable may have diluted U.S. psychiatric attrition statistics. This same author relates a "resistance to psychiatry in the submarine service" and exemplifies the resistance with a quotation from Admiral Rickover in speaking before a Subcommittee of the Committee on Appropriations:

> I view with horror the day the Navy is induced to place psychiatrists on board our nuclear submarines. We are doing very well without them because the men don't know they have problems. But once a psychiatrist is assigned, they will learn that they have lots of problems.[14(p583)]

The advent of the nuclear submarine ushered in a new gamut of missions and stressors for submariners. Submerged missions increased dramatically in length from 3 days during World War II to 60 to 90 days.

There have been few published reports of the incidence of psychiatric attrition during submerged missions. During 360 Fleet Ballistic Missile Submarine missions in the period from 1963 to 1967 there were some 192 psychiatric cases. This would be an incidence of about 4/1,000/y.[15(p1)] The proportion of crew members referred for psychiatric evaluation has been reported variously as 20/1,000/y in 1963,[14(p579)] 42/1,000/y in 1967,[16(p548)] and 50/1,000/y in 1968.[17(p26)]

One important problem is how many psychiatric cases require a medical evacuation at sea. Such evacuation may cause an entire mission to abort at relatively high strategic or tactical cost. Biersner[18] reported that from 1963 to 1967 there were no cases of mental disorders severe enough among submariners to require a medical evacuation at sea. From 1968 to 1973 there were only three cases severe enough to require evacuation at sea.[18]

U.S. submarine psychiatry began late in World War II with the assignment of a psychiatrist to the Submarine Base, New London, Connecticut. The psychiatrist was called upon to (*a*) decide whether volunteers with marginal aptitude test scores possessed compensatory traits predictive of later success and (*b*) apply therapeutic techniques to the few submariners who had met aptitudinal requirements but showed acutely maladjustive behavior during protracted war patrols.[14]

The Bureau of Medicine and Surgery made a decision shortly after the war to focus upon the selection of men with maximum adjustment potential rather than "salvaging" maladjustive crew members.[14] The use of empirically validated aptitude measures coupled with personality tests came into use. Those whose tests showed marginal aptitude or personality patterns were interviewed by the psychiatrist.

Insights gained from this process as to the dynamics underlying the decision to volunteer for the submarine service have shown that apart from increased pay for hazardous duty the most important motives are social in nature, that is, a person values highly the status coincident with the acquisition of the "dolphin" showing submarine qualification and acceptance in the "submariner culture." Also strong affiliative motives to establish highly affective-toned friendship relationships within the submarine crews are important aspects of the motivation.

Pathological motives such as counterphobic behavior demonstrated by volunteering in reaction to claustrophobic or other phobic impulses were postulated to be operating in some volunteers. Phobics who were not screened out initially were presumably eliminated during the training by failure to withstand 50 pounds per square inch pressure while in a recompression chamber and by failure to make an unassisted buoyant ascent to the surface of the training tank from an escape hatch in 50 feet of water.

Some volunteers appeared primarily interested in the possibility of fleeing domestic responsibilities. Obviously eliminated were those with "incipient psychotic trends." A "fair number" of antisocial characters were noted to slip through the intake "selection sieve" and later turn up as disciplinary problems usually resulting in elimination early in their submariner careers.

Medical Support for Submariners

Navy medical officers who volunteer are usually trained in undersea/diving medicine at the Naval Undersea Medical Institute (NUMI). The curriculum there contains a psychiatric syllabus. They are often assigned to a submarine squadron after training. The medical department aboard an individual ship is usually staffed by an independent duty corpsman.

Chapter 15 of the U.S. Navy *Manual of the Medical Department*[19] lists physical standards for selection for various duties. There is a specific section on screening volunteers for submarine service.

One current initiative in aiding the medical department aboard the submarine is a computerbased patient management system for isolated environments, called MEDIC. Four diagnostic modules are under development including abdominal pain, chest pain, psychiatric disorders, and dental problems.[20] The psychiatric module consists of a brief structured interview, with verbatim questions developed for use by medical corpsmen. Specific diagnosis and treatment suggestions were developed for each interview profile which make suggestions that are within the corpsman's trained skill levels. A computer-aided instruction component was also developed to provide the corpsman with initial training in some general emergency treatment principles.[21]

There is currently no psychiatrist assigned to the operational assets of the submarine service nor are there any assigned to the Naval Undersea Medical Research Laboratory. Psychiatric support to the operational forces is most often obtained through the psychiatrist assigned to the Naval Hospital near the home port. This contact is usually initiated by the independent duty corpsman or squadron doctor.

Merchant Mariners

Mission and Stressors

Although the Merchant Marine is not one of the uniformed services, it has great importance to any war effort. As any medical planner knows, "lift" is crucial to success and there is never enough "lift." Merchant ships have been called upon to deliver goods to invasion harbors and beachheads in the past and will be in the future.

The stressors imposed on crews of these shipping vessels during World War II by submarine warfare and bombing attacks were extreme. Sailors of the Merchant Marine were subjected to torpedo attack, bombs, mines, machine gun and shell fire, severe body wounds, long blacked-out voyages through submarine infested waters, and occasionally being cast adrift as a survivor of a ship sinking on the open sea with resultant exposure to cold, hunger, thirst, and exhaustion.[22]

Psychiatric Casualties

During the first year of American participation in World War II, more fatal casualties were recorded among American merchant seamen than among men in the combined armed services. The incidence of combat or "convoy" fatigue among survivors of torpedoed and bombed merchant ships was not clearly studied, for several reasons including seamen's unions, but it created such a serious drain on marine manpower that in January, 1943, the Surgeon General of the U.S. Public Health Service called a conference of leading military and civilian psychiatrists to discuss ways and means of preventing and treating this condition among merchant mariners.[23]

A program was formulated to be operated jointly by the U.S. Public Health Service, the War Shipping Administration, and the United Seamen's Service. The program centered on the need for convalescent homes set up at or near convenient ports of call along the Atlantic, Pacific, and Gulf coasts.

In attempting to evaluate statistics regarding Merchant Marine psychiatric casualties, as in attempting to evaluate all maritime psychiatric casualty statistics, there is one group of seamen with psychiatric disturbances who can never be studied or effectively counted—those whose acute reactions were so incapacitating as to prevent their making any effective effort to escape catastrophe. Many of these men were surely acute psychiatric casualties and just as surely buried at sea with their ships.

> [M]en showed blind confusion and panic, childlike states of terror, self dramatization, rage or stupor-like trance states. Some men clung to a red hot rail or buried their heads between their arms. Some leaped blindly into a blazing sea when there was no burning oil in some other direction or ran about with dangerous implements in their hands, striking blindly.[22(p401)]

The personality characteristics of Merchant Mariners have not been studied in any systematic way. Some impressions of the personalities of the survivors of torpedoing were that a majority had gone to sea early in life before age 18, and many of these had run away from home or gone in spite of parental objections. The sea as a vocation had only rarely been a tradition in the family.

Motivation for becoming Merchant Mariners seemed to derive from a strong, inarticulate need to get away from home and to get away from the disciplined social authority and regimentation of life on land. Several such sailors contrasted the regimentation and discipline of previous U.S. Army or U.S. Navy service with the freedom and informality of their life in the Merchant Marines. A large percentage had severed all contact with members of their families. Few were married.[22] Typical of the ships was the *Troubador*, a 5,808-ton tramp,

> a rusting steamer that had been scuttled by her truculent crew at Jacksonville when America entered the war, and now boasted a seventeen-nation crew of ex-convicts and the rakings of the U.S. deportation camps. While at anchor in New York harbour...the ship's ammunition magazine had been deliberately flooded 'by a person or persons unknown'. Eight Colt automatic pistols had been issued to the naval Armed Guard officers shortly before sailing: 'This was considered necessary in view of the conduct of the ship's crew.'...[I]n Iceland on 20 June, twenty members of *Troubador's* crew mutinied, having been told their ship was now bound for Russia. They sent a deputation up to their Master, the Norwegian Captain George Salvesen, and told him they refused to take the ship any farther. The Reykjavik port director ordered Salvesen to use his ship's Armed Guard to quell the mutiny. The American naval gunners rounded up the seamen and barred a dozen of them into a stinking hold in the forepeak area, in 'very crowded, foul conditions.' The seamen held out in there under armed guard for fifty hours and then surrendered. 'We didn't have any more appreciable trouble until the convoy reached Russia,' reported the Armed Guard officer, Ensign Howard E. Carraway, to his superiors.[24(p100)]

These sailors had an extraordinarily large pay, ($500 per month plus danger money) in defense of which it was pointed out that they were not maintained by a shipping company while on shore, did not receive a pension and had a high rate of casualties.[22]

Psychiatric casualties were not limited to unlicensed seamen. An increasing number of skippers, mates, and chief and assistant engineers were noted to be worn out nervously and physically as the war went on.

Chronic Sequelae

Margolin et al[22] studied 40 survivors of torpedoing who were continuing at sea. They found that 75% had persisting emotional reactions with 25% being categorized as severe or sufficient to make it impossible or inadvisable for the seaman to return to sea. Alcoholism or previous psychiatric history predisposed to severe and incapacitating reactions, both during and after any emergency. There was a suggestion that persons aged between 45 and 60 were especially susceptible to severe reactions. The incidence of severe reactions was particularly high among seamen from tankers; and there appeared to be little correlation between where a seaman was at the moment of attack and severity of the after effects.

Margolin et al noted that among seamen who were ambulatory and returning to sea there were surprisingly few psychosomatic disturbances. This was in sharp contrast to what had been reported among seamen who had been hospitalized. It was the authors' impression that the seaman in whom a severe psychosomatic disturbance developed had few qualms about "giving in" to the illness and accepting hospital care and to some extent felt that it was a legitimate reason for not going back to sea.

Askevold[25] studied Norwegians who had been sailors in the Merchant Navy during World War II. Of 35,000 who had sailed for the allied forces, 6,000 were killed by bombs or torpedoes. Most survivors had lived years during the war with a real fear of death. In examining a sample of these sailors some 30 years later, he found striking similarities between those with concentration camp syndrome (known as the "KZ" syndrome) and ex-war sailors.

He compared a matched group who were not war sailors for four symptom groupings: (1) asthenic symptoms (fatigue, irritability, lack of initiative, and emotional incontinence); (2) autonomic and somatic symptoms (dizziness, sweating attacks, dyspepsia, impotence, and somatic pain); (3) anxiety symptoms (nightmares, restlessness, disturbed sleep, and isolation); and (4) organic brain symptoms (impaired memory and concentration difficulties). The mean symptom load for ex-war sailors was 13.6 as opposed to 3.5 for the comparison group. There was also a higher relative frequency for each of the single symptoms in the war sailor group and a very similar relative frequency within each symptom group for both war sailors and concentration camp survivors.

It was evident to Askevold that of those still at work, the symptom load was high enough to warrant war pensions and their work capacity was marginal. He coined the term "War Sailor Syndrome" to describe the chronic effect on these sailors.

Treatment

Psychiatric treatment for American Merchant Marines during World War II was at rest centers established by the War Shipping Administration and the United Seamen's Service. A major part of the treatment at rest centers was conducted in groups. For the Merchant Marine at sea there were not only no psychiatrists, but no doctors at all. Treatment of the individual casualty as conducted at the rest centers was noted to be a "thin battle line tactic" given the resources available; "defense in depth" through the addition of preventive measures was recommended.[26] The preventive measures were to be through change of those factors external to the seaman and also by group education and treatment.

It was soon evident that many factors influenced the condition apart from actual battle experience. Factors external to the sailor himself included the presence or absence of adequate medical equipment, safety devices, food, convoy protection, sanitation, hours of work, and factors influencing morale including relations between officers and men and worries about personal affairs. Encouragement was given to captains to not fill a sick bay with paint and rope so that sailors might take a new interest in health because they had a clean sick bay used as a headquarters for sick call; for appetizing preparation of food and getting men to eat a balanced diet; for ensuring that the medicine chest contained supplies necessary to meet shipboard emergencies; and for adding pharmacists' mates (the World War II U.S. Navy rating equivalent to today's U.S. Navy corpsman) to the crews of merchant ships.

A second category of preventive focus was a recommendation to prepare sailors so that men would not be overwhelmed by fear. The idea was that when a man is taught to anticipate danger and to understand his reactions and how to deal with them, he is better prepared to cope with the danger and to meet the next experience. Seamen could be helped to understand ways of preventing and relieving their own nervous tension; commanders could be given training in the appreciation of the elements in a satisfactory psychological state and the methods by which it could be attained. Preconditioning by simulation was also considered.[26]

One preventive measure not discussed in relation to the Merchant Marine was screening, presumably because of the necessity of having crews to man ships and possibly because of the difficulties in instituting such a process for personnel who were not members of the armed forces. There is little to indicate that any preventive measures were instituted prior to the end of the war.

It is instructive to contrast these Merchant Marine casualties with those of the submarine service. They obviously differ as to the rates of casualties, and possibly to the chronicity of sequelae after wartime. Screening, personality type, motivation, and stressors appear to have been different.

It is possible to project that for merchant vessels subject to sinking in the future, there will be near universal acute symptomatology among the crew with some 25% developing symptomatology that will preclude going to sea under similar circumstances. With increasing exposure to possible death even higher numbers of incapacitated could be expected.

Surface Warriors

History

Surface warfare takes place among those ships and missions which are conducted on the surface of the seas. This is the traditional sphere of naval warfare. Prior to World War I the ships of the line of naval battle *were* the U.S. Navy and always had been psychologically. Older officers counseled:

"Stay in the big ships"; "work your way to the top in a big ship; that's where the real Navy is"; "don't waste your time in little ones"...."There always has been a mystique involving the self-contained little world of a large ship, combatting the far greater elements of wind and sky and the huge, trackless, sometimes malevolent sea. But not only did a big ship become a living, sentient being to those who served her, she was also a community of kindred souls, of men who thought alike and worshipped at the same shrine....Perfection of the ship becomes its own objective. Battle has nothing to do with it, although one always talks of battle, battle is harmful to the ship, and should be avoided if possible, though not so one can notice. To sailors of the old time, enlisted men and officers, their ship was their home and their religion."[27(pp422–423)]

After World War I most of the U.S. Navy's officers and men went to sea and most of the sailors were in either the "destroyer Navy" or the "battleship Navy." The "cult" of the battleship existed not just in the U.S. Navy but in the Royal Navy as well. Naval strategic thinking was described by Henry L. Stimson, President Taft's Secretary of War, as "the peculiar psychology of the Navy Department, which frequently seemed to retire from the realm of logic into a dim religious world in which Neptune was 'god,' Mahan his prophet, and the U.S. Navy the only true church."[28(p421)]

Destroyer sailors were of a different breed from the rest of the U.S. Navy. Their ships were faster and rolled more than the squat battleships and cruisers. And so the men rolled too, walking with a swagger on land, boasting of storms in which destroyers keeled so far that they took sea water in their stacks. Battleship sailors looked down at the ocean; destroyer sailors said they looked at the ocean in the eye. Destroyers were tactically used like bullets. A man aboard a destroyer in battle knew that he and his ship were expendable. That kind of knowledge gave a man a certain bravado.[29]

Psychiatric Casualties

Sailors see their ships as having a spirit and fatigue can affect not just individuals but entire crews and ships. In training prior to World War II, American crews were kept in condition watches (Condition 2 was one half of the crew in battle stations and Condition 1 was regular action stations) for days on end. Thus, they may have been up for General Quarters during morning and evening twilight and required to do ship's maintenance during working hours so they were in general deprived of rest. The British Navy had derisively said of the U.S. Navy that in the event of war with the United States they would keep their fleet safely in harbor for a couple of weeks, after which America would collapse from the unremitting strain of indiscriminate and unrealistic readiness at all times.

Case Study 2: Crew Exhaustion

On the night of 8–9 August [during World War II] a combined U.S. and Australian force of five fine cruisers was caught totally by surprise in the vicinity of Savo Island, off Guadalcanal, by a superior Japanese force. All hands in the American squadron, including those on watch, were exhausted from days on end without rest. Although technically in alert status, they were so tired as to be literally asleep on their feet....More than a thousand allied sailors were killed in the five cruisers....The Commanders of the ships involved were castigated for their individual lack of alertness. Yet...the fault lay in unrealistic demands for readiness at all times, with the inevitable result that although awake and on their stations, their crews were not truly alert....Commanders in the Pacific began to think more about the human demands being made on their eagerly willing crews.[27(p462)]

Comment: This example shows the validity of the concept of sleep and rest discipline in U.S. Navy combatants as has been shown in land troops.

Case Study 3: Stress in the Falklands

The scenario reported by the Royal Navy psychiatrist, who was with the Naval expedition during the 1982 Battle of the Falklands, can be seen as typical of U.S. Naval surface operations. As their task force approached the Falkland Sound:

"We were unsure before entry as to whether or not it had been mined. The rather ironical story is told of a frigate identified as an 'Irish Minesweeper' which was tasked to go in ahead of *Canberra* to determine whether or not any mines were present—apparently we would know whether or not this was the case if she blew up—fortunately she did not and we and the rest of the fleet had safe passage....All seemed calm and peaceful until about two hours after the assault began when suddenly the Argentinian aircraft appeared. From then on there was a succession of air strikes and we grew in our admiration of the skill and daring of the Argentinian pilots....We functioned as the major medical facility during the course of that day taking casualties direct from the ships which came under fire, including those that were sunk. Again, I found myself in a situation of dealing with a group of survivors from the aftersection of *Ardent* and during the course of the day, was in a position to support the nursing and medical staff who were busily engaged in their duties treating the wounded....The battle plan had to be changed rapidly when it became apparent how effective the Argentinian Air Force was. A mad scramble followed to put ashore the major medical logistics and at that stage it had not been allowed for the task force psychiatrist to deploy ashore on such short notice. So I found myself going out to sea with our survivors and wounded and there followed an intensive period of active intervention...dealing with the bereavement associated with the wounded and the survivors of the ships....The emotional needs of survivors can be dealt with under the following headings: There was initial relief of escape almost immediately followed through by the anxiety about the threat of further attack and fear of further trauma. Mixed with this was the anger not only directed at the enemy but at the units to which they belonged and the designers of the ships were found wanting in certain areas. There was the grief at the loss of companions and of course the ever familiar guilt at survival, this especially so amongst the single men who constantly queried why it was they who had survived and their companions, married men with young families, had been killed....After the fall of Stanley...we began our triumphant journey home. The fascinating feature of this journey for me was the amount of working-through people were doing all around me. The three weeks allowed a tremendous opportunity for reliving the battle scenes, making formal contact with critical figures and providing a setting for significant emotional catharsis....I am convinced this is one of the reasons why we have seen so few psychiatric casualties from amongst the Royal Marines in association with the Falklands crisis."[30(pp143–145)]

Comment: O'Connell[31] estimates that among the survivors of those ships that were lost there have been some 20 to 25 psychiatric casualties who developed chronic post-traumatic stress disorder. This from a crew of 230 to 250 would be a rate of 10% which would be in accord with the experience in the U.S. Navy after such incidents as suffered by the USS *Stark*.

Medical Organization

The medical department aboard a larger ship is headed by a medical corps officer who is designated as the ship's medical officer. That officer is responsible for maintaining the health of personnel, making medical inspections, and advising the commanding officer (CO) on hygiene and sanitation conditions. When no medical officer is assigned, hospital corps (enlisted) personnel run the department, but are assigned to the Operations Department for military and administrative functions. Currently, within the surface warfare community, it would be medical department personnel that would address psychiatric needs. It is thus crucial that the medical officer be trained in the principles of combat psychiatry, particularly of the importance of the support of the crew, including the medical officer, in assisting return to duty after acute reactions. The following case, one the author had the opportunity to review for the Board for Correction of Naval Records, is illustrative.

Case Study 4: A Missed Therapeutic Opportunity

The case was of a Lieutenant Junior Grade who had been aboard a destroyer during World War II throughout the Pacific campaign. He had generally performed well. During the battle of Leyte Gulf he was involved in escorting a convoy to Mindinao. During that escort, lasting some 3 days, several ships were hit by Kamikazi pilots. As they burned, the ships "disintegrated" causing the crew to realize that they were carrying ammunition. After some 72 hours of being on General Quarters, he was on the Bridge and had given his life jacket to a seaman who had forgotten his. This was in spite of the fact that he could not swim. A Kamikazi plane came directly at the Bridge. As it hit, he "found himself" going over the side of the ship, falling about 30 to 40 ft into the water. Fortunately he was not pulled through the ship's screws. He struggled in the water; and, just as he felt that he was going to drown, he was picked up by a small U.S. Army vessel. Subsequently, he was put into an U.S. Army hospital. A few days later his ship's medical officer came to the hospital. The officer hoped that the medical officer would come to talk to him; but he saw the medical officer glance at him with a "look of disgust" on his face. After that he developed increasing symptoms of combat fatigue and was never able to be returned to duty. Had the ship's medical officer been able to speak with him, he might have been able to return to ship's crew and not have become a chronic casualty.

Comment: A ship's medical department may have the option of brief admission to the sick bay for such "fatigue" cases. The ship's medical officer, as a member of the ward room, can communicate with other division heads and their chiefs to ensure that an individual sailor knows that he is needed back in the division. The medical officer aboard ship should not forget that he has more than just military authority in the eyes of the crew. The medical officer is also seen in the professional role of healer, one who cares, and mediator.

Naval Air Warriors and Carrier Battle Groups

History

As Beach[27] reports, new technology changed the conditions of battle at sea prior to World War II but U.S. Naval leaders were slow to change tactics:

> As the range of guns increased in battleships, spotting of the rounds became progressively more uncertain. This led to spotting by aircraft and each battleship was outfitted with small planes for that purpose. The idea of a ship devoted solely to handling wheeled aircraft on a long flat deck received little encouragement....Only aviators asked newly pertinent questions; what use was a battle line with weapons of 20 mile range if aircraft carriers could send weapons with greater accuracy 10 times as far? Or the antagonistic, ambitiously cynical one; why was a 20th century Navy still enam-

> ored of the 18th century line of battle? Did the psychological appeal of a line of great grey ships with glorious heritage from the days of sail, somehow affect the strategic thinking of the Fleet Commanders of the 1930s?[27(p446)]

During the later part of World War II battleships became relegated to a primarily shore bombardment role in support of amphibious landings. They were never in battle with similar ships, but became fleet escorts for the great number of aircraft carriers that were turned out after Pearl Harbor.

> The Queen of Battles of the Pacific war, lifting the crown from the battleship (which had never worn it in combat), was the aircraft carrier. In contrast to the long peacetime gestation of the battleship, the carrier leaped almost at birth into relentless combat. For years, Naval aviators had stressed the superiority of 3-dimensional combat over 2-dimensional strategy tied to the surface of the sea. Suddenly, war at sea in three dimensions took over from war in two dimensions and sea/air power dominated Naval tactics. Surprise became the basic ingredient of Naval combat. The slow inexorable confrontation of all available forces...was no longer germane to the ability to carry out a Naval mission quickly. To strike where needed and with stunning speed was the new way of war on the sea. In this outlook, Naval aviators and submariners were joined, for both groups had shared the 3-dimensional concept from the beginning....A plane came from nowhere in only minutes, did heavy damage, and disappeared....All the old ways of bringing ships into battle were outmoded; they now fought from places of invisibility, over the horizon, widely dispersed, or submerged.[27(p446–449)]

Psychiatric Casualties

The USS *Wasp*, an aircraft carrier, was torpedoed on the 15th of September 1943, while escorting reinforcements to Guadalcanal. The senior medical officer aboard was Commander Bart W. Hogan, a psychiatrist later to become the Surgeon General of the Navy. He surveyed survivors[32] and discovered the following reactions on board after the torpedo attack: 38% felt calm; 33% felt excited, nervous, tense, or shocked; 9% were very fearful; and 20% had no report. Twelve hours after the torpedo struck, 27% felt relief and thankfulness; 25% felt concern for shipmates; 46% were fearful, apprehensive, or nervous; and 2% had no report. Three weeks later, 46% expressed themselves as being normal and regretful; 37% stated that they were nervous, apprehensive, even jumpy; 80% were unaware of any physical change; 33% stated they were unaware of any emotional change; and 43% had a slight emotional change.[32]

Hogan related that during the service of the USS *Wasp* it had brought reinforcements to Malta and was then escorting reinforcements to Guadalcanal at the time that it was sunk. In all that time, only two minor neuropsychiatric cases developed. He called for tribute to the 18-, 19- and 20-year-old men who were winning the war and remaining stable. The crew on board at that time numbered over 1,080 with approximately 180 officers.

During a combat deployment to Vietnam, 121 U.S. Navy aviators were studied aboard an aircraft carrier.[33] Their illness patterns revealed a total of 116 illnesses amongst the 121 officers with 26% of the officers developing 73% of the illnesses. Five percent were responsible for 22% of the illnesses. Out of the 116 illnesses, 8 were noted to be neuropsychiatric in origin with the bulk of those being related to insomnia and one case each of hyperventilation, dizziness, and neuritis.[33] The illness rate was comparable to the overall rates for the enlisted crews of several other ships which had been previously studied. Illness rates were elevated during the combat periods compared to the in port periods with an exception being a sudden operational shift which occurred to another country.

A modern aircraft carrier with an airwing embarked accommodates about 570 officers and 5,720 enlisted men. From her decks operate nearly 100 aircraft—fighter, attack, electronic countermeasures, electronic warfare, reconnaisance planes, and helicopters.

When a carrier battle group left port in the 1980s with an airwing, escort and support vessels with amphibious landing capability from elements of the Fleet Marine Force, as many as 20,000 men accompanied it. It was usually during the first month out that most psychiatric morbidity occurred. Routinely, some 100 cases required psychiatric evaluation during a cruise.[34]

One psychiatrist[35] also designated as a U.S. Naval flight surgeon, who had been the senior medical officer aboard an aircraft carrier, contrasted two cruises that carrier made. One cruise was made to the Arabian Sea during a period in which hostilities might have started. That cruise lasted some 156 days. Prior to the cruise, in order to assist families, arrangements had been made to ensure that allotments or direct mail deposits for pay checks were taken care of because mail service could not be expected to be regular. Crews and families were informed that sailors would probably not be available for assistance and that emergency leave would be difficult. This cruise occurred during a period that a "reason to be there" was perceived by the crew. The carrier left the line briefly and returned for another 158 days. During a total of 256 days on line, there was one psychiatric medical evacuation. This was of a person who had fraudulently enlisted and had been getting Stelazine, an antipsychotic medication, by mail from a civilian general practitioner.

This was contrasted with another cruise lasting almost 200 days when the perceived purpose of the mission was not as clear. During that cruise, crew members felt continuing responsibility for what was going on at home and were "worried" quite often during that cruise. The average number of medical evacuations was some 2 to 3 per month.[35]

Medical Organization

The medical department aboard an aircraft carrier includes a senior medical officer who is also a U.S. Naval flight surgeon as well as additional general medical officers. There would usually be a general surgeon aboard during a cruise. An aircraft carrier has extensive sick bay capability including surgery and intensive care. When aircraft squadrons are aboard they usually bring their own flight surgeon and medical section aboard with them.

It is through the medical department that psychiatric services must generally be provided. These generally consist of those services the medical staff feels comfortable providing. Flight surgeons have an extensive psychiatric component to their training syllabus. For those diagnostic and treatment services beyond the expertise of the medical department, consultation is sought at the Naval Hospital, either in port or home port, or medical evacuation is initiated.

Marines: Amphibious Warriors

History and Doctrine

It is generally held as an axiom that the entire purpose of navies and seapower is to influence land. The most direct form of such influence is through the landing of troops. Historically, landings were rarely attempted in which troops were opposed during the landing and had to fight their way ashore.

The history of modern amphibious warfare began in Gallipoli in 1915 with disasterous results. In the United States, General John A. Lejeune was Commandant of the Marine Corps from 1920 to 1929. He was searching for a unique role for the U.S. Marine Corps and extensively studied the landing at Gallipoli. He ignored the maxim that developed after the operation which was that the advantage in such an operation was always with the defender. It was his opinion that the operation had failed for the more mundane reason of incompetence of execution. He set upon making the amphibious assault landing a U.S. Marine Corps specialty. Subsequent history in the Pacific campaign during World War II proved his foresight.

The culture and doctrine of the U.S. Marine Corps differ in general from those of the U.S. Army. The U.S. Marines more often believe that an all-out assault at the beginning of a battle will ultimately result in success with fewer casualties than the alternative which provides for a slower assault waiting for an overwhelming force to be brought to bear.

Psychiatric Casualties

Case Studies 5 and 6 relate different aspects of U.S. Marine operations in the pivotal battle of Guadalcanal. Case Study 5, contributed by Colonel Joe Fagan, discusses factors that protected U.S. Marines from becoming incapacitated from combat stress. Case Study 6 discusses some of the severe stressors faced by U.S. Marines and their psychiatric sequelae reported in the press at that time as "Guadalcanal nerves."

Case Study 5: The Protective Effect of Unit Morale

Generally speaking, the success or failure of military operations is more dependent upon group activity than on individual effort. Esprit de corps is often considered synonymous with group morale. It is high when individuals feel that they belong to a unit, place unit interests above their own, and are willing to strive for the goals of the unit.

"Creature comforts" (such as good food and post exchange [PX] availability)[36] are less essential for group success than unit identification and cohesion. Because individual morale is more volatile than unit morale, the unit, by providing a stable sense of group, can dampen and compensate individual morale fluctuations over a period of time.

To illustrate this concept, the Battle of Guadalcanal is studied because the success at Guadalcanal was related to the staying power of the U.S. Marines more than anything else. This staying power is a manifestation of leadership and morale.

The Battle of Guadalcanal was pivotal. Churchill concluded that Guadalcanal was one of those battles that, won or lost, would change the entire course of events in the world. Admiral Nagona, Chief of the Japanese Naval

General Staff, and General Kawabe, Deputy Chief of the Japanese Army General Staff, reported during an interview after the war that Guadalcanal was the turning point for them in the Pacific in World War II, marking their shift from the offense to the defense.

The amphibious invasion of Guadalcanal, 7 August 1942, was, fortunately, essentially unopposed. However, from that day on life was very difficult for the U.S. Marines. When the Japanese realized what had happened, their air and naval attack on the U.S. Navy task force supporting the U.S. Marines was so intense that the naval supply ships were forced to withdraw on 9 August 1942 without unloading a substantial amount of supplies needed by the U.S. Marines. Supplies present in insufficient quantities included barbed wire, radio batteries, medical supplies, and camouflage materials.[37,38] The Japanese air and naval forces subsequently enjoyed control of the sea and air around Guadalcanal. Consequently, the Japanese were able to land reinforcements and supplies as needed while the U.S. Marines received only a trickle of supplies and reinforcements.

A comparison of combat power of the U.S. Marines and the Japanese forces is difficult to quantify as accurate records are lacking and the situation was dynamic over time. Initially, the U.S. Marines landed 10,000 to 11,000 troops while the Japanese had a force on the island of 2,000 to 5,000 soldiers and laborers. The Japanese, upon realizing that the U.S. forces were confronting them in their drive to Australia, began to exercise their air and naval superiority to concentrate their forces to drive the U.S. Marines from the island. The Japanese were able to field a force of 26,000 to 29,000 troops which they maintained at that level despite substantial losses throughout the bulk of the campaign. The U.S. Marines gradually built up their forces so that by mid-October they had about 23,000 troops and by the time the 1st Marine Division was relieved in early December the level had reached about 45,000.[39]

The Japanese from August through November utilized about 37,000 men and sustained losses estimated between 20,000 and 28,000 troops. The U.S. Marines, utilizing fewer troops experienced substantially fewer losses. The 1st Marine Division during the 4 months of combat sustained about 2,736 losses. For a better comparison with the Japanese figures, the U.S. forces in all sustained about 6,000 losses.[37,39] The ratio of Japanese losses to U.S. losses is about 4 to 1. However, numerical comparisons do not tell the story of Guadalcanal.

Although the Japanese for most of the campaign enjoyed air and naval superiority in terms of combat power, the U.S. Marine pilots fought with the same will and determination as did the ground troops. Their force never exceeded 60 planes,[37] but their impact upon the Japanese planes and ships was substantial. The fighting on the island itself could but be described as a series of protracted small unit operations savagely fought in conjunction with a perimeter defense of Henderson Field. While each engagement was significant, a survey of the overall campaign will indicate those factors that allowed the Marines to defeat the Japanese.

Every man was critical with each unit deployed on the perimeter in an overextended front since there were no replacements or reserves. As the area of the perimeter was small, no spot could serve as a respite from the attacks, shellings, and bombings.[40] Henderson Field and the nearby hospital were constant targets and thus provided no greater safety than the front lines. When limited reinforcements did arrive on 17 September 1942, they permitted slight relief although they served to thicken the thinnest ranks and to permit the battle weary U.S. Marines to launch counterattacks as well as to maintain their perimeter defense. While the U.S. Marines were winning the battle, they were increasingly incapacitated by attrition, fatigue, and disease. The Japanese in a sense held the U.S. Marines in a constant state of siege.

Two weeks after the amphibious landing, the U.S. Marines turned back the first major Japanese offensive at the Tenura River. In mid-September, the Japanese again marshalled their forces although they were stopped at the Battle of the Ridge. A defeat for the U.S. Marines would have been devastating and was prevented by only the narrowest of margins. Near the end of October, the U.S. Marines held against the most furious of the Japanese attacks at the Matonikau River. Fighting these battles over and over sapped the strength and vitality of the men who were already suffering from malnourishment, fatigue, malaria, dysentery, and a host of other tropical maladies. However, they continued to fight and to fight well. From this point on, the tide of the battle swung toward the U.S. Marines although the actual fighting continued for some time. In lieu of tactical or logistical advantages, the U.S. Marines had utilized will, determination, and leadership.

The Guadalcanal Campaign can be examined within the framework of what many consider nine essentials for "individual" morale during combat.

1. *Good food.* The U.S. Marines landed, having lost weight while on board the transport ships. After landing, and largely because of the withdrawal of their supply ships, they again had a substandard diet offered only twice a day from 12 August 1942 on. Although their diet did fluctuate considerably over the course of the campaign, typically it was cold and consisted of combinations of beans, hash, rice, spam, and so forth, both for breakfast and supper. Captured enemy food supplies were the difference between a starvation diet and one above that point during the early phases of the operation.[38,41]
2. *Special rations and PX.* There were none.
3. *Physical comfort.* Prior to landing, the U.S. Marines had been confined in crowded troop transports for a minimum of 29 days.[37] Upon landing, they were met by a tropical climate with high temperatures and humidity. A shortage of water complicated their situation. Sleep and rest were effectively curtailed by Japanese float planes nicknamed "Louie the Louse" who dropped flares and "Washing Machine Charlie" who dropped impact fused bombs almost nightly. In addition, Japanese naval

forces shelled Henderson Field quite regularly. The Japanese were able to fulfill their purpose of denying the U.S. Marines any rest and to wear them down mentally and physically. Because of the nightly attacks the men generally slept in their foxholes which often had about 6 inches of water in them. Improving your foxhole was said to be the universal recreation on Guadalcanal.[37]

4. *Good health.* Malaria, dengue fever, and numerous fungal infections were endemic in Guadalcanal. In addition, an epidemic of dysentery required about a month to control. Estimates were that at any given time 20% of the U.S. Marines were incapacitated by the dysentery. As the epidemic was brought under control, severe fungal infections, aggravated by the men being generally without proper footgear and standing in water, severely limited the mobility of the men on an ongoing basis. The main health problem, however, was malaria.[38] It reached epidemic proportions shortly after the acute dysentery was brought under control. During the campaign about 7,000 U.S. Marines were hospitalized with malaria. Because of the manpower shortage, the criteria for hospitalization was a fever greater than 103 degrees Fahrenheit or about 4 degrees above normal. These conditions, of course, coexisted with malnutrition, fatigue, and battle wounds.[37]
5. *Clean and adequate clothing.* The military uniforms didn't stand up to the tropical environment and resupply was limited and sporadic. The men often fought barefoot with fatigue cutoffs. In mid-September they did receive about 20,000 pairs of boots so that the men wouldn't have to fight barefoot.[37] Bathing and washing facilities were quite limited.
6. *Dependable policy of rotation.* Rotation was not possible as every man was needed for the defensive positions.
7. *Combat relief.* The 1st Marine division experienced essentially constant combat from 7 August 1942 until relieved by U.S. Army forces 7 December 1942, when the worst of the battle was finished. Initially the U.S. Marines believed that they would have air and naval support and be relieved by U.S. Army troops in about 3 weeks and that they would be returning to New Zealand. When this did not occur, most despaired ever leaving Guadalcanal.
8. *Regular delivery of mail.* This certainly improved morale within the 1st Marine Division. Data are not available as to how often the mail was delivered. The first delivery of mail did occur 1 September 1942.[42] As one officer observed, each man seemed as happy as if he'd been given $100 at the mere thought of getting mail. Some said that mail should have priority over food.[42] The delivery of mail seems to have been a positive factor for morale. Presumably the mail was delivered on a sporadic basis but details are not available.
9. *Information.* This may have had the greatest impact in terms of improving morale. General Vandegrift used a billboard near the center of the perimeter to display a graphic representation of the perimeter defense of Henderson Field so that each man, and each unit, could visualize their part as well as the part played by others in their mission. They also knew that if they could hold Henderson Field the pilots would be able to provide some air protection for them. Consequently, there was a lot of pride in their "air corps." On the same billboard next to the baseball scores was a running account of the number of Japanese aircraft "their" pilots had shot down. Another example of the impact of command information on the men was their reaction when notified that Admiral Halsey was assuming command of the South Pacific Naval Forces. One officer reported that, "I'll never forget it—one minute we were too limp with malaria to crawl out of our foxholes—the next minute we were running around shouting like kids" upon hearing the news.[37] The men believed that he would send them assistance.

This appraisal of the nine elements finds that the U.S. Marines were substantially lacking in terms of good health, physical comfort, good food, PX and special rations, clean and adequate clothing, a dependable policy of rotation, and combat relief. They did possess adequate command information and benefitted greatly from delivery of mail. However, they were lacking substantially in seven of the nine essentials and yet maintained good morale.

The morale possessed by the 1st Marine Division was not expressed by happy or contented troops with the usual attention to dress, appearance, or protocol but by grim-faced U.S. Marines doing a very difficult and dangerous job but doing it well. As General Vandegrift observed, "They look like a bunch of Gypsies, but they'll fight because they've got it in here (tapping his chest)."[42] Possibly group morale in combat is best observed by noting how well the men carry out their mission.

Another perspective on morale in combat is gained by looking at the psychiatric casualty rate, sometimes used as a measure of morale.[43] A report by medical officers treating the wounded evacuated throughout the Pacific indicated that the 1st Marine Division on Guadalcanal had about the lowest rate of psychiatric casualties of any of the Pacific campaigns.[40] In general the Pacific theater had a higher ratio of psychiatric to wounded casualties than the European theater[43] with the exception of Guadalcanal. Perhaps more important, however, was the fact that even the nonpsychiatric casualties showed emotional reactions of a severity which would often have been considered incapacitating in other campaigns but not at Guadalcanal. Most of the men who were evacuated for psychiatric reasons had already been treated and returned to duty several times on Guadalcanal before it was necessary for them to he evacuated from the island.[40] This suggests excellent treatment of psychiatric casualties in combat, the need to conserve manpower wherever possible, and the feeling of the men that they didn't want to leave their fellow soldiers behind. This group cohesion prompted the men to continue under conditions that at other times, other places, would have resulted in evacuation. As previously noted, group morale is considered high when individuals feel like they belong to a unit, place unit interests above their own, and are willing to strive for the goals of the unit. This was seen on Guadalcanal where group morale sustained the U.S. Marines when individual morale, often dependent on "creature comforts," was lacking. The unit was able to keep the individuals going.

General Vandegrift took some other steps which also contributed to unit morale. He set up his personal tent and command post alongside his men and by sharing their hardships and risks he obtained immunity from criticism in regard to the hardships they endured. Their frustration was displaced to the "swab jockeys" who "hauled ass" and the "dog faces" who didn't relieve them. This allowed the men to avoid losing faith in their "own" chain of command.

General Vandegrift also recognized early on that his men in response to the "siege" conditions under which they were operating were "more than ready for a fight...they were aching for one."[37] This was because enforced passivity in the face of an ever present threat will lead to hopelessness if not countered by measures that allow for the channeling of the frustration into action. Thus General Vandegrift decided on a series of limited attacks on the Japanese to reduce the tension and to keep the Japanese off-balance.[41] The strategy worked quite well, in part because the experience of success against the Japanese helped to destroy the myth of the invincible Japanese soldier. On other occasions, General Vandegrift, in addition to genuine battlefield decorations, used mock awards ceremonies to break the misery and fear with humor using captured Japanese medals.[42]

In addition, from General Vandegrift on down the chain of command, the officers were expected to and did lead by example when necessary. There were examples of colonels and their staffs taking the "point" on river crossings when the men seemed to be holding back—ominously eyeing the forbidding dark woods. The colonels' effort was enough to resolve the situation. They also were able to convey to the men that they [the men] were capable of carrying out their mission despite the difficulties and that the officers fully expected them to do so in the tradition of U.S. Marines. The men were able to put forth second and third efforts that were essential for their defense to hold.

Comment: This study illustrates that morale in combat does not depend upon "creature comforts" but rather upon the quality of leadership and the cohesiveness of the small unit. In essence, it is not the hardships that the men endure that destroys morale, but rather that the unit itself can help them endure.

Case Study 6: Guadalcanal Nerves

The World War II amphibious campaign in which American doctrine would be tested began on 7 August 1942 when the amphibious assault on Guadalcanal began the island-hopping strategy which would mark the campaign in the Pacific. The assault was covered extensively by the press and brought the terrible realities of such warfare home to the American public for the first time. The landing was not opposed, so was not an assault landing in the sense of a frontal assault against a determined opposition. The stressors of the campaign were, however, unique and resulted in psychiatric sequelae labeled in the press as "Guadalcanal nerves."[23]

"Fear of all kinds entered the picture. Most men experienced fear as they approached the beach. Some tell you of their fear of being afraid and exhilaration as soon as they went into actual combat. But new attacks, new bomb near hits would relight fear—and all this was sure to take some toll. As the weeks passed, hope left most of these men—hope of winning the battle, hope of being aided or rescued. They were alone on the island and their expected relief did not come. They had no way of knowing why it did not arrive. Soon they were sure that none of them would get off the island—they were expendable, doomed. Soon this helpless hopelessness overwhelmed them and contributed in no small part to their final collapse."[43(pp94–95)]

Comment: Other factors in psychiatric breakdown included gross sleep deprivation from Japanese activities at night, weight loss as high as 45 pounds, rain, heat, insects, dysentery, malaria, and an exposure lasting months. Ultimately the result of exhaustion, fear, malnutrition, and disease in this jungle combat environment took a physical and mental toll. Numbers of psychiatric casualties evacuated are not uniformly recorded. One observer noted that aboard one ship which evacuated casualties 48 of 350 total casualties were psychiatric.[44] From his experiences in treating those casualties, he concluded that "By and large men were fighting to get home" rather than for some more abstract reason; that "Every unit should have an experienced Sergeant or Lieutenant with it"; that "Men should go into battle with a unit—not alone"; and that you should "Keep the feebleminded out of the jungle," recalling that when men with a mental age of 12 were sent into the jungle with their units they were more prone to "crack" and "then others around them would crack." This worry presages current concern about "contagion" of stress casualties in a unit.

Those psychiatric casualties evacuated to the United States from Guadalcanal seemed remarkably uniform to observers after their arrival. They suffered from

> headaches, lowered thresholds to sharp noises, periods of amnesia, of panic, sensory somatic complaints, marked muscular hypertonicity, tremors generalized or limited, functional palsies....Many arrived with cotton stuffed in their ears, and on the returning transport many of them required physical restraint if there was test firing....[T]hree weeks

> after combat, they had, according to their own statements, improved immensely....The fear that they would be thought 'yellow' was universal....We found one of our first duties to these newly arrived patients was to endeavor to relieve them of this thought of cowardice.[43(p94)]

One enlisted U.S. Marine rifleman lived to reflect and has written of his experiences in the amphibious assaults on Peleliu and Okinawa.

> As a Marine infantryman I was no better than average, I served through two major campaigns...I was wounded twice, cited for bravery once, and two times I was too frightened to do the job to which I was assigned...I know...that every man has his limit; but just as some men are taller and heavier, so some men can go longer and take more. Bravery is a fickle thing. It runs in some kind of cycle: it comes and it goes. One day a man is a lion in the fight: the next day a mouse...I have seen men who were brave when their feet were dry, cowards when they were wet; brave when they were warm, cowards when they were cold; brave when they were full, cowards when they were hungry; brave as long as they got their sleep, but cowards when they didn't. We often contrast bravery and cowardice. We think there is nothing between the two, but most men who know war know that there is.[45(pix,x)]

In preparing to board an AMTRAC (amphibious transport craft) prior to his first landing he recalled that,

> I caught fear from the men around me. I was deeply shamed for them and for myself. Later I got used to fear. It was like a scar or a limp that I had to learn to live with. I learned always to control what showed in my face, my hands and my voice. And I let it rage on inside. I never lost my fear, but I lost my fear of fear, because it became such a familiar thing.[45(p4)]

In commenting on motivation and loyalties during combat he notes that,

> In a war, loyalties shrink down past country and family to one or two men who will be with you. They become more important than anyone else in the world, more precious than father and mother, sister and brother, wife and girl. Only a few lonely men go though a war without buddies.[45(p9)]

Some months later Davis was assigned with an officer with whom he had many hours to talk and discovered the healing value of such recollection and retelling.

> [H]e was the one who finally cured me of my nerves. He had been in many campaigns, and he liked to tell 'sea stories.' He got me telling stories of what happened on Peleliu; and somehow, in the telling, the campaign didn't seem so bad. I began to sleep nights again.[45(p9)]

After the battle of Leyte Gulf had been won by the U.S. in late 1944, it had likely become clear to Japan that the ultimate objective of the U.S. operations in the Pacific would be an actual invasion of mainland Japan. Iwo Jima was anticipated to be a halfway station to provide fighter escort and emergency refueling for air raids of the Japanese home islands.

One of Japan's most capable generals was put in charge of the defense of Iwo Jima. As a result, the amphibious landing was one of the most heavily contested and deadliest operations in history. Of 23,000 Japanese troops who opposed the landing all but 200 died. The 60,000 Marines suffered 5,931 dead and 17,372 wounded.[39]

The Fifth Marine Division had a total of 2,779 killed in action. There were 1,285 wounded who needed evacuation. There were 590 hospital cases of combat fatigue, 369 of which were evacuated and 221 returned to duty. That number was closely approximated by the number of sick (nonbattle injury) of which 329 were evacuated and 252 returned to duty. Cases requiring evacuation for either combat fatigue or wounds would total 1,654 of which 22% would have been combat fatigue.[39]

Psychiatric Casualties in Medical Personnel

One group not often thought of in planning for battle fatigue casualties is the medical personnel. On Iwo Jima, 195 corpsmen were killed and another 529 were wounded. Seven doctors were also killed and 12 wounded.[46]

A battalion at that time consisted of some 900 U.S. Marines and the medical section had a battalion surgeon, an assistant battalion surgeon, a chief corpsman, 48 corpsmen and 16 assigned litter bearers. Litter bearers were thought to have the shortest life expectancy during amphibious operations as they had to stand upright to bear litters.

Case Study 7: Doctors in Distress

Dr. James Vedder was the battalion surgeon for the Third Battalion, 27th Marines with the Fifth Marine Division.[47] He described some physicians who became psychiatric casualties at Iwo Jima:

As he moved forward, he encountered another group of medics providing care and asked about one of the other doctors, who responded in a low monotone from from directly behind, "Here I am Jim. I'm doing all right."...He wheeled around to face Dr. Webber, who was standing stiffly upright, his face a frozen mask and his blank stare fixed on the horizon. Dr. Vedder continues, "We moved out into the open country, and I noted that Webber had not moved or spoken. His hands were still jammed into his pockets, and his immobile face was pointed in the direction of the western horizon."

The next day, D-Day +2, litter bearers brought Dr. Webber who had been with the First Battalion, 27th Marines to Dr. Vedder's aid station. After the litter bearers had deposited his large-boned, well-muscled body, a careful survey by Vedder discovered no recognizable wounds but all his muscles were contracted and his eyes were rolled upwards so that only the white sclera were visible. It was impossible to rotate him in any direction. As he lay there, breathing deeply at a normal rate with a ruddy color of good health on both cheeks, Vedder noted that "his bladder was functioning properly" as a large area in the crotch of his pants was soaked with urine. The accompanying medic noted that there had been no injury: "He just stiffened out like a plank during the night." Vedder wondered whether Webber could be feigning these unusual symptoms in order to get evacuated. To test this possibility, he gave him a jab in the thigh with the sharp point of a mosquito forceps. Webber uttered a loud grunt, his back arched up off the litter, but soon he settled back on the litter with a sigh, groaned and his bladder contracted.

After evacuating Dr. Webber, Dr. Vedder wondered what had caused the collapse:

"Physically he was stronger than most of us. But emotionally, he was far from strong. For weeks he had been living in a state of anxiety and terror that mounted daily as we neared the shores of Iwo Jima. Perhaps he had become a casualty long before he set foot on the black sands of this bloody island, with this paralysis merely the final stage."

The next morning, the Battalion Surgeon from the Third Battalion, 26th Marines wandered into Dr. Vedder's aid station in a state of acute agitation. Vedder commented:

"Between spells of sobbing, choking, and trembling, he managed to blurt out his unbearable problems. His unit had suffered heavy casualties when they had traversed our shell torn road the afternoon before. Their present aid station was located a few hundred yards to the northwest. They were working in open country without any suggestion of concealment. His men were being picked off at all too frequent intervals. His turn was sure to come soon. He just couldn't take it any more. He had felt like running off and hiding many times in the last 72 hours, but duty had forced him to stay on with his men. Now he did not care what happened....It was obvious that he was emotionally unfit to continue to function as a doctor at least for the time being. His evacuation tag was labeled 'combat fatigue.' Without further ado, he was loaded on a passing truck with two Marines who had also 'cracked up.'

"About a half hour after that evacuation, the Assistant Battalion Surgeon of the Third Battalion, 26th Marines "drifted into our aid station with the remnants of his medical section. Until the present, he had been an eager young physician willing to cope with the vagaries of military life. Now he appeared quite discouraged and despondent. Losing nearly half his men in the past 24 hours had been a severe blow. The recent collapse of his battalion surgeon was more than he could handle. He came to us for both help and companionship....He said 'Jim, I am all alone out there. Can I tie in with you until replacements arrive?' Several hours later, they were again functioning as a medical military team."

Dr. Vedder had to balance evacuation and other requirements in the case of a corpsman who had been sent up as a replacement.

"When I finally returned to my foxhole, I found De Wolfe still huddled up on his litter nervously gnawing on a 'K' ration biscuit. He presented a sad picture of total dejection. It seemed unlikely that he would ever become an asset to our medical section. My impulse at that moment was to sign him out as a combat fatigue and send him to the rear...but second thoughts ruled out this simple solution and the morale of the whole group had to be considered. After all, De Wolfe had yet to serve any front line duty. Many of his comrades, who were just as frightened as he, were functioning well under adverse conditions. If De Wolfe were sent back now, how many others would elect to follow the same course? So De Wolfe had to go back to H Company."

While going through the cemetery, after the campaign was over, Dr. Vedder chanced upon a grave marked with the name De Wolfe. He recalled how hard he had worked to persuade De Wolfe to overlook his fears. He knew that in his last days he had been an asset to the medical section serving his fellow men and felt certain that his mother and family would have been proud of him.

"A feeling of acute depression engulfed me as I walked out of the cemetery. I wondered if the price paid was really worth it. As I slowly headed back towards my jeep, one of the frequently used war slogans came to mind. 'Our Marines were willingly laying down their lives for their country'. This statement was sheer nonsense for the overwhelming majority of the men felt that they would be spared, and that it would be the next guy that would get killed or wounded. They had no intention of laying down their lives for their country or anything else. Each man believed he would be one of the lucky ones to return home. Those that lost or never did have this feeling of invulnerability would sooner or later crack up."[47(pp198,199)]

Comment: The psychological toll of combat will also be paid by medical personnel. These vignettes are particularly illustrative of that principle in the context of an amphibious assault against a motivated enemy.

During the Persian Gulf War reported psychiatric casualties were low in U.S. Marine Corps units. A classic amphibious assault did not take place although the threat of one riveted Iraqi attention.

The 2d Marine Division psychiatrist was located forward with the division headquarters and saw 25 referrals. He was able to return 22 of them to duty at the front. The 1st Marine Division Psychiatrist was able to personally educate over 7,000 personnel about combat stress and its management before the war started.[48]

Once again, reason to not forget about medical department personnel in planning for casualties was seen—particularly mental health personnel. One division psychiatrist developed disabling post-traumatic stress disorder on the first anniversary of the ground war. Interestingly, half of the mental health officers assigned to U.S. Marine Corps units in the first few months of the operation were returned to the continental United States before the ground war began—including one who was deployed while on antidepressant medication.

Medical Organization and Planning

Medical assets within Marine Corps Forces include organic support for all combat and combat-support organizations of battalion/squadron size or larger. At the battalion level each Infantry Battalion has organic medical assets that consist of two medical officers and 65 hospital corpsmen during combat. The Battalion Surgeon is a special staff officer. Within the battalion, a medical team of 11 corpsmen is assigned to operate with each rifle company in combat. The division medical section consists of a division surgeon, an administrative officer, an environmental health officer, and a psychiatrist. There are at present no specifically delineated duties for the psychiatrist who acts as an advisor and assistant to the division surgeon.

The division surgeon performs general duties under the cognizance of the G-4 (Assistant Chief of Staff [Logistics]) with respect to medical matters. Responsibilities include planning and supervising treatment and evacuation. The division psychiatrist must advise the division surgeon in these matters as they relate to psychiatric casualties.

Corresponding to the division surgeon are the wing surgeon for the Marine Air Wing and the group surgeon for the Fleet Services Support Group. Within the Fleet Service Support Group there is a medical battalion designed to provide second echelon (Echelon 2) support.

A medical estimate is prepared by the landing force surgeon and his staff and is intended to be a logical comparison of the medical requirements of each course of action. Casualty estimates are the doctrinal responsibility of the G-1 (Assistant Chief of Staff [Personnel]). Without this estimate, including numbers of psychiatric casualties, planning will be inadequate. The planner should be aware of the possibility of such casualties and outline courses of action with the division psychiatrist.

There must be close cooperation between the landing force surgeon and the amphibious task force surgeon on D-Day of an operation. Units will go ashore with their organic medical support. Handling of combat fatigue or combat stress reactions by personnel organic to the combat units going ashore would be optimal. Once ashore, evacuations rearward will usually be to a battalion aid station after triage by corpsmen working at the company level. Further to the rear, as time goes on, will be a beach evacuation station or Echelon 2 collecting and clearing company. These are points where combat fatigue or combat stress casualties can be pooled. The logistics of amphibious operations are such that it must be remembered that evacuation may bypass a lower echelon and end up at a much higher echelon—possibly at sea.

Those ships taking part in an amphibious operation have medical treatment capability as well. Amphibious assault ships include the LHA (landing ship, helicopter, assault) which resembles an aircraft carrier and is capable of transporting approximately 1,900 troops with the vehicles required to land them. They are normally designated as primary casualty receiving and treatment ships (PCRTS) in an amphibious operation. They have the largest medical capability of any ship currently in commission with medical spaces including two major and two minor operating rooms, 60 hospital beds, including an intensive care area and 225 to 230 overflow beds. It is possible for the LHA to be augmented with support personnel and the potential of receiving psychiatric casualties on these ships could be considered during the planning phase.

An LPH (landing ship, platform, helicopter) is designed to transport a battalion landing team utilizing vertical assault capability. They can carry about 900 to 1,000 troops and the medical spaces are limited to about 90 beds. They are not practical for use as primary casualty receiving treatment ships (PCRTS) although it is possible to use them in this capacity by using troop spaces as operating rooms and wards. They can be used as secondary casualty receiving treatment ships (SCRTS) and might be considered for psychiatric casualties. The medical department would require augmentation or training for such treatment.

Other ships [known as "L" class ships for their "landing ship" designator letters] have more limited medical capability such as Dock Landing Ships (LSD), Amphibious Cargo Ships (LKA), Tank Landing Ships (LST), and Amphibious Command Ships (LCC).

Currently there is no specific U.S. Navy doctrine that details the handling of combat stress reaction or psychiatric casualties. Such casualties will only be considered if included in the medical mission statement.

During the Persian Gulf War, The Medical Officer of the Marine Corps, Rear Admiral Dick Ridenour, himself a psychiatrist, requested that the author consult with the U.S. Marine Corps forces in theater on the handling of combat stress casualties as there were conflicting reports on requirements coming from different sources in theater.

There were several organizational problems encountered. One of the foremost was a senior staff surgeon who reported that he did not believe in the concept of stress casualties and did not like the fact that additional resources had been sent into theater to handle them despite his not requesting them. The second was fragmentation of command and control for medical services such that a "system" that would have to cross unit and echelon of care boundaries was next to impossible to coordinate because of a third problem, which was lack of doctrine.

Those additional mental health assets sent into the theater through the intervention of Rear Admiral Ridenour were nevertheless in place in four combat stress centers arrayed across the front at the beginning of the ground war. The four centers were under separate commands and had markedly differing philosophies for treatment based on preferences of the senior mental health officer assigned. Each had the capacity to handle 45 patients.

There was also difficulty coordinating requirements for treatment with the U.S. Navy who controlled the echelon 3 Fleet Hospital assets. Thus, mental health officers at each unit were essentially deciding what treatment mission they would perform without coordination. Despite these problems the tremendous dedication and talent of the U.S. Naval mental health personnel assigned, and sometimes their ingenuity in working around the organizational problems, resulted in successful performance of the mission. An interesting sidelight is that each psychiatrist involved in the Persian Gulf War was furnished drafts of five chapters of this volume, delineating combat psychiatry principles, by their respective surgeon general psychiatry consultants.

CARE OF CASUALTIES

History of Hospital Ship Operations

Spain appears to have been the first of modern nations to utilize the tactical advantages of hospital ships sailing with their fleet during the Armada. The British began using hospital ships sometime after an experience in 1626 when many men became sick and were distributed to the whole fleet, two to each ship, by which means, "the sickness was increased to such a degree that were scarce hands enough to carry the fleet home." The French toward the end of the 17th Century recommended that 100-bed hospital ships, devoted exclusively to the care of the sick and disabled be attached to the French Fleet in proportion of one hospital ship to every 10 ships of the line.

A real history of the modern hospital ship begins about the middle of the 19th Century when, during the Crimean War in 1854, England employed a fleet of transports to convey home the sick and wounded. In some 22 months over 100,000 patients were transferred home.

There is no record of the existence of hospital ships in the U.S. Navy prior to the outbreak of the Civil War when extensive use was made of hospital ships by the Federal forces operating on the Mississippi River. Also isolation ships made from former river barges were in use for smallpox patients.

The U.S. Navy's first hospital ship was the *Red Rover*, which was a side-wheeler that Union forces had captured from the Confederacy and converted to a hospital ship. The U.S. Navy's first volunteer nurses served aboard the *Red Rover*. Hospital ships were also used in the Spanish-American War and World War I. At the end of World War II, there were 12 hospital ships in the U.S. Navy. During the Vietnam conflict, two hospital ships, the USS *Repose* and the USS *Sanctuary*, were used offshore.

Lieutenant Commander Strange was aboard the USS *Repose* in 1966 off the coast of Vietnam.[49] The *Repose* had 500 beds, 48 of which constituted the psychiatric unit. The staff consisted of one psychiatrist, one psychiatric nurse, and nine hospital corpsmen. It was an open unlocked unit; patients were allowed freedom of movement aboard the ship commensurate with their degree of illness and responsibility. Patient census fluctuated greatly between 12 and 35. Stays ranged from overnight to 60 days or more.[49]

Mean length of inpatient care was 13.5 days. During that 7 months period, the *Repose* steamed in a scheduled pattern and received patients sent from major hospitals ashore at which time it functioned as a third echelon of treatment. Frequently, however, the ship furnished direct combat support with casualties being evacuated directly from medical units in the field with no previous specialty evaluation, placing the *Repose* in the role of second-echelon treatment.[49]

This fluctuation of echelons of care, depending on how a patient is evacuated, can certainly be expected in future operations. The availability of any medical support towards which helicopter or small craft evacuation is occurring can certainly bring casualties immediately to the hospital ship. During Lieutenant Commander Strange's tour, 143 psychiatric patients were seen with 54% referred to the ship by psychiatrists and 46% arriving aboard ship with no initial psychiatric contact elsewhere. Out of the patients, 67% were classified as character and behavior disorders, 20% psychoneurotic, and 13% as psychotic.[49(p37)]

The U.S. Navy today has two hospital ships, USNS *Mercy* and USNS *Comfort*. They are designed as 1,000-bed medical treatment facilities and have a psychiatrist assigned as a member of the medical treatment facility. During the Persian Gulf War each had a psychiatric ward prepared that could have handled 50 to 100 patients.

Rear Admiral H. James T. Sears, a psychiatrist, was assigned to the USS *Repose* early in his military career. He still recalls the formative influence of that tour on his decision to stay in the U.S. Navy.[50] He remembered the psychiatrist was often used as a triage officer when necessary. He also recalled the tremendous stress experienced by the crew of the hospital ship and the necessity of remembering to "care for the caregivers."

Rear Admiral Frances T. Shea, former head of the U.S. Navy Nurse Corps, served a tour as the Operating Room supervisor aboard the *Repose*.[51] She recalled that when adjusting to the initial shock of caring for casualties, people are not prepared for the catastrophic casualties that will come to the operating room. When her tour was up and she returned stateside, she felt guilty—that she didn't do enough, didn't care enough, that she left her shipmates and patients behind. She realized after returning to hospital work that she still couldn't talk to patients, particularly if she knew that they might die. That feeling went on for years compounding her guilt.

She found that the role of the nurse as comforter, consoler, and sympathetic listener heightened the stress she had already been experiencing. For her, understanding and admitting that she had been under great stress was therapeutic. She now relates that she has no difficulty visiting patients and can talk openly about experiences that were painful.[51]

In planning for future hospital ship operations, the tremendous stress of caring for casualties in a 1,000-bed medical facility should be considered and staff psychiatric support should be added to the mission. Some of this same emotional toll will be borne by psychiatrists. Perhaps it would be best that no psychiatrist be assigned in echelon 3 facilities without other mental health support.

Psychiatric Care of the Combat Injured

The combat wounded have psychiatric needs that must be addressed.[52] When someone is injured, their sense of personal invulnerability has been breached and they may become extremely reliant upon medical personnel for reassurance. Such reassurance can be of immense aid to those who have sustained minor injuries and it is essential for those who have major injuries. It is noteworthy that casualties may become anxious at each step of the evacuation chain. Many feel that the personnel where they are have kept them alive and they do not want to leave.

Traditionally, medical staff gather historical information about the injury itself but do not talk to the patients about their emotional reaction to the injury. Medical staff have their own need for denial about the carnage that they see and may rationalize not discussing injuries with patients on the basis that "They have suffered enough; they do not need to talk about it any more." At stateside medical facilities many medical staff will have their own fantasies about what the combat experience was like. Working with those staff in an educational way can be helpful.

Patients are more than willing to recount their experiences. They are primarily young and may be placed into semiprivate, if not private, rooms which can be equated with "good care." They tend to do better, however, in more open environments where they can see and support each other. Group therapy time can be built into ward schedules if the injured are grouped together in a specific ward environment. A group "debriefing" format can be most helpful. A strong need of the patients is to find out what happened to friends. There is usually much time spent trying to reconstruct what was happening at the time that they were injured. In facilitating the grief of these patients, particularly those who may have lost shipmates, a memorial service of some sort is essential.

Hospitals may be visited by dignitaries, family members, and the press, creating many time demands upon the injured. The families of those most severely injured may feel that the patient would be "better off dead." As time progresses, and they become used to the disability, those families often do not remember this initial reaction. Confronting that reaction is not helpful but providing education and structured experiences where they can help the patient in some meaningful way is. Some patients may consolidate their symptomatology into a classic post-traumatic stress disorder from some time about 6 weeks after injury and on.

Unusual situations can occur in the treatment of the combat injured. Care of the enemy injured and noncombatants may arouse different emotional responses in medical personnel. Injuries in combat may be self-inflicted. The psychiatric needs of those personnel may be unique. One suspected case of a self-inflicted injury, a U.S. Marine who was medically evacuated from Grenada, resulted in the patient ultimately being transferred to a psychiatric ward with what appeared to be a brief reactive psychosis. His behavior included reporting an atrocity (which he had not committed) to nursing staff, seclusion in his room, not eating, and hoarding his bandages. Interestingly, his treatment team consisted entirely of women including the mental health professional and a chaplain. Even though the other casualties suspected that he had a self-inflicted injury, this was never mentioned by the group members in therapy.

Experience shows that female therapists are accepted by male casualties and it appears they can reassure the male wounded about social acceptability better than male therapists can. One specific concern reported on clinical checklists is anxiety about sexual functioning.

There is no specific planning for the allocation of psychiatric resources to care for the needs of the combat injured. It was the author's experience that caring for 25 such casualties from Grenada and Beirut at the National Naval Medical Center consumed an immense amount of resources for approximately 45 days. The psychiatric consultant may be limited to liaison work with other medical staff in helping these patients.[52]

When examining the Grenada and Beirut casualties, some parallels and differences were found.[53] Both groups tried to reconstruct their experiences but they used different approaches. Casualties from Grenada were able to recall incidents with each other in reconstructing their experiences; however, those from Beirut, having been injured while asleep, had no ability to reconstruct. They felt initially that they didn't know what happened and then read about it as they would have about somebody else. They spent time talking to other casualties about where they were in the building and where they ended up: "How were you blown up?" This appeared to be a more passive reconstruction of events than that carried on by the casualties from Grenada.

There were sleep differences reported on symptom checklists. In group treatment, the Grenada patients who had problems with dreams reported nightmares about killing, thinking of dead bodies, touching dead bodies, and killing people. Those who were casualties from Beirut, where the headquarters had been blown up, had more problems with sleep initiation because they were fearful of returning to sleep. They would sometimes "play possum" and act as if they were sleeping to the nursing staff but not sleep. This was confounded by the fact that they had crossed several time zones.[53]

The casualties from Grenada had less survivor guilt at the time than the Beirut casualties. Beirut casualties already manifested survivor guilt. Group goals were different. The U.S. Marines who had been in Grenada wanted to get back to their units immediately as their units were going to Beirut. They had high morale and wanted to rejoin their units. The Beirut casualties primarily wanted to go home. Parenthetically, once they got home, they wanted to get away from home.[53]

The Grenadan casualties were more embarrassed by public attention. They did not want it or seek it out; they appeared to be comparing themselves with the Beirut casualties in the sense that they were only in combat for a day or a few hours and that the other casualties had been many months in Beirut. The Beirut casualties while in the hospital responded more positively to attention. When they went home and were afforded honors such as parades, they had great difficulty in tolerating that attention.[53]

SPECIAL PSYCHIATRIC RAPID INTERVENTION TEAM

History

Separate from the sequelae of stress in combat, psychiatrists in the U.S. Navy have long noted that there are psychiatric responses to disasters that affect sailors and marines long after the trauma itself. Often, personnel referred for evaluation with emotional or behavioral problems do not connect their problems or the onset of difficulties with a disaster they may have survived.

Disasters at sea are not uncommon nor are deaths due to operationally related training or other activities ashore. In November of 1975, the USS *Belknap* and the USS *Kennedy* collided, resulting in many deaths and extensive damage to the USS *Belknap*. Afterwards, the USS *Belknap* was towed to the Philadelphia Naval Shipyard with a portion of its crew, many of whom subsequently had outpatient psychiatric evaluations at the Philadelphia Naval Hospital. They had symptoms such as depression, sleepiness, poor concentration, and intrusive thoughts about the accident. These symptoms were noted to persist despite treatment. This was seen again after that psychiatry department moved to the Portsmouth Naval Hospital which was near the USS *Belknap's* home port.[54]

In January of 1977, a liberty launch collision in Barcelona Harbor in Spain resulted in some survivors who had long-term emotional problems that resulted in medical board action, early discharge, or psychiatric hospitalization. At that time, the staff at Portsmouth Naval Hospital felt that these problems appeared similar to those that were combat related. They formulated a clinical hypothesis that use of the same techniques proved in the combat setting might be useful in preventing or minimizing adverse psychiatric sequelae in disaster victims.

The first opportunity to test this hypothesis was in October of 1978 when a collision sank the USCGC *Cuyahoga* in the Chesapeake Bay offshore from Maryland. The U.S. Coast Guard requested that a team of mental health professionals work with the survivors. This occurred after the team leader had contacted them and informed them of the team's availability. That team saw themselves as following the basic combat psychiatry principles of immediacy, proximity, and expectancy in that the intervention was provided rapidly at the home port of the USCGC *Cuyahoga* with the 18 survivors. Furthermore, group cohesion and early return to duty were strongly encouraged.[55]

Preliminary clinical observations suggested that the intervention was successful and that survivors "appeared to be in much better physical and emotional health than would be expected based on the available literature on disaster victims." The special psychiatric rapid intervention team (SPRINT) concept was thus initially validated and the capability and need for a rapid contingency response was ultimately recognized. In February of 1983 SPRINT became one of the U.S. Navy's Mobile Medical Augmentation Readiness Teams (MMART).

Organization and Mission

These contingency response teams are located at U.S. Navy hospitals at Portsmouth, Virginia; San Diego, California; and Bethesda, Maryland. The composition of a full SPRINT is two psychiatrists, a clinical psychologist, a chaplain, a psychiatric nurse, and four corpsmen (neuropsychiatric technicians). They are required to be trained and immediately available in the event of a contingency, be it combat or disaster. There is no specific doctrine as to intervention methodology.

After-action reports and interviews after some 13 SPRINT deployments resulted in recurring observations.[54] A period of receptivity lasts about 24 to 72 hours after the initial tragedy. Anger is commonly expressed and is directed at any convenient focus such as lack of training, inanimate objects, adverse weather, and personnel up and down the chain of command. Loss of ships has special meaning for the survivors who lose not only shipmates but their unit identification, place of work, personal belongings, and abode. In those cases, salvaging part of the ship as a memorial is found to be beneficial. Team members dealt with survivor guilt, bereavement, and issues of death. Survivor guilt analogues were also seen in wives who felt guilty that their husbands had survived and were concerned about how to deal with the wives of the deceased in their community. There has also been a persistent denial of death by spouses when bodies recovered are not recognizable. Speculation, misunderstanding, and rumors tend to make all situations worse and disseminating accurate information is often essential prior to any resolution of symptoms.

Intervention Techniques

Successful interventions have had some common technical components. These involve the planning and training of team members; the notification process; arrangements for deployment and travel; and the structure of the intervention.

Planning and Training Phase

Team members must be selected, trained, and given an opportunity to work with each other. Given that the best training is that which is most realistic, they must train in environments similar to those where they will be expected to work. As they may have to go to sea, they need to have the skills that others expected to go to sea must have, such as fire fighting, and disaster control. They must be prepared to deploy within 24 hours of notification and will often be expected to leave sooner. This entails some detailed logistical preparation. Realistic training can also be seen as "service" when a team responds to incidents other than "disasters." This might include situations such as a suicide at a local command. They may also participate in disaster planning at local commands and may form liaisons in the community through such services as the provision of suicide prevention and stress management lectures. Through these activities, team members can develop a necessary attitudinal shift towards prevention rather than reaction to already developed pathology. A team without such a philosophy will seldom be requested. The team can also learn the useful "consultant's stance" as an appropriate approach to interventions of any size.

Notification Phase

At some point in time, team members will be notified that they are in an alert status to respond to a disaster or will hear through official or unofficial channels about a disaster. It is during this phase that some "systems" knowledge related to U.S. Navy organization is most helpful. After a large-scale disaster, the U.S. Navy community, particularly at higher echelons, is now sophisticated and understands the need for response teams. They conceive of such a team as being able to handle acute problems but do not often see the team in terms of prevention. Thus, liaison is needed with the appropriate commanders' staff, usually a staff surgeon or senior medical officer, to explain what assistance is available or has the potential to be most helpful. If the disaster has occurred at sea, the primary planning priority would be assistance to the crew of the casualty. A second planning priority would be aid ashore for families of victims and survivors. A third planning priority is ashore in support of the surviving injured who would be evacuated to local hospitals. The Bureau of Medicine and Surgery, Operational Readiness Division, is charged with ensuring execution of MMART, including SPRINT, deployments. (Some disaster responses may be handled by teams within local areas without activation; and, as long as they do not degrade SPRINT capability, they are usually considered a local command issue.)

This is the period of time during which the Specialty Advisor for Psychiatry and the officer in charge of the SPRINT can coordinate with line medical staff to ascertain preliminary data in order to plan the most effective intervention possible given resource, transportation, berthing, and other constraints. Liaison can also be initiated with local family service centers as well as hospital commanders where the injured may be evacuated.

Past experience indicates that the primary intervention sites will be with the crew, either at sea or in home port with the home port being an additional site for aid in the support of families. It is also necessary during this period to transfer patient care responsibilities of deploying team members safely and expeditiously. In those situations in which an entire SPRINT is not deployed, careful consideration must be given to which team members will be deployed.

For those teams that must operate somewhat independently, it is crucial that there be team members with professional and operational experience. Which professional disciplines are required for team makeup can create delicate questions. Everyone usually wants to go.

Deployment and Travel Phase

Some teams must travel to an intervention site away from their home port. Deployments are often on short notice and may require travel to sites where passports are needed. Loss of sleep and attendant fatigue can be degrading factors for team effectiveness once on site. Logistical coordination for berthing and local transportation can be time-consuming so that identification of points of contact prior to team departure can aid immensely.

From the time of departure until arrival at an intervention site there is rarely any new information available to team members so that the information they have when they depart will be dated by the time of their arrival. Some flexibility must be given to the officer-in-charge of the team for planning purposes. This also requires that the officer-in-charge have demonstrated flexibility in fluid situations. A team that travels with fewer members usually travels with greater ease.

In several recent interventions at sea, the team has been composed of three members. These "designer teams" have proved highly effective. They must utilize a triage system or prioritization of care once aboard ship. The officer-in-charge can usefully conceive team functioning in a utilitarian manner by trying to provide the greatest good for the greatest number of personnel as well as consulting to the unit itself. The mission that the team leader has as a goal is a limited one in attempting to restore the status quo ante as much as possible.

Intervention Phase

Interventions with military units should begin as soon as possible after arrival. The officer-in-charge must brief the commanding officer, executive officer, and senior medical officer as to team mission, capabilities, and intervention methodology. At this time the "consultant's stance" is most helpful. This allows the SPRINT members to handle the question, "Who do you work for?" by responding that they work for the commanding officer of the ship or unit. This will usually alleviate some anxiety as almost all disasters are associated with official investigations. All "outsiders" will be viewed with initial suspicion.

The concept of a "trauma membrane" surrounding the disaster victims and bonding them together is useful. Team members who come from a cultural background similar to those of the trauma victims can foster identification between the group victims and the SPRINT. With such identification, victims have an initial trust in those "there to help them" that helps separate the SPRINT members from investigators or other "outsiders."

This initial phase is also crucial in beginning to debrief the command structure of the ship. The "consultant's stance" has the team "learn" about what happened to the ship or unit. The team while doing this can, in essence, model for the commanding officer how the intervention will work.

Team members must also meet with members of the wardroom, which consists of all the commissioned officers aboard ship, as well as the Chief Petty Officer's Mess which consists of the senior enlisted leadership aboard ship. These groups will have the most information available and the team can begin to assess how much of that information is accurate and up to date. Such assessment is crucial and one of the first interventions that may be recommended is the dissemination of as much information to as many people as possible. This is helpful for two primary reasons: (1) rumor is always rampant and rumor may serve many separate functions in a unit—accurate information can lessen some destructive agendas; and (2) one of the initial steps in dealing with such trauma is the need for the victim to place himself in some context.

After meeting with these initial groups during which time the debriefing technique described below has been used, the team must integrate itself into the organizational structure of the unit in some way and begin further triage and intervention. If there is a medical department aboard ship, this provides a natural organizational placement for the intervention as well as clearly identifying the mission as a medical one. Triage is ongoing and gathering information from the leadership and medical department aboard ship will help in the initial identification process. Some individuals who are either dysfunctional or are considered by the crew as having suffered sufficient stressors that they should be dysfunctional are usually first identified through this process. These individuals can be provided individual assessment and treatment as necessary including recommendation for medical evacuation if indicated, although this would usually be the last resort as recovery could be expected to be most facilitated aboard ship, among shipmates and crew. It must be remembered that symptomatology for most individuals would be most acute immediately following the trauma.

The second triage task is to identify "at risk" individuals and groups. These are usually those individuals who were most intimately involved with the trauma. The first subset is those who were in danger of dying at the time of the initial trauma or who knew the casualties. A second "at risk" subset is those who were in danger during damage control or fire-fighting operations in the immediate post-trauma period. A third "at risk" group is those who handled bodies, body parts, or the more severely wounded. This last group must include the medical department personnel. These "at risk" groups should usually have a group intervention. Such groups are most effective if there are about 25 or less people in a group. Such groups should be planned to fall within the organizational structure of the ship so that people within similar divisions debrief together.

Those identified "at risk" individuals and groups as well as the wardroom and Chief Petty Officer's Mess would normally be provided with a debriefing. Evolution of this technique has stemmed from observations that there appear to be specific needs that can be addressed efficiently.

Techniques utilized successfully have included three basic components: the first component is cognitive or informational, the second component is related to identifying, experiencing, and validating emotions, and the third component is "educational" in nature.

Disasters are, in some respects, not much different from combat and, as S.L.A. Marshall[56] noted, those who participate in a combat action are likely to be confused by the events that took place. Marshall's interviews after combat with all members of a group who participated in an action were aimed at getting the "facts." His caveat that an interviewer must remember that he or she is not conducting a critique, takes part in no tactical debate, does not become personal or emotional, and avoids any reflection on any individual as he would the plague, is sound advice today. Through such reconstruction of events, cognitive errors and distortions can be corrected by the group and the individual can place himself or herself in a larger context.

The phase of the intervention dealing with emotions is more familiar to mental health professionals and usually coexists in part with the phase dealing with cognition. The debriefer must be ready to deal with emotional responses including anger. Generally, participants have a cognitive construct that they should not have experienced feelings or that they should be able to deal with their feelings without discussion with their shipmates. As individuals describe their emotional reactions or begin to experience emotional reactions during the session, other participants will identify with these reactions. It is important to validate and acknowledge their feelings. If there is any one crucial component of the intervention, it is in getting the message across that these are normal human reactions to extremely abnormal events.

In the "educational or teaching phase," material is presented that should aid the individual in current and future adaptation. Such information may include what the usual responses to overwhelmingly abnormal events are, what sort of symptom time course individuals can expect, and adaptive means of coping with symptoms. How to deal with families and children are always important questions for survivors. Caution should be exercised to some degree in description of potential sequelae which can become a suggestion that such sequelae will occur. An appropriate suggestion would be that acute symptomatology is normal and time limited.

A debriefing format, adapted from those developed by Marshall[56] for conducting interviews after combat and by Mitchell,[57] for Critical Incident Stress Debriefing, is shown in Exhibit 9-1. Utilization of this technique with those groups and individuals identified as being "at risk" also allows ongoing triage of individuals by the team. By dealing with groups from the same divisions within the ship, the team fosters bonding in the division amongst shipmates. The attitude of expectancy of recovery and return to the prior level of functioning is crucial to the success of this technique.

Another critical part of dealing with the aftermath of disaster is a memorial service. Such memorial services allow the team to "point" towards some concrete event and facilitate grief reactions. The military has great strengths in its rituals for handling such memorial services. Liaison with the pastoral care department can be most helpful. Usually such memorial services will be held ashore with families. Occasionally, they will be at sea or overseas. SPRINT members are invariably invited to participate in these ceremonies with the crew with whom they have bonded.

Termination with the crew needs to be considered. Interventions last for varying periods of time depending upon circumstances. It is a matter of judgment as to when to terminate the intervention. A good key is when crew members begin to talk about difficulties they had prior to the trauma. Too lengthy an intervention could be counterproductive. When a ship is ashore, ongoing liaison with gradual termination can be maintained through liaison with the medical department.

Interventions with U.S. Navy families must be considered. Past experience in this area has led the U.S. Navy to develop guidelines for commanders ashore in responding to these disasters. SPRINT members can provide a consulting role to activities tasked with providing services. SPRINT members can successfully advise the local base commander, through staff, on areas of intervention. The team can also coordinate with Family Service Centers as consultants and for the provision of individual services, when necessary.

Debriefing groups similar to those above have been used successfully with families as well as with staff at crisis centers on base. A common question is what to expect from spouses returning from sea. Training for casualty assistance calls officers (CACOs) is indicated.

Other anticipated problem areas will realistically include information flow. There are always expectations that more information will be available

EXHIBIT 9-1

PREPARING FOR AND CONDUCTING DEBRIEFINGS

Preparation

1. The debriefer should read everything available on the incident.
2. During this phase, the debriefer should identify the group, notify them, get space, arrive early, set up the room, meet the people to be debriefed, and talk informally with them. The debriefer should also listen for information and cues related to the incident.

Debriefing

1. Introductory Phase
   a. This phase should be controlled, slow, and designed to motivate participation by each member of the group.
   b. This phase is conducted by the team leader. Other team leaders are not identified at this time.
   c. The team leader introduces himself or herself, discusses why he or she is qualified to do a debriefing, discusses confidentiality, and emphasizes that discussions are designed to help them or others like them.
2. Fact Phase
   a. This is the transition between the introductory phase and the reaction phase.
   b. The debriefer should ask participants to go around the room to give the following information (and note that this is the only time in debriefing they will have to speak up and they do have the right to pass):
      who they are,
      their role at the event, and
      their perspective of what happened to them at the event.
   c. Other team members are interspersed in the circle. Their introductions of themselves can help participants maintain emotional control by periodically deescalating the rising tension in the room as their turn comes up for introduction while the event is discussed.
   d. During this phase the participants are guided in cognitively thinking about the facts and allowed to internalize them.
   e. Because thoughts are easier to discuss than feelings, this phase allows participants to feel more secure in dealing with the feelings that they are experiencing.
3. Reaction Phase
   a. During this phase reactions are sought more than just feelings.
   b. If a participant should cry, the debriefer acknowledges, validates, and moves on to the next person.
   c. Each participant is encouraged to talk about his or her own issues, not the overall operation and not other issues.
   d. This phase is usually very intense with a great deal of anger.
   e. This phase usually lasts 45 minutes to one hour.
4. Signs and Symptoms Phase
   a. There is some natural movement from the reaction phase into this phase.
   b. The debriefer asks questions such as, "How did you know your reaction was different than usual?"
   c. The purpose of this phase is to help participants identify symptoms within the four categories of physiological, cognitive, emotional, and behavioral, at the scene, later at home, and at the time of the debriefing.
5. Teaching Phase
   a. Incident-specific material is provided to the group.
   b. This phase is usually lengthy.
   c. Examples of material presented include how to deal with the spouse, children, stress reactions, grief, what to expect in the future in terms of feelings and thoughts about the event that might occur.
   d. This is not an appropriate time to teach stress management techniques such as deep relaxation or meditation.
6. Reentry Phase
   a. The atmosphere of the group now comes back around to normal.
   b. Debriefing should close when it seems natural.

sooner than is realistic. What people want appears to be information. Once the information related to casualty lists is known, emotion can escalate quite rapidly. Medically unstable cases can be expected because great stress can exacerbate already existing medical conditions. Examples include pregnant women or someone with a history of seizure disorder who begins hyperventilating. Medical assistance should therefore be available.

Before groups are notified of casualty lists, individuals are under great stress, extremely vigilant, and aware of any changes. It is therefore difficult, if not impossible, to unobtrusively locate and notify someone in such a group of the death of a loved one. Acute emotional reactions are not something with which crisis center workers, other than clinicians, necessarily have familiarity. Anger is an emotion known to accompany loss and can be expected. It may also be directed at authority figures. There are individuals who will be missed by usual methods of notification as they would not be listed in service records. A pregnant fiancée of a casualty, for instance, would not usually be known to assistance officers as someone who should be notified. This person may show up at a crisis center. The amount of mental health services demanded in these situations can be overwhelming and as many resources as possible will sometimes need to be mobilized.

Debriefing for the team members themselves is necessary. During the intervention, team members must debrief each other on an ongoing basis. Work days are seldom shorter than 20 hours during the acute phase of an intervention and fatigue rapidly sets in. The team also identifies strongly with the crew and must undergo their own emotional reaction. A more formal debriefing of the team members is most effectively performed after return to home port.

One phenomenon that team members have learned to expect is the feeling of others in their departments that they "left them behind" and that the assignment is perceived as "glamorous" while others must pick up the duties they have left behind. The team must reintegrate into the department. After-action reports from the team facilitate any changes that may be necessary and pass on lessons learned in a recorded format to future teams.

The media usually has intense interest in disasters. SPRINT members must realize that what the media seem to seek is a "human interest" story that will allow them to provide responses of "real people." Media requests are time consuming and may have potential for negative outcomes. They also provide great opportunity for public education about disaster response in general as well as dissemination of information to those who may be affected by the disaster. Interviewees should be aware that sensitive questions relating to policy may be raised. Public affairs officers can be helpful in preparing for such questions.

For those memorial services at which the President or other high ranking persons may be present, the Secret Service, whose mission is the protection of the President, may make inquiry about whether any individuals "debriefed" have made threats against the President's life. None have been encountered to date. The Secret Service may also request assistance should support be necessary for family members during a memorial service.

Outcomes of past SPRINT interventions have been generally determined to be successful based on broad criteria. There is a paucity of data as to outcome. An intervention with survivors of a fire aboard the submarine USS *Bonefish*[58] resulted in a 1-year outcome of no psychiatric medical board action; no disqualifications for submarine service, either voluntary or involuntary; no naval service attrition through a less than expected retention rate; and one individual known to be under psychiatric treatment. Outcome as judged by unit effectiveness could be judged by the record of the USS *Iowa* which deployed on a Mediterrean cruise and successfully completed that cruise, including contingency operations. The USS *Iowa* deployed some 2 months after the tragedy aboard and subsequent intervention. A similar outcome was experienced with the USS *Lexington* in November 1989 after a crash aboard the flight deck. The ship returned to its usual duties in a brief period of time after the intervention. The success of outcomes can, of course, not be attributed solely to SPRINT intervention, but must reflect directly on the commanding officers and crews of those particular vessels.

The SPRINT concept and techniques will continue to evolve as has U.S. Naval psychiatry. Applications to the many unique U.S. Naval subcultures and to the constantly changing world will be a challenge that will be met by U.S. Navy psychiatrists and mental health clinicians as they have met the challenges of the past.

SUMMARY AND CONCLUSION

Although the U.S. Navy has unique combat roles, the principles of combat psychiatry derived from World War I and World War II ground combat have found applicability in maritime combat. For combat stress breakdown, restoration of physiological deficits (rest, sleep, nutrition) in an atmosphere of expectation of return to duty and avoidance of evacuation usually suffices to restore the casualty to duty. Maintaining cohesive forces through good leadership while living and working together with shared hardships and dangers helps prevent breakdown in sailors and marines just as it does in soldiers.

There are unique "cultural" aspects to naval service. Some aspects of naval life prevent or promote psychiatric breakdown. Shipboard life reduces the potential for evacuation during combat and may account for lower rates of psychiatric casualties. Long separations from families during deployments in both peacetime and wartime result in increased social stress less often encountered in other services. Prolonged close living in small vessels, particularly submarines and amphibious transports, can exacerbate minor irritants into major confrontations.

Through experience, the modern U.S. Navy through methods of personnel selection, critical incident debriefing following disasters, and refined leadership has become an efficient force with minimal psychiatric casualties.

Modern naval forces are comprised of volunteers who meet rigorous entrance standards and are further screened psychologically for specific assignments, such as submarine service, before assignment. Naval personnel may be assigned combatant duties in surface, undersea, aviation, or ground combat environments, each of which presents a unique "cultural" milieu, requiring adaptation of the general principles of combat psychiatry. There is also some "plasticity" in the presentation of symptoms between these milieus. Through the use of rapid intervention teams in disasters and combat, naval services have been in the forefront of current paradigms of treatment and prevention.

REFERENCES

1. Duncan T, Stout M. *War Surgery and Medicine: Official History of New Zealand in the Second World War 1938–45*. Wellington, New Zealand: RE Owen; 1954.

2. Beach EL. *Submarine*. New York: Zebra Books; 1990.

3. Steyn RW. Retrospections: A system of nautical psychiatry through World War II. *Milit Med*. 1980;June:407–412.

4. White WA. Cited by: Steyn RW. Retrospections: A system of nautical psychiatry through World War II. *Milit Med*. 1980;June:407–412.

5. Braceland FJ. Neurosis and the war. *Proceedings of the 33rd Annual Meeting of the Medical Section of the American Life Convention*. Chicago, Ill, 22–23 June, 1944.

6. American Psychiatric Association. *Diagnostic and Statistical Manual of Mental Disorders*. (DSM-I). Washington, DC: APA; 1952.

7. Ursano RB, Holloway HC. Military psychiatry. In: Kaplan HI, Sadock BJ, eds. *Companion to Textbook of Psychiatry IV*. Baltimore, Md: Williams & Wilkins; 1985.

8. Gray E. *Submarine Warriors*. Novato, Calif: Presidio Press; 1988.

9. Beach EL. *Run Silent, Run Deep*. Annapolis, Md: Naval Institute Press; 1986.

10. Bughhein LG. *The Boat*. New York: Dell Publishing; March 1988. [Originally published as *DAS BOOT*. Munich, West Germany: R Barr & Co; 1973].

11. Duff IF, Shilling CW. Psychiatric casualties in submarine warfare. *Am J Psychiatry*. 1947;103:607–613.

12. Behnke AR. Psychological and psychiatric reactions in diving and in submarine warfare. *Am J Psychiatry.* 1945;May:720–725.

13. McHarg JF. The mental health of submariners with special reference to 71 cases examined psychiatrically. *J Ment Sci.* 1946;92:343–356.

14. Ninnow EH. Submarine psychiatry. *Arch Env Med.* 1963;6:579–588.

15. Wilken DN. *Significant medical experiences aboard Polaris submarines: A review of 360 patrols during the period 1963–1967.* Naval Submarine Medical Research Lababoratory. 1969. Report 460.

16. Satloff A. Psychiatry and the nuclear submarine. *Am J Psychiatry.* 1967;125:547–551.

17. Serxnon JL. An exercise in submarine psychiatry. *Am J Psychiatry.* 1968;125:25–30.

18. Biersner RJ. Mental health of submariners. *Undersea Biomed Res.* 1987;14:75–76.

19. US Department of the Navy. *Manual of the Medical Department.* Washington, DC: Bureau of Medicine and Surgery. NavMed P-117. 1951 [with periodic updates].

20. Ryack BL. *A Computer-Based Diagnostic/Information Patient Management System for Isolated Environments.* Groton, Conn: Naval Undersea Medical Research Laboratory; February 1987. Report NSMRL-1089.

21. Hedlund JL. *Development of Computer-Supported Assessment and Treatment Consultation for Emotional Crises (CATLEC) for a Submarine Environment.* Groton, Conn: Naval Undersea Medical Research Laboratory; March 1986. Report AD-A166588.

22. Margolin S, Kubie LS, et al. Acute emotional disturbances in torpedoed seamen of the Merchant Marine who are continuing at sea. *War Med.* 1943;3:393–408.

23. Deutsch A. Military psychiatry: World War II 1941–1943. In: Hall JK, Zilborg G, Bunker HA, eds. *One Hundred Years of American Psychiatry 1844–1944.* New York: Columbia University Press; 1944.

24. Irving D. *The Destruction of Convoy PQ.17.* New York: Simon & Schuster; 1968.

25. Askevold F. The war sailor syndrome. *Danish Med Bull.* 1980;27(5):220–224.

26. Blain D, Hoch P, Ryan UG. A course in psychological first aid and prevention: A preliminary report. *Am J Psychiatry.* 1944;101:629–634.

27. Beach EL. *The United States Navy: 200 Years.* New York: Hout; 1986.

28. Stimson HL as cited in Beach EL. *The United States Navy: 200 Years.* New York: Hout; 1986.

29. Polmer N. Allon TB. *Rickover.* New York: Simon and Schuster; 1982.

30. O'Connell MR. The Falklands experience 1982. In: Manglesdorf AD, King JM, O'Brien DE, eds. *Proceedings of the Fourth Annual User's Workshop on Combat Stress,* Consultation Report 85-002. Fort Sam Houston, Tex: US Army Health Services Command; 1985: 138–146.

31. O'Connell MR. Personal Communication, 5 June 1989.

32. Hogan BW. Psychiatric observations of senior medical officer on board aircraft carrier USS *WASP* during action in combat areas, at time of torpedoing, and survivors reaction. *Am J Psychiatry.* 1943;July:90–93.

33. Rubin RT, et al. Life stress and illness patterns in the US Navy: VI. Environmental, demographic, and prior life change variables in relation to illness onset in naval aviators during a combat cruise. *Psychosom Med.* 1972;34(6);533–545.

34. Yacavone DW. Personal Communication, June 1989.

35. Holtzman GR. Personal Communication, 30 June 1989.

36. Drucker AJ, Bradt KH. *A Survey of Opinions of Officers and Senior NCO's in Korea: Factors Contributing to Maintenance of Morale Under Combat Conditions.* Army Project Number 29535100. PRS Report 951, 1 April 1952.

37. Griffith SB, II. *The Battle for Guadalcanal.* Annapolis, Md: The Nautical and Aviation Publishing Company of America; 1963.

38. Zimmerman JL. *The Guadalcanal Campaign.* Washington, DC: US Marine Corps Historical Headquarters; 1949.

39. *The History of the Medical Department of the U.S. Navy in World War II, Vol 1, A Narrative and Pictorial Volume.* Washington, DC: U.S. Govt. Printing Office; 1950.

40. Lecke, R. *Helmet for my Pillow.* New York: Random House; 1957.

41. Werstein I. *Guadalcanal.* New York: Thomas Y Crowell; 1963.

42. Tregaskis R. *Guadalcanal Diary.* New York: Random House; 1943.

43. Smith FR. Neuroses resulting from combat. *Am J Psychiatry.* 1943;100:94–95.

44. Lidz T. Untitled seminar at Uniformed Services University of the Health Sciences, Bethesda, Md. 28 May 1987.

45. Davis R. *Marine at War.* New York: Bantam Books; 1988.

46. Simpson RW. Iwo Jima: A surgeon's story. *Leatherneck.* 1990;88(Feb):28–35.

47. Vedder JS. *Surgeon on Iwo: Up Front with the 27th Marines.* Novato, Calif: Presidio Press; 1948: 66.

48. Johanek M, Tullidge A. Personal Communication, 1991.

49. Strange RE, Arthur RJ. Hospital ship psychiatry in a war zone. *Am J Psychiatry.* 1967;134(3):37–42.

50. Sears HJT. Personal Communication, June 1989.

51. Shea FT. Stress of caring for combat casualties. *US Navy Med.* 1983;83(Jan–Feb):4–8.

52. Mateczun JM, Holmes-Johnson EK. The psychiatric care of the combat injured. In: Manglesdorff AB, et al, eds. *Proceedings of the Fourth User's Workshop on Combat Stress,* Consultation Report 85-002. Fort Sam Houston, Tex: US Army Health Services Command; 1985: 180–195.

53. Mateczun JM, Holmes-Johnson EK. Clinical differences between Beirut and Grenada casualties. In: Manglesdorff AB, et al, eds. *Proceedings of the Fourth User's Workshop on Combat Stress,* Consultation Report 85-002. Fort Sam Houston, Tex: US Army Health Services Command; 1985: 198–205.

54. McCaughey BG. US Navy Special Psychiatric Rapid Intervention Team (SPRINT). *Milit Med.* 1987;152:133–135.

55. Carlton TG. SPRINT: A psychiatric contingency response team in action. *US Navy Med.* 1979;70:11.

56. Marshall SLA, Atwood L. *Island Victory: The Battle for Kwajalein.* Washington, DC: Zenger; 1983: Appendix. [Reprint of 1945 ed].

57. Mitchell JT. Assessing and managing the psychologic impact of terrorism, civil disorder, disasters and mass casualties. *Emerg Care Q.* 1986;2(1):51–58.

58. Aitken JR, Bishop RJ, Dinneen MP. Personal Communication, May 1989.

Chapter 10

COMBAT STRESS CONTROL IN JOINT OPERATIONS

JAMES W. STOKES, M.D.* AND FRANKLIN D. JONES, M.D., F.A.P.A.†

*Colonel, Medical Corps, U.S. Army; Chief, Combat Stress Actions Office, Department of Preventive Health Services, Academy of Health Sciences, Army Medical Department Center and School, Fort Sam Houston, Texas 78234-6133

†Colonel (ret), Medical Corps, U.S. Army; Clinical Professor, Uniformed Services University of the Health Sciences, Bethesda, Maryland; Past President and Secretary and current Honorary President of the Military Section, World Psychiatric Association; formerly Psychiatry and Neurology Consultant, Office of The Surgeon General, U.S. Army

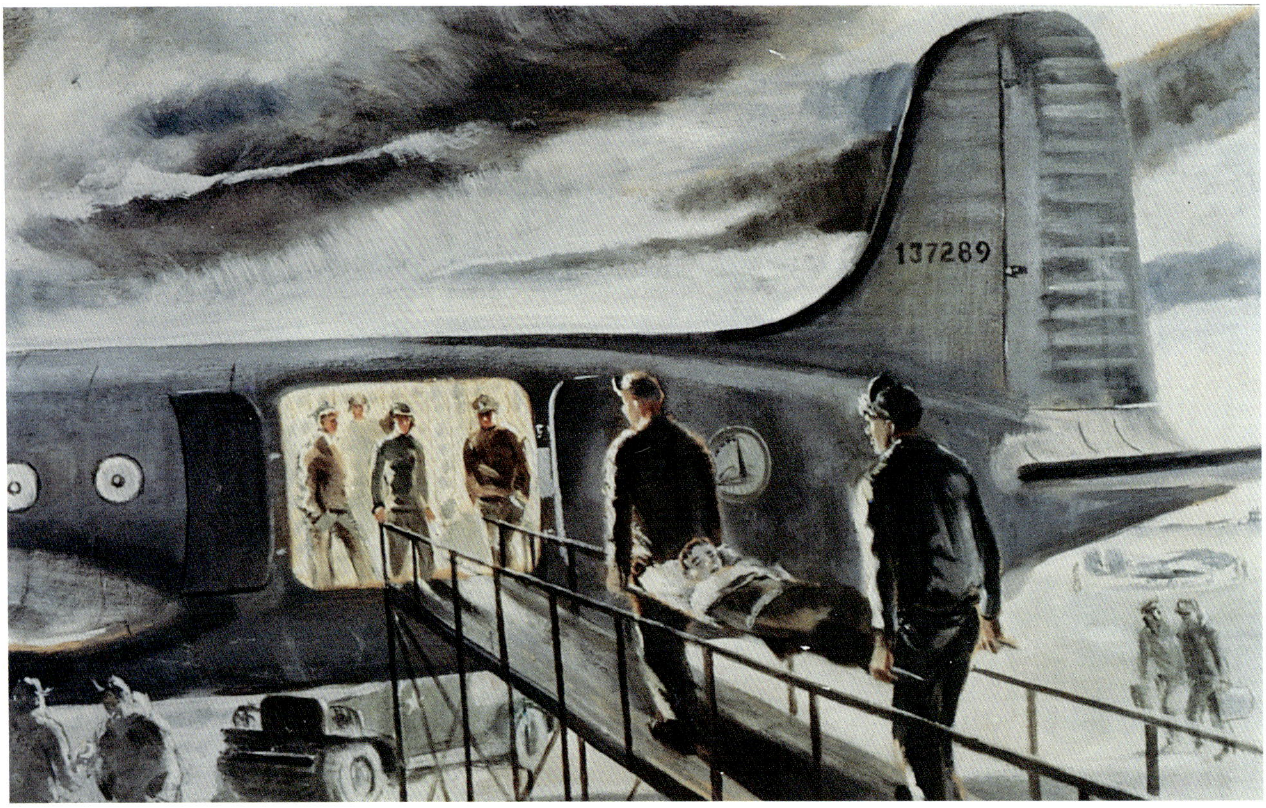

Hans H. Helweg *Patients Being Loaded on C-54, England* 1944

Air-evacuation of the wounded, as depicted in this painting by Hans H. Helweg from World War II, is a critical joint operation among the military services during combat. Of equal importance in a joint operations arena is the providing of restorative services to soldiers, sailors, and airmen suffering combat stress reactions.

Art: Courtesy of US Army Center of Military History, Washington, DC.

INTRODUCTION

As most recently seen in the Persian Gulf War and the peacekeeping mission to Somalia, U.S. Army combat operations in the post-Cold War will inevitably involve joint operations with the U.S. Air Force, and often with the U.S. Navy and U.S. Marine Corps.[1] Even peacetime power projections, such as humanitarian and civil assistance, foreign internal defense training missions, peacekeeping, and narcotics interdiction will commonly include members from several military services. Other federal and civilian agencies, such as the Federal Emergency Management Agency (FEMA), the State Department, the Central Intelligence Agency (CIA), the Federal Bureau of Investigation (FBI), Coast Guard, Public Health Service, Merchant Marine, Department of Veterans Affairs, Red Cross, and others, may also play important roles. In joint operations, U.S. Army Mental Health/Combat Stress Control (MH/CSC) personnel and units may be in a position to provide mental health support for personnel from other U.S. services. Conversely, U.S. Army personnel who are at risk to develop, or who are developing, stress disorders may benefit from assistance from another service.

INHERENT PROBLEMS IN JOINT OPERATIONS

Joint operations have proved difficult and dangerous down through history. Recent U.S. experience in the aborted Iranian hostage rescue attempt in 1980 and Operation Urgent Fury (Grenada) provided painful lessons learned when U.S. Army, U.S. Air Force, and U.S. Navy teams who had not previously worked and drilled together had to cooperate in complex, integrated operations. In part, the difficulties arose from incompatibilities of materiel: radios that could not communicate between the different service components even when frequencies were known, "incompatible" computer systems, and lack of spare parts and trained mechanics for each other's equipment. Difficulties also arose from the lack of shared standing operating procedures. To some extent, the services spoke different "languages"—service-specific vocabularies and especially acronyms which the users found so familiar that they did not even realize that their words were unintelligible to the other services or, worse, might have quite different meanings to them. Lack of a common training base raises doubts of the other's reliability and safety—these are not necessarily unrealistic when dealing with highly dangerous tasks requiring special skills such as landing U.S. Army medevac helicopters on ships in the dark. More subtle, and harder to counteract, are the suspicion and mistrust that arise from different nonverbal and verbal communication patterns, and different culturally-encouraged styles of leadership and comradeship. There is the natural human prejudice to favor one's own tradition and fellow service members. Even when leaders are trying to be impartial, subordinates may perceive favoritism. This resentment can further interfere with open communication, morale, and cohesion.

The Department of Defense, the U.S. Congress, and the civilian leadership have directed that serving in joint staff positions be an important criterion for promotion to senior command positions in each service, as well as to the joint major commands. Increased familiarity and experience may go far to resolve some of these inherent problems. Psychiatrists and other mental health professionals and noncommissioned officers (NCOs) who provide consultation to joint commands and staffs should use their behavioral science and communications skills to identify the problems and facilitate the solutions. Ideally, some mental health experts will become members of those joint staffs.

COMMON COMBAT PSYCHIATRY PRINCIPLES AND POLICIES

The medical support systems of all four services share the basic principles for the prevention and treatment of the dysfunctional combat stress reactions—"battle fatigue" and the disorders of frustration and loneliness, which are presented in greater detail in Chapter 1, Psychiatric Lessons of War. In all four services, control of stress and the prevention of stress casualties is a command and leadership responsibility. Psychiatric and other mental health expertise in the services' medical systems have the key role in supporting command with prevention and in evaluating and treating cases.

The U.S. Army expresses the basic principles for intervention for battle fatigue in the memory aid "Treat with PIES" (Proximity, Immediacy, Expectancy, Simplicity).

- *P*roximity: treat in or close to the service member's unit.
- *I*mmediacy: begin intervention immediately on recognition.
- *E*xpectancy: give positive expectation of rapid recovery and return to duty.
- *S*implicity: use straight-forward, nonmysterious interventions.

The U.S. Air Force and U.S. Navy often teach the same principles with the acronym "BICEPS" (Brevity, Immediacy, Centrality, Expectancy, Proximity, Simplicity). The additional concepts, brevity and centrality, are defined as:

- *B*revity: everyone involved knows from the beginning that treatment will be brief (hours to days).
- *C*entrality: stress casualties are treated at a central location separate from the sick and wounded and they are not evacuated until evaluated by skilled professionals to prevent inappropriate evacuations.

The U.S. Army also subscribes to brevity and to the clear separation of stress cases. However, the "central locations" (plural) will usually be dispersed, as far forward as possible (in accordance with the principles of proximity and immediacy), but under "central control." In addition, a central processing facility will reevaluate those being evacuated to determine whether they can remain in the combat zone.

The simple (austere) intervention methods for treating battle fatigue are summarized by the "Five Rs":

- *R*eassurance of normalcy.
- *R*est from extreme stress.
- *R*eplenishment of physiologic well-being.
- *R*estoration of confidence by treating the person as a service member, not a "patient"; by debriefing (retelling the stressful events); and by work activities.
- *R*eturn to duty, if possible, in the service member's own unit.

All cases of serious misconduct, *including* those that are attributable to combat stress (for example, substance abuse, insubordination, atrocities, absence without leave, and malingering) must be returned to the line units for administrative and disciplinary action in the theater of operations. They are evacuated according to "BICEPS" (brevity, immediacy, centrality, expectancy, proximity, simplicity) only if they have other medical, surgical, or psychiatric conditions that require medical treatment prior to administrative disposition.

True neuropsychiatric (NP) cases, for example major depression and persistent schizophrenic-type psychotic disorders, who have a poor chance for rapid return to duty should be evacuated as soon as they can be stabilized and reliably distinguished from battle fatigue. Post-traumatic stress disorder (PTSD) should be prevented by routine unit (team) debriefings. The debriefings should be accomplished as soon after trauma as is tactically feasible, and again during homecoming. Deployed service members can tolerate high stress best when they know that the unit, the service, and the government are assuring that their families are well cared for and informed.

Six Combat Stress Control Mission Functions

Six combat stress control (CSC) functions are defined by U.S. Army doctrine.[2,3] The relative requirement for each function varies depending on the scenario and mission, and especially on the type and intensity of conflict involved. The six functions, listed in usual order of priority, are as follows:

1. *Consultation-Liaison:* preventive advice, education, and interventions to unit leaders, staffs, medical personnel, chaplains, and troops.
2. *Reorganization/Reconstitution Support* to attrited units at field locations.
3. *Proximate Neuropsychiatric Triage:* sorting of stress and NP cases based on where they are best treated to maximize return to duty according to the PIES principles, where the "S" stands for safety—that of the soldier, the unit, and mission accomplishment.
4. *Stabilization* of seriously disturbed cases, for patient and unit safety and to evaluate return to duty potential;
5. *Restoration:* 1 to 3 days of holding treatment in forward, austere medical facilities.
6. *Reconditioning/Retraining:* additional 1 to 2 weeks of treatment at more secure (usually rearward) combat stress control facilities as needed by some cases.

All six combat stress control functions could call for joint operations, in somewhat the same order of priority as listed. Reconditioning is the least likely or desirable for joint sharing. Neuropsychiatric triage and stabilization may be especially important in some joint situations.

CSC Preventive Methods

The primary focus of combat stress control and mental health in a theater of operations (whether in combat or in operations other than war) is preventive. The mental health/combat stress control (MH/CSC) personnel must be proactive. They must diplomatically demonstrate their preventive value to line unit leaders. Specific methods include (but are not limited to) the following:

- Attending and providing input at staff meetings and planning sessions.
- Conducting frequent (routine) unit survey interviews.
- Keeping command informed of stress, morale, and leadership issues that concern the troops; advising and teaching stress control measures.
- Training and encouraging routine after-action debriefing by leaders of small units.
- Conducting critical event debriefings following any especially traumatic events.
- Training chaplains, medical personnel, and line personnel to do critical event debriefings, too.
- Coordinating and participating in end-of-deployment debriefings, memorial and closure ceremonies, and reunion preparation.

Limitations of and Need for Joint CSC Operations

Each service must have its own MH/CSC personnel, organic to its own structure (active and reserve) for the following reasons. MH/CSC personnel must have mutual positive identification and cohesion with the unit leaders and service members they support. More than any other medical specialty (except flight surgeons), they must know the mental and physical demands and stressors of the service members' mission duties in order to judge them psychologically able to return to duty. They must understand the organizational structure, individual and group dynamics, and leadership issues involved. Assuming equal training and experience within their own services, the MH/CSC person who is working within his *familiar* service can be expected to be significantly more effective than the one who is working with service members and organizations of a *different* service.

However, in joint operations, there will surely be times and places where each service will not have its own MH/CSC personnel on the spot when combat stress control support is needed. Immediacy and proximity are basic principles in combat stress control interventions. Another service may have combat stress control resources nearby. One service may also have a highly experienced combat stress control expert in the area of operation, while the other services may have only novices locally available. It is therefore important that there be contingency plans and, when feasible, standing operating procedures to permit efficient sharing of combat stress control resources. The cross-fertilization of ideas and techniques, as well as the professional moral support, will make all the participants more effective.

All stress casualties who are evacuated to another service's facility should receive the same treatment as that service's own cases: provide immediate reassurance, and initiate rest, replenishment, and activities to restore confidence. Successful 1- to 3-day restoration can probably be accomplished with mixed service groups. Care may need to be taken to assure that any interservice rivalry is used constructively, not destructively, in the program. The treatment is provided until the casualties can return to duty to their original units or be transferred to their own service's backup combat stress control facility.

In theory, longer-term reconditioning is best done by the casualties' own service, where it can maximize the common identity, traditions, and culture of that service. If limited resources require a single, joint reconditioning center, it would be best to have both (or all) services represented on the treatment staff. If the number of cases were sufficient, the cases could be organized into single-service working groups (squads). Here, especially, interservice rivalry and competition could be therapeutic, but would require careful modulation to keep it constructive. Joint reconditioning could also be applied to alcohol and drug rehabilitation in theater for cases with potential for useful return to duty.

This chapter will review the MH/CSC assets that the services may deploy to the theater. It will also suggest ways of using them jointly.

MILITARY BRANCHES IN JOINT OPERATIONS

Each of the four military services has its own applicable rules and regulations for the delivery of mental health care to its service members. These rules and regulations are "living" documents in the sense that they are modified through the course of time and experience. The following discussion of the structure and delivery of mental health care in the various services provides a snapshot view from the period immediately after the Persian Gulf War. The emphasis is not on the specific structure, although these structures are detailed for the reader, but rather on how the delivery of this vital care is coordinated between the various military services. It is expected that these configurations will change according to mission and available staff.

U.S. Air Force MH/CSC Capability

Overview

In World War II, U.S. Army Air Corps psychiatry was primarily concerned with "operational fatigue" in flight crews (especially bomber crews) who flew many high-casualty combat missions. The mental health of flight crews was (and is) the responsibility of the unit's flight surgeon.

In more recent wars, the flight crews have become increasingly "professional"—that is, highly selected, trained, and motivated officers and senior NCOs flying in highly sophisticated aircraft. Their living facilities (when they are not flying) and crew rest policies have usually been sufficient to minimize cumulative sleep loss and physiologic deprivation. Such factors have made these "elite" personnel relatively resistant to battle fatigue, even when flying high-risk missions over prolonged periods. However, they may still be subject to battle fatigue during surge conditions, or when there are serious problems at home, or as a "short-timer syndrome."

Recently, stress control concern in the U.S. Air Force has focused more on the ground personnel. These are potentially at high risk for stress casualties because they may work extremely long hours at complex, dangerous tasks. They may come under attack, including nuclear, biological, or chemical (NBC) attacks, unable to move from the center of the "bull's eye." They may receive little training in self-protection and have no way to strike back. The U.S. Air Force perspective on combat stress is described in *U.S. Air Force Combat Psychiatry*[4] and Chapter 8 of this volume, U.S. Air Force Combat Psychiatry.

U.S. Air Force Echelon II CSC

The U.S. Air Force Echelon II level of care is roughly equivalent to the U.S. Army's Echelon II (field medical treatment companies—with a surgical team added), but is less mobile on the ground. The Air Combat Command may deploy a 50-bed air transportable hospital (ATH) to provide Echelon II medical capability (or to reinforce existing air base dispensary medical personnel) at forward tactical air fields or air bases. The ATHs are each designated a numbered "Tactical Hospital."

Each 50-bed ATH includes a Combat Stress Unit (CSU) with one psychiatrist (*or* pediatrician with combat stress training, *or* clinical psychologist); one clinical psychologist *or* social work officer; and two mental health specialists (914s, equivalent to the Army's MOS 91G [social work technician]). This CSU is therefore similar to the U.S. Army CSC prevention teams in the CSC medical detachment and CSC medical company (previously described), except that it may not have its own vehicle.

The Combat Stress Unit is expected to provide consultation-liaison in the hospital and to nearby units. It may form a Disaster Response Team. It should be able to conduct outpatient treatment and a 1- to 3-day restoration holding treatment program. This program may be in tents collocated with the air transportable hospital's medical and surgical capability, in the hospital staff's quartering area, or perhaps separate from the hospital but still within the air base perimeter. This latter location would usually be in an available "building of opportunity." If there is an NBC threat, the building could be given some degree of collective protection. Cases who cannot be held at this echelon, or who fail to return to duty within 3 to 7 days (depending on the likelihood of return to duty and available space and personnel), would be transferred by air to Echelon III or IV.

U.S. Air Force Echelon III CSC

The U.S. Air Force Echelon III care is roughly equivalent to the U.S. Army's Echelon III (Combat Support Hospital) hospital care, but further to the rear, in the theater or communications zone (COMMZ). This care may be provided by a contingency hospital. This is a deployable medical systems (DEPMEDS) facility that, in some cases, may be in storage in the COMMZ prior to mobilization. Contingency hospitals can have over 250 beds and a neuropsychiatry section, staffed by psychiatrists, clinical psychologists, social work officers, and enlisted specialists (914s). The numbers of the specific professionals will vary according to the mission, the availability of staff, and evolving CSC doctrine.

This staff can provide consultation within and around the hospital, and deploy a disaster response team. It can supervise care of neuropsychiatric patients and medical/surgical patients who have psychiatric complications on the medical wards. If augmented with psychiatrically trained nursing personnel, it can staff a 16-bed neuropsychiatry ward. It could also establish a 1- to 3-day restoration program or a longer duration reconditioning program separate from the medical and surgical facilities. In a preestablished theater, Echelon III care might also be provided by a preexisting small base hospital; this might not have the combat stress control restoration/reconditioning capability unless augmented with MH/CSC personnel.

U.S. Air Force Echelon IV CSC

The U.S. Air Force Echelon IV is roughly equivalent to U.S. Army Echelon IV, general and field hospitals in the communications zone. For the U.S. Air Force, this care would be provided by large, fixed hospitals near major air bases. Approximately one in four such hospitals would have inpatient psychiatric capability. These might also have other mental health (psychology, social work, and occupational therapy) personnel. The other hospitals without the neuropsychiatric wards might still have some neuropsychiatric/mental health staff to provide consultation and triage. The neuropsychiatric-staffed facility should be configured to be able to conduct a reconditioning program which maintains a nonpatient care atmosphere.

U.S. Marine Corps and Navy MH/CSC Capability

Overview

Each U.S. Marine Corps Division is part of a task-organized Marine Expeditionary Force (MEF), whose medical planning is the responsibility of the MEF surgeon. All medical support in U.S. Marine Corps units is provided by U.S. Navy personnel. Each U.S. Marine Corps division has a U.S. Navy psychiatrist as division psychiatrist/assistant division surgeon, and a petty officer psychiatric technician. The psychiatrist is usually at the division's home base at Camp Lejeune, North Carolina; Camp Pendleton, California; or in Okinawa. On full deployment, he would deploy to the theater of operations. He might be augmented with a second U.S. Navy psychiatrist.

The U.S. Marine Corps can task organize into a Marine Expeditionary Force (MEF) which has an infantry division, a Marine Expeditionary Brigade (MEB) which has an infantry brigade, or a Marine Expeditionary Unit (MEU) which has an infantry battalion. The U.S. Marines deploy by way of ships at sea with a U.S. Naval task force, usually on a 6-month rotation; ships sailing directly from their base to the theater; and air transportation as reinforcements to the theater of operations where they rendezvous with units that deployed by ship to meet pre-positioned ships loaded with the equipment.

Each U.S. Marine Corps battalion has a battalion aid station (BAS) roughly similar to those of U.S. Army battalions. Within the MEF, additional medical support is task organized in the Force Service Support Group (FSSG) which includes the medical battalion.

U.S. Marine Echelon II Medical Battalion Assets

Each Marine medical battalion in a Marine Expeditionary Force has four surgical companies. The headquarters platoon of each company includes a combat stress platoon, each of which includes a U.S. Navy psychiatrist, two psychologists, and three psychiatric technicians.

These U.S. Navy mental health professionals only join the medical battalion on mobilization. As with the U.S. Army professional officer filler system (PROFIS) or Individual Ready Reserve fillers, such a late-arriving officer will take days to weeks to become a fully effective CSC consultant or treatment team leader.

If a MEF is at sea, the organic U.S. Marine Corps medical resources are controlled by the U.S. Navy's Commander, Amphibious Task Force (CATF) and function to some extent while aboard transport ships, caring for U.S. Marines. Once the amphibious force has established a beachhead, the CATF surgeon and the U.S. Marine Corps' Commander Landing Forces (CLF) surgeon meet to plan the landing of the beach evacuation station.

The troop transport ships have medical and surgical capability varying with size and type. Some ships (especially the helicopter assault ships or hover craft mother ships), would become emergency surgical or medical care sites (primary casualty receiving and treatment ships) in the first hours of an opposed landing. Any other transport or landing ship whose troops and cargo have disembarked could be used as a restoration site for stress casualties. It is recognized, however, that return to duty from a ship would be much more difficult than from a shore facility, both logistically and psychologically.

As the beachhead expands, additional medical assets are landed. A U.S. Marine brigade would usually be followed by one of the medical collecting and clearing companies as it moves further from the beach. The beach evacuation station might be expanded by landing the surgical support company.

There is currently no formal mental health doctrine as to whether U.S. Marine Corps battle fatigue casualties should be held/restored at the medical collection and clearing companies, the surgical support companies, or on the troop transport ships offshore. The U.S. Marine Corps division psychiatrist and the medical battalion's combat stress centers must train physicians, corpsmen, and other medical or line personnel to provide this treatment. The U.S. Marine Corps line units' Drug and Alcohol NCOs can be a valuable resource for cross-training.

Combat Stress Centers

When high-intensity conflict is expected and lead-time is sufficient, the combat stress platoon will implement a combat stress center. Four such combat stress center teams were improvised and fielded during the Persian Gulf War. Each such center was staffed by one or two psychiatrists, from one to three clinical psychologists, up to three psychiatric technicians, and corpsmen or nursing personnel who received on-the-job training. These teams were supplied with tents and cots at the surgical support centers to provide restoration, as well as providing preventive consultation and neuropsychiatric triage. In the Persian Gulf War, they did not deploy forward to augment the collecting and clearing companies.

U.S. Navy Echelon III/IV Afloat—Hospital Ship

A major U.S. Marine Corps or joint operation will be supported by a 1,000-bed hospital ship. Each hospital ship may have a neuropsychiatry ward and staff, including a psychiatrist, a clinical psychologist, two or more psychiatric nurses plus on-the-job-trained medical/surgical nurses, a social work officer, and petty officer psychiatric technicians plus on-the-job-trained corpsmen. The mental health/neuropsychiatric staff can staff a mixed medical/psychiatric ward on one of the ship's light care bays. They may establish a separate section of the ship for restoration of stress casualties who reach the ship. This section carefully avoids any patient care atmosphere. The hospital staff may also deploy task-organized teams, including special psychiatric rapid intervention teams (SPRINTs) to provide reconstitution support to ships which suffer heavy casualties from accidents or enemy action. The USS *Comfort* deployed such a team to the helicopter amphibious assault ship *Iwo Jima* following a boiler explosion with fatalities during the Persian Gulf War.

U.S. Navy Echelon III/IV Ashore—Fleet Hospital

The Combat Zone Fleet Hospital comes in two sizes—it can be a 250-bed or a 500-bed deployable medical systems (DEPMEDS) facility, roughly equivalent to the U.S. Air Force 250-bed Contingency Hospital and U.S. Army 500-bed General Hospital. These receive patients from U.S. Navy ships and U.S. Marine Corps units in the combat zone. The COMMZ Fleet Hospital (500-bed) has a convalescent mission which makes it roughly similar to the U.S. Army's 500-bed Field Hospital.

All fleet hospital staffs include a neuropsychiatry mental health team, consisting of one psychiatrist with the 250-bed facility and two psychiatrists with the 500-bed facility. No psychiatric nurses are specifically assigned, but a charge nurse and several ward nurses may be provided, and some could be psychiatric nurses. In addition there are three psychiatric technicians with the 250-bed facility and six with the 500-bed facility. There is also one clinical psychologist with the 500-bed facility only. This team staffs a neuropsychiatric ward. It can also establish a restoration or reconditioning program which maintains a nonpatient atmosphere, if provided with general purpose tents. Such a facility was established at two fleet hospitals during the Persian Gulf War, one in Saudi Arabia, and one in Bahrain.

U.S. Navy CSC Capability in Peacetime Disasters

For peacetime training accidents, airplane crashes, ship collisions, disasters, and other brief traumatic contingencies short of war, the U.S. Navy deploys SPRINTs, which are discussed in further detail in Chapter 9, U.S. Naval Combat Psychiatry.

Special psychiatric rapid intervention teams are task organized from a multidisciplinary pool of mental health personnel at large U.S. Navy hospitals. These personnel maintain a rotation in order to be available for deployment on 24-hour notice. Teams usually are led by a psychiatrist and may include a social work officer, psychologist, psychiatric nurse, chaplain, and enlisted technicians.

The SPRINT members provide on-site consultation to command. They assist local shipboard, port, or air station medical, mental health, and chaplain personnel with critical incident stress debriefing. The SPRINT concept is based on brief, immediate, proximate, positively expectant intervention following a critical incident. The teams have not been trained or equipped to provide restoration or reconditioning support to an ongoing combat operation.

U.S. Army MH/CSC Capability

U.S. Army Echelon II MH Sections

All divisions, brigades, and area support battalions have mental health sections. Each combat division's main support medical company or medical battalion has a mental health section consisting of a psychiatrist, a clinical psychologist, a social worker, and six or seven behavioral science specialists (91Gs). The Table of Organization and Equipment (TO&E) authorizes the mental health section three 1¼ ton vehicles. By doctrine, the section should deploy an NCO or an officer/NCO team to work consistently with each deployed maneuver brigade. The separate brigade's medical company has one NCO and two junior 91Gs (social work technicians) for a heavy (armor or mechanized infantry) brigade, and one NCO 91G for a light infantry brigade. Armored Cavalry and Ranger Regiments currently have no organic mental health personnel. Future U.S. Army plans will make a mental health officer/NCO team organic to all maneuver brigade and armored cavalry regiment medical companies, while keeping the division psychiatrist at division level to supervise all combat stress control operations. Each area support medical battalion in the corps has a psychiatrist, a social work officer, and eight 91Gs (E-3 to E-7) The section has one 2½ ton and three ¾ ton trucks. It should routinely assign a 91G NCO to each of the three area support medical companies. These are supervised and, when needed, reinforced by the officers from the area support medical battalion's headquarters and medical support company.

U.S. Army Echelon II/III CSC

The medical CSC detachments and companies provide U.S. Army Echelon II/III care. The medical detachment CSC has 9 officers, 14 enlisted, one 2 ½ ton and six 1¼ ton trucks with trailers. Basis of allocation is one per division or one per two or three separate brigades. It is composed of three CSC prevention teams (each with a psychiatrist, social work officer, two 91Gs); and one CSC restoration team (each with a psychiatric nurse and two psychiatric technicians, an occupational therapist and two occupational therapy technicians, a clinical psychologist and three 91Gs, plus a patient administration specialist).

The CSC prevention teams usually reinforce the brigade support areas to prevent stress casualties and unnecessary evacuation, and to assist the return to duty of recovered cases and unit reorganization efforts. The CSC restoration team usually provides neuropsychiatric triage, stabilization, and 1- to 3-day restoration at a medical company in the division rear or forward corps. This team also provides consultation and reorganization support there, and reinforces forward as needed. These multidisciplinary teams are not unbreakable atoms. Their specialist personnel should be combined or cross attached flexibly to make mission-specific "task-organized CSC elements." In operations other than war, the CSC detachment may be only partially deployed, and support the echelon-above-division units as well as reinforcing the division MH assets.

The Medical Company, CSC has 27 officers, 58 enlisted, one ¼ ton, six 2½ ton, and ten 1¼ ton trucks. Basis of allocation is one per two or three divisions for high-intensity war, or one per corps or theater for prolonged low-intensity conflict. The CSC company has a company headquarters; six CSC prevention teams (psychiatrists, social work officers, 91Gs); four CSC restoration teams (psychiatric nurses, psychologists, occupational therapists, technicians). Personnel from these teams should be switched flexibly across the CSC prevention and CSC restoration teams to tailor for specific missions.

The company headquarters (HQ) assists medical brigade or medical group HQ with CSC planning and with command/control and administrative/logistic support of its dispersed teams and the CSC detachments. The cook and vehicle mechanics are usually divvied out to the dispersed CSC working elements. The CSC HQ has a staff chaplain to provide the religious/spiritual perspective to the

MH/CSC team and to help coordinate with the chaplain network of unit ministry teams, HQ staff chaplains, and hospital chaplains.

The company's six CSC prevention and four CSC restoration teams are task organized into larger elements to provide comprehensive CSC support behind each division. The CSC elements can staff reconditioning centers (usually collocated with combat support hospitals); deploy teams to reinforce the area support medical battalion mental health section in corps; detail teams to provide direct CSC support to the corps' brigades or to units undergoing reconstitution; deploy its personnel or teams forward by air ambulance or ground vehicle to rapidly reinforce or reconstitute the CSC detachments at the divisions and brigades as needed.

U.S. Army Echelon III Corps-Level Hospitals

Each 300-bed combat support hospital (MedForce 2000 model) in the corps is a DEPMEDS facility which has a neuropsychiatry ward and consultation service. This service has a social work officer, three psychiatric nurses and one medical/surgical nurse, seven psychiatric ward aids (MOS 91F), one behavioral science specialist (MOS 91G), and an occupational therapy specialist (MOS 91L). The section provides consultation throughout the hospital and to nearby units. They staff a 20-bed intermediate care ward module which may also treat medical cases.

The current 60-bed (and the future 30-bed MedForce 2000) Mobile Army Surgical Hospitals and the current 200-bed combat support hospitals (CSHs) have no MH/CSC staff, although a psychiatric nurse could be filling a vacant medical/surgical nurse slot. The current 400-bed evacuation hospital has a psychiatrist, a psychiatric nurse, and two psychiatric technicians (MOS 9lFs). It will be replaced by the MedForce 2000 CSH.

U.S. Army Echelon IV General and Field Hospitals

The 500-bed general hospital and 500-bed field hospital (MedForce 2000 models) are DEPMEDS facilities which will usually be established in the communications zone. Each has the same neuropsychiatry ward and consultation service as the MedForce 2000 model CSH described above. The field hospital also has a clinical psychologist with two 9lGs, and an occupational therapist with two 9lLs. The mission of the MedForce 2000 field hospital is to be a convalescent facility which returns soldiers to duty in the theater within 30 days. It should have a reconditioning facility, kept separate from the "patient care" area. It may also provide a drug and alcohol rehabilitation program for soldiers with good return to duty potential (the current field hospital has no neuropsychiatry staff). The mission of the MedForce 2000 general hospital is primarily to prepare soldiers for safe evacuation to the continental United States (CONUS), including the severe neuropsychiatric disorders who cannot return to duty in theater.

U.S. Army CSC in Medical Command/Control Headquarters

The MedForce 2000 organizational structure provides for mental health staff sections in the theater and corps-level medical headquarters units. The medical command and the medical brigade each will have a psychiatrist, a social work officer or psychologist, an occupational therapy officer, and a 91G NCO. The subordinate medical groups each will have a psychologist, a social work officer, and a 91G NCO.

These MedForce 2000 positions will not be officially implemented until 1995. However, the precedent has been established for having some neuropsychiatry staff at headquarters level. In the Persian Gulf War, the U.S. Army Central Command Surgeon requested and received a staff neuropsychiatry consultant from the Office of The Surgeon General as an interim measure. Seventh Corps also requested and deployed to the Persian Gulf with a staff corps psychiatrist. The medical brigade at Fort Bragg, North Carolina, requested and received a psychiatrist (rank of colonel) for their relief mission in South Florida following Hurricane Andrew, and now has PROFIS staff on post. The Medical Group headquarters at Fort Lewis, Washington, took its authorized social work officer, psychologist, and 91G NCO to Somalia, then sent them home early. The Medical Group in Europe has directed its PROFIS social worker to plan contingency CSC support for Bosnia peace enforcement.

Situations for CSC Cooperation Between the U.S. Army and Air Force

A number of situations have occurred or will occur in which U.S. Army and U.S. Air Force personnel must cooperate in the treatment of stress psychiatric casualties, as well as in preventive stress control activities.

U.S. Air Force Liaison Personnel in U.S. Army Units

U.S. Air Force personnel routinely work as air liaison officers in U.S. Army headquarters units down to the brigade level. Under special circumstances, they might function further forward as observers calling in air strikes.

These personnel should receive preventive consultation support along with their U.S. Army headquarters. If these personnel develop battle fatigue, they should be treated in the same way and in the same facilities close to their units as their U.S. Army coworkers, with positive expectation of return to their same duty in 1 to 3 days. If they fail to respond to treatment, they should be transferred to U.S. Air Force facilities.

Downed U.S. Air Force Pilots

U.S. Air Force forward air controllers (FACs) fly small aircraft above the battlefield and guide high performance attack aircraft against ground targets close to U.S. units. Other U.S. aircrews attack targets far behind enemy lines. Both FACs and attack aircrews may be forced to crash-land or bail out, and may subsequently show symptoms of battle fatigue which could harden into post-traumatic stress disorder (PTSD). Transport aircraft crews could crash or be disabled while making air drops or flying into forward U.S. Army air strips. Some U.S. aircrews may be shot down behind enemy lines and reach U.S. lines only after extended periods of escape and evasion under conditions of extreme physical and mental stress. Other downed airmen may be extracted from behind enemy lines by U.S. Army helicopters or Special Operations. Some may be brought to U.S. Army medical facilities after being rescued or exchanged as prisoners of war.

The line unit leaders and medical personnel who encounter U.S. Air Force aircrews first should automatically apply all of the principles and methods of treating battle fatigue: reassurance; rehydration; nutrition; sleep; restoring hygiene; opportunity to talk about and ventilate the experience; and appropriate self-care duties that restore confidence. It is important *not* to predict psychopathology, and to instead convey the quiet expectation of return-to-duty. The airman should be transported (not "evacuated") back as soon as possible to their unit's air base or to the U.S. Air Force medical facilities (described earlier) which support that base.

If more serious signs of battle fatigue develop or persist while the airman is awaiting transportation, combat stress control personnel talk with the airman to reinforce the initial crisis intervention. They emphasize the normality of the symptoms and the likelihood of their rapid improvement.

U.S. Army Units Stationed near U.S. Air Force Bases

U.S. Army units, especially combat-support/service-support units, may be located on or close to U.S. Air Force bases. These may lack organic mental health support and be distant from U.S. Army combat stress control unit elements. The combat stress unit of the U.S. Air Force's tactical hospital should provide proactive consultation and mental health support to the U.S. Army units. For example, in the Persian Gulf War one combat stress unit provided such outreach support to a U.S. Army transportation battalion whose drivers drove very long, dangerous convoys on the Tapline Road and a Patriot air defense artillery battalion under heavy stress defending against the Scud missiles.[5]

Forward U.S. Air Force Bases under Attack

U.S. Air Force bases will be located in the corps and communication zone, and perhaps even in division areas as the battle progresses or in unconventional counterinsurgency conflict. The air bases' ability to function may be severely degraded in high-intensity conflicts. Air bases are natural targets for air and long-range missile attack, including time bombs, cluster bomblets, persistent chemical and/or nuclear weapons. Even in low-intensity conflicts, they are targets of mortar, short-range rocket and sapper attacks. Because of their stockpiles of munitions and fuel, even small attacks on air bases can produce catastrophic disasters. Even in peacetime, air crashes can also produce sudden mass casualties and widespread devastation.

U.S. Army units will be located next to air bases, both in the corps areas and communications zone, and may be detailed to reinforce their organic ground defense (air police) and antiair/antimissile defense capability. Forward air bases, especially those that do not have an area theater hospital, will have very limited medical/surgical resources, and may need routine support from nearby U.S. Army medical units. This could include combat stress control consultation and neuropsychiatric triage/stabilization from the MH/CSC personnel of the area support medical battalion; CSC company; or CSH, field, or general hospital. Only after careful coordination might U.S. Army combat stress control units provide restoration or reconditioning for air base personnel, in preference to evacuation to rear echelon U.S. Air Force facilities.

In the event of mass casualties at the air base, U.S. Army combat stress control teams, along with other medical units, could provide emergency triage and reconstitution support. As soon as possible, these teams would be joined by (and continue to work with) additional U.S. Air Force combat stress unit (CSU) disaster response teams sent to the site. As suggested above, mass casualties or traumatic crashes can occur in peacetime. The following case history illustrates support by U.S. Army Combat Stress Control teams to a U.S. Air Force base.

Case Study 1: Mass Murders at a U.S. Air Force Base

A disgruntled ex-airman who had been discharged from the U.S. Air Force on psychiatric grounds entered the hospital of Fairchild Air Force Base (Spokane, Washington) with an automatic weapon. He killed the psychiatrist while the doctor was providing therapy to a patient, killed the psychologist, then stalked through the hospital, randomly shooting patients and staff in the corridors and waiting rooms. He was finally shot and killed in the parking lot by U.S. Air Force security police. On hearing the news, the psychiatrist commander of the U.S. Army's 98th combat stress control detachment (Fort Lewis, Washington) contacted the surviving members of the Fairchild mental health section and offered to send a team to assist. The hospital commander concurred, but the initial reaction at a higher U.S. Air Force echelon was that the U.S. Air Force was sending its own teams and a U.S. Army team would be superfluous. The Fairchild and Fort Lewis mental health personnel mobilized general officer support to reemphasize the potential mutual value of the U.S. Army team's participation, and approval was quickly granted. A four-person CSC preventive team (a psychiatrist, social worker, and two enlisted personnel) deployed by commercial air within 2 days. Their orders had been pushed through the system by their higher TO&E headquarters over a weekend, and their travel funding provided by the medical activity.

At Fairchild Air Force Base, the U.S. Army team interfaced well with, and provided debriefing support to, the surviving U.S. Air Force social work officer and behavioral science technicians. While reinforcing U.S. Air Force stress teams worked in consultation and debriefing with other hospital staff, patient, and community groups, the U.S. Army team was given responsibility for assisting the U.S. Air Force Security Police who had been involved in the incident. They also assisted the mental health section in scheduled and special psychotherapy for their outpatients, who were deeply distressed by the deaths of their therapists. Those sessions were conducted in a temporary clinic away from the hospital, which was closed for forensic evidence collection and necessary cleanup and repairs.

While these activities were still ongoing, a B-52 bomber crashed on base while practicing low-altitude stunt maneuvers. All the crew were killed. A second four-person team of the 98th CSC detachment was hastily deployed from Fort Lewis, Washington. It assisted with debriefings of the emergency crews and others who rushed to the crash site and recovered the bodies. Upon completion of their work, both teams returned to Fort Lewis.

Comment: The nature of the horrible mass murder was such as to impact on the entire Fairchild Air Force Base community and the surrounding retiree outpatient population. While the U.S. Air Force could have mobilized sufficient stress and mental health teams from other bases and medical centers, that would have put a greater strain on quality of care elsewhere in the U.S. Air Force system. It made tactical and economic sense to include in this relief effort the teams from a relatively nearby U.S. Army unit that had been trained in the mission of quick deployment to deal with critical events. The tragic opportunity provided excellent clinical experience for the U.S. Army teams. It also provided administrative experience in coordinating a rapid joint operation in the peacetime, garrison force. When the B-52 crash compounded the trauma for the Fairchild Air Force Base community, it was simple to reinforce the effort.

Initial Rapid Deployment Contingency Operations

In rapid deployment contingency operations, such as Operation Just Cause (Panama, 1989), medical care at the airhead may at first be provided only by the U.S. Air Force personnel of the Aeromedical Evacuation Squadron (operating a mobile aeromedical staging facility). These may be augmented by U.S. Army surgical squads (forward surgical teams). None of these units have organic MH/CSC personnel, although psychiatric nurses may have been assigned to fill surgical nurse vacancies. Battle fatigue and neuropsychiatry cases for all services will probably be brought to this facility along with the seriously wounded, ill, and injured. Many cases may have had no prior MH/CSC evaluation.

The ability of this facility to prevent the overevacuation of simple stress casualties (including battle fatigue, minor heat exhaustion, mild concussion, and other conditions) is severely limited by its preoccupation with the seriously injured. However, training the triage officers and other patient care providers in combat stress control principles can enable them to hold and return to duty stress casualties. This is normally accomplished after the initial rush of surgical cases has been treated. In Operation Just Cause, the U.S. Air Force nursing personnel did hold and return to duty a U.S. Army battle fatigue casualty on the third to fourth day of the operation. The following case is taken from the Persian Gulf War.

Case Study 2: Chaplain's Assistant

In the Persian Gulf War, the medical company of the U.S. Army armored brigade had moved into Kuwait close behind the armored battalions. Battles against Iraqi armor and infantry were still going on. Several kilometers away, U.S. air power attacked Iraqi forces that had dug in around a mosque. In the aftermath, it was discovered that Kuwaiti civilians had taken refuge in that mosque, and some had been killed or wounded by the "collateral damage." The medical company hastily sent a mass casualty response team, which included the brigade's U.S. Army psychiatrist, the forward support battalion chaplain, and the chaplain's assistant. The psychiatrist remembers vividly the image of the chaplain's assistant coming out of the wreckage carrying two very young girls, one dead and the other seriously injured. Over the next several hours as the surviving casualties were transported to the medical company and given emergency care, there was no time to conduct an immediate debriefing. The chaplain's assistant became silent and preoccupied, withdrew from the group, and finally began to shake uncontrollably, barely able to communicate. The psychiatrist would have preferred to treat him on site, but armored battles were still occurring nearby and there was the possibility of another mass casualty or emergency move. He could neither devote full attention to this one stress casualty nor trust that casualty to respond appropriately and safely in an emergency. Reluctantly, he sent him with the other casualties on a truck going back to the U.S. Marine surgical support company (and combat stress center) in Saudi Arabia.

Several days later, the chaplain's assistant was returned to duty in the forward support battalion. By this time, the ground campaign had concluded, but the unit was still occupied with the dangerous and often gruesome process of securing the battlefield. The chaplain's assistant was able to participate in the unit's new missions in his original role, and demobilize and return home with it.

Comment: This case illustrates the constraints that the tactical situation can impose on preventive and treatment intervention at far-forward medical facilities. The U.S. Marine Corps/U.S. Navy backup system was able to function and return the soldier to duty quickly. This reduced (if not eliminated) the risk of PTSD developing from what was a highly traumatic event for all the medical personnel, and arguably an even higher psychological trauma for a young man in the chaplain corps.

The capability to return stress casualties to duty at a forward deployed aeromedical evacuation squadron and U.S. Army surgical team task force could be greatly improved at little cost. This could be accomplished by providing one or two NCO or officer personnel (preferably with MH/CSC training), plus some very spartan "sheltering" (not formal "patient holding") and supplies. Local buildings, hangers, or improvised shelter may be sufficient. The supervisory personnel could be either from a U.S. Army unit mental health section, from a U.S. Army medical combat stress control detachment or company, or from a U.S. Air Force unit. To be fully effective, this augmentation must be present at the outset of the operation. If it arrives later, the majority of stress casualties who arrived with the first, second, or third rush of badly wounded cases will already have been evacuated.

In addition to preventing the loss of "pure" battle fatigue cases, this austere restoration capability could also permit holding and return to duty of some minor disease nonbattle injuries whose over-evacuation could result in psychological harm. Such cases include members of elite units (such as U.S. Army Airborne, Ranger, and Special Operations Forces, and U.S. Navy SEALS [SEa Air Land commandoS], descendants of the World War II Underwater Demolition Teams) who tend to regard evacuation for minor orthopedic jump injuries, heat exhaustion, dehydration, or mild concussion as dishonoring. Such patients may often volunteer to be allowed to remain at the mobile aeromedical staging facility (MASF) for one to three days, eating meals-ready-to-eat (MREs), sleeping on ground pads, providing local security, and helping out within the limits set by their minor disability, rather than be evacuated far from their comrades. This could be medically permissible, provided the delay does not increase the risk of death or permanent disability from an inadequately diagnosed condition. If such selected cases *are* held, and later evaluation indicates that they can still not return to limited or full duty in their units, they could then be evacuated without feeling shame or guilt. The MH/CSC personnel who supervise such cases would also initiate stress debriefing for those wounded in action (WIA) who were awaiting evacuation and for the medical staff.

Ongoing Combat Operations

As the theater stabilizes, the aeromedical evacuation squadrons will continue the primary role of staffing mobile air staging facilities. These facilities, located at air bases and simple landing strips, receive patients from the combat zone hospitals. They hold the patients for several hours, providing continuity of care until the patients can be loaded onto aircraft for air evacuation to the communications zone or the continental United States (CONUS). Some of the airframes may be dedicated medical aircraft; however, most aircraft that depart from the combat zone will be general purpose cargo aircraft (C130s, C141s, a few C5As, the future C17) hastily reconfigured with litter sets. The MASF also serves as the rest and staging area for the in-flight nursing personnel.

The MASFs will deal with three types of patients who pose stress or psychiatric issues:

1. *True, severe neuropsychiatric patients.* By doctrine, these will arrive and be transported on litters, in restraints, well medicated and sedated. Only if departure is delayed by weather or other mishap will these patients pose problems.
2. *Wounded or injury cases with significant psychological distress or organic mental disorder.* These may create a considerable strain on the MASF staff and the in-flight nursing crews. Both the patients and the staff could benefit from special MH/CSC advice regarding their psychological and pharmacologic management.
3. *Battle fatigue cases who have not responded to restoration or reconditioning and who are being evacuated to COMMZ or CONUS for further reconditioning or treatment for PTSD.* These soldiers should be ambulatory, but may have been given long-acting antianxiety medication (such as diazepam) for the flight. It is important that the MASF and in-flight personnel maintain the sense of positive expectation of full and rapid recovery. They, too, should treat these cases as service members being transferred temporarily to the rear, not as sick or "mental" patients. However, unless the flight personnel have been thoroughly briefed and reassured by the neuropsychiatry or MH/CSC consultants, they may insist that these battle fatigue cases be restrained on litters, causing some psychological harm. (If that *must* be done, it should be explained as giving the service member better opportunity to sleep on a long and possibly bumpy flight.)

Personnel from the combat support hospital's neuropsychiatry ward and consultation service, the area support medical battalion mental health section, and/or the medical combat stress control detachment or company should maintain regular contact with the MASF personnel. This is important both to assure the correct management of the stress and neuropsychiatric evacuations and also to assist the MASF and in-flight U.S. Air Force nursing staffs with processing their own, high-stress experiences.

During a Major Buildup

In the buildup phase of a rapidly developing contingency theater, one or more airfields will be major points of entry for U.S. Army (and perhaps Marine) forces into the country. The U.S. Air Force 50-bed air transportable hospitals at the airfields are likely to be the first U.S. Echelon II/III hospitals set up in the country. U.S. Army clearing companies and mobile army surgical hospitals, if they arrive by air, will probably move quickly off the airfields to support the maneuver units. U.S. Army unit medical and CSC personnel should determine what U.S. Air Force medical facility is supporting the airfield and its vicinity. If possible, this information should be provided before the units leave CONUS. As U.S. Army units continue to pour into the points of air debarkation, any soldiers who develop serious stress, physical, or neuropsychiatric symptoms in flight or soon after landing could be brought to the U.S. Air Force facilities for evaluation and care.

If feasible after landing, the U.S. Army medical and combat stress control personnel should visit the U.S. Air Force facility to review basic doctrine for the triage and treatment of stress casualties. They should coordinate the procedures for returning *duty* battle fatigue cases to their units immediately (prior to the unit's departure from the airfield or temporary assembly area). They should coordinate where restoration battle fatigue (*rest* battle fatigue) cases can be sent for 1 to 2 days' light duty with the soldier's unit's own combat service support elements. Depending on staffing and workload, it may be possible for the area theater hospital's combat stress unit to provide 1- to 2-day observation and restoration for any *hold* battle fatigue cases. Here, too, coordination for how to return recovered cases to their units (which are themselves in transit) will be critical.

In the unlikely event that many stress casualties developed in flight or soon after arrival, it may be useful for the U.S. Army division mental health section, area support medical battalion mental health section, or combat stress control detachment or company to temporarily reinforce the U.S. Air Force combat stress unit at the area theater hospital while many units are flowing through the airhead.

Every reasonable effort should be made to apply the principles of PIES and the method of the Five Rs to prevent the unnecessary evacuation of stress, fatigue, jet lag, and minor somatic and orthopedic overuse syndromes from the theater soon after their arrival. Most of these cases will present with physical, not emotional, complaints. Over-evacuation may cause permanent psychological harm to the patients. It may also grow into an "evacuation syndrome" (see Chapter 1) as other new arrivals under stress consciously or unconsciously develop the same symptoms. Malingerers, who are deliberately faking or self-inflicting symptoms, should be returned to their units in the theater for disciplinary action.

During Redeployment Home

To a lesser extent, U.S. Army units may also need to rely on U.S. Air Force area theater hospitals or contingency hospitals at the airheads during some phases of redeployment to CONUS after the conflict is over. In this case, the stress issue will not be apprehension over impending battle but rather impatience to get home, perhaps mixed with apprehension in some soldiers over what they will find there.

U.S. Air Force and U.S. Army medical/combat stress control personnel should coordinate their preventive consultation and triage practices to discourage the tendency for some soldiers and airmen to develop stress syndromes in the unconscious or conscious wish to get home before the rest of their unit. The MH/CSC personnel may also provide or facilitate prereunion briefings and discussion groups to defuse potential homecoming stress. Coordination with the chaplains of both services is essential to this effort.

Post-traumatic stress symptoms may also be present, but are more likely to be mentally suppressed by the focus on putting the unpleasant experiences behind one and going home. U.S. Army and U.S. Air Force MH/CSC personnel may be able to cooperate and pool dwindling resources (along with the chaplains) to provide preventive after-action stress briefings or critical event debriefings to individuals, groups, or units at special risk.

Situations for CSC Cooperation Among the U.S. Army, Navy, and Marine Corps

As with the U.S. Air Force, a number of situations will require cooperation between U.S. Army, U.S. Navy, and U.S. Marine Corps personnel.

U.S. Navy/Marine Corps Liaison Personnel in Army Units

In combat actions close to the ocean, where U.S. Army units can receive close air support or gunfire support from U.S. Navy ships offshore, the U.S. Army headquarters units may be augmented by U.S. Navy or U.S. Marine Corps air liaison teams and naval gunfire liaison teams. If these personnel develop battle fatigue, they should be treated in the same way as the U.S. Army and U.S. Air Force personnel and in the same facilities close to the U.S. Army unit.

Downed Pilots

If U.S. Navy or U.S. Marine Corps aviators are shot down over U.S. Army territory or are recovered from behind enemy lines, they should be treated as indicated above while they are being returned to their units or to U.S. Navy/U.S. Marine Corps medical facilities. Conversely, U.S. Army aviators who are recovered or rescued by U.S. Marine Corps or U.S. Navy units should receive similar treatment from their rescuers and, if necessary, from U.S. Marine Corps/U.S. Navy MH/CSC personnel until returned to the U.S. Army.

Neighboring Units

If U.S. Marine Corps and U.S. Army units are fighting alongside each other, as happened in the World War II Pacific Theater, Korea, Vietnam, and Southwest Asia, they may use each other's medical/surgical facilities. This would most likely occur as a result or side effect of the air evacuation of serious surgical wounded cases.

The U.S. Marine Corps/U.S. Navy medical battalion does not have dedicated medical evacuation vehicles. Evacuation of any casualties by air must use general purpose helicopters or request U.S. Army "dustoff" medevac. In the latter case, they may be brought to U.S. Army medical treatment facilities. Ground evacuation must be coordinated using ground vehicles in backhaul. This latter is the U.S. Army's doctrinally preferred way to transport *all* battle fatigue cases. Stress casualties traveling by truck will naturally be brought to their own service's medical clearing facilities. However, in the confusion of real operations, doctrine restricting the air evacuation of stress casualties may be set aside. In crisis situations, line commanders and forward medical personnel will seek to clear the battlefield of all noneffective casualties.

Those stress cases who show symptoms of amnesia, loss of motor or sensory functions or agitation (in particular), may be sent immediately by air or ground to a hospital to rule out serious physical causes. This could be the hospital of the other service. It will be necessary to extract any such stress cases from the evacuation chain and return them to suitable battle fatigue restoration facilities. In this situation, it is important to get the service member back to his own service as soon as possible.

In a large-scale operation near the ocean, a U.S. Navy hospital ship is quite likely to reach the theater before U.S. Army combat surgical hospitals have arrived and been set up. On one hospital ship in the Persian Gulf during Operation Desert Shield/Storm, 9% of psychiatric admissions were U.S. Army personnel and 5% were U.S. Air Force personnel.[6]

While the hospital ship's neuropsychiatric ward provides a suitable place to stabilize true neuropsychiatric cases for further evacuation, it is not well suited to restoring U.S. Army battle fatigue casualties to duty. The shipboard environment, even of the non–patient-care combat stress control bay, would be both unfamiliar and seemingly remote from the soldiers' units. Extra effort would be necessary to maintain positive expectation and the sense of proximity. The potentially recoverable U.S. Army soldier should be transferred to a restoration and reconditioning center ashore as soon as possible. The same concerns are probably relevant to U.S. Air Force stress casualties evacuated to a hospital ship.

The shipboard setting may be less significant for U.S. Marines treated for stress on the hospital ship's combat stress center, as they are accustomed to going directly from ships to ground combat. It may be even less a problem for U.S. Navy shipboard sailors who are recovering from battle fatigue incurred in ship disasters or combat. Prompt return to the service member's original unit or ship remains crucial to maximizing recovery.

Cross-Attached Units

U.S. Army battalions or brigades may be cross-attached to U.S. Marine Corps task forces or divisions, and U.S. Marine Corps elements may be cross-attached to U.S. Army units. For Operation Desert Storm, a U.S. Army armored brigade was attached to a U.S. Marine Corps division to give it M1A1 (Abrams) tank capability. The U.S. Army Operations and Sea Force concepts for the post-Cold War world make such cross-attachment increasingly likely.

U.S. Army personnel who are evacuated to a U.S. Marine Corps/U.S. Navy/U.S. Air Force facility, such as to the psychiatric or combat stress center at an MH/CSC should receive the correct treatment for battle fatigue there. In the Persian Gulf War, a U.S. Army combat stress control officer/NCO team (from the division mental health section) with the U.S. Army armored brigade had to refer four combat stress casualties back through U.S. Marine Corps/U.S. Navy channels. One, who proved to have additional neuropsychiatric problems, was evacuated to a U.S. Air Force hospital in England. Three returned to duty with their U.S. Army unit in days, proving that joint combat stress control interventions can work.

Case Study 3: Light Battle Fatigue

During the Persian Gulf War, a soldier arrived at night by helicopter, along with several wounded soldiers. He had the 1,000 yard stare, sat passively, and responded slowly to questions in one or two words only with firm prompting. He knew his name, rank, serial number, and unit, but was unable to describe what had happened. The medical/surgical nurses who triaged him knew the principles of BICEPS, and it was feasible to hold him for the night because the initial surge of surgical mass casualties had slowed and a holding tent with cots had finally arrived. The orthopedic surgeon they consulted trusted their triage judgment. The soldier was given verbal reassurance and taken to lie down and sleep. The next morning the nurses found the soldier at the mess line, wolfing down breakfast. He said he was "fine," and had to get back to his unit. He was still unclear about what had happened when the unit had "taken heavy flak," and only vaguely remembered being brought by helicopter and talking with someone in the night. He was assigned to performing work details around the MASF while waiting for his unit to pick him up. Indeed, he complained so much about the menial duties that the U.S. Air Force nurse reminded him that she was the officer and he the enlisted soldier, that one of them had to do these duties, and she said it was to be he. Both were happy when his unit's truck arrived to take him back to duty.

Comment: Had this soldier been evacuated to San Antonio, Texas and home base, it is quite likely that he would have become a true psychiatric casualty, left the U.S. Army, and perhaps developed long-term disability.

Battle fatigue casualties in U.S. Marine Corps combat units that are working under U.S. Army command/control should be transported to their own medical units if such units have been included in the task force from the Force Service Support Group. These medical units could be augmented by combat stress control personnel or teams from the U.S. Army division mental health section, combat stress control detachment, or combat stress control company. If no U.S. Marine Corps medical battalion companies are included, U.S. Marine Corps stress casualties should be sent to the nearest U.S. Army brigade, division, or area support clearing company with combat stress control capability.

During a Major Buildup

The U.S. Army now has cargo ships with preconfigured unit sets of equipment pre-positioned strategically around the world. These are a seagoing version of the European theater's "POMCUS" (pre-positioned overseas material configured unit sets) sites. The ships can sail to a suitable port at the threatened host nation, to which the soldiers can be flown from their units in CONUS. Other U.S. Army units will load their heavy equipment onto fast cargo ships at ports of embarkation in CONUS (or Europe, as in the Persian Gulf War). The ships sail to the theater, while the troops finish predeployment preparation at home station and fly to the theater in time to meet the ships at the port of debarkation. U.S. Army transportation units have the mission and equipment to unload these ships at the port. If hostilities have begun, the port is likely to be the target of a long-range missile, air, or terrorist attack, adding to the stress of very long, hard working hours in crowded spaces.

Initial U.S. Army units assembling at a seaport of entry could utilize the combat stress unit of a U.S. Air Force air-transportable hospital at the airfield. Alternatively, they might utilize the medical collection and clearing company or surgical support company of a U.S. Marine Expeditionary Force if any of those have been landed. Those facilities could have the U.S. Navy psychologist and/or psychiatric corpsmen. The U.S. Army contingent in the port could eventually receive echelon II medical support from a U.S. Army area support medical company, which should have a 91G NCO and perhaps the social worker or psychiatrist of the area support medical battalion. These could also support the U.S. Navy, U.S. Marine Corps, and U.S. Air Force units.

Later in the buildup, U.S. Army troop units that are landing from ships at a port of embarkation or awaiting the arrival of their equipment by ship could receive MH/CSC consultation and treatment support from a nearby Fleet hospital if no U.S. Army MH/CSC or combat support hospital neuropsychiatric assets are available. In the Persian Gulf War, the fleet hospital in Bahrain did provide the neuropsychiatric ward capability for a nearby U.S. Army combat support hospital which (having the pre-MedForce 2000 TO&E) had no organic mental health/neuropsychiatry personnel. Conversely, a U.S. Army combat support hospital's neuropsychiatric ward and consult service could care for U.S. Navy and U.S. Marines (and U.S. Air Force) cases if no fleet hospital had arrived.

During Redeployment Home

Some U.S. Army combat service support units may have to remain longer in the theater than other units to load equipment on ships for transport home. These units should be supported by U.S. Army combat stress control teams, but could also be supported by personnel from the U.S. Navy fleet hospital if it has not already been redeployed. This will work best if the fleet hospital neuropsychiatry personnel practice preventive outreach consultation. Conversely, the U.S. Army combat stress control teams could provide proactive prevention and treatment as needed by U.S. Navy dockside or shipboard personnel in the port, if the fleet hospital or other U.S. Navy combat stress control is not available or needs reinforcement.

Joint SPRINT Operations

In peacetime or military operations short of war, joint special psychiatric rapid intervention teams may be hastily task-organized to support a major U.S. Navy, U.S. Marine Corps, or U.S. Army reorganization/reconstitution support mission. For example, following the Iraqi Exocet missile attack on the *USS Stark*, a joint U.S. Navy-U.S. Army team was deployed to debrief surviving crew members. Crew members were debriefed as they worked on the damaged ship next to a tender at Bahrain. The team consisted of U.S. Navy SPRINT personnel out of Spain, plus members of a U.S. Army stress management team from 7th Medical Command, Europe. The U.S. Army team had had extensive experience in responding to terrorist and hostage incidents. The activities of that joint team have been published.[7]

JOINT OR COMBINED OPERATIONS OTHER THAN WAR

Overview

The post-Cold War world will continue to call upon the U.S. armed forces to conduct peacekeeping, humanitarian civil assistance (international disaster relief), and nation assistance (public health, engineering, and other projects) in which no combat is anticipated. Alternatively, the unstable situation may call for peace enforcement ("peacemaking"), noncombatant evacuation operations, or foreign internal defense training missions to countries that are experiencing terrorism or insurgency warfare. In these situations, U.S. forces are at higher risk of having to fire in self-defense, but with very restrictive rules of engagement. While some of these operations may be of brief duration and clear objective, others may be greatly prolonged, with no clear endpoint. Most such operations will be joint operations, and many may be coalition operations under multinational or United Nations auspices.

CSC Mission Priorities

The combat stress control mission in stressful operations other than war (in usual order of priority because of relevance) is to:

1. *Prevent post-traumatic stress disorder (PTSD).* This is a risk for the service members who must encounter extreme human suffering, victims of injustice or atrocity, and perhaps confused combat under ambiguous, restricting rules of engagement. Preventive activities are indicated routinely, because stress or PTSD symptoms may not be evident at the time.
2. *Prevent misconduct stress behaviors.* Stress-induced misconduct can be due to tension, high ambiguity of friend vs foe, reaction to atrocities seen or casualties sustained, cultural friction, frustration, boredom, tedium, and let-down. There may be special temptations for alcohol or drug abuse, because of local availability, lack of routine urine screening as a deterrent, and casual use of substances by coalition allies or the local population. Unless prevented, weakening discipline could escalate to use of excessive force and even commission of atrocities. Such misconduct would invalidate the humanitarian mission in the eyes of the local population, the media, and U.S. and world opinion. Because criminal violation of the Uniform Code of Military Justice and international law *must* be publicly investigated and punished, combat stress control preventive advice to leaders in how to recognize and defuse early signs of stress is critical to success.
3. *Prevent and treat (return to duty) battle fatigue or contingency fatigue.* This is done in the usual ways. In static operations other than war, it is expected that most such cases can be helped in their own units while still on duty, or be rested for a day or two in a nonmedical support element. Few will normally need medical holding, and very *few* should be evacuated.
4. *Prevent, diagnose, stabilize, and evacuate or return to duty any neuropsychiatric disorders (environmental or substance-induced organic ones, and the endemic functional disorders).* These may include cases with psychiatric disorders who were on medication from civilian sources without wanting it on their military records. They may relapse when supply runs out, or have medication side effects aggravated by the local climate. If feasible, they should be tapered off medication or shifted to drugs that can be continued safely in theater. In some soldiers, the situations observed in the operation may activate PTSD from prior combat, childhood, or inner city experiences. If PTSD is reactivated from prior traumatic exposure it would be best to treat in the theater, working through past and current trauma simultaneously, if that is feasible.

CSC Staffing

The CSC support for an operation other than war should be tailored to the specific mission, the expected stressors and the size and mix of forces deployed. This will have to be determined by experience and perhaps at first by trial and error. For instance:

Vignette 1: Sinai peacekeeping missions involve about 1,000 U.S. troops in a multinational coalition on 6-month rotations in desert observation. Conditions are stable, with no combat, but occasional accidental injury or deaths occur. While no mental health support is required, having a mental health/combat stress control NCO, an officer or an officer/NCO team on site significantly reduces problems in the unit. These personnel are frequently requested by command. Social workers, psychologists, psychiatrists, occupational therapists and 91G behavioral science NCOs have filled these assignments.

Vignette 2: Medical support for U.N. peacekeeping troops in Croatia involved a U.S. mobile army surgical hospital (MASH) augmented with a social worker/91G team, located in Zagreb. These provide MH/CSC services to sick, injured, or wounded peacekeepers from many countries, often working through translators. They also support the hospital staff and cooperate with allied (British, Dutch) mental health personnel. A 50-bed U.S.

Air Force air-transportable hospital staff replaced the U.S. Army MASH in the rotation plan. Six months later, staff from a U.S. Navy fleet hospital took over the facility, including a psychiatrist, psychiatric nurse, and psychiatry technicians.

Vignette 3: Operation Restore Hope in Somalia was initially "front-end loaded" to support about 28,000 troops with a U.S. Army light infantry division's mental health section of a psychiatrist, social worker, psychologist and several 9IGs supporting one brigade (plus) at several locations; a U.S. Army medical group headquarters with a social worker, psychologist, and 91G; a U.S. Marine Corps medical battalion (minus) with a filler U.S. Navy psychiatrist, psychologist, and corpsman. No shipboard mental health neuropsychiatric personnel were involved. A U.S. Army medical combat stress control detachment's preventive section with three psychiatrists, three social workers, and six 9IGs (social work technicians), was deployed. A U.S. Army combat support hospital (minus) with a psychiatrist, psychiatric nurse, and two 9IFs (psychiatric ward aids) was also deployed. No U.S. Air Force mental health personnel were deployed to Somalia with the U.S. Air Force's MASF team. A 50-bed air-transportable hospital with a social worker supported the staging facility at Cairo West, Egypt.

The various elements coordinated activities to provide mental health outpatient and brief inpatient therapy, mobile preventive consultation and education, and critical event debriefing (CED). The CEDs followed deaths of unit members, deaths of Somali civilians under stressful circumstances, and other highly traumatic events. The U.S. Army CSC teams debriefed U.S. Marine Corps companies following two combat deaths and a suicide. (They also debriefed an Australian unit following a death by accidental weapons discharge.) They provided consultation to the U.S. Air Force AeroMedical Evacuation Squadron.

As the situation in Somalia became clearer, the U.S. Navy/U.S. Marine Corps and the U.S. Army Medical Group quickly sent their mental health personnel home. The U.S. Army division mental health section and combat stress control detachment sent their personnel home later by increments, each replacing them eventually with one social work officer each and one 91G each as the force in country sank below 4,000. The U.S. Army combat support hospital neuropsychiatric section rotated home with the hospital, being replaced by a field hospital with no mental health/neuropsychiatric personnel.

Vignette 4: Operation Continue Hope (in Mogadishu, Somalia under United Nations auspices) began with the two U.S. Army social workers and two 9IGs as above, supporting 4,000 U.S. Army troops plus a few U.S. Marines, U.S. Air Force, and U.S. Navy personnel in the U.N. headquarters. The division social worker was then recalled home on compassionate grounds.

The combat stress control detachment social worker and 91G worked out of the field hospital, providing case evaluation and treatment plus active preventive education and critical event debriefing to units. Workload increased as ambushes caused mass casualties among the coalition allies and sporadic injuries and eventually deaths to U.S. service members. Nocturnal mortar and rocket attacks also harassed the five United Nation's cantonment areas in the city. The combat stress control officer also assisted with debriefings and prebriefings of the Swedish hospital's personnel, and of coalition wounded at the U.S. Army CSH.

Efforts to reinforce the combat stress control detachment officer and NCO rapidly with an occupational therapist and NCO were frustrated. Eventually, after 3 months, the combat stress control detachment team rotated, replaced by two social workers and two 9IGs, while fighting and U.S. casualties continued to escalate. The 10th Mountain Division replaced its one 91G with two. The new U.S. Army combat stress control team later provided training and debriefing supervision to the U.S. Navy corpsmen supporting a 50-man U.S. Marine Corps detachment at the United Nations headquarters after three U.S. Marines were wounded and a Somali interpreter was killed by a command-detonated mine. There were still only the two U.S. Army mental health social work officers and three 9IGs in Somalia when U.S. casualties escalated markedly in early October 1993, followed by a rapid U.S. Army troop buildup. These worked as best they could to provide mobile, preventive consultation and debriefings until rotating home late in the withdrawal of U.S. troops.

Lessons Learned from Recent Experience

1. Joint coordination in planning total combat stress control staffing capability in theater can be improved.
2. It is relatively easy to "front end load" MH/CSC personnel into operations other than war, when the combat arms aren't dictating that their personnel and warfighting logistical needs require all the transport capability.
3. It is relatively easy to send people or increments home early.
4. It may be almost impossible to reinforce the theater rapidly with more CSC assets (at least by the U.S. Army). Therefore don't send too much home too soon.
5. U.S. Army CSC detachments can be deployed in increments and maintain a rotation schedule. There is still resistance (prejudice) against sending occupational therapy and psychiatric nursing expertise on CSC missions, which must be overcome.
6. Preventive workload estimate is that there should be no less than two MH/CSC officers and two NCOs for a brigade-sized (joint) force; and sufficient officer/NCO

teams to visit each company-sized unit (approximately 100 men) for 1 hour weekly, and more often and longer when critical event or end-of-tour debriefings are needed.

Joint Special Operations

Overview

Special Operations Forces prepare for and support battle in all levels of open conflict. They also play a major role in military operations other than war, including nation assistance ("building") and humanitarian civil assistance, disaster or refugee relief, counternarcotics, counterterrorism, intelligence gathering, peacekeeping/peacemaking, search and rescue (open and covert), strikes and raids, and noncombatant evacuation operations. While some of these operations may be well-publicized after the fact, most of them (and especially the Special Operations aspects of them) generally keep a low profile and avoid attention. Some are covert, and some are deeply covert.

Special Operations Forces

The U.S. Army has Special Operations Forces ranging from the well-known Airborne Ranger Battalions and the Special Forces ("Green Berets" of the 1960s) to the secretive but highly publicized Delta Force (counterterrorist team), the Psychological Operations (PSYOPS) units which provide printing and broadcasting capability, the Civil Affairs units, Long Range Surveillance Companies, and a special helicopter aviation unit. The U.S. Navy has the SEALs, and the U.S. Marines have Force Recon. The U.S. Air Force has Special Operations Forces aviation units. There may be other military and government intelligence and covert operations units whose very existence is a secret.

Mental Health Capability in Special Operations Forces

Because of the strict requirement for secrecy, Special Operations Forces (SOF) units have their own psychologists and perhaps other mental health personnel, who also avoid publicity. The psychologists have an important role in screening applicants for suitability for special operations, monitoring the high stress training and selection process, and providing ongoing personnel reliability and readiness-for-duty evaluations. They may debrief SOF teams after critical events. Many of these tasks cannot be done by regular MH/CSC personnel who lack the necessary organizational trust and security clearances. The SOF MH personnel presumably also provide or arrange mental health psychiatric treatment for whatever neuropsychiatric disorders arise among their highly selected but highly stressed and somewhat atypical populations. The families of the SOF personnel (and SOF personnel in nonsensitive positions) are presumably cared for by the routine mental health/medical system.

Contact Between Special Operations and Conventional MH/CSC

In deployments and combat, Special Operations Forces personnel can develop disabling battle (conflict) fatigue, misconduct stress behaviors, posttraumatic stress disorders, and stress-induced functional or organic neuropsychiatric disorders. They may then be brought to conventional MH/CSC personnel or facilities because they need urgent management or care, and the few Special Operations MH/CSC personnel are not immediately on hand. Wounded or sick Special Operations Forces personnel will usually be evacuated through conventional channels. This can create a problem for those in highly covert units because they and their organizations go to great lengths to maintain secrecy (even to the extent of deleting the cases from the medical record and patient flow statistics).

The conventional MH/CSC clinician (U.S. Army, U.S. Navy, or U.S. Air Force) could find himself trying to diagnose whether the service member who refuses to tell him anything about himself or his unit (or who is rambling deliriously about his "secret mission") has a paranoid or grandiose delusion, is deliberately faking for personal reasons or to get over on the system (malingering), or really does belong to the Special Operations Forces. The answer may not be easy to get quickly.

If the latter case is true, it would be best to get the service member back under the care of Special Operations Forces specialists. Like the downed U.S. Air Force, U.S. Navy, or U.S. Army pilots who are best returned to their own roots, the return to the Special Operations Forces environment may be more therapeutic than keeping the case further forward among strangers. This may be a situation where SOF-trained MH/CSC personnel of a different service could be more effective than non-SOF personnel of the same service.

For less dramatic SOF cases that qualify as routine battle (conflict) fatigue, the Five Rs should still work to get the service member back to his own forward-deployed unit in 1 to 3 days. The primary modification would be not to push the debriefing phase to the point of describing a secret mission in great detail. The main effort is to restore and build on the SOF ethic of resilience and elite reputation. Because of that SOF elite identity, SOF personnel may be more likely to present with the loss of physical abilities forms (somatoform disorders) of battle fatigue than with the overtly emotional forms. This adds to the problems of differential diagnoses.

Joint Prisoner of War or Hostage Repatriation

Prisoner or hostage repatriation is often a joint operation. The prisoners of war (POWs) may come from two or more services. The U.S. Air Force is likely to fly the survivors from their release point to one of the service's hospitals for a thorough physical examination and treatment of any injuries or illnesses. There, they will be subjected to intensive intelligence debriefings whose primary purpose is to document facts about their captors and captivity. They will also be the subject of intensive media interest and perhaps interviews. Their families may also be involved in the nationwide or worldwide attention and may be flown to the medical facility.

U.S. Army stress management teams have had extensive experience in hostage release scenarios, such as:

- A cruise ship and airliners briefly seized by terrorists (with loss of life).
- Military and civilian embassy personnel held by Islamic fundamentalists for over a year.
- Individual hostages held for years under extreme hardship and deprivation.
- POWs repatriated at the end of the Persian Gulf War.

The stress control challenge in this hectic process is to provide therapeutic critical incident stress debriefing (CISD) and reunion assistance in the midst of conflicting demands while minimizing secondary trauma from the repatriation process itself. The principles of PIES apply. Contact with an MH/CSC team should begin as far forward as possible. Ideally, the same MH individuals will travel back with the victims to complete the process. If that is not possible, the "hand off" to a second team should be clear and positive to the victims. Joint coordination and participation in this process is essential.

This chapter has thus far discussed various administrative structures and programs to prevent and treat psychiatric casualties. A main theme has been that unit troop morale and cooperative coordinate interservice efforts are critical in both prevention and treatment of combat stress reactions. Chapter 16 provides additional information regarding interventions with POWs.

Civil Disaster Relief and Civil Disturbance Response

Similar cooperation between military and civilian agencies is seen in disaster relief efforts. National Guard units (U.S. Army, U.S. Navy, U.S. Marine Corps, and U.S. Air Force) have often been called up by their state governors to maintain law and order and provide emergency medical and engineer support following natural disasters. Experience after Hurricanes *Hugo* and *Andrew* suggests that the active component of military services will also be increasingly called upon to provide quick and massive response following major disasters in the United States.

Case Study 4: Hurricane Andrew

After Hurricane *Andrew* (1992), a joint task force (JTF) was given extensive responsibility for coordinating and implementing emergency relief and cleanup activities. It included active component U.S. Army divisional and corps assets, U.S. Marine Corps units, U.S. Navy ships, U.S. Air Force aircraft, and ground personnel. The mission included setting up and running tent cities to house and feed homeless victims, and clearing wreckage to restore essential infrastructure, providing medical and preventive medical support. All of this was in complicated relationship to state, local, volunteer, and other federal agencies, the media, and the victims themselves.

The U.S. Army medical brigade commanded the medical task force. It requested and received an experienced neuropsychiatry consultant. U.S. Army division mental health section personnel from three divisions deployed with their division units to the disaster area with the following functions:

- To provide stress control support to the corps-level units along with those of their divisions.
- To train U.S. Army personnel who were canvassing areas block-by-block to identify potential mental health problems and cases.
- To relay this information every evening from the medical brigade to the state mental health authorities who directed civilian mental health teams to fill the need.

A U.S. Navy SPRINT team was initially requested by the U.S. Coast Guard to provide critical incident stress debriefing to U.S. Coast Guard families, and later it became a joint task force resource. U.S. Air Force stress teams deployed to assist at Homestead Air Force Base which was heavily damaged by the storm, but did not later join the JTF. U.S. Army combat stress control personnel from a corps-level detachment were standing by to deploy but were not required as civilian mental health assets became available. U.S. Army Reserve combat stress control units were also preparing to send volunteer teams on temporary tour active duty if called upon. (A U.S. Army Reserve combat stress control company did activate 12 persons to assist the Red Cross at refugee shelters following the January 1994 Los Angeles, California earthquake. The organizational, cross-cultural, and language skills of the U.S. Army reservists proved especially helpful.)

Comment: The JTF that responded to Hurricane *Andrew* provided a coordinated response, in conjunction with the efforts of the civilian community, to alleviate the various hardships that survivors were experiencing. These responses lessened long-term problems for these communities.

Mass Casualty Disasters

In a disaster that kills and injures thousands, as well as devastating property, additional military mental health/combat stress control would be needed as follows:

- To provide or supervise stress debriefing and follow-up of the service members who are pulling the bodies of living and dead from the ruins and providing emergency care.
- To provide combat stress control support to mobilized service members (especially those in the local National Guard units) whose own families are in the disaster area, and whose fates may be unknown for some time.
- To assure stress control support to those service families, once located.
- To coordinate the military effort with the many other agencies and resources.

Effective coordination under high stress conditions is the key to success. U.S. Army corps-level combat stress control detachments and companies (both active and reserve components) should have this as a contingency mission with written standard operating procedures.

In a major mass casualty disaster that devastated all medical facilities over a large area, U.S. Air Force area theater hospitals and contingency hospitals, U.S. Army medical companies and CSHs, U.S. Marine Corps surgical support companies (SSCs), and perhaps U.S. Navy Hospital ships might also be deployed, bringing their additional neuropsychiatric/mental health personnel.

While physical trauma cases may have to be evacuated some distance for definitive surgery, any civilian stress cases (and secondary military ones) should be kept close to their homes or displaced families (or their units). As with battle fatigue, these cases need to be treated according to PIES and the Five Rs in a non–patient-care atmosphere.

Recovery of Dead Human Bodies

One mission that is common across the services, in war and in many operations other than war, is the requirement to recover and process dead human bodies. These may be the bodies of fellow service members, perhaps even personal friends. They may be the bodies of enemies killed in combat, either by oneself or by other combat forces. They may be civilians, including children, adult men and women, and elderly people with whom one naturally identifies and empathizes. The number of bodies may range from intimately few to appallingly many. Depending on the cause of death, time elapsed, and weather, the state of the bodies may be grossly mutilated and decomposed (as in the Jonestown massacre) or unnervingly intact and seemingly unharmed ("as if only asleep"). The sights and smells (and perhaps touch) in the work of processing human bodies invoke an arguably innate horror and revulsion, especially on first exposure. Prolonged exposure may produce cumulative horrors or a numbing of all feeling. The intense sensory experiences, often combined with emotion-provoking thoughts, can form extremely vivid, painful memories that become the seeds of post-traumatic stress disorder.

Extensive studies have been conducted on military and civilian units that were unexpectedly required to recover human remains, and on mortuary affairs personnel and other specialists who process human remains on a routine basis.[8,9] Even the latter can be adversely impacted by special individual bodies or by mass casualties. The research has focused on what specific aspects of the task cause the greatest distress. It has recorded the ways that those recovering and processing the bodies have found to protect themselves. Exhibit 10-1 summarizes and condenses recommendations from a number of sources, most notably McCarroll et al[8] and Ursano and McCarroll.[9] This was prepared in pocket

EXHIBIT 10-1

WHEN THE MISSION REQUIRES RECOVERING DEAD HUMAN BODIES

HOW TO PREPARE YOURSELF, YOUR BUDDIES, AND THE UNIT

THE MISSION

One consequence of many humanitarian and peace support missions, as well as of war, is coming in contact with bodies which have died under tragic or horrible circumstances. All soldiers, in all types of units, may be assigned the mission of recovering, processing and perhaps burying human remains.

- We may collect the bodies of fellow service members so that the Mortuary Affairs specialists can return them to the United States for identification and burial.
- We may gather and perhaps bury the bodies of enemy or civilian dead, to safeguard public health.
- The numbers of dead may be small and very personal, or they may be very, very large.
- The victims may include service members much like ourselves, or young men and women, elderly people, small children and infants for whom we feel an innate empathy.
- Being exposed to children who have died can be especially distressing, particularly for individuals who have children of their own.

Extensive experience has been gained during such missions, and in working with the body recovery teams afterwards to help them cope with the memories. This experience can help you, your buddies and your unit take such a difficult mission in stride. You can complete the mission proud of what you have done, and return to your usual duties, career and family life without being unduly troubled by the memories, even when those memories include some very sad, unpleasant or distressing details.

WHAT TO EXPECT

Some body recovery missions involve situations where there are no living survivors. Other situations are in concert with ongoing rescue, emergency medical care, and survivor assistance activities. In the latter case, the reactions of the living victims may include grief, anger, shock, gratitude or ingratitude, numbness or indifference. Such reactions may seem appropriate or inappropriate to you, and may interact with your own reactions to the dead.

In some situations, the bodies may be distorted or mutilated. Seeing mutilated bodies invokes an innate horror in most human beings, although most of us quickly form a kind of tough mental "shell," so that we won't feel so badly. To some extent, we come to see the remains simply as objects, without reflecting that they were once people.

- The dead bodies may be wasted by starvation, dehydration, and disease (eg, Rwanda refugees or some POW and concentration camp victims).
- They may have been crushed and dug out from under rubble, (eg, the Beirut barracks bombing or earthquake victims).
- They may be badly mutilated by fire, impact, blast or projectiles (eg, the victims of the air crashes at Gander, Newfoundland, and Sioux City, Iowa; the civilians killed by collateral damage and fire near the Commandancia in Panama City, or the Iraqi army dead north of Kuwait).
- They may be victims of deliberate atrocity (eg, the Shiites of south Iraq, or any side in Bosnia).

Sometimes, however, the cause of death leaves few signs on the bodies (eg, the mass suicide with cyanide at Jonestown, Guiana [South America], or victims drowned in floods). The caregivers often say this is harder to adapt to, because it is harder to form that "shell."

Of course, the degree of decomposition of the bodies will be determined by the temperature and climate, and by how long it has been before you can reach them and begin collection.

In addition to seeing mutilated or nonmutilated bodies, you will often have to smell the bodies and other associated strong odors. You may have to touch the remains, move them, and perhaps hear the sounds of autopsies being performed, or other burial activities. These sensations may place a strain on your capacity to do the work, and may trouble you in memories. We will list below things you can do to help this.

Being exposed to large numbers of dead bodies is not a normal part of human experience. Therefore, when you are exposed to bodies, you should not be surprised to be feeling things you are not used to.

- When you are exposed to bodies, you may experience sorrow, regret, repulsion, disgust, anger, and futility. REMEMBER, THESE ARE NORMAL EXPERIENCES GIVEN THE SITUATION IN WHICH YOU HAVE BEEN PLACED.

In fact, it would be surprising if you did not have at least some of these emotions.

- You may start to see similarities between yourself (or others you love) and those who have died. This could lead to feelings of guilt ("Why wasn't it me?" or "Why can't I do more to stop it?") or anxiety ("It could have been me"). Again, these feelings are NORMAL given the situation.
- Humor is a normal human reaction or "safety valve" for very uncomfortable feelings. In body handling situations, it naturally tends toward what is aptly called "graveyard humor." Don't be surprised at finding this in yourself or others.

GUIDELINES FOR HOW TO WORK WITH HUMAN REMAINS

Prepare yourself, as much as time and access to information allows, for what you will be seeing and doing. It is better to be prepared for the worst and not have to face it than to be underprepared.

- Learn as much as you can about the history, cultural background, and circumstances of the disaster or tragedy. How did it come to happen? Try to understand it the way a historian or neutral investigating commission would.
- Look at videos and photographs of the area of operation and of the victims. The television news networks and news magazines may be sources. If pictures of the current situation are not available, look up ones from previous similar tragedies in the library archives. Share them as a team, and talk about them.

Understand the importance and value of what you are doing.

- Remember that you are helping the deceased to receive a respectful burial (even if in some cases, it must be a hasty and mass burial). You are saving their remains the indignity of simply being left on the ground to decay.
- In some cases, you are helping survivors know their loved ones have died, rather than remain for years in uncertainty. Those relatives or friends can then take the bodies for private burial, or at least know where they are buried.
- By collecting or burying the bodies of those who have already died, you are providing a safer, healthier environment for those individuals still living.

EXHIBIT 10-1 (continued)

When you are seeing or working with the bodies, think about the larger purpose you are serving, without attempting to relate to each individual who has died. By not focusing on each individual, you will be able to do your important job more effectively.

- Remember that the body is not the person, but only the remains.
- Some people who have done this important work have found it helpful to think of the remains as wax models or mannequins (as if in a training exercise), or as memorial models to which they were showing the respect due to the original person who was no longer there.
- If your job requires you to collect personal effects from the bodies for identification, intelligence or other official purposes, do not let yourself look closely at or read those personal effects. (The people who need to examine those effects are advised to do so remote from, and preferably without having seen, the body.)
- Needless to say, do not desecrate or take souvenirs from the bodies. Those are criminal acts.
- Humor, even graveyard humor, is helpful if it remains on a witty and relatively abstract level. It is unhelpful when it becomes too gross, too personal (eg, comments or practical jokes which pick on members of the team who need support, not ridicule), or too disrespectful of the individual dead. Some members of the team may become upset at excessive graveyard humor, and even the joker may remember it with guilt years later.
- Each of you can say prayers for the dead, and conduct whatever personal ceremonies your own beliefs and background recommend. The unit chaplain and/or local clergy may also conduct rites or ceremonies. Even very brief rites at the time can help, perhaps to be followed by larger, formal ceremonies later.

Take steps to limit exposure to the stimuli from the bodies.

- Have screens, partitions, covers, body bags or barriers so that people don't see the bodies unless it is necessary to their mission.
- Wear gloves if the job calls for touching the bodies.
- It may help to mask the odor with disinfectants, air-fresheners, or deodorants in some locations. Using other scents such as perfume or aftershave lotions is of limited value in the presence of the bodies, and is perhaps better saved for when taking breaks away from the work area. Don't be surprised if the scents bring back memories of the experience for a while thereafter.

Take care of yourself and each other.

- When the mission allows, schedule frequent short breaks away from working with or around bodies.
- Drink plenty of fluids, continue to eat well, and especially maintain good hygiene. To the extent possible, Command should assure facilities for washing hands, clothing, and taking hot showers after each shift. (If water must be rationed, Command should make clear what <u>can</u> be provided and how it should be used and conserved.)
- Hold team after-action debriefings frequently to talk out the worst and the best things about what has occurred, sharing thoughts, feelings and reactions with your teammates.
- A mental health/stress control team or chaplain may be able to lead a Critical Event Debriefing after a particularly bad event or at the end of the operation.
- Plan team as well as individual activities to relax and get your mind off the tragedy you are helping to correct. Do not let yourself feel guilty about this, or about not being able to fix all the tragedy immediately. YOU MUST PACE YOURSELVES FOR THE TASK, AND DO WHAT CAN BE DONE WITH THE RESOURCES AVAILABLE, ONE STEP AT A TIME.
- Stay physically fit.
- Keep your Unit Family Support Group fully informed about what is happening, and make sure your family members and significant others are included in and supported by it.
- Take special care of new unit members, and those with recent changes or special problems back home.

If the stress caused by working with the dead bodies begins to interfere with your performance or your ability to relax, or if you feel that you are becoming overwhelmed, TAKE ACTION. Do not ignore the stress.

- Seek out someone to talk with about how you are feeling. This might be a buddy or someone else. Other people are likely to be feeling the same things you are. The important thing is not to withdraw from others and become isolated.
- The unit chaplain, medic, or a combat stress control/mental health team member can often help.

Likewise, it is important to help your buddy, coworker, subordinate or superior if he or she shows signs of distress.

- Give support and encouragement, and try to get the other person to talk through the problems or feelings that they are having. By working with each other, you both will be better able to cope with the situation in which you must work.

After you have completed your mission and are no longer working around the bodies, you may experience a variety of feelings. These may include feeling bad about not treating each body as an individual, and needing to express the emotions that were pent up while you were doing the work of body recovery. DO NOT KEEP THESE EMOTIONS INSIDE. They are normal, and are best worked through by talking with your fellow unit members.

- Take an active part in an end-of-tour debriefing and pre-homecoming information briefing within your unit prior to leaving the operational area.
- Follow through with Family Support Group activities which recognize and honor what the unit has done and shares the experience (and the praise for a hard job well done) with the families.
- Don't be surprised if being at home brings back upsetting memories from the operation. You may find it hard to talk about the memories with family or friends who weren't there. This is very common. Try to talk about them anyway. Also stay in touch with your teammates from the operation.
- If you still find yourself upset, don't hesitate to talk with a chaplain or with the community mental health or stress control team in your area. This is just wise preventive maintenance.

Reprinted from Combat Stress Actions Office; HSHA-PO, Department of Preventive Health Services, AMEDD Center and School, Fort Sam Houston, Texas 78234-6142.

card format for the Rwanda refugee relief mission. The card was subsequently used by the commander of the second of two National Guard medical companies activated and deployed to conduct body recovery and processing at a civil airline crash site and nearby armory. In initial follow-up, the company reported that the recommendations had proved very helpful. The first National Guard medical company deployed to the same site had not had the card, and within a month of demobilization it had made seven referrals for treatment of PTSD. Follow-up of both companies is continuing.

RECOMMENDATIONS

The U.S. Army, U.S. Air Force, U.S. Marine Corps, and U.S. Navy are all working to improve their capability to prevent stress casualties across the continuum of operations. Their efforts are directed toward providing immediate intervention close to the battle or high-stress activity and the service members' units. The organizational and written doctrine are still evolving, but all recognize and adhere to the basic time-proven principles. Because cooperation and coordination are the guiding principles of combat stress control, the following actions should be taken to achieve an effective Joint Operations CSC capability.

Joint Coordination. For any joint operation, combat stress control (neuropsychiatric, mental health) personnel from each service should seek out and coordinate with their counterparts in the other services. The following actions should occur:

- Coordination should be initiated by the joint command staff early in the contingency planning and operations. Each joint command surgeon should have triservice (multidisciplinary) CSC consultants. These should be on staff or available by telecommunication or temporary duty, even in operational security (OPSEC) situations.
- Each service should be encouraged to deploy sufficient MH/CSC personnel to support its own major contingent.
- Arrangements should be made for MH/CSC backup from other services to support small elements that do not bring their own CSC assets.
- All headquarters and MH/CSC personnel being deployed should be informed about all the other CSC personnel on the way as quickly as possible (consistent with operational security).
- Coordination should be continued and fostered by the joint headquarters during mobilization and deployment.
- Coordination must be an important mission for U.S. Army mental health staff sections of major command or medical command headquarters, medical brigade (combat zone and communications zone), and medical group.
- Coordination must be actively considered and, when feasible, be accomplished by the mental health section or neuropsychiatric ward/section of U.S. Army divisions (mental health section of main support medical company or medical battalion); U.S. Marine Corps divisions (psychiatrist of division HQ, psychologist of surgical support company); U.S. Air Force tactical (air-transportable) hospital (combat stress unit); area support medical battalion (MH Section); U.S. Army medical CSC companies and detachments; U.S. Army combat support, field, and general hospitals; U.S. Air Force contingency hospitals; U.S. Navy field hospitals; and U.S. Navy hospital ships.

Initiative at the Operator Level. In the spirit of joint operations, direct coordination between junior MH/CSC officers and NCOs in the theater of operations should be actively encouraged by all higher headquarters. The MH/CSC personnel at the operator level should take the initiative to make such contacts even in the absence of coordination from higher echelons. They should, of course, inform their higher HQ of all such contacts as soon as possible.

Conferences and Symposia. When the tactical situation allows, formal conferences or symposia should be scheduled to bring together representative MH/CSC personnel from all the services in the theater of operations (plus allies and the host nation) to share their experiences. Joint participation should also be actively sought in peacetime conferences and continuing health education courses.

Doctrine Development. In preparation for joint contingencies, doctrinal material on joint CSC operations should be drafted, staffed through all necessary channels, and incorporated into the relevant manuals and training programs of all services. Joint CSC involvement should be practiced whenever possible in field exercises and training deployments. The lessons learned in these, and in true contingency deployments, should be systematically staffed and incorporated into the evolving doctrine.

Periodically, the lessons learned from recent conflicts are reviewed to facilitate doctrine development and more productive operations in the future. Such reviews commonly consider the substantial logistical assets, including medical services, in a combat zone. The usual rationale for the establishment of medical assets (aside from moral and morale considerations) has been that returning medically noneffective service members to duty is the most efficient way to mitigate losses due to attrition, that is, to conserve the fighting strength.

Conventional medical support in the theater of operations, however, is a substantial undertaking—the hospitals are heavy, require huge spaces, and are difficult to move; they are staffed by a large number of personnel; and they have extensive requirements for food, fuel, and unique equipment and supplies not usable by any other component of the deployed force. Thus their setup occupies significant quantities of personnel, space, time, and "lift."

The most likely future war-fighting scenarios for the U.S. military describe discrete combat actions of strictly limited duration fought by small elite forces. Only a small portion of the full spectrum of medical support is likely to be available at the onset of an unexpected war, or an operation other than war, that is likely to be of short duration. Furthermore, in these future scenarios, few service members who become medically noneffective for more than 1 to 3 days are likely to return to duty before the fighting ends and the unit withdraws. Thus, there is little need, from the viewpoint of many in the line, to establish extensive medical support in the combat zone for the purposes of returning medically noneffective service members to duty.

A possible medical operational scenario following from these scenarios would be to immediately evacuate all service members who become medically noneffective to existing bases outside of CONUS or to CONUS where they would be treated. The only service members who would receive medical treatment in the combat zone would be those with critical injuries who would not survive evacuation. Small, rapidly deployable surgical hospitals would be available to provide resuscitative surgery. What little additional medical support present in the combat zone would be at the unit level and except for treating the most minor medical and surgical problems, would be used for triage and preparation for evacuation. Almost all of the conventional third echelon medical support would be absent.

These review processes periodically suggest that mental health personnel not be deployed for supposedly brief combat scenarios and that any combat stress casualties and lightly injured casualties be rapidly evacuated from the combat zone, perhaps as far as CONUS. In such scenarios, service members manifesting combat stress reaction would not be kept at the unit level as required by existing doctrine but would be evacuated. The proponents of such scenarios maintain that although less than optimal from the standpoint of the current tenets of military psychiatry, the number of such service members expected would be minimal; first, because only elite units, the members of which seem to have a greater tolerance to combat stress, will be deployed, and second, because the expected duration of combat will be short.

There are substantial fallacies in this argument. First, the mental health personnel who are organic or attached to the critical combat and combat support units can be crucial in their primary mission of helping leadership sustain and enhance combat performance. They will exercise primary prevention by reducing the negative impact of stressors and by prophylactic debriefings to minimize PTSD and other post-deployment difficulties. These delayed problems can occur in service members who show no dysfunction during the operation. Avoidable attrition of combat-experienced service members, due in part to post-traumatic stress, was observed following the successful 1983 Grenada and 1989 Panama operations (see Chapter 1, Psychiatric Lessons of War). The mental health personnel in theater will also exercise secondary prevention by enabling temporarily overstressed service members to regain optimal effectiveness without leaving their tactical teams or their organic combat service support elements. There the overstressed service member is aided by his own buddy, immediate leader, medic, chaplain, or a general medical professional. These helpers must receive technical supervision and mentoring from a mental health officer or NCO. Mental health expertise is required to triage and make initial interventions in some cases. In a pinch, the battalion surgeon, if already well-mentored and knowledgeable, can subsume the mentoring role. The service members who are restored to effectiveness in this manner within their own units never become medical casualties because they are not absent from duty.

Secondly, some overstressed service members will require 1 to 3 days of restoration activities before return to their units. It must be emphasized that these combat stress cases, although casualties because they are temporarily absent from their units, are not medical patients. The forward-deployed mental health personnel will perform neuropsychiatric triage to identify and stabilize the small number of true neuropsychiatric patients for prompt evacuation. Of major significance to the issue of deployment of assets in a theater of operations, the support for combat stress casualties is minimal: a sleeping bag, MREs, and a trained helper. These stress casualties can be temporarily assigned to a combat service support unit, if no level II medical company is suitable. At the combat service support unit, these stress casualties remain under the technical supervision of mental health personnel or the CSC team. This practice is in accordance with the doctrine of some North Atlantic Treaty Organization (NATO) countries. Years of hard experience have confirmed the importance of not evacuating overstressed (or minimally injured) service members from the theater without a brief (1- to 3- day) period of restoration. The restoration program poses minimal logistical burden beyond the subsistence of the participants who pay for their keep by performing necessary labor. The entire program is deliberately not medical, and has no necessary relationship with large hospitals.

Finally, and most importantly, any behavior that allows an honorable exit from combat can become an evacuation syndrome, no matter how elite the troops. In addition, combat stress casualties would likely occur in greater numbers in combat support troops, which are necessary to any deployment, as was seen in the 1973 Yom Kippur War, the 1982 Lebanon War, and the 1989 invasion of Panama. Lightly wounded casualties react much the same as combat stress casualties when evacuated. The point most often overlooked by the line, and by many in the medical profession, is that nonevacuation of combat stress casualties *is* the treatment. An evacuated combat stress casualty may become a chronic mental cripple. His best chance for recovery is in the early proper management of the syndrome.

Any proposed deletion of psychiatric support brings to mind the World War II psychiatrically disastrous early North African campaign. A few brief battles resulted in large numbers of psychiatric casualties, many of whom were evacuated to CONUS to fill VA hospitals for years after the war ended. Such a policy, seemingly compassionate, is medically inhumane.

CONCLUSION

The U.S. Army, U.S. Air Force, U.S. Marine Corps, and U.S. Navy are all working to improve their capability to prevent stress casualties. Their efforts are directed toward providing immediate intervention close to the battle and the service members' units. The organizational and written doctrine are still evolving, but all recognize and adhere to the basic time-proven principles.

REFERENCES

1. US Department of the Army. *Operations*. Washington, DC: DA; 1993. Field Manual 100-5.

2. US Department of the Army. *Health Service Support in the Theater of Operations*. Washington, DC: DA; 1 March 1991. Field Manual 8-10.

3. US Department of the Army. *Combat Stress Control in a Theater of Operations*. Washington, DC: DA; 29 September 1994. Field Manual 8-51.

4. US Department of the Air Force. *U.S. Air Force Combat Psychiatry*. Washington, DC: USAFSAM-TR-85-83; January 1986.

5. Pierce MI. Personal Communication, 1992.

6. Dinneen M. Interventions aboard the Iwo Jima following a fatal boiler explosion. In: Belenky GL, Martin JM, Sparacino LR, eds. *The Shield in the Storm: Mental Health Operations During the Persian Gulf War*. Westport, Conn: Greenwood Press; in preparation.

7. Sokol RJ. Early mental health intervention in combat situations: The USS Stark. *Mil Med.* 1989;154(8):407–409.

8. McCarroll JE, Ursano RJ, Wright KM, Fullerton CS. Handling of bodies after violent death: Strategies for coping. *Am J Orthopsychiatry.* 1993;63:209–214.

9. Ursano RJ, McCarroll JE. Exposure to traumatic death: The nature of the stressor. In: Ursano R, McCaughey B, Fullerton C, eds. *Individual and Community Responses to Trauma and Disaster.* New York: Cambridge University Press; 1994: 46–71.

Chapter 11

DEBRIEFING FOLLOWING COMBAT

RONALD J. KOSHES, M.D.*; STEPHEN A. YOUNG, M.D.†; AND JAMES W. STOKES, M.D.‡

*Chief Psychiatrist, The Center for Mental Health, Washington, D.C. 20020; Guest Scientist, Division of Neuropsychiatry, Walter Reed Army Institute of Research, Washington, D.C.; Assistant Clinical Professor of Psychiatry, Uniformed Services University of the Health Sciences, Bethesda, Maryland; President, Society of American Military Psychiatrists
†Major, Medical Corps, U.S. Army; Department of Psychiatry, Walter Reed Army Medical Center, Washington, D.C.; formerly Chief of Psychiatry, Gorgas Army Hospital, Panama
‡Colonel, Medical Corps, U.S. Army; Chief, Combat Stress Actions Office, Department of Preventive Health Services, Academy of Health Sciences, Army Medical Department Center and School, Fort Sam Houston, Texas 78234-6133

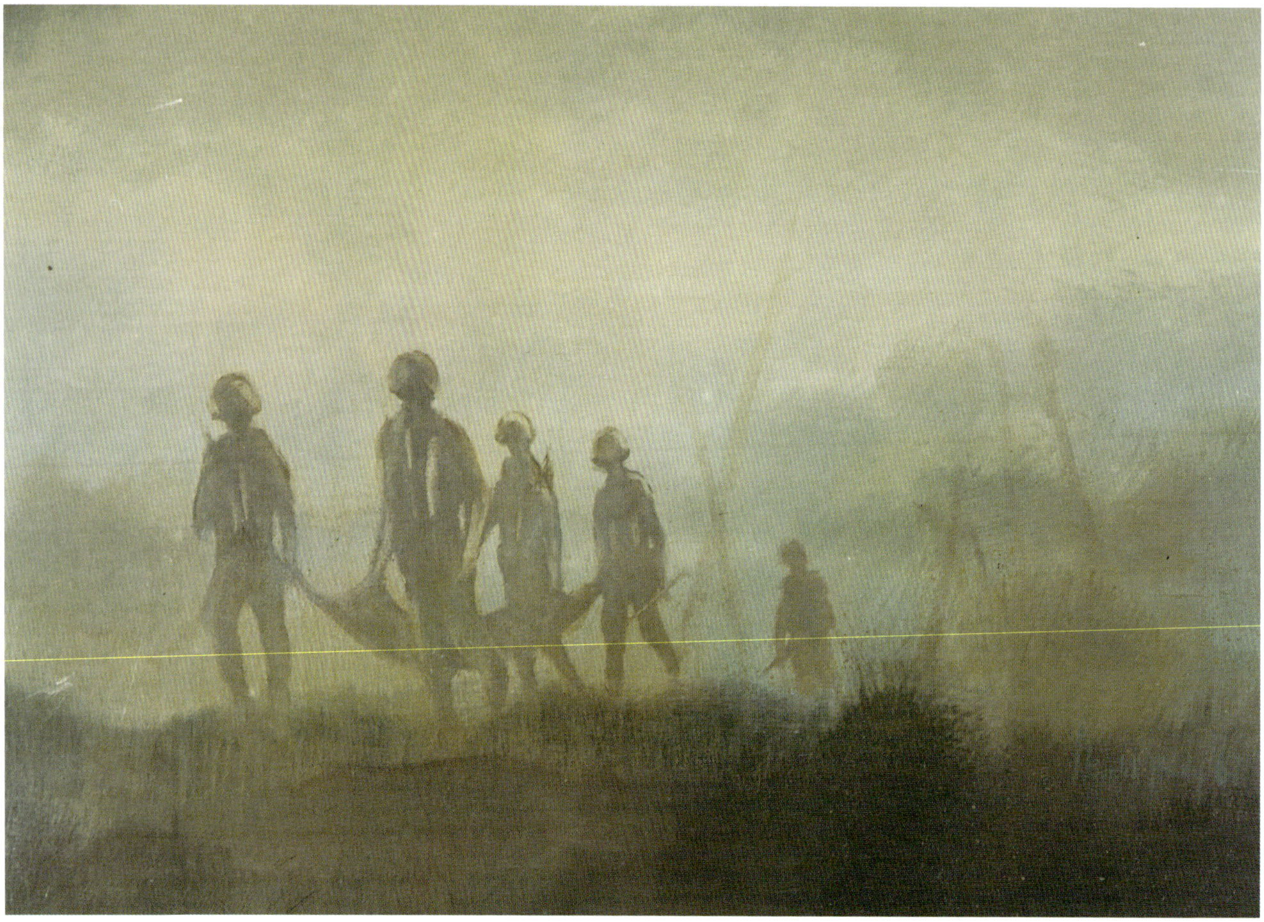

Burdell Moody *Killed in Action* 1968

Burdell Moody, with U.S. Army Artist Team #4, starkly portrays a squad returning to base camp in Vietnam, carrying the body of one of their soldiers. Perhaps the most stressful aspect of combat for a soldier, other than pondering his own death, is the death of another, especially a member of his own unit. Witnessing death is a critical event in the life of any soldier and his unit, one warranting immediate debriefing to lessen the likelihood of developing post-traumatic symptoms in the future.

Art: Courtesy of US Center of Military History, Washington, DC.

INTRODUCTION

Emergence of post-traumatic stress disorder (PTSD) as a clinical condition presupposes the experience of an overwhelming trauma and consequent biopsychosocial adaptation. By the criteria of the Diagnostic and Statistical Manual, 4th ed.[1] (DSM-IV), the individual must reexperience the event, perhaps through intrusive recollections, distressing dreams, and avoidance of stimuli associated with the event, and may have persistent symptoms of increased arousal manifesting as hyperalertness, vigilance, and irritable behavior. The symptoms must last for at least 1 month. The stress of combat does not inevitably result in PTSD; debriefing following combat is an intervention that appears to interrupt the causal connection.

Often, at some later point in life, the person exposed to trauma, be it a natural disaster, terrorism, war, or other highly emotionally charged lethal or life-threatening events, will reexperience feelings associated with the original trauma because of an environmental or emotional trigger. In the case of war, PTSD can occur in as many as 15% of those individuals exposed to combat.[2] In natural disasters, terrorists attacks, and devastating industrial accidents (the so-called civilian critical incidents—CCI), PTSD rates are more variable, depending on the meaning attributed to the stressor and the possibility of legal damages.

Trauma, however severe, is likely to be an organizing factor in a person's life, defining for the individual adaptation that can be both attributed to and dated by the event. Perhaps the most useful intervention is the help provided by families, friends, church groups, military units, and others in stabilizing the individual in the community, allowing for the ventilation of feelings, and validating the role of the individual in the communities to which he or she belongs.[3]

Psychological trauma following civilian critical incidents has been similarly studied. Erikson[4] documented the importance of tending to basic needs of survivors when the dam on Buffalo Creek broke and devastated a whole Appalachian community. Long-term distress was exacerbated when families were separated, homes relocated, and roads were built without direct community involvement. As a result, rescue workers learned the importance of enlisting survivors in their own recovery process, a principle that has been utilized in CCI training and actual experience.

For combat, various models have been proposed and studied to reduce the incidence of PTSD and other acute psychiatric reactions. Most models rely on the assumption that unit cohesion, training, and leadership are important in helping soldiers adapt to traumatic or adverse conditions. The decreased incidence was striking in subsequent psychiatric casualties experienced by an elite paratrooper unit when compared to ordinary combat units in the Israeli Army during the 1973 Yom Kippur War.[5] Significant differences in the units highlight the role of trust toward the immediate commanders, unit identity, and professional soldiering knowledge.[2,5] Moreover, the community support and effective integration of soldiers returning from battle into their units or homes appears to have the greatest influence on the development of long-term psychiatric sequelae.[6–9]

THE HISTORY OF POST-TRAUMA DEBRIEFING

One process by which individuals can reduce untoward effects of trauma (eg, natural disasters, war, civil unrest) is called debriefing.[10] Simply put, the individual or group meet at the request of a larger supervisory body to begin a process of integrating the trauma into their individual and group experiences. Debriefing is a process that has been described by mental health workers attendant to natural disasters,[10] terrorism,[11] combat,[12] and military accidents.[13,14] It involves a structured meeting designed to allow for ventilation of feelings, fears, and the telling of stories of the traumatic event. It is not the end, but rather the beginning, of the healing process during which the reentry of individuals into the community at large is facilitated.

The concept of group debriefing grew out of the work of S.L.A. Marshall[15] during World War II when he attempted to record accounts of small unit military operations for historical purposes. Marshall noted that when a person could describe what happened to him during a harrowing experience this served not only an abreactive purpose but allowed colleagues to correct misperceptions and render social support. This appeared to decrease the development of combat stress reactions. Marshall observed that these historical debriefings or "reconstructions" restored unit cohesion and readiness to return to combat. He considered this one of his most important contributions to the U.S. Army. Marshall continued to conduct official historical debriefings for highly selected units throughout the Korean and Vietnam conflicts. To the knowledge of the authors, the technique was not used at that time by clinical mental health personnel.

In 1978, the debriefing process was incorporated by Navy psychiatrists in developing the Special Psychiatric Rapid Intervention Teams (SPRINT), which have been discussed in Chapter 9, U.S. Naval Psychiatry). In the 1980s, the U.S. Army's 7th Medical Command in Heidelberg, Germany used debriefing techniques on their Stress Management Team deployments in response to a number of terrorist attacks. A joint U.S. Navy-U.S. Army team deployed to the Persian Gulf to assist the U.S. Navy frigate *Stark* after it was damaged by an Iraqi Exocet missile.[12] The air show disaster at Ramstein Air Force Base in Germany also required extensive debriefing of survivors, witnesses, and caregivers.

Critical incident stress debriefing (CISD) has also been utilized in the civilian world.[16] Some volunteer CISD teams are now active in most of the United States and in other countries including Canada, Great Britain, the Netherlands, Norway, and Australia. These teams respond to critical incidents involving police, fire, and emergency medical departments. Some governmental and nongovernmental agencies have their own debriefing teams and policies.

During and after the U.S. invasion of Panama and the Persian Gulf War, U.S. Army mental health teams conducted a number of unit debriefings, although there was no formal doctrinal mandate or training program. With the deployment to Somalia in January 1994 of U.S. Army division mental health and combat stress control detachment teams, critical event debriefings became common practice. They were conducted following deaths in a unit from enemy action, accident or suicide, or after other distressing events involving deaths of civilians or mass casualties of multinational force allies at U.S. medical facilities.

U.S. Army critical incident debriefings have been conducted following training deaths at the National Training Center (NTC) in California and the Joint Readiness Training Center (JRTC) in Louisiana; the Green Ramp disaster at Pope Air Force Base in North Carolina; the mass murder followed by a B-52 bomber crash at Fairchild Air Force Base in Washington state; and many other traumatic incidents. The U.S. Navy's SPRINT teams continue to deploy on call, as have U.S. Air Force teams. U.S. Army doctrine[17,18] establishes critical event debriefings as doctrinally appropriate after especially traumatic events. Allied countries have also accumulated extensive experience with military debriefings following critical incidents and difficult tours of duty.

TYPES OF DEBRIEFING

A number of models or types of debriefings have evolved from this extensive experience. These include (but are not limited to) the types summarized below:

- After-Action Review (AAR)
- After-Action Debriefing (AAD)
- Historical Group Debriefing (also called Historical Event Reconstruction Debriefing—HERD)
- Civilian Critical Incident Stress Debriefing (CISD)
- Critical Event Debriefing (CED)
- Psychiatric Debriefing
- Large Group Debriefings
- End-of-Tour Debriefings

After-Action Review

After-action review (AAR) is the standing operating procedure for all U.S. Army teams and small units following any training exercise. The training cadre bring the team together immediately after each training event and have them talk through what happened. The cadre share their own observations. The product is positive lessons learned, not blame. Further, AARs may bring together the leaders of all the participating small groups to give the wider perspective and derive lessons learned on command control, communication and coordination. All U.S. Army leaders are expected to conduct their own AARs routinely, without cadre, when conducting their own training exercises. They are encouraged to continue this practice in real world missions, including combat.

The AAR is designed for nonlethal training, and focuses cognitively on the operational lessons learned. It does not explicitly encourage emotional ventilation or sharing of feelings and reactions. However, effective leaders and supportive cohesive teams do recognize, and work through, the sometimes intense feelings that arise. Mental health personnel are not normally present at AARs, except in their own training. However, it is valuable for the mental health personnel supporting combat units in field exercises to be transported to the AARs of units that have experienced simulated critical incidents, to hear what the combat units do, be seen, and exercise the ability of command to get them to units to assist after real traumatic events.

After-Action Debriefing

After-action debriefing (AAD), in U.S. Army doctrine, is an extension of the routine AAR.

> The after-action debriefing process shares the after-action review's concerns with details of what happened. It goes further by actively encouraging the team members to share and even talk out their emotional responses to the event. After-action debriefings should also be routine during training, operations other than war, war, and following any difficult or unpleasant event. Doing after-action debriefing routinely will make them second nature following any especially traumatic event. The objective of after-action debriefings following traumatic incidents is to promote "healing" by opening up, "cleaning and draining" any unpleasant or painful memories.[17(pp6-6,6-7)]

Exhibit 11-1 lists the key steps of the after-action debriefing process. More detailed guidance on how to lead an AAD is also available.[17(Appendix A)] The critical components for leader actions are shown in Exhibit 11-2. The AAD is led by the small unit's own leader(s). Mental health personnel, chaplains, and other trusted outsiders who were not participants in the event would attend only by invitation, and purely as observers. Furthermore,

> Combat stress control/mental health personnel should always be notified whenever serious psychological trauma has occurred in a unit. They can assist command in assuring that the after-action debriefing process is done correctly.[17(p6-7)]

The mental health personnel might intervene subtly during the processes only if they saw that the AAD was ending without having reached a generally positive outcome on issues of guilt, blame, anger, or other disruptive emotions. More often, they would be available to the team members afterwards, who would know that they now shared comprehensive knowledge of the event.

EXHIBIT 11-1

KEY STEPS IN AN AFTER-ACTION DEBRIEFING

- Explain the purpose and ground rules to be used during the debriefing at the outset.
- Involve everyone in verbally reconstructing the event in precise detail.
- Achieve a group consensus, resolving individual misperceptions and misunderstandings and restoring perspective about true responsibility.
- Encourage expression (ventilation) of thoughts and feelings about the event.
- Validate feelings about the event as normal and work towards how they can be accepted, lived with, atoned.
- Prevent scapegoating and verbal abuse.
- Talk about the normal (but unpleasant) stress symptoms unit members experience and which may recur for a while, so they, too, can be accepted without surprise or fear of permanence.
- Summarize the lessons learned and any positive aspects of the experience.

Reprinted from US Department of the Army. *Leaders' Manual for Combat Stress Control.* Washington, DC: DA; September 1994. Field Manual 22-51: 6-7.

EXHIBIT 11-2

LEADER ACTIONS TO OFFSET BATTLE FATIGUE RISK FACTORS

Leader Actions

Conduct small team after-action debriefings after every difficult action (in training and in combat). An after-action debriefing is an extension of after-action reviews which are routine in training. Reconstruct what really happened so that the team benefits from the lessons learned. At the same time, this releases bottled-up emotions and inner conflict that can lead to decreased unit cohesion, battle fatigue, and perhaps even to PTSD. This is the purpose of the after-action debriefing. Feelings of anger and mistrust may go away on their own once the soldier sees how things looked to the others. At least the feelings are out in the open and can be dealt with honestly. Soldiers' natural emotions of loss and grief come out, too, when buddies are wounded or killed in combat. Guilt or shame may come out when soldiers make mistakes. Such soldiers can be comforted and helped to put things into perspective by the rest of the team. The mistakes can be acknowledged and forgiven or atoned for. When conducting the after-action debriefing, the leader must

1. Select a location that is relatively safe from enemy attack.
2. Set the ground rules.
3. Reconstruct the action from everyone's memories.
4. Share thoughts and reactions to the action.
5. Encourage talk about any physical or mental signs of battle fatigue anyone may be having if the action was a high stress event.
6. Bring the focus back to the mission after the feelings have been recognized and ventilated.
7. Use after-action debriefings to orient new unit members. These debriefings familiarize them with the unit's most recent history, introduce them to the veterans' roles and personalities, and acquaint them with the unit's Tactical Standing Operating Procedure (TSOP). It also helps when merging survivors of two units into one, with or without other new replacements.

Adapted from US Department of the Army. *Leaders' Manual for Combat Stress Control*. Washington, DC: DA; September 1994. Field Manual 22-51: A-7–A-9.

Historical Group Debriefing

Historical group debriefing (also called, historical event reconstruction debriefing—HERD), patterned after the work of S.L.A. Marshall, involves all participants of a preexisting unit in processing a brief (up to several days) chronological reconstruction of a significant event. That event may, but need not, involve traumatic events. Shalev,[19] in Israel, has revised the original S.L.A. Marshall protocol and demonstrated its therapeutic effectiveness in traumatic military unit settings where more "clinical" approaches often encounter resistance. This technique may be less suited for ad hoc groups, such as random survivors of an accident, because it concentrates on filling out a timeline of fact that random "victims" might not care about and does not explicitly work through thoughts and reactions that strangers might be unwilling to share. Exhibit 11-3 (adapted from Shalev's work) summarizes the historical reconstruction technique.

Civilian Critical Incident Stress Debriefing

Civilian critical incident stress debriefing (CISD) is the debriefing format developed by Mitchell and used and taught by the Critical Incident Stress Foundation. Its key points and the seven phases of the debriefing are summarized in Exhibit 11-4. The CISD was designed for brief, traumatic incidents involving preexisting civilian teams, but is also usually applicable to ad hoc groups. The debriefer does elicit thoughts, reactions, and symptoms after a relatively brief survey of each participant's perspective on the "facts" of the event. The debriefer also provides some education at the end. The CISD format has been learned and used by military debriefers in military contexts.

Critical Event Debriefing

For the Somalia deployment, a prototype pocket card was developed and fielded to facilitate train-

EXHIBIT 11-3

HISTORICAL EVENT RECONSTRUCTION DEBRIEFING: SUMMARY OF S.L.A. MARSHALL'S DEBRIEFING TECHNIQUE

1. Debriefings are conducted as soon as possible after the action.
2. Prior to the debriefing session, the debriefer collects information about the unit's background, structure and role in the battle, and the outcome of the action.
3. The participants are told that the debriefing consists of a chronological reconstruction of the event in its most minute details (to understand and learn from the action, not as fault-finding).
4. All those who took part in the action participate in the session. No others are allowed to participate (although new replacements to the unit can be allowed to listen if the veterans agree).
5. The debriefer emphasizes that all ranks are put aside during the session and all participants have equal status as witnesses.
6. After initial "modeling" by the historical debriefer, the debriefing is led by the unit's own commander.
7. The entire group takes part in the reconstruction of the action in all its details. Each soldier is encouraged (but not forced) to add his own version to the other soldiers' accounts.
8. *All* the information and *all* points of view *on each stage* of the action are collected from the participants.
9. Ambiguous information and contradictory statements are recorded by the interviewer as illustrating the complexity of human interactions during an event.
10. Criticism and attempts to teach are discouraged. No open disbelief in any witness's testimony is expressed by the interviewer.
11. No attempt is made to reach agreement among participants. Premature conclusions and closure are avoided.
12. The debriefer creates and maintains a congenial atmosphere and facilitates communication and openness throughout the session.
13. Emotional reactions are recognized and validated, but are *not* emphasized. No deliberate psychological intervention (eg, clarification, interpretation) is attempted by the debriefer.
14. The session is not limited in time, and continues for as long as it takes to reach the comprehensive description of the event. It may adjourn temporarily for breaks, and resume after food and sleep.

Adapted from Shalev A. *Historical Group Debriefing Following Combat: A Study of SLA Marshall's Debriefing Techniques. Final Report.* [Coordinated by Department of Military Psychiatry, Walter Reed Army Institute of Research and Department of Mental Health, Medical Corps, Israeli Defence Forces.] Jerusalem, Israel: Department of Psychiatry, Center for Traumatic Stress, Hadassah University Hospital; 1992.

ing in debriefing techniques. The card drew extensively on the CISD 7-phase model, differing primarily in greater emphasis on filling in an unbroken timeline in the Fact Phase. While calling for an agreement on confidentiality (as in CISD), it also reminds everyone of their obligations to the Uniform Code of Military Justice if material on violations of that code are raised in the debriefing. By agreement with Mitchell, this military modification of CISD is being referred to as critical event debriefing to avoid confusion over the necessary differences in applying the CISD format in the context of ongoing U.S. Army field operations and organizations. According to U.S. Army doctrine,

> When indicated, the unit should arrange for combat stress control/mental health personnel to conduct a critical event debriefing. Critical event debriefings are similar to after-action debriefings but differ in the following ways:
> The critical event debriefing is led by a trained debriefer who is not a member of the unit being

EXHIBIT 11-4

CRITICAL INCIDENT STRESS DEBRIEFING: KEY POINTS AND PHASES

Points

The CISD should be conducted after an *exceptionally* distressing event.

The CISD is conducted by a specially trained team.

The participants are normal persons who have survived an abnormal, severe stressor.

Stress debriefing is *not* therapy or counseling. It is basic wise *preventive maintenance* for the human mind.

Phases

1. Introductory Phase: to introduce the team and explain the process.
2. Fact Phase: to reconstruct the event in detail, in chronologic order, as an unbroken "historical time-line," viewed from all sides and perspectives.
3. Thought Phase: to personalize the event and shift focus; to transition from factual to emotional focus. Participants are asked to share what "thoughts" they had at key times.
4. Reaction Phase: to identify and ventilate feelings (emotions) raised by the event.
5. Symptom Phase: to normalize personal physical stress responses. The leader guides transition back from emotional to factual focus, legitimizing participant's physical symptoms and behavioral reactions.
6. Teaching Phase: to reassure by educating that the feelings and stress symptoms are normal reactions to abnormal conditions; they may last a while, but can be expected to resolve normally.
7. Reentry Phase: to complete and close the debriefing.

It is important to ensure that participants have follow-up options as individuals or as a group.

Adapted from US Department of the Army. *Debriefer's Guide to Critical Event Debriefing*. Fort Sam Houston, Tex: Combat Stress Actions Office, Department of Preventive Health Services, Army Medical Department Center and School; 1993: 1–4.

debriefed; the after-action debriefing is led by the small unit's own leader.
The critical event debriefer explicitly defers issues of operational lessons learned in order to focus on the stress aspects and stress responses; the after-action debriefer does seek to capture relevant operational lessons learned in positive terms.[17(pp6-7,6-8)]

U.S. Army doctrine[17] also cautions leaders regarding preventive intervention after traumatic stress.

(1) The analogy between PTSD preventive interventions and traumatic wound surgery suggests a cautionary warning. If the surgery is not done skillfully, it can cause more harm than good, leaving dead tissue and bacteria in the wound. It may cut away tissue that did not need to be sacrificed, or realign the broken bones incorrectly. The same is potentially true for poorly executed after-action debriefings or critical event debriefings.

(2) The problem for early prevention efforts is to forewarn of possible post-traumatic stress symptoms without glamorizing them or advertising them as a reimbursable long-term disability. To do the latter invites malingering. It also subtly encourages those who do have real but not disabling post-traumatic symptoms to magnify them. This will be especially likely if they have other psychological issues or grievances which the symptoms also address, such as feeling unappreciated for the sacrifices suffered or guilt at having left their buddies.

(3) As with the treatment of acute battle fatigue, it is essential that all persons involved in preventive or treatment interventions for PTSD express positive expectation of normal recovery. At the same time, they must indicate that continuing or recurring symptoms can and should be treated, still with positive expectation of rapid improvement. They should advise that post-traumatic stress symptoms may recur in the future at times of new stress. Successful treatment after future episodes should deal with the ongoing, new stressors as much as with the past trauma.[17(p 6-8)]

Case Study 1: The Medic and the Resuscitation

In the evening of 28 February 1991 (the cease fire ending the Persian Gulf War had gone into effect at 0800 hours that morning), as two cavalry units were moving into captured territory, the headquarters troop was establishing camp for the night. They had moved their vehicles into a coil, which is a circular defensive arrangement with tanks and fighting vehicles facing outward. The men were digging foxholes in front of their vehicles. One young soldier, a member of a fighting vehicle crew, was digging his foxhole when his vehicle commander called him back to his vehicle. The soldier turned, shouldered his shovel, and stepped on an unexploded Dual Purpose Improved Conventional Munition (DPICM), which exploded. The soldier was carrying rifle grenades in a bandoleer across his chest. These exploded as well. The soldier was in all probability killed outright.

Two young medics (both inexperienced and just out of school), who had only a few months earlier joined the unit, and only a few weeks before joined this particular troop, tried to resuscitate the soldier. The resuscitation was gruesome. As they tried to ventilate the soldier, air escaped from his cheek, so someone put a hand there. Then air escaped from his chest, then his abdomen, and finally even from one eye socket. The medics continued their efforts for approximately 20 minutes at which time a physician from the medical troop arrived, assessed the situation as hopeless, and called off the resuscitation.

Two days later a combat stress control (CSC) team was asked to see one of the medics because he was clearly troubled by what had happened. The team members responded that they would see him, but that if he was obviously distressed there was probably significant distress in others who had been involved in the resuscitation, as well as the soldier's comrades, and his immediate chain of command. The team proposed assembling all involved to do a debriefing and reconstruction of the accident and resuscitation, along with relevant events before and after. The chain of command agreed.

The group was assembled in the open air and arranged cots in a circle for everyone to sit on. The briefing was begun with the suggestion that for the purpose of reconstructing events, ranks be set aside and that all participants be accorded the status of equal witnesses.

In the course of the debriefing, the details of the resuscitation were presented. The medic the team had been asked to see twice got up and stood in the center of the group, with his eyes focused far away from the group, and described what he had seen and done during the resuscitation. The other medic contributed details as well. The soldier's vehicle commander described the events leading up to the accident. The soldier's friends initially expressed reservations about the competency of the medics and whether all that could have been done had in fact been done. At that point the distressed medic stood back up in front of the group and provided graphic details of the resuscitation. It was then obvious to the dead soldier's friends who had not seen the accident and the resuscitation efforts that the medics had done all that could be done. The medics had done more than the soldier's friends could imagine themselves doing. As he recounted the resuscitation, the medic became less distressed and gained confidence and self-assurance. Concerns of the soldier's friends over the quality of the resuscitation quickly receded.

The dead soldier's chain of command raised another issue before the group. By regulation, the soldier could have been granted emergency leave to go home to visit his wife and new baby just before the ground war had begun, but he had decided to stay with the unit and go to war with his friends. After some discussion, the group consensus was that he had made the correct decision to stay with his group even though they were all sorry that he was dead.

One other issue was raised by the group. The soldier had been wearing a rifle grenade bandoleer when he stepped on the DPICM. The explosion of those grenades probably contributed to his injuries. The fact that he was carrying these grenades at all had been a concern to some of his friends and to his chain of command. He had no compelling reason to be carrying them once the cease fire went into effect, but no one had pushed him to give up wearing the grenades. In retrospect, the participants wished they had taken a firmer stance with respect to the grenades.

By the end of the debriefing the participants had a clearer view of the accident, its antecedents, and the resuscitation. For the distressed medic, the debriefing was clearly a turning point in terms of how he viewed himself and how his comrades viewed him. By the end of the debriefing he was clearly free of distress and his comrades viewed him with new respect.[20]

Comment: This case report demonstrates the value of group debriefing after an especially traumatic and gruesome event. It was clear from the participants that most members of the unit, not just the distressed medic, had been affected by the accident and subsequent death. Clarifying the sequence of events and responses to them allowed the unit to put the event into perspective, thus facilitating the reintegration of the medic into the unit.

Psychiatric Debriefing

Psychiatric debriefing (as presented further in this chapter) begins the debriefing process with an education briefing about normal stress and the prevention of PTSD. This may be delivered to large audiences. Groups of participants are then led by psychiatrically trained debriefers in an active process of ventilation (abreaction), sharing, and normalizing of stress reactions. This includes further interpretation and education about psychological defenses (the adaptive and the maladaptive ones). While participants are told that they are not "patients," this technique comes close to being psychotherapy. It may be the most expedient method for assisting a large, ad hoc group that will disperse after the debriefing and not have the protective benefits of continuing in a cohesive, working organization.

Large Group Debriefing

Large group debriefing[17] is an umbrella term for expedient debriefings involving large numbers of people (100 to 500 or more) where it is impossible to actively involve everyone. The organizational leaders of the sub-elements of the group (for example the platoon leaders, company commanders, first sergeants) perhaps supplemented by natural leaders or "key players" from the enlisted ranks, review and reconstruct the facts of the critical event or longer operation while the remainder watch and listen. Large group debriefings are of limited use for critical traumatic events, except for further integrative processing after the most traumatized elements have been debriefed in their own smaller groups. They can be very effective as end-of-tour debriefings.

Case Study 2: Troop by Troop

An armored cavalry regiment fought effectively in the ground offensive of the Persian Gulf War, but suffered losses from friendly fire and from unexploded ordnance. During and immediately after the battle it had the benefit of an expert combat stress control (CSC) team that had been requested by the regimental commander from the corps. That team conducted several small group debriefings during and after the campaign. On returning to home base, one of the squadron commanders followed the advice of the CSC team and conducted debriefings with the entire squadron, a troop at a time. The squadron commander, assisted by each troop's commander, conducted debriefing reconstructions of the entire battle with the assembled troops. Concerns that the process might scapegoat or place guilt and blame on only a few individuals were unfounded. It was clear to all that the confusion and fatigue of a rapid advance through desert winter weather and the snowballing consequences of many small glitches in communication, coordination, and alertness spread the blame. Further, it was clear that when things went well, it wasn't just one person doing the right thing, but a whole series of correct and timely actions that led to a good outcome.

Comment: Postcombat reconstructive debriefings are something that not only mental health personnel but every commander should have in his hip pocket and be ready to use after any significant action.

End-of-Tour Debriefing

End-of-tour (or demobilization) debriefings summarize all the significant events in an entire, prolonged operation. It begins by soliciting memories (good and bad), thoughts, and reactions during initial alert and mobilization. When everyone has had their say on that, discussion proceeds step by step through the good and bad memories and lessons learned of the actual deployment, the first days, middle and final phases of the operation, up to the present. The operation may or may not have involved traumatic events, but is likely to have caused many frustrations and perhaps resentments that can be ventilated and not carried home. The process should end with a positive sense of closure.

These debriefing categories are not rigidly fixed, and can merge into each other. The debriefing team must choose the appropriate type and format for the specific traumatic incident. For example, natural disasters may require different debriefing styles than do combat or human-caused incidents. Debriefings of impersonal, mass-casualty disasters should differ from those for small but highly personalized or traumatic incidents. The characteristics of the participants should influence the choice of format. Even in the same traumatic event, debriefings conducted with surviving victims must differ substantially from debriefings of the immediate response rescuers, or of the second-echelon caregivers. Debriefings of senior leaders and their staffs will differ from the debriefings of the junior leaders and the troops. Debriefings of elite, cohesive, and "macho" units must differ from debriefings of ad hoc assemblages of victims, rescuers, or survivors. End-of-tour debriefings (EOTD) that do not involve traumatic events must differ from those that do.

Available resources will often limit (but should not dictate) the type of debriefings that can be accomplished. Some of the factors that influence the choice of debriefing format are the number of experienced and partially trained debriefing personnel, access to safe and reasonably comfortable facilities, the total number and internal organization of the population to be debriefed, the other conflicting mission or treatment demands, and, especially, time.

The remainder of this chapter presents the first and second authors' experience in conducting psychiatric debriefings and end-of-tour debriefings during and after the U.S. invasion of Panama and the Persian Gulf War. Other information on debriefings is provided in Chapter 9, U.S. Naval Combat Psychiatry, and Chapter 12, Postcombat Reentry.

PSYCHIATRIC DEBRIEFING TASKS

Predebriefing

A model of community consultation which had been developed in the wake of the Korean conflict is useful in setting the stage for the psychiatric debriefing.[21] Because the debriefing is intended to initiate the reintegration process, the mental health personnel must make contact with the command structure of the unit being debriefed.

If possible, a working relationship with the command structure should be developed prior to any trauma. The contact is intended to educate the leaders of the group about the importance of psychological debriefing in the prevention of PTSD and other sequelae of mobilization and reentry. The process of command contact has been described in Chapter 9, Command Consultation, in *Military Psychiatry: Preparing in Peace for War*,[22] a companion to this volume. This process applies whether the mental health team is organic to the higher headquarters of the supported unit (for example, the mental health section in a division) or is providing area support (for example, the mental health section of an Area Support Medical Battalion or U.S. Army CSC Detachment in the field or the Community Mental Health Service or Departments of Psychiatry, Psychology or Social Work of a post's Medical Activity in garrison). The same skills have been practiced by U.S. Army psychiatrists working in civilian homeless shelters. In this instance psychiatrists prepared the shelter staff for the introduction of direct delivery of psychiatric services[23,24] by building relationships with the shelter leadership over a 3- to 4-month period. The objective of this approach is for the commanders to give permission to soldiers (or civilian workers, family members, and others) to voice their concerns without fear of repercussions. Their experience is validated as a necessary part of their job during difficult circumstances.

Thus, predebriefing tasks are

- Preparing commanders.
- Conducting higher command or installation briefing.
- Maintaining liaison with chaplains and other medical and mental health support agencies.
- Conducting mental health activity training.

Military authorities higher than the unit command structure or installation directly involved may have to be briefed concerning the necessity for psychiatric debriefing of soldiers. This is because soldiers can be negative about the command structure during the debriefing itself, and the work of the mental health team may be seen as divisive and undermining. A simple explanation of the facts concerning the prevention of PTSD and the helpfulness in maintaining unit cohesion in the face of trauma is usually all that is necessary.

Chaplains, mental health and social support services, emergency, and other medical personnel will become involved in the debriefing process or its follow-up, and it is necessary to educate and coordinate activities with them. When services are not coordinated, other workers may label individual soldiers as patients and thereby increase their psychiatric morbidity. This phenomenon was seen most strikingly during World War II, when soldiers were evacuated to the rear and developed prolonged emotional symptoms.[25,26] This has been found to be a sequela of the "evacuation syndrome."

Training of mental health staff is especially important during this phase prior to the debriefing. Mock debriefings may be helpful in providing staff an opportunity to practice interventions that encourage the expression of feelings and discourage the tendency to overemphasize the reaction to the trauma. In the experience of the authors, staff training is ongoing and involves mock debriefings, follow-up information, and dissemination of data on the efficacy of psychiatric debriefings. Work of this nature is likely to decrease the incidence of worker burnout as well as provide for more effective delivery of care.[27] Ideally, members of a debriefing team should first observe a real debriefing led by an experienced debriefer; second, lead a debriefing while being observed and mentored by an experienced debriefer; and, finally, observe and mentor a new debriefer. This is the "see one, do one, teach one" method. However, this ideal requires a steady succession of local traumatic events which will not always be available for training.

Debriefing

When the debriefing begins, it is essential that commanders provide an introduction to lend credibility to the event. A model that has proven beneficial includes the large group setting initially for relaying information about the risk factors for the development of PTSD and potential problems associated with reunions with families and communities. Of special importance is the message that the feelings and symptoms, which can be emotional or physical, are normal responses to an abnormal situation. Often this is enough to relieve the anxiety of the soldiers affected.

If time permits, small groups of 8 to 10 participants can then be formed with one or two workers from the mental health staff, who facilitate a discussion of events encountered by the soldiers.

The tasks of the debriefing are

1. Utilizing large-group setting for information sharing and discussion of normal reactions to trauma.
2. Utilizing small groups (8–10 participants, 2–3 facilitators) for exploration of issues (if sufficient staff is available).
3. Maintaining confidentiality.

Confidentiality appears to be a major theme in these discussions. During the small group sessions soldiers may be reticent to describe their experiences because of possible repercussions. They have to be assured that the purpose of the debriefing is not to point out blame or to solve administrative problems. Therefore, they can be encouraged to share their feelings with impunity. Also, silence, sometimes encouraged in therapy, is not helpful in these groups. The facilitators have to be aggressive and ask the soldiers to recall stories and hear about their concerns. The time limit for the entire debriefing can vary from 90 to 120 minutes.

Common defenses during this phase may be denial, anger, and guilt, which have been described elsewhere.[28,29] As in the experience of any traumatic event, the psychological mechanisms which mollify the experience come into play almost immediately. The debriefer must be aware that supporting these defenses, by allowing for ventilation at an early stage, can make the use of these defenses less important as time goes by.

Postdebriefing

It must be remembered that debriefing is the beginning of a process of reintegration for soldiers involved in combat or other trauma. Therefore, the debriefers must set the stage for further supportive work if needed, without predicting negative reactions or fostering dependency. This includes identifying and contacting individuals who show signs of needing psychiatric referrals, without stigmatizing them. It includes continued consultation to commanders who may require guidance in matters such as giving passes, leaves, and reassignments.

It is also crucial that the administrative/clinical head of the debriefing process debrief his or her own staff. Feelings of anger, denial, and guilt present in the soldiers can also be overwhelming for the debriefers. Because war can be horrifying, involving the death and mutilation of friends, comrades, and even family members, it is important to take care of the workers involved in helping the soldiers integrate the experience.

After-action reports also serve to organize one's thoughts, and serve as a "clinical" record of the proceedings of the debriefing. They are extremely useful in understanding some of the basic themes experienced by soldiers and the data from after-action reports can guide remarks in the opening moments of the debriefing.

Thus, the postdebriefing tasks are

- Conducting follow-up and referrals as needed.
- Conducting command/community consultations.
- Debriefing staff.
- Completing after-action reports.

ISSUES AND PITFALLS OF DEBRIEFING

There are several issues and pitfalls in debriefing. First is a lack of support on the part of the command or leadership structure of the unit. This is often due to misunderstanding of the value of the debriefing to future readiness. The command may view the debriefer as creating problems rather than preventing them or even of being divisive and subversive. Because so many feelings are part of the experience of trauma, and there is a tendency to project blame onto leadership, commanders can feel that their authority is being undermined. Contact with commanders early on alleviates the responsibility of blame from them. When presented with the historical data suggesting increased unit cohesion, and a decrease in psychiatric symptomatology following debriefing, commanders are ready to utilize debriefing services.

Debriefers may find that there is a tendency to provide easy solutions and to assign blame for the problems of the unit. It is easy enough to agree with soldiers or victims that their commander's lack of leadership abilities was responsible for their waiting in the desert for 2 weeks without an assignment. In fact, the assignment may have been beyond the commander's ability to influence, but angry feelings are nevertheless present. An exploration of these feelings is the proper intervention, rather than blaming the commander or encouraging that the unit initiate an investigation into his ability to lead.

The timing of the debriefing is of vital importance. While certain groups may be too emotionally and cognitively exhausted to process information, immediacy is a factor in the theory and practice of debriefing. Often, groups have already begun to process the traumatic event in a destructive manner, and the large groups involved (eg, U.S. Army, civilian communities) may act pro forma and without regard to long-term consequences by dispersing groups exposed to trauma in a rushed fashion. Reflexive defenses start to work almost immediately as the individuals begin to deny and project anger, so many groups can and should be debriefed as soon as possible. The clinician has to assess if they are able to do so at the time.

However, when debriefing is done too close to the traumatic event, victims may feel further traumatized and vulnerable. A period of rest and regrouping is preferable (but in the "real world," sometimes not possible) prior to debriefing. Some researchers feel that when a person is in a state of physiological arousal (1–5 d) after the trauma, debriefing may be harmful.[30] Others cite the tendency of individuals and groups to form a "trauma membrane" (a mental scab) after about 3 days; prior to then they may be eager and even driven to talk of the event. After then they may avoid and resist being reminded. In this formulation, 1 to 2 days after the event is optimal for debriefing. This area is controversial and will require further study. The following case example shows how debriefing a combat unit too soon might have caused an increasing psychiatric pathology. The case is disguised to protect the anonymity of the unit.

Case Study 3: The Helicopter Crash

Company A, deployed to Saudi Arabia prior to the start of Operation Desert Shield in 1990, suffered the loss of 15 of its 60 members during a helicopter crash. While on nighttime maneuvers, part of the unit being transported by helicopter crashed into the desert sands. All members on board the aircraft were killed by the impact and badly burned in the ensuing fire.

When the unit commander learned of the crash, he informed his superiors and subordinates in the chain of command. On orders from the senior commander, a psychiatrist and social workers were sent within 4 hours to gather the remaining soldiers in the unit and begin a debriefing. During this period, the psychiatrist provided information about stress-related psychiatric disability and predicted the possibility of intrusive nightmares, thoughts, and angry feelings. Soldiers at the meeting, which lasted about 2 hours, were generally quiet, and appeared dazed and startled. Others looked angry, while still others were sad, immobile, and worried.

After the mental health personnel left, the soldiers met independently in their barracks and discussed how angry they felt towards the psychiatrist and social worker because of the invasion of privacy they felt. "They don't even know what we do, who we are, or how we feel," some members of the unit stated.

A follow-up on this unit revealed an increased incidence (compared with other units) of disciplinary actions, and alcohol-related incidents 4 months after returning to the United States.

Comment: In effect, this intervention was a stress briefing, not a debriefing. It may have inadvertently "pathologized" rather than "normalized" the predictable stress symptoms. Also, it lasted too long. The Critical Incident Stress Foundation[16] recommends brief (10–15 min) "defusings" immediately after the critical event to normalize the immediate reactions and set the stage for a debriefing in 1 to 3 days. A debriefing might have been more effective if it had asked unit members to describe how they were involved or heard about the crash and encouraged them to share their feelings rather than listening to theories about stress.

Mental health staff can become overwhelmed by the debriefing process. War, because of its intensity and disregard for human life, may bring forth a variety of feelings from those individuals who work with combat veterans. The staff must have a period of decompression themselves in order to put the experience into perspective. Most individuals in the helping professions would rather take care of a problem when it arises; during the debriefing process, taking care of the problem involves a reticent, supportive, and encouraging stance.

Thus, the issues and pitfalls of the debriefing process are

- Lack of command understanding and support of the debriefing process.
- Tendency to assign blame.
- Tendency to provide "easy" solutions.
- Inappropriate timing.
- Failure to debrief mental health staff.

IMPLEMENTATION OF PSYCHIATRIC DEBRIEFING

The following case studies are provided for illustration of key concepts in the process of psychiatric debriefing. In Case Study 4, attention is paid to the psychiatrist's efforts at following the correct debriefing process. Although no relationship was built with the affected unit prior to the trauma, the psychiatrist used the medical facility as a familiar site and medical demobilization as a familiar process to aid in developing rapport with the soldiers. In Case Study 5, a disguised case example, the importance of eliciting feelings is demonstrated. Both examples are taken from military experience, but may be adapted easily to the management of civilian critical incidents. Case study 4, drawn from the authors' experience, is of a delayed post-trauma and end-of-tour debriefing.

Case Study 4: Explosion in the Desert

Company B is a reserve unit of about 70 members who were called to active duty in preparation for an overseas military mission. Prior to deployment, the commander of the unit assisted soldiers in developing family care plans, organized spouse groups, and rallied community support. Most soldiers were new to the unit and in their 20s.

When the unit arrived at the deployment site, the commander suffered an exacerbation of physical complaints that had been long-standing. He required hospitalization, evaluation, and eventually was given a medical profile that restricted him from deploying with the unit. The executive officer of the unit assumed command. The first sergeant arrived late because of family problems and was unable to assist in the reorganization and stabilization of the unit. Additionally, the unit, which was originally scheduled to deploy within 3 days of arrival at the mobilization site, was delayed for departure by 2 weeks.

During this time, the chaplain assigned to the unit noted high levels of stress and uncertainty about the details of deployment in the unit. He reported high levels of anxiety and apathy as calls to family members exacerbated unit members' sense of helplessness in dealing with family issues back home.

When the unit finally deployed, family members arrived at the deployment site to wish the unit well. Although there was a ceremony with speeches from political as well as military officials, unit members reported feeling scared and overwhelmingly sad about leaving.

Upon arriving in the war zone, the unit was housed in temporary quarters awaiting its mission in the war effort. Soldiers reported feeling useless and anxious about the uncertainty of their jobs in the overall mission.

Two weeks after arriving, a fuel tank exploded and nearly one half of the soldiers were killed and most of the others were wounded. Most of the living and wounded soldiers suffered ruptured eardrums and acute anxiety reactions.

After the explosion, the soldiers were evacuated to a safe area, given clothing (as some were in night clothes and most uniforms had been destroyed), and were given permanent housing. The surviving soldiers met briefly with a "stress team" consisting of a chaplain, psychologist, and psychiatrist, who described some of the aftereffects to be expected from this tragedy and attempted to elicit feelings and fears.

The Persian Gulf War ended so soon after the explosion that the surviving unit was redeployed to the continental United States without ever having been reconstituted to perform their mission. The psychiatrist at the deployment site explained to the medical command the need for debriefing and began training the mental health staff in preparation for this task. Initially, there was not much support for debriefing the soldiers because the process was seen as another time commitment with logistical problems for the hospital staff. As a compromise, the debriefing was streamlined and "married" to the out-processing medical examination.

When the hospital command learned of the return of Company B, there was already pressure from political and installation officials to rapidly process the remaining soldiers for return to home in civilian life. A parade was planned as was a reception by the post commanding general.

The soldiers were met at the airport by high-ranking military officers and the chaplain originally assigned to the unit. The soldiers were to be examined that evening and returned home in the morning. However, because the medical staff reemphasized the importance of rest and debriefing, examinations were rescheduled for the following morning.

The debriefing almost did not occur. The debriefers planned to meet the group after the medical examinations for 15 to 30 minutes and break into smaller groups for 1 hour. Some officials said that the debriefing already occurred in Saudi Arabia. In fact, the hospital commander was told by a representative from the installation that the examinations were taking too long, the doctors were not working fast enough, and that "all these soldiers need is a hug from their families ... so hurry up."

The authors, as the debriefers, however, insisted upon conducting the debriefing but were given only 30 minutes. The meeting opened with introductory remarks describing the usefulness of debriefing as well as the difficulties that soldiers might face upon reentry into their communities. One soldier said, "We don't need this, we are all friends and don't want to talk." Most were able to talk about their feelings, however, which centered around anger and helplessness. There were attempts to place blame on the unit's leaders as well as on those not injured in the attack, or were absent at the time of the bombing. Soldiers described various somatic complaints: hearing problems, gastritis, muscle aches, and headaches. They said that communication was poor in the war zone, they did not know who had been killed, where the unit members were, or who was in charge. A second lieutenant was given command in the war zone and despite his eagerness and enthusiasm, he was the object of some ridicule for not being able to solve problems such as clothing and shelter.

They described especially their reaction to the stress team. Many soldiers felt that the team was intrusive, invasive, and offered solutions to problems too prematurely. They experienced the stress team as chiding them for poor behavior in the face of a crisis.

After the debriefing, the staff met to talk about the experience. Most had never participated in a debriefing of this type. The overall sense was one of helplessness and a need to place blame and find solutions. The installation commander was blamed for hustling these troops, the hospital commander for lack of support, the soldiers for being inarticulate and childlike, and the staff blamed itself for opening up emotional wounds. The need for blame was again interpreted and at that time, the process of debriefing was better understood.

One week later, an after-action report was forwarded to the hospital commander and the Office of the Surgeon General recommending training in debriefing and greater support of this endeavor. After the soldiers of Company B returned home, several of the soldiers made an official protest regarding the rushed treatment they received during the demobilization process. Many wanted to spend time as soldiers in a nonthreatening environment after combat, but were quickly returned to civilian life. As a result, some actually had to be brought back onto active duty to continue with psychiatric treatment and other debriefing activities.

Comment: This case study highlights the importance of communication with the command structure and the role of debriefing soldiers who have been involved in combat. Several pitfalls were avoided when the psychiatrist enlisted the support of the medical and administrative staff of the hospital to authorize the debriefing. The debriefing of the mental health staff was essential in their understanding the whole process of debriefing as well as to clear any possible feelings of guilt and responsibility in the endeavor.

The following case example, also drawn from the authors' experience, describes the importance of team work in debriefing and demonstrates the effectiveness of debriefing in eliciting feelings and emotions related to the combat situation. It involves a delayed post-trauma debriefing and end-of-tour debriefing.

Case Study 5: After the Battle

When Company C returned from Saudi Arabia, one of us (RK) was asked to debrief this reserve combat unit. The debriefing was conducted 4 months after return from the Persian Gulf. The unit was from the area adjacent to the mobilization post, so the preparations for deployment were familiar. The unit had begun preparations about 1 month prior to the start of the ground war by combat training in the United States. Three weeks prior to the ground war, the unit arrived in Saudi Arabia. They continued their combat training and suffered some psychological hardship of having no mail and no phones available for approximately the first 2 months.

Company C participated in the beginning of the ground operation and actually preceded the infantry into Kuwait. One service member was injured in his face by fragments but suffered minimal long-term effects. A second service member was killed while he was attempting to clear bunkers and apparently stepped on explosives. He lost a limb immediately and then died two days later in the hospital.

When the participants of the debriefing were allowed to comment freely, the following is a sampling of what they said:

"After we got back home, it was hard to get back into the flow of things. We had a terrifying experience for a short period of time, but now we feel like we want to use our time wisely."

"The period after the war was perhaps more psychologically disturbing than the war itself, since we had so much time on our hands and nothing really to do. We played volleyball, ate beans and rice and were really lonely. Phones were then available for the first time but they were expensive to use and there were long lines."

"We had trouble getting back into the flow, especially changing from military to civilian life. We didn't have any drills for the first 2 months after we got home."

"We tried to eat all the good food we had missed and drink all the good alcohol we had missed for 6 months."

"Although this unit returned to this country in May 1991, this debriefing (September 1991) is only the third Reserve meeting we have held."

"Routine matters like paying bills do not seem to matter much."

Comment: As the soldiers spoke, it was clear they were describing the frustrations of reentry into usual military life or civilian life. It was tempting for the team members to help them with suggestions, but the team members resisted and allowed the soldiers to tell their stories.

"We were promised that we would have a job waiting for us when we got back but some of us really had slots waiting and not regular jobs, and some of us had to move to another state."

"The main problem was that for 4 to 5 months we had one purpose and one purpose alone, then we came back to civilian life and we had absolutely nothing to do. We asked what is the meaning of life."

"Many of us were angry, especially for the first 2 weeks."

"After we were angry, nothing phased us. Overdue bills would bring this kind of reaction—Gee, this is all they've go to do?"

"There was poor attendance at Reserve drills for the first drill or two in contrast to before combat where drill attendance had been 95%."

"Much of the equipment has not arrived back to the unit even as of yet."

"The morale was good up to the cease fire."

"The service member killed in combat was 21 or 22 years old. He was a college student who was going to be a unit leader. He was a member of the company for about a year. He was well-known and well-liked."

"One of our members died in a street accident. It was a case of 'mistaken identity,' although drugs may have been involved."

"Being without money was not a big deal because it was expensive and there were long lines to buy things. Being without mail for 2 months was very upsetting, we could see no reason for having our mail come to us late. We were simply told that there were not enough people to sort the mail."

"There were many problems with pay, both active duty and reservists. The active duty had one pay system and the reservists had another. Some of us got no pay at all, some got double pay, and some of us had much more taken out later than we had imagined."

"Some of us felt, and still feel annoyed when people walk up to us in shopping centers and ask if we killed anybody. The support is strong but sometimes results in constant nagging and asking questions that upset us."

"Why did it take them so long to get us home? We waited for 35 days to have our chance to get onto an airplane and come home. One of our senators came to visit us but he did not know where we had been or what we had done."

"When we arrived in the desert, which took us only a day to get there, we were treated warmly by the active duty units, but when they left, they left us taking our equipment and leaving us with no feeling that we had been appreciated because they left us there alone."

"The activation process took too long. It created a great deal of stress. We were within several hours of home but we could not go there for more than a month. We said good-bye to our families and then went just several hours away and stayed there for a month, creating a lot of stress that we could not deal with. We feel that we should have had some psychological debriefing at that point."

Comment: Many soldiers were angry concerning their service in the Persian Gulf War. They spoke about the inefficiencies they encountered and when returning did not feel they were treated "special" for their efforts.

"One of our greatest stressors was not knowing one day to the next what is going on. This was not due to our leadership. The officers were also uninformed. We were not informed. A major problem was communication. We especially needed to improve communication between active duty and reserve units."

"The active duty often put us down, even though we were in front of them in the battle."

"Another major problem was false information."

One service member said PTSD stands for "pissed, tired, and sick of drills" without knowing he was very close to the actual meaning of the symptoms of PTSD, and that his anger, difficulty sleeping, and substance abuse were early stages.

"The government got us geared up for high expectations for combat. We were not let down because we were not in combat much and yet we had a great deal of energy created within us and it had no where to go. We have not yet found a way to release this energy. The energy is stopped up inside of us. Working out or exercise helps a little bit. We really don't know what to do with the extra energy."

"Back home after combat, everything seems trivial. Dealing with others is very difficult now."

"Some people seem to hold it against us for going to war, especially if we try to say anything about it. We don't want to hurt the feeling of those who didn't go, yet some of us are very mad at those 18 members of our unit who lied about reasons for not being sent to war."

"We are sick and tired of being compared to Vietnam."

"Some people who watched the war on TV said 'You didn't really fight a war, you just sat around in the sand.'"

"I am involved at home with my wife and child, I have calmed down only a little bit."

"I was just married and sent overseas 6 months after I was married. It has been hard to get back into the relationship since I got back, it just doesn't seem right any more. I have to get out of the house and I usually go somewhere and drink."

"People ask stupid questions like, 'Did you kill anybody, or who was the first person you killed?'"

"We did our job, we are back in the real world, and it is hard to get back into the flow of things."

"Jobs and things that used to worry us, don't really seem that important any more."

"Money is a problem. The military didn't pay us as much as we made on the outside. Some of us didn't pick up any help either."

"Our unit still feels a little bit disorganized. We are getting things done, but we don't seem like we were before we went to war."

"We feel the reserve unit should stay together longer to support each other." (The group was encouraged to exchange phone numbers and stay in close contact with each other.)

"What pissed me off the most was getting ready to go over there and then getting over there and feeling like we didn't get the job done completely and the fear we may have to go back."

"We need psychological debriefing before deployment."

Comment: These sentiments are fairly typical of the several dozen debriefings the authors conducted during the demobilization phase of Operation Desert Shield/Storm. The debriefing demonstrated that many personnel in a unit can experience significant and persistent distress from the circumstances of the deployment and return home, unrelated to any specific critical (life-threatening) event. Many of the problems discussed and the persistent bad feelings they engendered could have been prevented had the unit been encouraged and mentored to conduct routine after-action reviews and after-action debriefings throughout the entire deployment.

There is an interesting follow-up regarding Company C. Approximately 9 months following the debriefing where the above comments were made, two soldiers were killed in automobile accidents that involved alcohol. Several others had not yet procured jobs, while others had been referred for alcohol and drug treatment. Another debriefing of the reserve unit was requested. Comments from this debriefing centered around the sense of helplessness and abandonment by families, friends, and the community. A commitment was made to continue work with this reserve unit, who found it helpful to have the opportunity to express feelings and frustrations regarding the effects of deployment on their lives.

Finally, the process of developing a multidisciplinary team prior to combat or trauma is described in the following case, which involved a critical incident psychiatric model debriefing.

Case Study 6: Death in the Jungle

Prior to any battle during Operation Just Cause, the Chief of Psychiatry at the U.S. Army Hospital in Panama assembled a crisis intervention team. The purpose of this team was to provide immediate mental health intervention during and after disasters related to combat. The team consisted of a team chief who was a military psychiatrist trained in crisis intervention and debriefing. Virtually all other military mental health providers in Panama were included on the team (psychiatrists, psychologists, social workers, nurses, and enlisted mental health specialists). This all-inclusive concept was considered critical to ensure that enough trained personnel were available when needed.

The second key element in staffing was to utilize U.S. Army, U.S. Navy, and U.S. Air Force personnel. Training accidents and natural disasters could affect any of the three service populations. A team member from that service could act as a valuable liaison, especially in the initial phase of trust-building between the affected personnel and the crisis team members.

Finally, it was important to utilize enlisted personnel in these interventions in order to promote the building of rapport. Many affected enlisted individuals might have difficulty relating to officers during a time of crisis.

Training in mental health interventions in combat and natural disasters was conducted on an ongoing basis. Discussions were held on the main tenets of crisis intervention therapy, victimology, and command consultation. Specific topics at such meetings included: the unique psychodynamics of individuals who have had to face life-threatening situations themselves, or who lost a friend to sudden, violent death. Additionally, any actual disaster interventions were reviewed with special attention to lessons learned.

Command sponsorship was especially important. Because the team was organized prior to any actual combat, enough time was available to brief commanders about the importance of mental health intervention during combat or disasters. The previous state of haphazard referral promoted anxiety among commanders about the consequences of allowing mental health personnel into a disaster scene, and kept troops in need of help out of reach. In order to ensure that command sponsorship became a reality in Panama, a detailed proposal was forwarded to the military command in Panama explaining the need for the team and the critical importance of the command's formally incorporating the mental health mission.

During the early morning hours of 22 February 1990 (approximately 6 to 7 weeks after Operation Just Cause), two helicopters flying a night training mission were lost in a northern province of Panama. The night was moonless and severe weather added to the difficult flying conditions. Once the aircraft were reported missing, an intensive search was begun. The search parties included personnel from the same unit that had suffered the losses. Due to the triple canopy jungle, poor weather, and wide search area, the downed aircraft were not found for nearly 36 hours.

The searchers located the two helicopters destroyed in the separate accidents that had caused the immediate deaths of 11 U.S. Army soldiers. There were no survivors. The affected units included aviators (the air crew) and infantrymen (the passengers). Due to the unexpected and massive nature of the tragedy, there was considerable emotional fallout in the community. Notably, the disasters took place during a period of high morale in the local population. The long-anticipated invasion of Panama 2 months earlier had inspired a feeling of a "job well done." The community was much better prepared for the potential loss of life during combat than at the time of the above-described accidents.

As the situation developed over the 36 hours after the accidents, it became clear that an aggressive mental health intervention was needed. Local mental health providers became aware of the tragedy later that day and began immediate efforts to contact the commanders involved. This effort was hindered by the fact that many of the affected individuals were involved in the search and were unavailable and the commander of the infantrymen involved had been killed in the crash. Nonetheless, by the second day, the mental health team chief accompanied those personnel tasked with identification of the dead. In addition, team members, including a psychologist and five enlisted behavioral science specialists, were on standby status. Aggressive negotiations with commanders resulted in the team arriving at the unit barracks on Sunday morning, 25 February 1990. After initial briefing interviews with the command, the team then held two group sessions of approximately 90 minutes each with all available members of the affected units. The following sections describe the specifics of that intervention in these areas: education, identification, process, and follow-up.

Education. The education process was begun with a brief overview of the history of combat psychiatry. The emphasis here, and throughout the intervention, was on the normal responses to psychic trauma. The team explained the evolution of thought in this area (eg, how in previous conflicts soldiers suffering psychological symptoms in the face of trauma were sometimes evacuated and treated like mentally ill patients). Team members explained that modern day mental health providers think of psychologic symptoms as a normal response to trauma, and expect that most soldiers will recover fully. They were pointedly told, "You are not patients."

In addition, an explanation of the psychology of victims was presented. Victimology classifies various levels of individuals affected by a disaster primarily by psychologic proximity to the event. This concept was very useful in helping soldiers understand their affective responses, even though many were not directly involved in the accident.

Team members also discussed the classic acute responses to trauma: anxiety, sleep disturbances, irritability, increased alcohol use, and somatic complaints.

This initial portion of the session (approximately 20 min) provided a cognitive framework for the soldiers to begin thinking about their varied and intensely emotional responses.

Identification. From the outset of the intervention, the group was told that some people may need or want individual attention. The soldiers and commanders were given the location and phone numbers of the two military mental health clinics several times throughout the day.

Additionally, the debriefing team members were instructed to watch for individuals who seemed especially affected. During breaks, providers approached smaller groups of soldiers and individuals with this idea in mind. A small number of people were identified in this fashion and later seen on an outpatient basis.

Process. Those affected individually were encouraged, at times, and even called on, to discuss the events of the previous 2 days. Predictably, many of the group members were feeling angry, guilty, or were in a state of denial of symptoms. Team members were instructed to allow discussion and be able to tolerate silences. Appropriate interpretations were made, especially in the areas of displacement, regression, and denial.

The almost universal incidence of some degree of guilt and denial warrants further description. A phenomenon observed numerous times involved individuals inappropriately accepting responsibility for elements of the tragedy. This was consistent with Schwartz's[31] observation, "The patient becomes unable to discern where his will ends and fate begins." While this construct allowed them the solace of not having to face their powerlessness, the accompanying guilt for action not taken was in some cases overwhelming.

The presence of "survivor guilt" during acute crisis reactions was evident in this group. Members showed almost no denial of the actual events, but many initially denied emotional symptoms, so called "inhibited grief." According to Raphael,[3] inhibited grief is a common syndrome and "usually combines psychological numbing, over control, and containment of all feelings related to the death and the disaster." This syndrome is generally considered to be maladaptive and likely to be associated with future impairment. Therefore, efforts were made to gently confront and interpret this defense.

Follow-Up. One message that the crisis team emphasized was the availability of follow-up. Recognizing that individuals integrate psychologic input at different rates, the team members informed the soldiers that some might have symptoms during the days and weeks after the event. A mental health technician was placed at the local troop medical clinic on a daily basis during the week following the incident. The mental health clinic phone numbers were posted in conspicuous places in the unit work and living areas. A small number of individuals were identified and followed up via input from these two sources.

An unexpected outcome in the area of follow-up occurred several weeks later when another unit experienced a similar, but smaller scale event. The commander of this second unit was referred to the crisis team by command elements in the units involved in the incidents described above. This can be taken as indirect evidence of positive reaction to the first debriefing. Follow-up efforts were limited by troop movement, denial within the system, and by the inability of the providers to arrange on-site follow-up treatment groups over the days and weeks that followed.

Comment: The psychiatric debriefing format illustrated here begins with a general information and education briefing for all participants. As this must establish the debriefer's credibility, and rapport for the subsequent debriefing, the material must be properly focused for the specific participants. It must not use technical jargon which will turn them off. It is especially important that it not pathologize the process or the participants, even by inference. The identification of participants who may need individual therapy must be done in low-keyed fashion, without creating an expectation that many will need such care, without turning people who could manage on their own into patients, and without spotlighting and stigmatizing those who do seek further mental health assistance. The ideal of stress debriefing is not to generate referrals or follow-up cases, but rather to make them unnecessary. However, a temporary increase of patients who thereby gain mastery over acute stress symptoms is clearly preferable to a delayed stream of chronic, difficult-to-treat PTSD cases. The process phase of psychiatric debriefing (unlike S.L.A. Marshall's HERD or CED/CISD) is less concerned with eliciting facts and more active in eliciting participation in abreaction. It actively interprets the psychological processes involved—here, too, the vocabulary used must be carefully calibrated for the participants and not alienate them with psychiatric jargon. Follow-up must not be so aggressive as to create negative expectations of successful self and buddy care.

SUMMARY AND CONCLUSION

Debriefing in one of its several forms is an important part of demobilization from any combat situation or stressful operation other than war (OOTW). Debriefing is crucial to quickly restoring unit effectiveness and preventing post-traumatic stress problems following critical (traumatic) events. Research from management of mental health issues in natural and manmade disasters, personal trauma, and war indicate that when a group is allowed to ventilate fears, frustrations, and feelings about the event, and its individuals receive the support of their comrades, the likelihood of PTSD is decreased. The lessons learned from various armed conflicts and disaster management are preparing mental health practitioners to exercise preventive care for potentially large numbers of combat veterans before they develop psychiatric symptomatology.

Acknowledgement

The authors thank COL Robert S. Brown, for help in preparing Case Study 5.

REFERENCES

1. American Psychiatric Association. *Diagnostic and Statistical Manual of Mental Disorders*, 4th ed. (DSM-IV). Washington, DC: APA; 1994.

2. Steiner M, Neumann M. Traumatic neurosis and social support in the Yom Kippur War returnees. *Milit Med*. 1978;12:866–868.

3. Raphael B. *When Disaster Strikes*. New York: Basic Books; 1986.

4. Erikson KT. *Everything in its Path: Destruction of Community in the Buffalo Creek Flood*. New York: Simon & Schuster; 1976.

5. Levan I, Greenfeld H, Baruch E. Psychiatric combat reactions during the Yom Kippur War. *Am J Psychiatry*. 1979;136(5):637–641.

6. Silsby HD, Jones FD. The etiologies of Vietnam post-traumatic stress syndrome. *Milit Med*. 1985;150(1):6–7.

7. Holloway HC, Ursano RJ. The Vietnam veteran: Memory, social context, and metaphor. *Psychiatry*. 1984;47:103–108.

8. Borus JF. Reentry: Facilitating healthy readjustment in Vietnam veterans. *Psychiatry*. 1973;36:428–439.

9. Rahe RH. Acute versus chronic psychologic reactions to combat. *Milit Med*. 1988;153:365–371.

10. Division of Education and Service Systems Liaison, Emergency Services Branch, National Institute of Mental Health. *Prevention and Control of Stress Among Emergency Workers: A Pamphlet for Team Managers*. Rockville, Md: US Department of Health and Human Services; 1988.

11. Laskow GB. Intervention strategies for victims of terrorism/disasters: USAREUR [US Army Europe] scenario. Proceedings of the Conference on Military Applications of Clinical Neuropsychology and Health Psychology. Presidio of San Francisco: Letterman Army Medical Center; 1987.

12. Sokol RJ. Early mental health interventions in combat situations: The USS Stark. *Milit Med*. 1989;154:407–409.

13. Wright KS, ed. The Human Response to the Gander Military Air Disaster: A Summary Report. Washington, DC: Walter Reed Army Institute of Research; 1987.

14. Taylor AJW, Frazer AG. Psychologic Sequelae of Operation Overdue Following the DC-10 Air Crash in Antarctica. Wellington, New Zealand: Victoria University of Wellington Publication in Psychology, No. 27; 1981.

15. Marshall SLA. *Bringing up the Rear: A Memoir*. San Rafael, Calif: Presidio Press; 1979.

16. Mitchell JT. Demobilizations. *Life Net* (Newsletter of the American Critical Incidents Stress Foundation). 1991;2(1):8–9.

17. US Department of the Army. *Leaders' Manual for Combat Stress Control*. Washington, DC: DA; 29 September 1994. Field Manual 22-51.

18. US Department of the Army. *Combat Stress Control in a Theater of Operations*. Washington, DC: DA; 29 September 1994. Field Manual 8-51.

19. Shalev A. *Historical Group Debriefing Following Combat: A Study of SLA Marshall's Debriefing Techniques. Final Report*. [Coordinated by Department of Military Psychiatry, Walter Reed Army Institute of Research and Department of Mental Health, Medical Corps, Israeli Defence Forces.] Jerusalem, Israel: Department of Psychiatry, Center for Traumatic Stress, Hadassah University Hospital; 1992.

20. Belenky GL, Martin JM. Debriefings and battle reconstruction following combat. In: Belenky GL, Martin JM, Sparacino LR, eds. *A Shield in the Storm: Mental Health Operations During the Persian Gulf War*. Westport, Conn: Greenwood Press; in preparation.

21. Bushard B. The US Army's mental hygiene consultation service. *Symposium on Preventive and Social Psychiatry*. Sponsored jointly by the Walter Reed Army Institute of Research (WRAIR), Walter Reed Army Medical Center, and the National Research Council. Washington, DC: WRAIR; 1957.

22. Jones FD, Sparacino LR, Wilcox VL, Rothberg JM, eds. *Military Psychiatry: Preparing in Peace for War*. In: *Textbook of Military Medicine*. Washington, DC: Office of The Surgeon General, US Department of the Army and Borden Institute; 1994.

23. Koshes RJ. Psychiatric care of the homeless mentally ill: An opportunity for military psychiatry training. *Milit Med*. 1991;156:121–126.

24. Koshes RJ, Clawson LD. Working with the homeless: The psychiatric resident's experience. *Jefferson J Psychiatry*. 1989;7(1):60–66.

25. Jones FD, Crocq L, Adelaja O, Rahe R, Rock N, Mansour F, Collazo C, Belenky G. Psychiatric casualties in modern warfare: I. Evolution of treatment. In: Pichot P, Berner P, Wolf R, Thau K, eds. *Psychiatry, The State of the Art*, Vol 6. New York: Plenum Publishing; 1985: 459–464.

26. Jones FD. Lessons of war for psychiatry. In: Pichot P, Berner P, Wolf R, Thau K, eds. *Psychiatry, The State of the Art*. Vol 6. New York: Plenum Publishing; 1985: 515–519.

27. Burkle FM. Coping with stress under conditions of disaster and refugee care. *Milit Med*. 1983;148:800–803.

28. Young SA, Holden MS. The formation and application of an overseas mental health crisis intervention team. Part I: Formation. *Milit Med*. 1991;156:443–445.

29. Young SA, Holden MS. The formation and application of an overseas mental health crisis intervention team. Part II: Application. *Milit Med*. 1991;156:445–447.

30. Ursano RJ. Personal Communication, 1993.

31. Schwartz HJ, ed. *Psychotherapy of the Combat Veteran*. New York: SP Medical and Scientific Books; 1984.

Chapter 12

POSTCOMBAT REENTRY

FARIS R. KIRKLAND, Ph.D.*

**Lieutenant Colonel (ret), Field Artillery, U.S. Army; Senior Research Associate, University City Science Center, 3624 Market Street, Philadelphia, Pennsylvania 19104; Guest Scientist, Department of Military Psychiatry, Division of Neuropsychiatry, Walter Reed Army Institute of Research, Washington, DC 20307-5100*

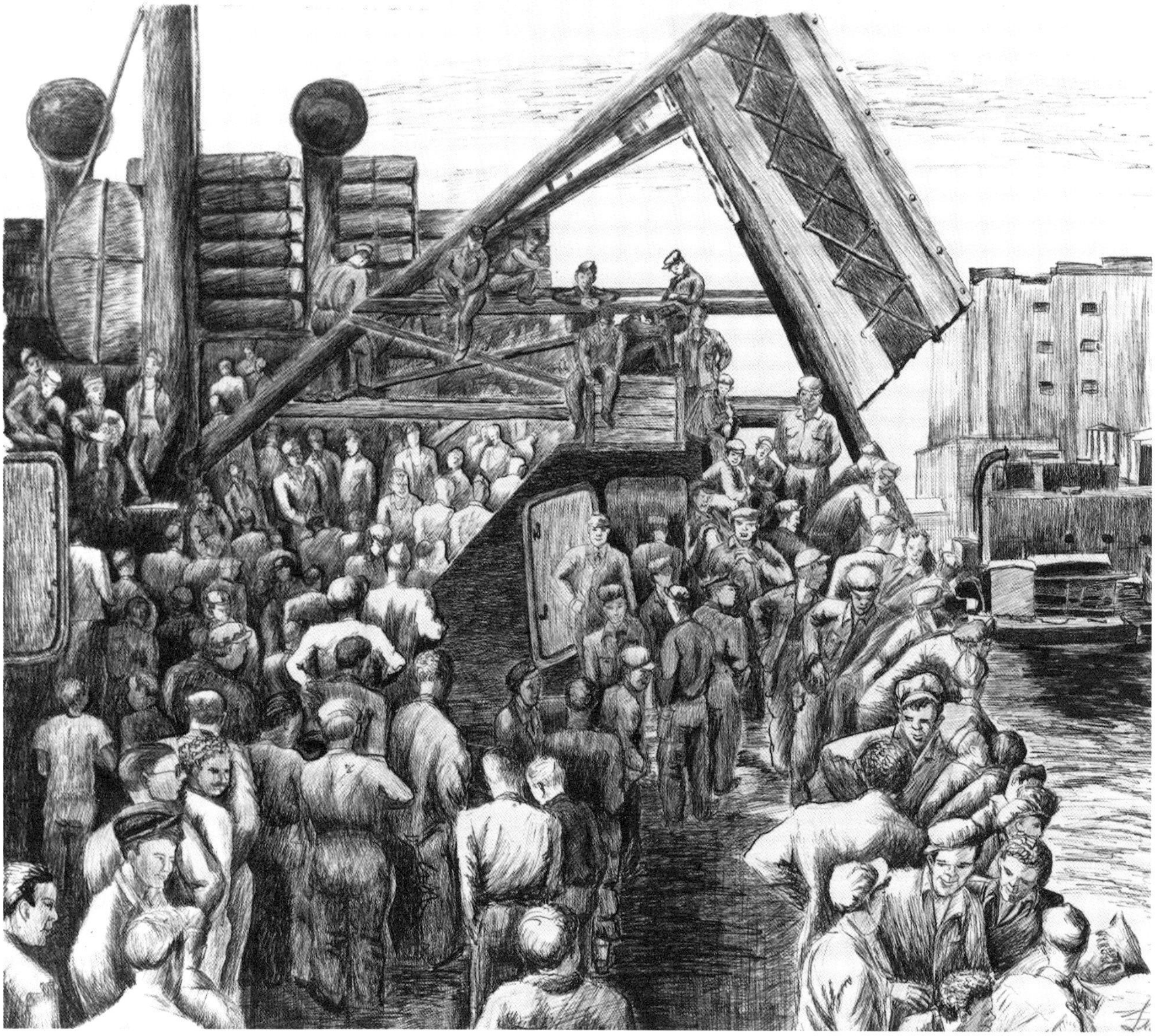

Leslie Anderson *Troops Boarding Homebound Ship* 1947

Captain Leslie Anderson, who joined the U.S. Army Combat Art Section toward the end of World War II, depicts troops boarding a ship to head for home. The return home is a greatly anticipated event for all soldiers, sailors, and airmen, especially after combat. With the increased range of air transports in the 1960s, these trips were shifted from ships to planes, resulting in less time to decompress from battle and prepare oneself mentally for return to civilian life.

Art: Courtesy of US Center of Military History, Washington, DC.

INTRODUCTION

Major wars in the 20th century have usually comprised indoctrination of populations with the grievances against potential adversaries, a period of mounting tension vis-à-vis a particular adversary, years of combat, and involvement of the populace in enduring hardships and contributing to the war effort. Throughout this process individuals who are members, or who are likely to become members, of the armed services have time to get used to the psychological roles they will be playing as delegates of the population. They learn that they will be called upon to take great risks as champions of their people in a generally agreed-upon cause,[1] (eg, David representing the Israelites against the Philistine Goliath[2]). Civilians and military personnel alike have time to cultivate a set of perceptions that the enemy is an evil pseudospecies whose people may be killed and whose property may be destroyed without inhibition.[3,4] The development of wartime mind-sets helps military personnel not only to carry out their combat duties but also to manage the attendant trauma and guilt so they can reenter the peacetime world when the war ends.

The attitudinal adjustments necessary to define a group as enemy are easy to learn, but they require time, social support, and certain sociocultural prerequisites.[5,6] Similarly, the transition back to peace—relating to families, friends, and coworkers; dealing with social and material situations from a civilian rather than a military perspective; and perceiving the former enemy as neutral or even friendly—requires time and social support.[7–9] Among the strongest social supports that can help the individual soldier make the transition from war to peace is a national consensus about the war that legitimates his behavior in combat and validates the suffering, deprivation, guilt, and fear that he experienced. Not all service members have been able to manage to put their wars behind them and get on with their lives. In many cases lack of a positive consensus has played a role in these failures[10–12] Further discussion of this may be found in Chapter 16, Chronic Post-Traumatic Stress Disorder; Chapter 17, The Prisoner of War; and Chapter 18, Follow-up Studies of Veterans, in this volume.

Some campaigns required only fractional commitment of national resources and did not put national survival in jeopardy (Boer War 1899–1902,[13] French Indo-China War 1945–1954,[14] Korean conflict 1950–1953,[15] French Algerian War 1954–1962,[16] Vietnam conflict 1963–1973,[17] Soviet intervention in Afghanistan 1980–1990). These wars were conducted in a different psycho-political climate from that obtaining in major wars, and produced different reentry issues. Governmental assertions about the national interests that were at stake were not particularly credible, and the longer the wars went on the more threadbare became public support. Civilian inconvenience and involvement were modest, and because casualties were few and affected but few families, there was little pressure in the society as a whole for validation of the war effort to reduce dissonance arising from public distress (Table 12-1).

Soldiers participating in these limited wars had time prior to induction, during training, and during deployment voyages to adjust to the prospect of combat, but reentry presented a number of problems. The most serious of these was that the absence of a national consensus in support of the war made legitimation of the soldiers' actions and validation of their suffering problematic. Moreover, return from the two limited wars waged by the United States was on an individual basis. The returnees were not able to process their experiences with the comrades with whom they had trained and fought. Various kinds of acting out by veterans resulted. The effects of post-traumatic stress disorder on vet-

TABLE 12-1

CASUALTIES AMONG GREAT POWERS IN LIMITED WARS

War	Dates	Deaths
Boer War	1899–1902	21,942 British
French Indo-China War	1945–1954	29,685 French
Korean Conflict	1950–1953	33,629 U. S.
French Algerian War	1954–1962	12,000 French
Vietnam Conflict	1963–1973	56,737 U. S.

Data sources: [Boer War] Amery LS, ed. *The Times History of the War in South Africa*, Vol. 7. London: Sampson Low, Marston; 1909: 24–25. [French Indo-China War] O'Ballance E. *The Indo-China War: 1945-54, A Study in Guerrilla Warfare*. London: Faber & Faber; 1964: 249. [Korean Conflict] Blair C. *The Forgotten War*. New York: Times Books; 1987: ix. [French Algerian War] O'Ballance E. *The Algerian Insurrection: 1954-1962*. Hamden, CT: Archon Books; 1967: 201. [Vietnam Conflict] Westmoreland WC. *A Soldier Reports*. Garden City, NY: Doubleday; 1976: 299.

erans of the American troops who fought in Vietnam are discussed extensively in this volume (Chapter 3, Disorders of Frustration and Loneliness, and Chapter 16, Chronic Post-Traumatic Stress Disorder). The lack of consensus in France about the wars in Indo-China and Algeria led to military challenges to the regime in 1958 and 1961.[18,19] The stress imposed on the weakening fabric of the Soviet Union by the intervention in Afghanistan was one of the factors in the collapse of the communist union. Regimental officers were sufficiently alienated from the national leadership that they would not order their troops to fire on demonstrators opposing a military coup to restore the regime.

A third kind of conflict has emerged during the Cold War era—rapid deployment, short duration interventions such as the British reconquest of the Falkland Islands (1982), the U.S. invasion of Grenada (1983) and Panama (1989), and the Persian Gulf War (1990–1991). The psychological sequelae of such conflicts differ from those encountered in longer wars, especially wars in which there was time to prepare psychologically in advance. One might expect that a soldier who is involved in a short period of fighting would experience less psychic distress than one who endured prolonged combat, and that has proved to be the case, as discussed in Chapter 1, Psychiatric Lessons of War.

Several other factors warrant consideration. The most important of these is that when a state is defended by a small, long-service professional armed force, the same personnel are likely to be involved in several armed interventions. The soldiers are not, as was the case with the majority of soldiers in wars fought by mass conscript armies, discharged to the civil sector for management of their reentry problems; they stay in the service. It is essential that reentry issues be understood so that steps can be taken to capitalize on those aspects of combat experience that strengthen a service member's competence and confidence, and to mitigate traumatic or depressing aspects.

A second factor that merits consideration is that rapid deployment to combat can deprive service members of opportunities to develop clearly defined attitudes about the virtues of the American cause, the evil nature of the adversary, and the importance of the campaign to values that are important to them. As a consequence, military personnel participating in rapid deployment operations may have but little psychological armor to help them manage the experience of killing, the loss of comrades, or the pain and shock of wounds to themselves. A psychologically informed effort must be made before combat to prepare personnel for these experiences. Similarly, postbattle action is necessary to facilitate recovery from these traumata both to alleviate suffering and to preserve the combat potential of units.

The purpose of this chapter is, first, to review the experiences of participants in rapid deployment campaigns, and second, to describe the action by command and by mental health professionals that supported reentry processes and strengthened the psychological integrity of individuals and units. The first section will be a historical summary with a view to identifying policies and behavior relevant to reentry from rapid deployment campaigns. The second section is a catalogue of issues that have emerged from research on such campaigns. The third section is a discussion of the roles of mental health professionals, operating in support of, and in collaboration with, command in managing the reentry process.

HISTORICAL REVIEW

Between 1775 and 1992 the armed forces of the United States have waged seven major wars—six against foreign powers and one nationwide civil war. They have conducted more than 30 limited wars or armed interventions that entailed the use of substantial forces, and carried out hundreds of military operations that included combat or the threat of combat. Following each campaign there have been reentry processes. Of interest to the mental health community are those that provide guidance for policy and conduct in the future. This historical review will focus on reentry processes that affected the postwar active army. It has three parts: (1) major wars, (2) limited wars, and (3) rapid deployment wars.

Major Wars

The American solution to reentry following its seven major wars has been demobilization. After the Revolutionary War the army was reduced to 718 men. Following the War of 1812, 71% of the army was demobilized; after the Mexican War, 77%; the Civil War, 94%; the Spanish-American War, 62%; World War I, 94%; World War II, 93%.[20] Demobilization made reentry a societal, not a military problem. The former soldiers went home to the approbation and welcome of their friends and families; the Regular Army went into hibernation. Many potential problems were solved by units staying together during long trips home by sea, foot, and horse-drawn vehicle from Vera Cruz (1849), from the Philippines (1902), and from France (1918–1919). Soldiers and leaders could process their experiences together, reassure each other, agree on acceptable myths that validated their behavior and feelings. World War I was the last—until the invasion of Panama (1989–1990) from which units made the journey home as units.

World War II was totally different from the standpoint of reentry. Though units to a large extent trained, deployed and fought with the same men—less casualties and plus replacements, when it was time to go home it was every man for himself. In spite of the national consensus that World War II was a "good" war,[8] there were numerous manifestations of hostility and episodes of indiscipline in connection with the processes of returning home, demobilizing, and reentry into civilian life. A system was devised by which each soldier could earn points for time in the service, time overseas, time in combat, wounds, and decorations. Those with the most points were to be sent home first. The design of the point system was based on research among military personnel.[21]

An unforeseen consequence of the point system was that it transformed the serviceman from a member of a social unit to an isolated individual. He no longer had the support of the comrades and leaders with whom he had trained and fought, and who had given his deeds and discomforts meaning. Because there was a finite number of ships and aircraft with which to bring personnel home, many of them were frustrated by having to wait. In 1946 there were reports that the Pentagon intended to slow the demobilization process. Servicemen "took to the streets and demonstrated in more than a dozen countries."[22] In some embarkation camps soldiers left without authorization, did not report for guard duty, and misbehaved in local civilian communities.[23,24] In the camps, the soldiers were a mob of angry individuals deprived of the fabric of trusted comrades, leaders whom they knew, and the networks of missions, trust, and mutual obligations that had given psychological substance to the authoritarian structure of the armed services. That fabric was necessary to sustain, orient, and support soldiers' self-control. Without it, they acted out their feelings of helplessness and frustration.

The effects of the predischarge period of alienation were to focus and solidify the feelings of discontent that had accumulated during the soldier's service, attenuate the memories of effectiveness and comradeship, and send many home from the service with a bitter sense of denigration and impotence. The veterans of World War II, though they participated in a much longer struggle and won a more comprehensive victory than did their forbears from World War I (1917–1918), were not the committed and cohesive advocates for the armed services that the older veterans were.

Another consequence of the bitterness engendered by the individualized return and demobilization process was a series of complaints about the behavior of officers. The criticism provoked an investigation by a commission chaired by Lieutenant General James Doolittle. The commission found that many officers had behaved inappropriately, and proposed sweeping reforms.[25] The reforms, oriented toward removing arbitrary distinctions in dress and privileges between officers and enlisted personnel, did not address the fundamental issue—which was how to build mutual respect up and down the hierarchy. The reforms proved to be a source of confusion and alienation that complicated relationships between officers and enlisted personnel for more than 30 years.

Postcombat alienation, acting out, and hostility to the armed forces differed from symptoms of combat stress disorders or nostalgia, but they were still part of the psychological aftereffects of a mid-intensity traditional war. By comparing the reentry policies employed after World War II and their consequences with the policies and consequences following other conflicts it is possible to identify actions that are most adaptive.

Limited Wars

Between 1783 and 1940, the United States engaged in 14 limited war campaigns—an average of one every 11 years, as shown in Table 12-2. The guerrilla wars, like the major wars, were fought mainly with volunteers. When the job was done, the volunteer regiments went back to the United States and were disbanded. Return from the combat zone was by ship or on foot, and provided plenty of time for soldiers to talk through their experiences with each other. The regular officers and noncommissioned officers (NCOs) had to look for places in regular units, usually several ranks lower than those they had held in the regiments of volunteers.[26]

TABLE 12-2

LIMITED WARS 1783-1940

War	Dates	Type
Quasi-war with France	1798–1800	Naval
Barbary Coast wars	1801–1805	Naval
Seminole War	1817–1818	Guerrilla
Second Seminole War	1835–1842	Guerrilla
Philippine Insurrection	1899–1903, 1910–1913	Pacification
China Relief Expedition	1900–1901	Pacification
Cuban Pacification	1906–1909	Pacification
Nicaraguan Pacification	1912, 1926–1933	Pacification
Haitian Expedition	1915, 1919–1920	Pacification
Santo Domingo	1916	Pacification
Mexican Border Campaign	1911–1919	Pacification

Most of the pacification operations were carried out by Regular Army or U.S. Marine Corps regiments that remained intact after the operation. Though deployment and return were slowed by the transportation technology available, combat was often intense and brief. These operations were small-scale forerunners of rapid deployment campaigns such as the U.S. invasions of Grenada and Panama and the Persian Gulf War. Unfortunately they took place before the era of interest in the psychological dimensions of warfare, and little has been written that is helpful in understanding the dynamics of the reentry process.

Between 1945 and 1992 the United States intervened more than 15 times in other countries with substantial forces: Korea (1950–1953), Lebanon (1958), Quemoy and Matsu (1958–1963), Cuba (1962–1963), the Congo (1964), the Dominican Republic (1965–1966), Vietnam (1963–1973), twice in Cambodia (an evacuation in April 1975 and the *Mayaguez* battle in May 1975), Vietnam evacuation (1975), Lebanon again (1982–1983), Grenada (1983), Honduras (1988), Panama (1989), the Persian Gulf region (1990–1991), Somalia (1992), and Haiti (1994). None of these operations involved the survival of the United States, and the levels of popular support varied from almost total approval (Persian Gulf, Grenada) to high levels of disapproval (Vietnam after 1968). The forces varied in size from less than a division of ground troops to the bulk of American combat strength. Most involved land, sea, and air forces. Those before 1973 were supported by conscription. Those after 1980 resemble expected future operations most closely in being carried out by professional forces, in the rapidity with which forces were projected and the brief time deployed, and in their frequency—an average of one major operation every 2 years.

Reentry following the two largest limited conflicts—Korea and Vietnam—resembled that following World War II in that service members left the combat zone as individuals. Because most of them were discharged shortly after completing their obligated tours, reentry was a matter for the civil sector to handle. But the conflicts in Korea and Vietnam were not supported by a solid national consensus. The country was apathetic about the Korean conflict, especially after the first year when armistice negotiations began and progress at the bargaining table attracted more attention than combat operations. Casualty rates were high during the first year, but total casualties were so low that too few families were affected for them to become a matter of widespread concern. Three years of combat in Korea killed only about one tenth as many Americans as 4 years of World War II. Returning soldiers were ignored by the populace, but often received a hostile reception from their own service.[27]

Service members returning from the conflict in Vietnam were for the most part met with indifference until 1968.[28] From 1969 on they stood a good chance of encountering savage abuse.[11,28,29] The widespread post-traumatic stress disorders (PTSD) reported among veterans of the conflict in Vietnam have been partially attributed to absence of validation and legitimation from the civilian population. Another factor, one that is rarely cited, was the absence of support and validation from comrades and leaders—who either came home before or were still in Vietnam. The veteran of Vietnam went from the battle zone to the United States in 48 hours. He did not have time to think and talk through what he had seen and done, and in any event he went back with strangers, not the men he had served with. He had to confront reentry to the civilian world completely alone, and often it was a hostile world.

The record of reentry following World War I, World War II, the Philippine Insurrection, the Korean conflict and the Vietnam conflict are of limited relevance for the future. Either the units demobilized, or they stayed in the field and men rotated through them. The units never reentered until the war was over; the individuals left the service at the end of their obligated service. The problem for the future is reentry in which a unit deploys, fights, and returns—as a unit. The unit and its members will continue to stay together, and must remain ready for the next deployment. Only the most recent history is directly relevant—the history of rapid deployment wars with short periods of combat.

Rapid Deployment Operations

In 1982, 13,000 Argentinean troops seized and garrisoned the British Falkland Islands. In 7 weeks a British multi-service task force assembled and moved 8,000 miles to put ashore a force of 10,000 men to recapture the islands. In 24 days of bitter land, sea and air fighting 252 British soldiers were killed, 6 ships were sunk, and approximately 1 dozen aircraft were destroyed.[30] The reentry processes for the British units are useful for this study because the British attack resembled the type the United States has used since and probably will continue to use, and because the British used regular units, not conscripts.

The British units stayed together after the battle, preparing for the next one. Reentry problems rarely emerged for two reasons. The more important reason is the supportive nature of the British regimental system. It assures the soldier that he will always be with the same unit, the same comrades and leaders, and the same traditions. He partakes of, contributes to, and derives significance as a person from the regiment.[31,32] The honor of the regiment requires him to behave in certain ways. He follows the traditions, feels proud of living up to them, and is cloaked with their dignity. He never experiences reentry alone.[33,34]

The second reason that reentry problems rarely emerge is the British tradition of undemonstrativeness and reluctance to express emotions. These cultural behavioral characteristics limit the range of communications and can mask psychological distress. Ritualized manifestations of loyalty to the regiment distract men from their fears and help them through difficult moments, but they also make it hard for leaders to detect incipient problems in time to take action to alleviate them. Probably some leaders are only too glad that discipline, honor, and the stiff upper lip protect them from having to become aware of, and deal with, psychological pain in subordinates that they are working hard to deny in themselves. Often the first hint of combat stress reaction is serious acting out or decompensation.

The United States conducted rapid deployment operations involving combat in Grenada in 1983, Panama in 1989, Saudi Arabia in 1990, and Somalia in 1992. Many units train continuously for the rapid deployment mission. They know they could go into combat any day on short notice. They know that the mission is real, because their units have gone into combat on 24-hours notice.

The classic rapid deployment operation was Operation Just Cause (OJC)—the invasion of Panama in December 1989. A force of about 4,000 combat troops was on the ground in Panama. An additional 16,000 were air-dropped and airlanded over a 24-hour period, and within 48 hours the entire Panamanian military structure was destroyed. Rules of engagement were strict: U.S. soldiers could fire only at enemy personnel who could be seen firing at them. No suppressive fire was permitted, and no indirect fire by artillery or mortars was used. Only two aerial bombs were dropped, and they were in remote locations. As a result, the action by U.S. forces caused few civilian casualties and minimal collateral damage. Unfortunately, a much larger number of civilians were killed and one barrio destroyed by fire as a result of action by Noriega's Dignity Battalions and of personal vendettas carried out during the collapse of the Panamanian government.

The Department of Military Psychiatry of the Walter Reed Army Institute of Research (WRAIR) conducted extensive research into the human dimensions of OJC. The WRAIR team interviewed more than 800 soldiers of all ranks from ten infantry battalions and two military police companies. The research caught the units in the midst of the reentry process just after they returned to their home stations in the United States, or in Panama in the case of units permanently stationed there. The findings from that study have provided much of the empirical data on which the analyses that follow are based.[35]

The data from the study done by WRAIR indicated that few soldiers suffered from traditional combat stress reactions or disorders of loneliness or frustration (nostalgia), but that rapid deployment, short-duration campaigns provoked specific types of stress reactions in some soldiers, and most units reported some difficulties in coming down from combat to the mundane routines of training. It is these kinds of issues that commanders and mental health professionals need to understand. Properly managed, they can preserve the psychological readiness of units that have taken part in a rapid deployment combat mission. If they are treated with benign neglect because no one knows how to handle them, or because other matters appear to be more important, morale and cohesion can languish and the unit can lapse into a degraded state of psychological readiness.

REENTRY ISSUES

The 10 infantry battalions studied by the team from WRAIR were cohesive and competent. Three had been in Panama for several months before Operation Just Cause was launched. Members of the battalions lived and trained together 24-hours-a-day, week in and week out. They patrolled constantly and provocatively, and had frequent hostile encounters, with loaded weapons, with members of General Noriega's Panamanian Defense Force (PDF). These battalions became cohesive in conditions that were not far removed from combat. Two others were elite Ranger battalions in which cohesion was developed by continuous high-intensity training, free from distractions not related to the mission. Five battalions, including one of those already in Panama, were COHORT (cohesion, operational readiness, training) units. Their first-term soldiers had gone through initial entry training together and stayed together for 3-year tours in their battalions. The last battalion, though neither Ranger nor COHORT, was a part of the division that has been on the highest alert status in the army for decades.

Several of the battalions that were not in Panama when OJC was initiated were on relaxed alert status. Two had sent most of their personnel on Christmas leave. Nonetheless they assembled, packed their equipment and were airborne en route to combat in about 24 hours. Three parachuted into combat; four were airlanded. Official after-action reports and the findings from the WRAIR study indicate that all of the battalions performed their missions effectively. Most of the action was at squad or platoon level, though some company commanders were able to control all of their platoons some of the time.

Six of the battalions studied engaged in severe combat. Between them they suffered 10 killed and 116 wounded in action. In addition there were 6 men killed in accidents. Only one of the 10 battalions studied had no fatalities. OJC is an appropriate case study because it is a prototype of future military operations, and because it was an unqualified success with minimal friendly casualties. As a consequence, the reentry problems that emerged were few in number and easy to recognize and study. From the 10 battalions studied it is possible to describe the range of problems that may arise and the techniques used by commanders and mental health professionals that were most effective in dealing with them. The issues fell into three categories: (1) acute reactions to combat, (2) postcombat validation, and (3) reintegration into the postwar world.

Acute Reactions to Combat

Veterans of OJC reported three kinds of emotional reactions to combat: (1) distress over killing PDF soldiers; (2) a complex mix of grief, guilt, and rage over losing comrades; and (3) generalized patterns of anxiety, irritability, and nightmares.

Distress over Killing

Casualties that the soldier inflicted himself on enemy soldiers were usually described as the most stressful events. A first sergeant described the reactions of soldiers who had killed PDF in close combat: "They don't feel good having a confirmed kill." A company commander said: "Shooting people has been harder for most soldiers to come to grips with than the death of a friend." A squad leader said of one of his men: "He killed two. That night he was punching the wall and crying. He has a bad feeling." His comrades described a soldier who had killed a PDF in a fire fight: "Joe was wound up, talked a mile a minute. He kept asking us what we thought. We told him he had done a good job. He was a pain in the ass, wouldn't shut up. Finally they sent him to the rear to decompress. We never heard from him again." The platoon sergeant of a platoon that had riddled a bus full of fleeing PDF officers said: "There was blood running out the door. People were screaming and bleeding to death. I'll never forget that sight."

Evidence was more often indirect than direct; many of those who had killed were reticent about it, and their distress sometimes took the form of withdrawal or denial: "He was dazed after shooting a PDF soldier three times in the neck—a perfect shot. But he didn't want to talk about it." The squad mates of a one soldier said: "After he killed two guys hand-to-hand he got real quiet. He has since gotten out. He should have gotten counseling." One squad leader described one of his men who had killed two PDF at close range: "He was the most upset guy. He got very quiet." A company commander reported that he had hoped to make a soldier who had two confirmed kills an institutional hero: "He kept to himself. He got out. He said he never wanted to be in a situation where he would have to do that again."

Confronting feelings proved to alleviate stress to some extent. A platoon sergeant said: "Then there's the burden of killing people. I can't reconcile it, I just carry it." A private reported: "I hit an adult and a child. That bothered me." A group of squad leaders distressed by the fact that they and their men had killed a number of PDF said: "We consoled each other." A sergeant major encountered a group of soldiers who had been in a fire fight: "They had killed some people and wanted to talk. It was an impromptu session with 14 guys."

Compassion for the PDF was an issue. One soldier said: "When we saw how terrified they were, we felt sorry for them." Another noted when describing dead PDF: "They were just soldiers, doing their job." A Spanish-speaking soldier told his squad mates that their prisoner had said, "He doesn't like Noriega, but he has five kids and needed a job."

Some soldiers had no apparent negative reaction to killing. After a car full of civilians had failed to stop at a road block and one of the occupants was killed a soldier said, "Better one of them than one of us." A private described the mood of himself and his comrades: "We were very excited. We had been in the country 2 days, killed people, and had no casualties. We were hyped up, felt invincible." When a soldier was killed accidentally, his comrades said of their killing some PDF: "It was gratifying to get some kills. It made us feel better." One soldier who killed a PDF said: "It was like a video game. He was shooting at me." A squad leader who had encountered a PDF ambush said: "It didn't mean anything to me. I shot one, the team leader got the other." A spokesman for a squad that had killed two and wounded two PDF said: "It was a relief. We didn't know how we would react, and we had done okay."

There were three factors that made it difficult for the soldiers who fought in OJC to manage the psychological aftereffects of killing PDF soldiers. The first and most obvious is the aversion most mammals have to killing conspecifics (members of their own species).[36,37] This aversion does not preclude killing in all cases, but it does constitute a threshold the strength of which varies with species and among individuals within a species.[38–40] Pseudospeciation, the ability of humans and some other primates to classify certain members of their own species as "other," can neutralize the threshold of inhibition so they can kill conspecifics.[41–43] While pseudospeciation makes it possible to kill, it does not include processes to neutralize the affect associated with an action against which there are phylogenetically strong inhibitions. The soldier who kills is left with his psychological afterburn.

The second factor was ambivalence. The soldiers who fought in OJC had had opportunities to adjust their perceptions to classify the Panamanian dictator Noriega and his henchmen in the PDF as "bad," as inhuman enough to kill. But the pseudospeciation process was partially vitiated as a psychological support by the identification U.S. soldiers had with PDF personnel as soldiers, and as frightened human beings.

The third factor was isolation. The afterburn U.S. soldiers experienced was exacerbated by the fact that comparatively few U.S. soldiers killed anybody. Those who did were alone with the conflict between having done something inherently aversive, and having done a praiseworthy deed in the context of their social group. Their ability to communicate with and derive support from their group was apparently inhibited to some extent by this conflict. Because the combat phase was brief, there was not enough time for killing to become routine, for it to become an experience most of the soldiers shared. Those who had killed were likely to remain a breed apart.

Reactions to Casualties Among Comrades

Soldiers and leaders reacted to casualties among their own comrades in patterns that were fairly constant irrespective of whether the casualties were caused by enemy fire, friendly fire, or accident. The intensity of their reactions was a function primarily of how well they knew the victims. There were six emotional themes evident within these response patterns: (1) anger, (2) grief, (3) horror, (4) guilt, (5) bonding, and (6) dependency on the mission.

Soldiers expressed anger toward the PDF even if they had nothing to do with causing the casualties. The following are responses by soldiers whose comrades were killed by friendly fire support systems: "We were more aggressive toward the enemy." "It helped to return fire." "If we hadn't been able to shoot at the PDF we'd have fallen apart." Their reactions were about the same when the PDF killed an American. When one soldier was killed, his platoon sergeant said: "People got mad. They wanted revenge." A squad leader observed: "It was hard to enforce the rules of engagement after Joe was killed. The guys did what I told them, but I sensed that they were close to getting out of control." Another squad leader said: "They were eager to kill someone. One guy was especially eager to kill. I said, 'Let's get it under control, get Panama squared away.'" The essence of the emotional state of the comrades of dead Americans is evident in a description of a junior NCO whose best friend was killed in action: "He was freaked out, angry and frustrated." Their complete helplessness in the presence of the totality of death was extremely difficult for these young soldiers. They were in the early years of their manhood, they had chosen the U.S. Army as a means to achieve a sense of potency, of instant adulthood, and instead they were faced with a loss about which they could do nothing.

The second theme, grief, took two forms: (1) immediate shock, and (2) a deeper feeling that men experienced later. The immediate response was a compound of refusal to believe and a wish to undo the death. A company commander who had just lost a man said: "I wanted to be alone with him for a while. I closed his eyes. Then the medics pushed me away, and I lost it." Another officer expressed a similar feeling: "He's yours and he's lost and there's a family." Describing a death that was reported over the company command radio net, a soldier said, "The platoon went batshit over the radio." A soldier who observed a platoon in which two soldiers were killed and two others wounded said: "The squad froze when the squad leader was hit. The platoon leader got them going again with words and by touching them. He said to the team leader, 'You're one-one [the radio call sign of the fallen squad leader] now,' and the team leader took charge." Several soldiers expressed a sense of time rushing by: "It all happened so fast. We couldn't stop." "If you stop to mourn, you make mistakes." "There was so much going on. We really didn't have time to be sad then." "It happened so fast. It was deeply sad, but it went through so fast we didn't have time to grieve then." One soldier recalled a succession of thoughts flashing through his mind: "His wife is pregnant. Am I going to get home? I was nervous. Oh my God."

The longer-lasting grief responses were often delayed. A private who had lost a comrade experienced his grief most acutely at a memorial service in the continental United States (CONUS): "It hit me when I saw his family and I realized how much he had lost." A platoon leader described his men's grief: "You could see in their eyes that they were missing something." A soldier who saw another killed beside him reported, "I still see it in my mind and think about it every day." A squad leader described the members of his squad after a man had been killed: "They were sad. I was sad. His best friend was real quiet." A commander who met another who had lost men said, "I'm sorry about your guys." The other replied, "Yeah, it's rough." Expression of grief was sometimes possible, sometimes not. In some companies soldiers reported that during memorial services: "There wasn't a dry eye in the place." "The company commander spoke, and he broke down. That helped." But in another unit a soldier said: "I'm sure people were sad, but we all felt it would be a sign of weakness to cry." A company commander reported, "I was really sad, but I didn't think it would be right for the men to know it."

Though OJC was limited in time and scope, some soldiers experienced or witnessed a full measure of horror. A soldier who looked into a comrade's face just after he had been mortally wounded in the head said, "I'll never forget his look of terror; he was still alive." The members of a mechanized infantry squad told how their machine gunner had been hit: "When daylight came we saw the track and the gun were covered with his blood. It stank." A platoon sergeant said that casualties affected the least experienced soldiers most: "The newbies were overwhelmed." A soldier described what happened when a rocket hit a soldier from behind: "It set off an explosion in his ruck. There were parts of him all over Bill." A soldier who witnessed the wounding of his comrades said: "I couldn't forget about the wounds, how bad they were. It could have been me. I felt weird, wanted to be alone." The best friend of a man who was accidentally killed by a gunshot in the head was angry and tearful as he described cleaning up the mess.

Guilt was a particular burden of leaders and medical aidmen—those who saw keeping others alive to be their responsibility. A company commander who lost a man in a well-planned and executed operation said: "I was so stunned I couldn't believe it. Could anything have been done better?" A squad leader who had lost men insisted, "I would rather it had been me than them." In another unit a squad leader felt responsible for casualties, but his platoon leader reported, "The squad helped the squad leader to stop blaming himself." A team leader who had been near his squad leader when he was mortally wounded kept saying, "He took my bullet." One medic who tried to treat a man whose arms had been blown off was distressed to admit, "I felt a moment's hesitation about touching him." Another medic was dropped by parachute at a considerable distance from where men were hit: "I wasn't where I should have been." There were also a few who expressed survivor guilt: "Why was it him and not me?"

When a unit suffered casualties, soldiers tended to cling to each other emotionally. One squad leader expressed a feeling shared by others: "There was tighter bonding. We tried to give more as squad leaders." A seriously wounded platoon sergeant ignored his own injuries in his anxiety about his men: "All my soldiers are still out there. You've got to get to them." After casualties were evacuated a survivor said, "The squad huddled together all night." A medic reported that in the aid station: "The wounded guys kept asking each other, 'Are you all right?'" The friend of a man who was hit said, "After he was wounded he wanted to stay with the unit but it was better that he was evacuated." A platoon sergeant had a man hit near the end of an operation: "I hugged him after he was hit, and told him to squeeze my hand if the pain got too bad."

After sustaining casualties, most units persevered in the mission, but with heightened care and caution. A squad leader spoke for many, saying: "Everyone acted different. Functioned better. They worried about each other. They paid attention to detail. They kept going; no one gave up." A soldier whose friend had been killed said, "We were prepared for this; we expected casualties and we had a job to do." Another soldier who had lost a squad mate said, "We were nervous, alert to each other; we still had a mission to do." A platoon sergeant described his men as: "Looking for reassurance in their tactics. They knew it could be them next." One company commander who was grief-stricken by a death described his soldiers: "They put their loss behind them. They haven't forgotten but they continue to perform." A soldier who had had a comrade killed beside him said, "We didn't want to go on, but we did."

Anxiety, Irritability, and Nightmares

Witnessing the death or maiming of a comrade heightened the survivors' awareness of their own vulnerability. In these cohesive units they looked to each other for reassurance and for a restored sense of strength. They also used the mission to distract them from becoming fully aware of their feelings at the time of the event. These responses were adaptive both for the accomplishment of the mission and for the mental well-being of the soldiers. They provided both time and opportunities to talk through, or share silently, the losses they had suffered, the horrors they had seen, and the fears they had experienced.

But neither time nor comrades erased the memories of killing, losing friends, guilt, shock, and fear. Several soldiers reported post-traumatic stress symptoms. Flashbacks and nightmares were a problem for some: "I had insomnia, and I was irritable." "I was angry at battalion, I jumped a lot, had nightmares, and I kept a weapon within reach." "I keep dreaming that I see him explode." "Several times I have woken up and found myself low-crawling on the floor." "I keep getting pictures in my head; I wonder what could I have done to keep from getting wounded." Almost all of the soldiers who described stress symptoms said they kept them to themselves: "We never mention nightmares or none of that stuff. It could hurt your career." "In this outfit they think you're pussy if you have psych stuff." "My wife listens, but she doesn't have any idea what I'm talking about."

Chaplains and commanders reported that there were increases in both maturity and acting out. There was a rash of marriages and of conception of children in some units after return. In other units there was increased drinking and fighting. Soldiers had not only to manage their acute reactions to their experiences, they had to readjust to peacetime training and routines, and the married ones had to readjust to living with their families.

Reintegration to Peacetime Garrison and Family Life

Historically many men who went through combat have found that there were aftereffects that complicated their return to peacetime pursuits. Research conducted on veterans of World War I found that even those who had the best postwar outcomes—those who were in good health, self-supporting, and happy—reported they were irritable, quick to anger, excitable, nervous, forgetful, restless, and plagued by headaches and dizziness.[44]

Reintegration processes for veterans of short wars, who stay in the armed services and have to prepare for the next intervention, have three characteristics that distinguish them from the processes associated with long wars. First, the intense emotional experience of combat has not been blunted by time and the erection of defenses. This makes the letdown from war to peace more intense.

Second, service members who remain on active duty after combat lose the sense of personal significance and potency associated with a "real world mission" and do not have it replaced by a qualitative change in identity from soldier to civilian. They are still in the service, but instead of being on the cutting edge of national policy they are involved in simulation, make-believe, and bureaucratic procedures. Several soldiers made comments such as, "Down there we were men; back here they treat us like children."

A third factor is that there is no perception that the job is done, the misery is over, and there is an end to terror. Professional military personnel know that there is a high probability that they will be called into combat again, probably soon. These factors did not affect many servicemen at the ends of the big wars or those who finished tours of duty in Korea or Vietnam. The research team from Walter Reed found several clusters of long-term issues associated with reentry. They can be grouped under five rubrics: (1) horizontal cohesion, (2) vertical cohesion, (3) command behavior, (4) persistent stress reactions, and (5) relationships with families.

Horizontal Cohesion

Military personnel who fought together were tightly bonded with each other. They trusted one another and felt safe with each other after having survived dangerous situations together. One commander described his men: "They're closer after the stress plus 50 days of propinquity plus the satisfactions of participating successfully in an important event. People feel better about working together." A senior NCO noted:

"Now we are real relaxed. The men talk about their experiences and joke. The mood is lighter, there is less bickering, and they tolerate each other better. They know the other guy will watch their back. They don't hold grudges. Everybody is a little bit closer after 74 days of hell."

From privates' perspectives: "We pull for each other, we check one another. It's live or die." "The squad is tight, real tight. We were close before we went, but it is really a different kind of closeness now. We know we can depend on each other."

Soldiers varied in their responses to returning to combat from, "I never want to go through anything like that again" to "I'd go back in a heartbeat." But they were almost unanimous in saying, "If I have to go back, I want to be with these guys." This medley of feelings led to a congeries of psychosocial issues as replacements came in and veterans either left the service or were transferred. The salient themes were: "I trust the guys I went to combat with, but not the new guys" on the one hand and, "We train with the new guys and help them; everyone has a battle buddy; we need them and want them, so we do for them" on the other. In some squads there was a feeling of loss and despair as trusted comrades transferred out and clumsy rookies took their places: "They came from no-stress basic training. They're weak and don't want to learn." "It's too bad we can't stay together. We could mature together but instead each guy who leaves takes some experience with him."

The receptions for new men were generally positive: "Peers help the newcomers out a lot." "Nobody is lording it over the new guys." "Most of us don't even wear our CIBs [Combat Infantryman Badges], except on our Hollywood uniforms." "Oh, there was a little hazing, but it was good-natured. The new guys are okay." "The squad hasn't changed. We still bullshit around. The new guys are fitting right in." The new men saw things differently: "It was awesome joining a squad where everybody had been in combat." "This COHORT unit was harder to break into than either of the other two units I have been in. The major reason was that I had not been to Panama with them." "They let me in, but I really had to show them that I would put out."

Because of the life-or-death nature of combat, men who did not do well found themselves extruded. Squads bonded tightly with all of the members keeping the one perceived to be a slacker on the outside. "There were some guys who didn't do their share. They're isolated by the rest of the unit." "When we attacked, he hid under a boat. Nobody talks to him anymore." A platoon leader said, "I had some guys who failed in combat. It was their big chance, and they blew it. What do I do with them?"

Vertical Cohesion

Postcombat turnover among junior leaders had the heaviest impact on vertical cohesion. A battalion commander reported, "We had 8 new NCOs waiting for us when we got back, and we're turning over 40 more in the next couple of months. The new ones may have trouble getting accepted. It will work out if they can do their jobs. I worry more about the NCO turnover than anything else."

From the privates' viewpoint the worries were justified: "We have had four squad leaders in 4 months." "The sergeant who replaced our squad leader who was killed is too familiar; he is trying to fit in too fast." "Since all the NCOs were wounded, we have all new squad leaders." "A sergeant came in from another division that had also been in Panama. We advised him to take off his combat patch from that division." These problems could involve many NCOs in the same unit.

> Sergeant X isn't here half the time, he's at school. Sergeant Y was our best team leader and now he's

> a squad leader in another platoon. He takes time to talk about our problems, he shows us how things work. Instead of writing you up, he squares you away. Sergeant Z knew his shit, how to navigate, what needed to be done, how to take care of soldiers. He was busted and transferred. Sergeant Q, who cracked in Panama, is still a sergeant.

New officers joining a unit that had been in combat had problems, but they were less severe. One lieutenant said:

> I told them I was depending on the veterans to train the new guys. That was all it took. I guess they were pleased that their experience was being recognized. Of course, I was one of the new guys. They trained me but nobody said that in so many words.

Command Behavior

It is difficult to separate vertical cohesion from command behavior because the former is a product of the latter. The essential distinction in this argument is that under the section on vertical cohesion new leaders' problems of being accepted were discussed, whereas in this section the behavior of leaders, whether new or veteran, is the topic. The most critical issue facing commanders upon reentry is engaging the veterans' interest and effort for training after they have done the job in combat. A company commander complained: "I'm having a hard time playing the game. I'm tired of retreading the same territory." A lieutenant said: "It is like starting spring training after you have been to the Super Bowl."

Soldier after soldier echoed these sentiments, but with more pungency: "Why are they putting us through this Mickey Mouse bullshit when we've shown we can do it?" "The highers are actually serious about training for NTC [National Training Center]. Can you believe it? As if it was something real." "The training is bad. We go charging off 100 miles per hour in the wrong direction. It's more like being disciplined." "Battle drill may be needed, but they're going about it wrong. Instead of building on Panama they are like saying, 'Forget Panama.'" "It's the same old horseshit. Ever since we got back we've had people on our backs about barracks arrangement, micromanaging, telling us things we want are impossible when we know perfectly well they are possible." "This so-called training is nothing but repetition of things we already know. No one is reenlisting." "We don't feel we're doing any useful mission here. We felt fulfilled in Panama, but not here." "Training doesn't have the same seriousness or level of importance it did before."

Not all units had problems getting troops interested in training. A lieutenant said: "Things can't just stop. You owe it to the soldiers to train them to be as proficient as possible. But you have to be sensitive about Panama, too." Privates in another battalion reported: "Panama was the highest gear we had been in. We went home, showed off, and came back ready to get back to training, get ready for the SQT." "I have a different attitude toward training. We got back because we knew our shit." "I'm more serious. I train harder now." "There's no pressure in this battalion for unrealistic standards. You try to beat your own standard." Squad leaders in the same battalion added: "We've had no problem converting back to training because we need to work on our weak points. We have a meeting at 1600 each day on what we'll do tomorrow. I stay a little while with the troops to see if they have any problems." "After Panama there was a different attitude toward training; it had been hard, but it registered on them that if you got it right, your chances of coming back are better."

Another issue was the question of time off for decompression. There was general agreement that there should be time off, that the soldiers should go on leave, and that the pace of training should be less intense. But there was wide variation in how much was enough. Commanders expressed satisfaction; a typical comment was: "The battalion went on block leave as soon as we had recovered our equipment. When we came back I declared a number of 4-day weekends, and we held to those rigorously." The rank and file had different perceptions: "Other battalions got 10 days administrative leave; we had to use our own leave time." "Ten lousy days is all we got. We had missed Thanksgiving and Christmas and New Years." "Who the hell wants block leave in February?" "We had been down there 4 months and been on duty 7 days a week and all we got was 14 days leave." A thoughtful officer described the dynamic in his platoon:

> There should be a policy that after combat or a prolonged, stressful deployment soldiers get time off. They need to dream, filter away the combat. They should maybe be allowed to take more leave if they need it. It takes a couple of months. When we got back we got one day off and then back to work. Is training that critical? Stuff builds up—administration, housework, kids. They need to feel the establishment is behind us.

Persistent Stress Reactions

The flashbacks and nightmares described under acute reactions to combat were a continuing problem for some soldiers. NCOs were most articulate in describing their own symptoms. They tried to deal with them by keeping busy—for distraction and so they could sleep at night. When asked about increased irritability, they reported being angry but not at any specific persons or situations. They were mad at "leaders," mostly at battalion level, for "dog and pony" shows and having to "buy new fatigues to look nice." Paratrooper sergeants reported fears of jumping, especially at night.

Comparatively few privates reported having symptoms. Some of their NCOs said they were concerned about them. Most said they had not had time to ask their soldiers how they're doing. They agreed that the "quiet ones" seem to have more problems. They think that many soldiers on their return from Panama had problems with what they had seen and done. No one had debriefed them or provided them information about combat reactions. (For a further discussion of debriefings, see Chapter 11, Debriefing Following Combat.) They think this would have been helpful and a good idea. They would have heard that others shared their feelings and experiences. A platoon sergeant described a soldier who had intrusive memories and who thought he was crazy. Another told of a soldier who had nightmares about having a dead soldier's blood all over him. No one had told them that nightmares and flashbacks are normal.

There was evidence of a need for mental health services in theater in connection with the operation and its aftermath. A psychiatrist reported, "We had two combat stress casualties." A first sergeant said, "Three of our guys had symptoms—nightmares and such. They had all been hurt and evacuated away from the unit." Another told the team, "One soldier cared for a dying comrade for several hours; he went to the psych unit after his friend died."

But most soldiers and leaders in line units shunned mental health services after their return to home base. There were several apparent reasons; fear of the unknown realm of psychological functioning was one. One company commander said, "Psychologists don't go over well in my unit. They're too 'touchy-feely.'" Another officer noted, "In the religious community, Freud equals evil." A perceptive sergeant major observed, "People fear mental health workers. They might make them look at themselves."

Another reason was anxiety about having their thoughts probed by a staff officer from higher headquarters. A platoon sergeant told the team, "The psychiatrist offered to come to the unit, but command dragged its feet." Another reported, "A mental health team came to the unit. Someone told them to give the information to the chaplain. They didn't want a stranger in the unit."

There were also practical issues such as worry about the impact of a psychiatric report on a service record, and concern about possible psychological malingering. To even mention a psychological problem was seen as a potential black mark. Several NCOs said they thought their men would not go to the troop medical clinics for fear of being labeled "a psychiatric case." With respect to malingering, one platoon sergeant noted that there had been an article in the post newspaper from the division psychologists about availability of assistance for those with Post-Panama Stress Syndrome: "I didn't approve; I thought it would just put thoughts into guys' minds." In one unit a thoughtful group of NCOs expressed a worry that talking with the team from Walter Reed would "Just bring it all back."

Relationships with Families

The deployment and combat put severe strains on wives and children. When the soldiers returned, the role adjustments the wives had made while their husbands were away had to be renegotiated. These strains were exacerbated by the irritability and tension the men brought back with them and, in some units, by their disillusionment with the return to military garrison routine and an uninspired training regimen. The results were an increase in the incidence of divorce, the return of some wives to their parents, and a few cases of spouse abuse. The principal buffers that facilitated soldiers' reintegration with their families were family support groups, a period of uninterrupted leave together, and, in a few units, more predictable on-duty and off-duty schedules.

Family support groups provided information, practical assistance with the tasks of living and raising families, and social support. The more effective family support groups were successful in strengthening wives' morale and mitigating their hostility toward the U.S. Army and their husbands while they were away and upon their return. These factors were important determinants of the ability of the soldier and his family to reintegrate. The effectiveness of family support groups was in turn a function of the degree to which they were democratically organized, open in communications, and focused on the wives' needs rather than on matters of interest to the U.S. Army.[45,46]

There was a positive side to the experience of combat with respect to soldiers' ability to reintegrate with their families. Several soldiers reported to the research team or to their chaplains or comrades that their feelings about fundamental issues had undergone changes that put higher values on their families. One sergeant major said: "A lot of these kids grew up. They don't sit around and drink and waste time anymore. They don't want to embarrass the unit or themselves." Several chaplains reported a sudden upsurge in marriages, and there was more subtle evidence in the form of an increase in the numbers of children conceived. One chaplain said: "They went through a life and death experience; now some of them are making decisions for life." The accuracy of his analysis was born out by the statements of several privates: "I see life as more special, valuable. We should spend time doing what matters." "I have, like, a reverence for life." "I've changed emotionally; my buddy died." "When I came, I questioned things. Now I'm more pliable, serious. I dig in." "I learned a lot about myself."

There were other behavioral changes—besides marrying and conceiving children—to implement the changes in values. Several soldiers opted to leave the service to, as one new father put it, "Not put myself and my family in jeopardy." A group of platoon sergeants described their struggles with whether or not to stay in the military after encountering the "life and death moral dilemmas that have to be addressed in combat." A substantial proportion of the soldiers interviewed gave evidence of moral growth during the brief period of the invasion of Panama. In some cases they outgrew their need for the U.S. Army; in others that portion of the U.S. Army with which they were associated matured along with them to meet their new patterns of needs. One of those needs was validation—which is the topic of the next subsection. On a broader level, the process by which military mental health professionals can contribute to the institutional maturation of the U.S. Army will be the subject of the concluding section of this chapter.

Validation

Soldiers in combat experience a plethora of unpleasant emotions that can cause post-traumatic stress disorders unless they are managed intelligently. Validation of their experiences, behavior, and feelings is an essential part of the management process. Comrades, leaders, subordinates, friends, families, the public, and members of the mental health/spiritual health community play roles in validation.

The painful emotions that follow combat include reactions to physical distress—hunger, fatigue, cold, heat, prolonged exertion, heavy burdens, wounds, and injuries. They include psychological distress—fear, loss, shame, and guilt. Fear takes more forms than can be counted: fear of death or injury, fear of making a mistake, fear of abandonment, fear of leaving loved ones in the lurch, fear of cowardice, fear of being afraid and showing it—each soldier has his personal closet of terrors. Losses include friends, one's own innocence and idealism, one's fantasies about oneself. Shame is more often for feelings than behavior; most soldiers perform well, but remember how much they wished they could escape from having to perform. Guilt has many facets—what they did, who they hurt, and hurts that befell others but not them.

No one can escape these feelings; repressed they can fester and give rise to future psychopathology. Validation makes it easier to bring them out and confront them, and can detoxify some of them. The veterans of Panama reported three categories of validation that were useful when they were available, and that they longed for when they were absent. The first is symbolic validation—gestures by people or institutions that defined the soldier's miseries and actions as virtuous. The second is validation of losses by expiating guilt and reconciling the loss. The third is substantive validation—interactions that integrate the individual soldier's sufferings into a stronger unit or army.

Symbolic Validation

Approval expressed by a remote, depersonalized entity such as the U.S. Army, the media, or the public is an important source of validation because it is perceived as absolute, as independent of human judgment or prejudice. Herein lies the power of medals, television coverage, and welcome-home banners. Soldiers dealing with the shock and horror of what they have seen and what they have done or failed to do feel better if an "Olympian" voice proclaims their deeds meritorious and their cause worthy. Infantrymen often feel that the hardships of their branch set them apart, and that no one has the right to pass judgment on what they do. Sometimes they turn up their noses at awards. But a medal is a statement by the U.S. Army that what the soldier did was good, and to that extent it helps in the reentry process.

Many soldiers who had fought in Panama felt that they and their comrades were denied medals because there had been a furor after the invasion of Grenada in 1983 because the press reported that more medals were awarded than there were people participating in the operation: "We got short-changed on awards because the [U.S.] Army was embarrassed over Grenada." Though the cultural ethic is that "medals don't mean shit," there was bitterness in most units over the paucity of awards: "The only guys who got awards were the ones who got hit." "PFC W spoke Spanish, so he was out in front on every patrol. He never knew where the bullet would come from, but he knew it would be aimed at him. But he kept going out because we needed him. He got zip." "The first sergeant was the most important person in the success of our company. He was put in for a bronze star, but got nothing." "I was given a quota of four awards for the company." "I put in 47 guys for awards. We got six. The colonel said the descriptions showed that my people deserved the medals I had recommended, but there was a quota." "The medals bit was all politics. We didn't have a general to fight for us so we got very few." Awards are the most effective symbolic aid to validation the military has at its disposal. Overdoing is a mistake, so is underdoing. Because awards support successful reentry, a liberal policy is less likely to do harm than a restrictive policy.

The services have less control over the validation provided by the media than they do over their own system of recognition. A certain division may get a disproportionate share of media coverage for any number of reasons, including the influence the reporter covering it has with his superiors or the interest his editors have in military affairs. Soldiers in most of the units in Panama perceived that battalions from only one division got television coverage, and that the others "might as well not have been there." Service members in Panama and the Persian Gulf watched television and knew which units were covered and which were not. Many soldiers expressed the feeling that because the activities of their units were not reported in the visual or the print media, their efforts had no significance. This perception was not trivial; not to be covered was not to exist. The impact of television as a source of validation in American culture needs to be taken into consideration.

Public opinion is a force yet less under the control of the armed forces than are the media, but it is the third "Olympian" source of validation. The high incidence of successful postwar adjustments following World War I and World War II was probably a result of the intense national support for the wars and the men who fought them. The prevalence of post-traumatic stress disorders following the Vietnam conflict is most often said to be a result of negative attitudes among the public toward returning veterans. It is interesting to note that the single most pervasive and gratifying source of validation involved in Operation Just Cause was neither the American people, nor television, nor the Army; it was the grateful and admiring behavior of the Panamanians.

Validating Losses

The most difficult psychological problem veterans have to cope with is the death or maiming of comrades, especially close friends. There is the helpless feeling of loss: "I was looking at him and it kept going through me, 'He's *dead*!" "I was giving him CPR, and the medics were saying, 'He's gone.' 'You can stop now.' They tried to pull me away but I shook them off. I couldn't let him go." Equally difficult is survivor guilt: "He took my bullet." Leaders and medics had a particular kind of guilt about not having done their utmost: "I keep going over it in my mind, what could I have done differently so it wouldn't have happened."

Of particular importance from the reentry standpoint is that the dead should not have died in vain, and that they not be forgotten. These are difficult issues, because a death in battle is obscenely and obviously a waste. Soldiers realize that it is all too easy to forget those who are gone. They are horrified at the prospect that they, too, could die in vain and be forgotten. Soldiers in Panama found memorial services and physical memorials to be important to them: "We had a memorial service the next week. The guys in the squad organized it with the chaplain and the first sergeant. It helped us to realize that we didn't have him anymore." "We had a last role call and taps. There wasn't a dry eye in the company. We had to go through it, and it helped." "His best friend and his squad leader spoke. There wasn't no brass in it. It was our service." Most units that lost members put together monuments or trophy cases in the company to commemorate their fallen comrades. "Each time we go in the dayroom we'll think of him. It's sort of like he's still in the company." "We're going to have a plaque on a rock in front of the barracks. It'll look real sharp."

Senior commanders had different perspectives about memorial services compared to enlisted men and officers in companies. Junior personnel opined, "The company service in Panama was healing. But then we had another back here, and another for his folks. What is all this?" "The colonel wanted another memorial service back in the States. He said it was for his friends back here to say good-bye to him, but it looks like a photo opportunity. All the senior brass came, and the press." "The battalion commander didn't come to the memorial service in Panama, he said his feet hurt. Then he made us turn out for a formal service back here with photographers and all. The general came. Bunch of PR bullcrap."

The fates of wounded soldiers were a matter of concern that had an impact on reentry. Soldiers who were wounded but conscious often did not want to leave the unit, and their comrades did not want them to leave. Good sense always prevailed and those whose injuries were serious were evacuated. But their comrades worried about them and were persistent in their efforts to find out what had become of them. Finding out was difficult because they were evacuated by air to Texas, and there was no direct way of getting word about them: "He was evacuated and that was it. No one knew where he was or how he was. It really bugged us." Their absence and condition remained an open point of anxiety for the men in their units, and those who returned were welcomed back.

Many soldiers who were too seriously injured to stay in the service visited their units, or came back to outprocess: "He came back. He was in a wheelchair. Christ, that was hard to take. He loved the [U.S.] Army. But at least we could say good-bye." These reunions were important. The best situation was when recuperating soldiers were on the same post as their units, and they could visit each other. One lieutenant said, "They're going to be medically discharged, but they're still my men. I visit them whenever I can, and they come do things with the platoon when they're able."

Substantive Validation

Substantive validation not only helps the soldier to manage his feelings and reenter the peacetime world with minimal psychological distress, but also strengthens the unit by reinforcing cohesion and exchanging information gained through combat experience. The primary process of substantive validation is talk—talk among peers, between leader and subordinate, and among the members of a squad or platoon. The talk can be formal or informal, it can be about military matters or about feelings. For it to be effective it has to be forthright and honest. It can only take place in a climate of trust.

The most important sources of substantive validation for a soldier are the men who shared the battle with him. Foremost are his comrades in his primary group; if his squad mates approve of his behavior most soldiers can survive psychologically, though they may be embittered that the approval is not more general. There was a case in Panama in which a soldier accidentally killed one of this friends. He was devastated by the loss and horrified that he was the agent of his friend's death. In addition, he was placed under arrest, interrogated by the criminal investigation authorities, and faced a court-martial. There were no sources of support from outside his squad. But his squad mates, though they had liked the dead man, still stuck up for him, insisted that it was an accident, and maintained their bonds with him. This support facilitates the psychological process described as "concurrence," which helps the soldier see that he and his squad mates are alike and that he is not an isolate. Concurrence is essential to psychological survival.[47–50] It illustrates the power of the primary group bond. If his squad mates reject him, a soldier is in a psychologically vulnerable situation. External sources of validation can provide some support, and it is essential that they be mobilized fully and quickly.

Leaders who participated in the battle are usually the second most important source of substantive validation. Their effectiveness in the validation process is a function of the esteem in which they are held and the degree to which they shared their subordinates' danger and privation. Leaders who are perceived as trustworthy and genuinely interested in their subordinates are credible sources of validation. Together with primary group members, they can alleviate much of the guilt and shame soldiers bring with them out of combat. The mechanisms are listening, talking the battle through, sharing feelings: "We sat around with Sergeant P and went over what we did. He'd say things like 'That must have scared you,' and I'd think, 'Yeah,' and somebody else would say he felt scared and then it would seem okay, I wasn't any more yellow than anyone else." "We had a secret place for the platoon and we fixed it up. We'd go there at night and talk it through. The lieutenant always came. Little by little I got less uptight."

The system of after-action reviews (AARs), that is standard procedure after any operation to bring out the military lessons to be learned, is also an important validation mechanism. Intended to enhance performance by a frank, mutual review of what everyone did, AARs serve to get the sources of guilt and shame out in the open. One soldier said: "I thought I had really blown it when Smitty got hit, but we went over it in the AAR and everybody said they would have done the same thing I did." The AAR, conducted routinely by the team leader, will be discussed later in this chapter.

Mental health professionals and chaplains can provide substantive validation by helping veterans to interpret their experiences in psychological or spiritual terms through debriefings or religious observances. In a way, these validations partake of the symbolic in that the chaplains invoke the blessing of the deity and the mental health professionals invoke psychological processes, all of which are remote from the day-to-day world of the soldier.

THE ROLES OF MENTAL HEALTH PROFESSIONALS

Successful reentry following the invasion of Panama was the result of teamwork between line leaders and members of the helping professions. Because the concept of reentry is new, few members of either community had worked out comprehensive plans for it. Inevitably, successes were episodic, but lessons can be derived from failures as well as successes. This section is a compilation of the positive and negative lessons that may lead to a provisional program of mutually supportive action by command and the helping professions.

Because of the paucity of mental health professionals in the armed forces, they are limited in the number of soldiers they can help with reentry through individual or group therapy or counseling. Their effectiveness can be multiplied by sensitizing chaplains, commanders, and unit medical personnel to reentry issues and their management. It is of the utmost importance that the mental health staff of a division or comparable headquarters respect the battalion, squadron, or ship's surgeon. The unit medical staff shares danger and discomfort with the combatants, and enjoys their trust. There is no quicker way for a mental health team from a higher headquarters to lose all influence than by treating the unit medical staff—which is often headed by a physician's assistant or by a lieutenant or sergeant without professional medical education—as inconsequential. On the other hand, if the mental health team earns the respect and endorsement of the unit medics, its acceptance by the combatants is much more likely.

During peacetime training there are opportunities for the command mental health staff, unit medical officers, and NCOs to get to know each other through case referrals and ongoing education programs. It is important for the mental health professional to be active and supportive in these interactions. Whenever possible, the division mental health and supporting corps-level combat stress control (CSC) unit teams should deploy to the field with the line units. For on-post exercises this could be as simple as an overnight, 2-day visit. Even better are scheduled deployments to the combat training centers (National Training Center [NTC], Joint Readiness Training Center [JRTC], and the Combat Maneuver Training Center [CMTC]) during which the mental health teams provide active mobile consultation. The mental health personnel in the Medical Department activities (MEDDACs)—the Community Mental Health Services (CMHS) and the Departments of Psychiatry, Psychology, and Social Work may not be able to deploy to the field, but can conduct education and consultation activities in the supported units' work areas in garrison.

The program laid out here is designed to maximize the ability of military psychiatry to exert a positive influence on successful reentry through a combination of command consultation, participation in unit reentry programs, and direct psychiatric treatment.

Consultation on Command Action

Most of the work leading to successful reentry is done by leaders from senior command (division, corps, theater/fleet/air command) down through squad and work group supervisors. Further, most of the work that leads to successful reentry is part of the normal routine of leadership and command. The role of mental health professionals is to advise commanders and to monitor those aspects of leadership behavior that are conducive to successful reentry to see that they are not neglected or off-track due to the leaders' own stress or personal issues. In the process of advising, military psychiatrists and mental health workers can make themselves part of commanders' teams at every level and work toward undermining the antipsychiatry bias they are likely to find in most military units. There are four spheres of command activity on which the psychiatrist and his staff should focus: (1) debriefings (called after-action reviews [AARs] in the U.S. Army), (2) dissemination of lessons learned, (3) memorial services for deceased members, and (4) decompression leave. (See Chapter 11, Debriefing Following Combat.)

After-action reviews are prescribed techniques in the U.S. Army for learning from mistakes and successes. In training exercises, an AAR is to be conducted following each phase of activity. In combat, it should be conducted as soon as it is safe for the leader to bring the team together. The AAR is informal, solicits input from all participants, and is nonpunitive. It has as its immediate purpose finding out what worked, what needs to be improved, and how to improve it. A broader purpose is to so improve the fighting capacity of units that they can accomplish missions with minimal loss. Along the way several intermediate purposes are achieved such as strengthening cohesion, cementing trust, and opening communications. Members of units in which AARs are a normal part of life are accustomed to admitting when they were confused, uncertain, or frightened, having their human weaknesses accepted, and getting help from comrades and leaders on how to manage, overcome, or compensate for them. AARs following combat provide superb forums for reliving and getting support for the inevitable fears, failures, and guilt with the people whose acceptance and approval are most important. They provide firm foundations for successful reentry. Prior to combat, military psychiatrists and technicians should support commanders in requiring open, honest, fear-free, professional AARs. They can train the leaders to expand the routine AAR into a team after-action debriefing (AAD) which deliberately works through the emotional as well as operational issues, as discussed in Chapter 11, Debriefing Following Combat.

The process of disseminating lessons learned by combat veterans to new members of the unit or to other units provides a means for validation as well as enriching the combat know-how of those who were not participants in the action. The combatant's perception that what he did is sufficiently important that it merits the attention of the service as a whole goes a long way toward alleviating aversive emotions attendant on combat. Because the future of military operations is likely to include fairly frequent short-duration, force-projection operations, only parts of the armed services will be involved in each of them. Those not involved will be eager to learn what went on and what worked so that they will be better prepared when their turns come. Again the role of the military psychiatrist and mental health worker is to support commanders in their resolve to use veterans in cross-pollinating other units. It is good for the service, and it helps resolve reentry problems for the veteran.

Memorial services are helpful for veterans in coming to terms with losses. As noted above, they can backfire if they are perceived as opportunities for senior commanders to be photographed expressing their grief. Memorial services that were perceived by the rank and file as public relations events drove deep wedges between commanders and subordinates, including subordinate commanders. They were perceived as obscene exploitation of subordinates' deeply felt losses. Memorial services must be for the service members who knew and loved the deceased. Memorial services offer opportunities for the mental health workers and chaplains to cooperate in a sphere in which their interests are congruent. Their combined influence can support commanders in using memorial services to solidify vertical cohesion and facilitate the management of grief.

In this connection it is worth mentioning that chaplains outnumber psychiatrists in a division by a ratio of about 20:1, and the entire division mental health team by 2:1. The chaplains are likely to have much higher credibility in companies and battalions. The battalion chaplain is there for the soldier in emotional and spiritual distress. He is part of the unit, not some staff officer from division. Most of them have won some measure of trust and acceptance in their units. They help soldiers' families, show up in the field, and are the channel for action and solace when family tragedies strike. The folklore about chaplains includes heroism on the battlefield rescuing the wounded and comforting the dying. Complimentary comments about chaplains in Panama ranked just behind the almost worshipful love for company combat medics: "The chaplain must have balls of solid brass to parachute into combat without a weapon."

On the other hand, no one had ever heard of a "shrink" on the battlefield. A visit to the psychiatrist was usually perceived as a way station en route to chapter action. When psychiatrists compete head to head with chaplains for influence in military units, the psychiatrists lose. On the other hand, an alliance between the two enhances the effectiveness of both. They can catch a commander who tends toward being indifferent to his subordinates' needs between two fires. Chaplains are usually easier to get time with than commanders, and can provide access to commanders through the chaplains' already established channels. Memorial services are only one of many ways in which chaplains and psychiatrists can help commanders bring their units through reentry stronger than they were before.

The mental health team has an important role in supporting the chaplains, who are themselves subjected to extreme stress by the nature of their pastoral duties, especially in combat. The mental health professionals can mentor and train the chaplains to recognize serious psychiatric disturbance and know when to refer soldiers for medical/mental health evaluation. The mental health personnel and chaplains can debrief each other, to share the emotional burden.

Decompression is the process by which soldiers separate themselves progressively from the tension, fear, and horror of the battlefield. It includes AARs, talking about combat experiences with comrades and with others who were not there, dreaming, and doing things totally different from combat. After Panama there was a great deal of urgency on the part of several commanders to get back into training. (As the researchers talked to veterans of Panama they recalled the British Regular Army major who on 11 November 1918, was quoted [in reference to the end of World War I]: "Well, at last that's over. Now we can get back to some real soldiering.") The longest leave identified in any battalion was 14 days. A number of senior NCOs and junior commanders were of the opinion that a longer period would have brought the unit back together with more zest for the next phase of training. One platoon leader said:

> The battalion should have shut down for a month, and part of the leave time should have been nonchargeable administrative leave—a kind of "thank you" from a grateful nation. Personnel who felt unready to return after a month should have had the option of taking additional leave.

The short decompression leaves after Panama left a number of soldiers feeling badly used. Further, they were still so keyed up from combat that they saw the training as boring and beneath them as veterans of real combat. Chaplains, company medics, junior officers, and senior NCOs are in the best position to judge the burned out state of their people and how much leave they should have for the unit to return most quickly to peak psychological readiness. The role of the mental health technicians and psychiatrist is to support commanders in getting the leaves authorized using psychological arguments.

Participation in Unit Recovery Processes

Mental health professionals can assist in the reentry process directly by limited participation in some of the programs undertaken by units to facilitate the management of postcombat emotions. The small number of mental health professionals available makes it impossible for them to participate regularly in most of the programs, but they can provide some direct support according to the guidelines in this chapter. There are three functions that are within the capability of the mental health staff: (1) short-term concentration on small units, (2) initiation of some group processes, and (3) occasional participation in after-action reviews, end-of-tour debriefings and prehomecoming information briefings. Their effectiveness in all of these functions will be enhanced in scope and in duration to the extent that they can sensitize and train the battalion medical staff in psychologically supportive processes.

End-of-tour debriefings (EOTD) should be conducted by all small units before deploying home. The unit leaders lead a discussion which reviews all phases of the operation—notification or alert, mobilization, deployment, and the significant actions up to the present. All participants are encouraged to talk about what went well and what did not, the good times and bad, noting lessons learned and working through unresolved, painful, or controversial issues. Like the AAR, this must be well-led to assure a positive sense of completion or closure at the end. Trusted chaplains and mental health personnel can facilitate the process.

Prior to redeployment from the theater, all units and soldiers should receive a prehomecoming briefing. This reviews what changes and expectations are commonly encountered when soldiers, spouses, and children are reunited after a prolonged separation. It provides tips on how to deal with these predictable stresses. The families at home should receive their version of the same briefing. Pocket cards summarizing the briefing have proved useful for both the service members and the families. Sample cards are provided in Exhibits 12-1 and 12-2. These briefings are often conducted by the unit chaplains in the theater, and by the unit support groups at home base, with input and attendance by mental health personnel.

When units return from combat one at a time, the mental health professionals should focus on them for a week or at least a few days. Mental health technicians should be informally available for soldiers to talk to. They should hang out in the mess

EXHIBIT 12-1

HOMECOMING AFTER DEPLOYMENT DEALING WITH CHANGES AND EXPECTATIONS

With deployments come change. Knowing what to expect and how to deal with changes can make reunion more enjoyable and less stressful. Below are some hints you might find helpful.

Expectations for soldiers

- You may want to talk about what you saw and did. Others may seem not to want to listen. Or you may not want to talk about it when others keep asking.
- You may miss the excitement of the deployment for a while.
- Some things may have changed while you were gone.
- Roles may have changed to manage basic household chores.
- Face to face communication may be hard at first.
- Sexual closeness may also be awkward at first.
- Children have grown and may be different in many ways.
- Spouses may have become more independent and learned new coping skills.
- Spouses may have new friends and support systems.
- You may have changed in your outlook and priorities in life.

Expectation for spouses

- Soldiers may have changed.
- Soldiers, used to the open spaces of the field, may feel closed in.
- Soldiers also may be overwhelmed by noise and confusion of home life.
- Soldiers may be on a different schedule of sleeping and eating (jet lag).
- Soldiers may wonder if they still fit into the family.
- Soldiers may want to take back all the responsibilities they had before they left.
- Soldiers may feel hurt when young children are slow to hug them.

What children may feel

- Babies less than 1 year old may not know you and may cry when held.
- Toddlers (1–3 years) may hide from you and be slow to come to you.
- Preschoolers (3–5 years) may feel guilty over the separation and be scared.
- School age (6–12 years) may want a lot of your time and attention.
- Teenagers (13–18 years) may be moody and may appear not to care.
- Any age may feel guilty about not living up to your standards.
- Some may fear your return ("Wait until mommy/daddy gets home!").
- Some may feel torn by loyalties to the spouse who remained.

Source: US Department of the Army. Homecoming after Deployment: Dealing with Changes and Expectations. US Army Medical Department Center and School, Combat Stress Actions Office, Fort Sam Houston, San Antonio, Texas. Modification of materials prepared by 101st Airborne Division Mental Health Section for the Persian Gulf War (1991).

hall, day room, and barracks, for example, and initiate conversations. Their purpose should be to validate feelings and experiences. When opportunities present, these informal conversations could expand into group discussions with the mental health worker as facilitator. The psychiatrist should dedicate his time to the battalion for the week, and should focus on sensitizing leaders and working with those individuals and primary groups that experienced the most severe traumata.

When the simultaneous return of several units precludes concentration on a single battalion, the mental health staff should focus all its assets on initiating group processes in squads and other primary groups in several battalions simultaneously. The ease with which this can be done will be a

EXHIBIT 12-2

HOMECOMING AFTER DEPLOYMENT TIPS FOR REUNION

Reunion is part of the deployment cycle and is filled with joy and stress. The following tips can help you have the best possible reunion.

Tips for soldiers

- Support good things your family has done.
- Take time to talk with your spouse and children.
- Make individual time for each child and your spouse.
- Go slowly when reestablishing your place in the family.
- Be prepared to make some adjustments.
- Romantic conversation can lead to more enjoyable sex.
- Make your savings last longer.
- Take time to listen and to talk with loved ones.
- Go easy on partying.

Tips for spouses for reunion

- Avoid scheduling too many things.
- Go slowly in making adjustments.
- You and your soldier may need time for yourself.
- Remind soldier he is still needed in the family.
- Discuss splitting up family chores.
- Stick to your budget until you've had time to talk it through.
- Along with time for the family, make individual time to talk.
- Be patient with yourself and your partner.

Tips for reunion with children

- Go slowly. Adapt to the rules and routines already in place.
- Learn from how your spouse managed the children.
- Be available to your child, both with time and with your emotions.
- Let the child set the pace for getting to know you again.
- Delay making changes in rules and routines for a few weeks.
- Expect the family will not be the same as before you left; everyone has changed.
- Focus on successes with your children; limit your criticisms.
- Encourage children to tell you about what happened during the separation.
- Make individual time for each child and your spouse.

Source: US Department of the Army. Homecoming after Deployment: Tips for Reunion. US Army Medical Department Center and School, Combat Stress Actions Office, Fort Sam Houston, San Antonio, Texas. Modification of materials prepared by 101st Airborne Division Mental Health Section for the Persian Gulf War (1991).

function of the level of trust and openness already developed in the various units, in the degree of hostility toward mental health professionals preexisting in the unit, and in the quality of the relationships between members of the division mental health staff and the battalion medical platoon. The objective of the mental health staff is to get the groups up and talking, and then turn them over to their own leadership. With more than 30 primary groups in each battalion it is imperative for the mental health workers to move on as quickly as possible. In battalions with strong traditions of AARs conducted throughout the deployment, there may be little for the mental health staff to do—members of those battalions will already be working through their feelings. In battalions with weak traditions of AAR and unit medics who are not psychologically oriented, the mental health people will have to come back to the same squads repeatedly. The psychiatrist will have to divide his time among all the battalions to keep up to date on problems identified by the chain of command and to maintain access for his teams.

Mental health workers can assist units conducting AARs or end-of-tour debriefings to expand their scope to include feelings as well as behavior, making them after-action debriefings. The psychiatrist will usually have to solicit invitations to AADs or EOTDs by explaining to commanders the importance of the emotional dimensions for the successful reentry of the unit. The role of the mental health worker at an AAR is to listen to the process, and when given an opportunity, assist members who appear to be repressing strong emotions to express them. He can explain the potential of AADs to help individuals manage their feelings and to help units achieve a higher state of psychological readiness. The presence of mental health personnel can be explained as an opportunity for the latter to learn what real combat involves so that they can be helpful to other combat soldiers in the future. By emphasizing the readiness component it is sometimes possible to convert the perception of emotional expression from the realm of unmanly and unmilitary "touchy-feely" to the realm of military competence. If after AARs, AADs, and EOTDs, it is clear to the unit leaders that there are still unresolved issues and bad feelings, those leaders can be encouraged to schedule a critical event debriefing (CED), to be led by mental health personnel trained in debriefing. While such debriefings are best conducted within days of the critical event, even weeks later may be better than not at all. The acceptability of CEDs, like that of the critical incident stress debriefing (CISD) which are now widespread among civilian police, fire, and other emergency response agencies, has improved as they have become common practice and proved their worth. If at all possible, the CED should be conducted while the unit is still in the theater, even if the mental health team needs to be flown in for it. Such activities are unlikely to be well received if they must compete with reunions with families at the home station.

Psychiatric Treatment

Though the emphasis so far has been on assisting the relatively stable members of units to avoid serious psychiatric distress by seeding primary groups with knowledge of how to conduct their own group therapy, there will be individuals and units that require concentrated support, or long-term support, or both from mental health professionals. The reasons are legion: particularly horrifying experiences, heavy casualties, inept leadership, poor precombat intragroup trust or communications, or preexisting psychiatric vulnerabilities. The reason does not matter. The goals are to restore the unit to a state of psychological readiness, and in the process to relieve psychic suffering. The methods are standard group therapy and individual therapy.

The critical issue is creating a climate of readiness to look to psychiatric staff for help. Sometimes the distress is masked by various forms of denial or acting out. The tasks of the psychiatrist are to alert commanders to be on the lookout for aberrant conduct in individuals or primary groups, and to develop in commanders a readiness to support psychiatric intervention. In many cases it may be advisable to seek the participation of all of the members of a squad if one of them is in particular distress. The individual may be the "designated sickie" for the squad, or he may simply be the one who was most affected. The task of the mental health worker will be facilitated, and probably shortened, if he can engage the squad in the recovery of one of its members.

SUMMARY AND CONCLUSIONS

The most common missions of the armed forces of the United States have been and are likely to continue to be rapid force projection operations of short duration. Because history indicates that the frequency of these operations is likely to increase, the Army Medical Service must anticipate repeated commitment of the same units and personnel to combat.

Generally speaking, combat veterans function more effectively and suffer fewer casualties than green personnel, so repetitive commitment is not fundamentally a problem. However, rapid deployment operations entail rapid transitions from peace to war and back to peace, and these transitions have been found to cause stress reactions that vary with the individual and with the nature of his experiences. It is the task of military mental health professionals to take the lead in managing the emotional aspects of short wars in ways that preserve and strengthen the psychological readiness of units so that they can perform with peak efficiency in the next encounter.

Successful reentry following force-projection operations has been the product of a partnership between commanders, chaplains, the unit medical staff, and mental health professionals. The psychiatrist and his staff are likely to understand the dynamics of reentry most clearly, but they are few in number and they do not always enjoy acceptance among military personnel. To gain acceptance, mental health professionals should endeavor to work with commanders, battalion surgeons/physician's assistants, and units before combat. Alliances with the chaplains and the battalion medical staff are effective ways to gain entry, and are essential if the mental health staff is to win the trust of the combatants. But some chaplains will perceive the mental health staff as competitors for the souls of the members of the unit, and some unit medical personnel will have negative attitudes toward psychiatry and all its works. If this cannot be overcome by positive education and commitment, the mental health staff may do better to devote its limited resources to other units and let word-of-mouth testimonials from those who have been helped by the mental health team's good work convince the suspicious.

To compensate for their small numbers, the members of the mental health staff can transfer some of their skills and understanding to chaplains, commanders, junior leaders, and unit medics. The best time to do this is before combat during training and practice deployments. Assisting commanders in developing mutual trust and confidence across ranks, in including emotional material in after-action reviews, and in restoring troubled soldiers to productivity can create a climate of readiness to confront mental health issues honestly and without fear. When such a climate exists in a unit, or in some of its subelements, many leaders and medical aidmen will be able to acquire quickly many of the supportive skills of mental health professionals.

A second way to make the most of limited resources is to dedicate all of the mental health staff to one unit for a restricted period of time—primarily to transfer skills to leaders, but secondarily to alleviate anguish among members of units that have been severely traumatized. This approach is feasible in peacetime, following a war in which only a portion of the units in a command were committed, or when committed units return on a staggered schedule.

The psychiatrist and the other mental health professionals can be most effective when they operate concurrently on three levels—staff, unit, and individual. On the staff level the psychiatrist supports senior commanders (flag and general officers) in policies that facilitate the management of reentry processes: (*a*) decompression leave, (*b*) cross-pollination of lessons learned, and (*c*) validation through awards, media coverage, and public information programs. Advocacy of constructive reentry policies is likely to entail conflict with other staff officers with equally compelling agendas. The psychiatrist must be prepared to demonstrate that his colleagues' objectives are more likely to be achieved if reentry is managed effectively.

On the unit level the mental health staff supports intermediate commanders (brigade, group, battalion, squadron, and ship) by advising them on how to develop trust and cohesion before commitment to combat, and helping them work constructively with postcombat reactions. These reactions are often contradictory: heightened anxiety in some, new levels of confidence in others; indifference to training, or total commitment to training; abuse of spouse and children, or decisions to marry and conceive; reluctance to ever be in combat again, or insatiable zest for combat. Different types of behavior are required of commanders, chaplains, junior leaders, and members of primary groups to ameliorate the dysphoric reactions and foster the positive reactions.

The mental health staff can be most effective in helping members of units sort out their postcombat emotions if they have helped the unit in peacetime to develop habits of open communications and readiness to deal with feelings during their AARs. After combat, the mental health staff can support commanders in keeping primary groups intact, validating combat behavior, conducting memorial services that promote rather than undermine cohesion, and organizing training that manifests respect for the combat achievements of the veterans.

On the individual level the psychiatrist and the mental health staff assist individuals and groups that have responded in dysfunctional ways to the experience of combat with individual therapy, group therapy, and unit therapy. Some of these interventions may be prolonged; others may lead to medical separation. Their objective is to restore the psychological readiness of the individual and the unit for combat. This does not mean brainwashing personnel to get them back into action at whatever cost to their mental health. It does, however, add some dimensions to classic psychotherapy. In the first place, the therapist has allies not usually present in a therapeutic setting—the service member's comrades and leaders. In most cases these people will have both a practical and an emotional interest in restoring the patient's effectiveness and balance. If they are not interested in him, it is unlikely that he will ever be able to function satisfactorily in the service, and discharge is indicated. Another dimension is that military life is a rough business. Each individual has his limit, and some reach it early. The psychiatrist does neither the individual nor the service any good if he returns to duty a service member who is likely to decompensate in the presence of further stress.

One final word about unit therapy. Whenever possible it is helpful to treat a soldier who is distressed in the context of his primary group. The methodology partakes of family therapy, and appropriately so; a small military unit functions emotionally as a family—and the unit medic is usually a member of that family. However therapeutic the goal of the intervention, the mental health practitioner must avoid the use of the term. Military personnel do not take kindly to being labeled sick—especially sick in the head. Euphemisms such as "debriefings" or "development workshops" might be seen through, but they are better than "group therapy." The approaches that have been most successful emphasized strengthening combat readiness and psychological preparation of the group for combat. Before battle, a soldier who describes himself, or who is defined before the group, as psychologically weak, will be extruded. His comrades would feel that they could not depend on him; they could not predict his behavior. After combat, manifestations of combat stress are accepted and the group will participate in "helping Joe." But the other members of the group will not accept being classified at the outset as having psychological problems—even when most of them do.

Mental health professionals have a decisive role to play in managing reentry in ways that preserve the emotional integrity of military units. Their success will be a function of their sensitivity to fighting men's fears of emotional vulnerability, and of their ability to help combat soldiers accept themselves and their vulnerabilities. It is a particularly challenging facet of mental health work; it is one that will pay immediate dividends in trust and intimacy within units, and in lives saved.

REFERENCES

1. Ardant du Picq CJJJ. *Battle Studies.* Greely JN, Cotton RC, trans. Harrisburg, Pa: Stackpole Books; 1958: 46–47.
2. 1 Samuel 17.
3. Fussell P. *Wartime.* New York: Oxford University Press; 1989: 116–126.
4. Volkan VD. *The Need to Have Enemies and Allies.* Northvale, NJ: Jason Aronson; 1988: 99–100.
5. Shalit B. *The Psychology of Conflict and Combat.* New York: Praeger; 1988: 83–85.
6. Boulding KE. *Conflict and Defense: A General Thesis.* New York: Harper & Bros; 1962: 162, 285–286.
7. Coser LA. *Continuities in the Study of Social Conflict.* New York: The Free Press; 1967: 42–43.
8. Terkel S. *The Good War.* New York: Pantheon Books; 1984: 117–118, 123–124, 127, 137–138.
9. Orwell G. *Nineteen Eighty-Four.* New York: Harcourt, Brace; 1949: 35–36, 189–200.
10. Atkinson R. *The Long Gray Line.* Boston: Houghton Mifflin; 1989: 324–330, 360–361, 526–527.
11. Van Devanter L. *Home Before Morning.* New York: Beaufort Books; 1983: 208–212.
12. Hendin H, Haas AP. *Wounds of War.* New York: Basic Books; 1984: 5–13, 240–241.
13. Amery LS, ed. *The Times History of the War in South Africa.* Vol 7. London, England: Sampson Low, Marston; 1909: 24–25.
14. O'Ballance E. *The Indo-China War: 1945–54, A Study in Guerrilla Warfare.* London, England: Faber & Faber; 1964: 249.
15. Blair C. *The Forgotten War.* New York: Times Books; 1987: ix.
16. O'Ballance E. *The Algerian Insurrection: 1954–1962.* Hamden, Conn: Archon Books; 1967: 201.
17. Westmoreland WC. *A Soldier Reports.* Garden City, NY: Doubleday; 1976: 299.

18. Kelly GA. *Lost Soldiers: The French Army and Empire in Crisis, 1947–1962.* Cambridge, Mass: The MIT Press; 1965: 54–55, 70–72, 206–232, 254–286.

19. Ambler JS. *The French Army in Politics, 1945–1962.* Columbus, Ohio: The Ohio State University Press; 1966: 208–260.

20. Weigley RF. *History of the United States Army.* Bloomington, Ind: Indiana University Press; 1984: 599–600.

21. Stouffer SA, Lumsdaine AA, Lumsdaine MH, et al. *The American Soldier. Vol 2: Combat and its Aftermath.* Princeton, NJ: Princeton Univ Press; 1949: 520–524.

22. Kennett L. *GI: The American Soldier in World War II.* New York: Warner Books; 1989: 224–225.

23. Faubus OE. *In This Faraway Land.* Conway, Ark: River Road Press; 1971: 654–660.

24. Rossetti LE. *APO 451.* New York: Carlton Press; 1969: 69.

25. United States. War Department. Report of the Secretary of War's Board on Officer-Enlisted Man Relationships. Washington, DC: War Department Bureau of Public Relations; May 1946.

26. Millett AR. *The General: Robert L. Bullard and Officership in the United States Army 1881–1925.* Westport, Conn: Greenwood Press; 1975: 206, 210, 222–223.

27. Hackworth DH. *About Face.* New York: Simon & Schuster; 1989: 286–288.

28. Cohen R, Gatti C. *In the Eye of the Storm.* New York: Farrar, Strauss & Giroux; 1991: 93.

29. MacDonough JR. *Platoon Leader.* New York: Bantam Books; 1985: 197.

30. Middlebrook M. *Operation Corporate: The Story of the Falklands War. 1982.* London, England: Viking; 1985: 382–384.

31. Vaux N. *Take That Hill! Royal Marines in the Falklands War.* Washington, DC: Pergamon-Brasseys; 1986.

32. Jolly R. *The Red and Green Life Machine.* London, England: Corgi Books; 1983.

33. Baynes J. *Morale: A Study of Men and Courage.* London, England: Cassell; 1967.

34. Dietz P. *The Last of the Regiments.* London, England: Brasseys; 1990: 118–119, 124–125.

35. Kirkland FR, Ender MG. Analysis of Interview Data from *Operation Just Cause.* Washington, DC: Working paper available from the Department of Military Psychiatry, Walter Reed Army Institute of Research; June 1991.

36. Lorenz K. *On Aggression.* New York: Harcourt Brace & World; 1963.

37. Eibl-Eibesfeldt I, Mosbacher E, trans. *The Biology of Peace and War.* New York: Viking Press; 1979: 68, 91–93, 102–104.

38. Fossey D. *Gorillas in the Mist.* Boston: Houghton Mifflin; 1983: 66–72, 218–221.

39. Goodall J. *The Chimpanzees of Gombe: Patterns of Behavior.* Cambridge, Mass: Harvard University Press; 1986: 503–534.

40. Nishida T, Hiraiwa-Hasegawa M, Hasegawa T, Takahata Y. Group extinction and female transfer in wild chimpanzees in the Mahale National Park, Tanzania. *Zeitschrift fur Tierpsychologie.* 1985;67:284–301.

41. Erikson EH. *Identity, Youth, and Crisis.* New York: Norton; 1968: 41–42.

42. Erikson EH. *Toys and Reasons: Stages in the Ritualization of Experience.* New York: Norton; 1977: 73.

43. Bernard VW, Ottenberg P, Redl F. Dehumanization: A composite psychological defense in relation to modern war. In: Schwebel M, ed. *Behavioral Science and Human Survival.* Palo Alto, Calif: Science and Behavior Books; 1965: 64–83.

44. Fenton N. A postwar study of a typical group of war neurosis cases in 1919–20 and 1924–25. In: Bailey P, Williams FE, Komora PO, Salmon TW, Fenton N, eds. In: *Neuropsychiatry.* Vol. 10. In: *The Medical Department of the United States Army in the World War.* Washington, DC: Office of The Surgeon General, US Department of the Army; 1929: 443–474.

45. Kirkland FR, Furukawa TP, Teitelbaum JM, Ingraham LH, Caine BT. Unit Manning System Field Evaluation, Technical Report 5 (ADA 207193). Washington, DC: Walter Reed Army Institute of Research; September 1987: 34–44.

46. Kirkland FR, Katz P. Combat readiness and the Army family. *Milit Rev.* 1989;69(4):69–70.

47. Bushard BL. The US Army's mental hygiene consultation service. *The Symposium on Preventive and Social Psychiatry.* Washington, DC: GPO; 1957: 431–443.

48. Jones FD, Stayer SJ, Wichlacz CR, Thomes LJ, Livingstone BL. Contingency management of hospital-diagnosed character and behavior disordered soldiers. *J Behav Ther Exp Psychiatry.* 1977;8:333.

49. Poirier JG, Jones FD. A group operant approach to drug dependence in the military that failed: Retrospect. *Milit Med.* 1977;141:366–369.

50. Wichlacz CR, Jones FD, Stayer SJ. Psychiatric predictions and recommendations: A longitudinal study of character and behavior disorders. *Milit Med.* 1972;137:54–58.

Chapter 13

BEHAVIORAL CONSEQUENCES OF TRAUMATIC BRAIN INJURY

EDWIN A. WEINSTEIN, M.D.*; ANDRES M. SALAZAR, M.D.†; AND FRANKLIN D. JONES, M.D., F.A.P.A. ‡

*Consultant in Neurology, National Naval Medical Center, Bethesda, Maryland; Consultant in Psychiatry, Walter Reed Army Medical Center, Washington, D.C.; Formerly Chief, Fifth Army Neuropsychiatric Center (World War II)

†Colonel, Medical Corps, U.S. Army; Professor of Neurology, Uniformed Services University of the Health Sciences, Bethesda, Maryland; Director, Defense and Veterans Head Injury Program

‡Colonel (ret), Medical Corps, U.S. Army; Clinical Professor, Uniformed Services University of the Health Sciences, Bethesda, Maryland; Past President and Secretary and current Honorary President of the Military Section, World Psychiatric Association; formerly Psychiatry and Neurology Consultant, Office of The Surgeon General, U.S. Army

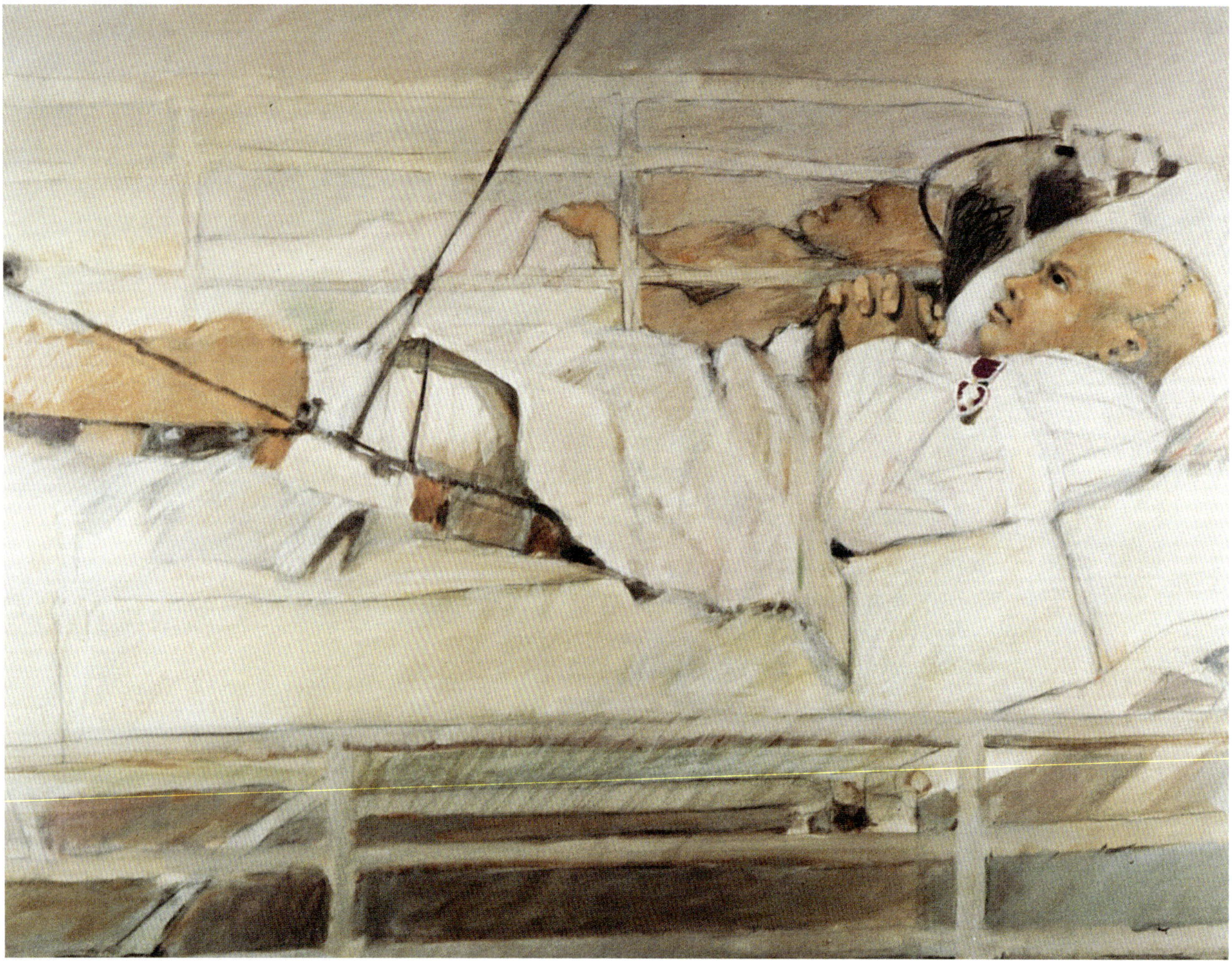

John O. Wehrle *Purple Heart* 1966

John O. Wehrle depicts a serviceman in Vietnam who has received his Purple Heart in a Surgical Intensive Care Unit. In combat settings, traumatic brain injury often occurs in conjunction with other injuries, as shown in this painting.

Art: Courtesy of US Center of Military History, Washington, DC.

INTRODUCTION

Traumatic brain injury (TBI) is the leading cause of death and disability in young adult Americans today.[1] The incidence of TBI requiring hospitalization is approximately 200/100,000/y; about 75,000 persons die and another 75,000 are permanently disabled each year. Similarly, in the Vietnam conflict, head and neck wounds accounted for 40% of all battlefield fatalities, and for about 11% of all surviving casualties. Yet, largely because it affects the young and can result in prolonged convalescence and a lifetime loss of earnings, the impact of TBI is greater than most other injuries. The total peacetime economic cost of TBI in the United States has been estimated at over $25 billion per year.

A number of underlying themes will be emphasized in the following discussion of TBI, particularly as a basis for understanding its neuropsychiatric consequences. First, it must be recognized that TBI represents a spectrum of disorders, with regard to mechanism of injury (penetrating vs closed-head injury), severity of injury, and pathology (see below). Secondly, TBI is a dynamic process. The acute evolution of secondary cellular injury and brain swelling in the first hours post-trauma offers a therapeutic window of opportunity that is the subject of intense study and rapid development in the field at present. Postacutely, the natural history of TBI is one of recovery, often to a remarkable degree in young adults. However, this recovery often represents compensation for functions lost, and its pace should not lull health care providers into ignoring the long-term behavioral deficits and maladaptations commonly seen in these patients. Third, "outcome" should be considered a summation of a variety of factors, including not only physical and cognitive recovery but behavioral and psychosocial reintegration as well. Fourth, preinjury status is a major determinant of final outcome after TBI; this has been reemphasized in a recent study showing that preinjury intelligence was the single most important determinant of cognitive performance in a large cohort of head-injured Vietnam veterans.[2] In this chapter, the current understanding of the pathogenesis of TBI will be briefly reviewed, with some comments on experimental treatment. The phenomenology and the cognitive, neurobehavioral, and psychosocial outcome of head injury will be discussed, as will be the behavioral and pharmacological aspects of therapy.

PATHOGENESIS

Closed-head Injury

Given that TBI results in a spectrum of pathologies, all of which can affect outcome, it is relevant to review the various components here. Over the past decades there has been movement from conceptualizing the pathology of closed-head injury (CHI) in terms of hematomas and "coup-contrecoup" contusions to a four-component classification.[3] Three parallel components were initially identified: (1) focal injury, (2) diffuse axonal injury (DAI), and (3) superimposed hypoxia or ischemia. More recently, (4) diffuse microvascular injury with loss of autoregulation has been implicated as playing an important role in the acute stage of moderate and severe head injury. All of these pathological features have been reproduced in animal models of angular acceleration without impact; and possibly except for diffuse axonal injury, all are also features of penetrating head injury (PHI).[4]

Focal Injury

Focal tissue disruption, swelling, contusions, or hematomas at the site of impact or penetration result in focal cortical neurologic deficits referable to that area (eg, aphasia, hemiparesis). By far the most common location for contusions after deceleration injury is in the orbitofrontal and anterior temporal lobes, where the brain lies next to bony edges. This is also an area rich in limbic connections governing mood, emotions, and memory. Thus, a relatively typical pathological picture is often seen in most closed-head injuries (CHIs). Among its most troubling clinical sequelae are attentional, memory, and behavioral abnormalities, which may be referable to the frontal and temporal lobe injury. Subdural hematomas are most common with rapid decelerations such as occur with impact after a fall, especially in the aged, and are usually due to rupture of bridging veins; they appear to be much less common after penetrating head injury. Delays longer than 4 hours in the surgical management of hematomas appear to worsen prognosis significantly. Delayed hematomas as well as bleeding into contusions are particularly important in the so-called "talk and die" patient, who may initially appear to be at low risk but then deteriorates unexpectedly.[5]

Diffuse Axonal Injury

Diffuse axonal injury (DAI) is one of the most important causes of prolonged coma and persistent severe neurological deficit in CHI. Originally described as a "shearing" injury of axons, it was characterized by axonal "retraction" balls microscopically in the hemispheric white matter, corpus callosum, and brain stem.[6,7] Recent work with mild to moderate fluid-percussion injury in animal models, however, shows that the typical light microscopic histopathology of DAI showing axonal shear may not emerge until 12 to 24 hours postinjury. The only early abnormality is a relatively subtle focal intraaxonal disruption seen on electron microscopy, with an intact axon sheath. This leads to a disturbance of axonal flow, accumulation of transport material with axonal ballooning proximal to the injury, and then eventual delayed severing of axons 12 to 24 hours later.[8,9] The role of alterations in calcium metabolism at the injured site on the axon may be particularly important. One obvious clinical implication of these findings is that *there may be a potential 12 to 24 hour window of therapeutic opportunity* postinjury during which future treatments may prevent total axonal disruption. Another important conclusion is that DAI can be demonstrated even after "minor" head injury, and occurs even in the absence of morphopathologic change in any other vascular, neural, or glial elements. This confirms earlier uncontrolled pathological studies in humans and makes such axonal damage a possible organic basis for the "postconcussion syndrome" and perhaps for the cumulative effects of repeated concussion, as seen in some boxers.[10]

Interestingly, a major feature of the pathology of *dementia pugilistica* is the presence of neurofibrillary tangles (NFT). NFT in Alzheimer's disease and in other conditions such as Guamanian amyotrophic lateral sclerosis, have been postulated to result from abnormalities in axonal flow, in the latter case probably related to aberrant calcium metabolism.[11] While classical Alzheimer plaques are not seen in this condition, recent studies show plaquelike structures that stain with monoclonal antibody to the beta amyloid precursor protein both chronically in boxers and acutely after severe head injury.[12–14] It is unknown whether repeated trauma might alter the secretion, metabolism, or structure of the amyloid precursor protein in such a way as to lead to plaque and NFT formation or whether the phenomenon of lipid peroxidation, which is discussed further in this chapter, may also play a role in this process.

Hypoxia-Ischemia

The classical pathology of hypoxia-ischemia, involving mainly the hippocampus and the vascular border zones of the brain, is frequently superimposed on the other pathological features that are more specific for TBI. The traumatized brain is particularly sensitive to hypoxia-ischemia.[15] When present, such pathology, including the concomitant hippocampal necrosis, can obviously become a major determinant of ultimate clinical outcome, particularly with regard to post-traumatic memory disorders. Recent improvements in the survival of the TBI patient have largely resulted from recognition of the importance of this component and its prevention, especially through the development of emergency resuscitation and transport systems.

Microvascular Change

Diffuse microvascular damage has also been recently implicated as a major component of both closed and penetrating TBI. Depending on the severity of the trauma, early physiological changes include an early loss of cerebrovascular autoregulation with a decreased response to changes in CO_2 and perfusion pressure, and an initial transient systemic hypertension (probably related to release of catecholamines).[16,17] The loss of autoregulation makes the brain particularly susceptible to fluctuations in systemic blood pressure. For example, systemic hypertension can increase the risk of vascular dilatation with hyperemia and brain swelling, or otherwise tolerable hypotension can result in ischemic damage. In addition, altered vascular sensitivity to circulating catecholamines or acetylcholine can lead to vasoconstriction and further focal ischemia or reperfusion injury ("no-reflow" phenomenon). Recent blood flow studies have confirmed a relative cerebral ischemia in a large proportion of TBI patients acutely.[18] Such changes may be susceptible to pharmacological interventions.

The pathology appears to be biphasic, with an early, transient alteration of the blood-brain barrier (BBB), and a more delayed (6 plus h) endothelial change.[19,20] Diffuse perivascular damage with astrocytic footplate swelling is a prominent feature at both the light and electron microscopic levels within minutes of high-velocity gunshot wounds as well as after acceleration injury in nonhuman primates. The basic cause of this swelling was initially thought to be a break in the endothelial BBB, but recent studies have demonstrated an increased pinocytotic transfer of horseradish peroxidase marker with intact endothelial tight junctions.[21] The astrocytic swelling is usually maximal at 30 to 60 minutes and is much reduced by 6 hours postinjury; it is thought to represent an initial reaction to the altered transport across the BBB. It should be emphasized, however, that the classic concept of BBB breakdown and cerebral edema post-TBI is undergoing radical revision, particularly in the absence of evidence for increased brain water after either uncomplicated PHI or CHI.[22] Cerebral edema, per se, may become more of a factor when hypoxia, ischemia, or both complicate the injury.

The second microvascular phase is one of endothelial change, including formation of intraluminal microvilli or blebs, which then break to form endothelial craters. This peaks at about 6 hours postinjury but usually persists as long as 6 days. Although the clinical significance of these changes is still not known, they are probably related to the altered microvascular sensitivity to circulating neurotransmitters, to the loss of autoregulation, and perhaps to secondary brain swelling. Recent studies have shown an associated loss or inhibition of various endothelial hormones including endothelium-derived relaxing factor (EDRF).

EDRF was first described almost a decade ago and has recently been identified as nitric oxide.[23] Inhibition of EDRF may be responsible for prolonged vasoconstriction and perhaps the so-called "no reflow" phenomenon leading to secondary focal ischemia, while loss of other factors may have the opposite effect. One of the principal inhibitors of EDRF in TBI appears to be the superoxide radical, which has also been shown to have a vasoconstrictive effect in experimental models.[24,25]

Application of free radical generators (such as xanthine-xanthine oxidase) to the intact pial surface of nontraumatized animals reproduces very similar changes to those seen after TBI.[26,27] Superoxide dismutase will prevent or reverse this vascular hyperactivity experimentally, suggesting that the vasoconstrictive effect is mediated through the superoxide radical itself.

Secondary Tissue Injury

The picture of a TBI patient who is initially relatively stable and awake or in light coma and then deteriorates and dies is all too common. While some of these cases represent delayed hematoma amenable to surgery, most are probably related to an uncontrolled brain swelling that does not respond to conventional management. Over the past decade, delayed secondary injury at the cellular level has come to be recognized as a major contributor to this phenomenon and to the ultimate tissue loss after TBI.

Understanding of the pathogenesis of secondary injury is thus particularly important to the present-day management of the head-injured patient. As suggested above, a cascade of biochemical and physiological events is set in motion in injured tissue. This includes changes in arachidonic acid metabolites such as the prostaglandins and the leukotrienes,[28] the formation of oxygen free radicals,[16] changes in neuropeptides,[29] electrolytes such as calcium and magnesium,[30] neurotransmitters such as glutamate or acetylcholine,[31,32] lactic acid,[33] various kinins, and a leukocyte response with release of lymphokines such as interleukin-1.[34]

These products can result in progressive secondary injury to otherwise viable brain tissue through a number of mechanisms: (*a*) by altering vascular reactivity and producing further ischemia, (*b*) by producing brain swelling (hyperemia, edema, or both), (*c*) by injuring neurons and glia directly or activating macrophages that result in such injury, or (*d*) by establishing conditions favorable to secondary infection. In other words, much of the ultimate brain loss after PHI may be due not to the injury itself, but to an uncontrolled vicious cycle of biochemical events set in motion by the trauma.

Oxygen Free Radicals and Lipid Peroxidation

Perhaps the most important path of cellular injury in TBI involves oxygen free radicals. These are produced early in ischemic and traumatic tissue injury, both in the central nervous system and elsewhere.[16,35,36] The superoxide radical ($O_2^-\bullet$) is formed through a variety of mechanisms, including normal mitochondrial respiration, the xanthine oxidase and arachidonic acid pathways, or by activated leukocytes. The phenomenon of receptor-mediated phospholipase activation may play an important role in the initial release of arachidonic acid after both trauma and ischemia.

The superoxide radical results in tissue injury in its own right through its effect on the microvasculature. However, when combined with its own metabolite, hydrogen peroxide, in the presence of free iron, it forms the hydroxyl radical (OH•). This reacts with the abundant lipids in the brain in the process of lipid peroxidation, with further release of arachidonic acid and a vicious cycle in which more free radicals are produced through the cyclooxygenase pathway (along with prostaglandins), overwhelming natural free radical scavenging mechanisms. There is a marked rise in lipid peroxidation markers as early as 2 hours postinjury, and lasting at least 5 days in severely head-injured patients. This confirms the ongoing nature of delayed secondary cellular injury in the postacute period, as well as the possibility that the postinjury therapeutic window of opportunity may be considerably longer than has been thought until now.[37]

Pharmacological intervention to reduce the formation of free radicals, or to scavenge those already formed, or both would thus be expected to reduce ultimate tissue injury. Animal models have confirmed this potential benefit in several systems. Because free radicals are formed through a number of biochemical pathways, a variety of drugs or drug combinations may be useful to control them. These include the use of steroids to inhibit lipid peroxidation and the release of arachidonate (megadose methylprednisolone and especially the nonglucocorticoid 21-aminosteroids or "lazaroids");[38] α-tocopherol (Vitamin E) and its analogues;[39,40] cyclooxygenase inhibitors to block prostaglandin formation; xanthine oxidase inhibitors such as allopurinol;[41,42] iron chelators such as desferrioxamine;[43] enzymes such as superoxide dismutase and catalase;[27,44] and various other free radical scavengers such as mannitol and dimethyl sulfoxide.

Superoxide dismutase (SOD) may be particularly attractive as therapy because it scavenges all superoxide radicals regardless of their source. In a particularly relevant model using intracranial balloons in dogs to mimic subdural hematoma, SOD in doses equivalent to those being used in current clinical pilot trials practically eliminated BBB breakdown and postdecompression pathological change when compared to conventional therapies, and decreased mortality from 80% to 0%.[44] Clinical pilot studies have shown a 50% decrease in mortality in severely head-injured patients treated with SOD, but final conclusions must await a larger controlled study.[45]

Penetrating Brain Injury

The majority of casualties with penetrating head wounds who survive long enough to reach the hospital level have been injured by fragments from explosive munitions.[46] Penetrating wounds, as noted, share a number of the features of moderate and severe closed-head injuries. These include the frequent involvement of more than one lobe; contusions, hematomas, and hemorrhages, some distant from the point of penetration; edema; hypoxia, ischemia, or both; and diffuse microvascular injury with loss of auto-regulation. There are, however, some important clinical differences.

Whereas the soldier with a moderate or severe acceleration/deceleration closed-head injury is by definition unconscious, and the severity of the injury can be graded by the Glasgow Coma Scale, a slight majority of the men who suffered a penetrating head injury in Vietnam did not lose consciousness, or did so only briefly. Of 342 subjects in the Vietnam Head Injuries Study, 53% had no or only momentary unconsciousness, and only 15% had prolonged unconsciousness.[47] While retrograde and anterograde amnesia are almost invariably present in moderate and severe closed-head injury, 121 of the 342 patients in the Vietnam study reported having had no amnesia. Penetrating head injuries have a much higher incidence of seizures with figures up to 50%. The rate in closed-head injuries in which the dura mater has not been pierced runs from 2% to 11% depending on the complications.

The neurological deficits following penetrating brain injuries are more focal and variable, depending, as most do, on the particular cortical area involved. The deficits include aphasia, hemiplegia, and hemiparesis; cortical sensory disturbances; visual field defects; and impairments in visuospatial processing. Closed-head injury patients with damage to frontal and temporal limbic structures are more apt to manifest long periods of disturbed consciousness and impairments of memory, attention, personality, perception of reality, and social behavior. These differences are not absolute. Patients with closed-head injuries may have focal signs depending on the point of impact, and penetrating injuries of the basilar and other deep structures can result in prolonged unconsciousness and memory loss.[47]

POST-TRAUMATIC STRESS DISORDER

The potential interaction between traumatic brain injury and post-traumatic stress disorder (PTSD) remains unclear. The second author has had the opportunity to address this issue in a large cohort of head-injured Vietnam veterans and a group of uninjured Vietnam combat veteran controls participating in the Vietnam Head Injury Study.[48] The data indicate that 15% of head injured and 8% of controls fit the criteria previously established for post-traumatic stress disorder in non-brain-injured subjects on the Minnesota Multiphasic Personality Inventory.[49] Neither total brain volume loss, nor lesion location, nor post-injury cognitive change showed a relationship with PTSD scores.

Head-injured PTSD subjects reported relatively decreased psychological support from community and government upon their return from the Vietnam theater, whereas control PTSD subjects complained more often of a general negative impact of the war on their lives. As expected, PTSD correlated with other measures of psychopathology, especially depression, in both controls and head-injured men. The findings suggest that while many factors may contribute to the development of PTSD, the brain injury itself may play a less important role than other psychological variables. Treatment of PTSD is addressed in Chapter 16, Chronic Post-Traumatic Stress Disorders.

MILD HEAD INJURY

Mild head injury (concussion) has been defined as an acceleration/deceleration closed-head injury, almost always associated with a period of amnesia, usually with a momentary interruption of, or brief change in, consciousness, and followed by a characteristic group of symptoms, including headache, dizziness, poor memory and concentration, fatigue, and irritability.[50] The injuries are incurred mainly as the result of motor vehicle injuries, assaults and falls.

The term concussion has been largely replaced by the designation mild or minor head injury because over the past 20 years it has been shown that such injuries may be associated with neuroanatomical and neurophysiological abnormalities, and with deficits in neuropsychological tests. Concussion, on the other hand, had been thought to involve a shaking up of the contents of the skull without any structural lesions. Animal models of concussion, however, have shown diffuse axonal damage, and magnetic resonance imaging (MRI) as well as positron emission tomography (PET) and power-spectral electroencephalogram (EEG) have repeatedly demonstrated structural, metabolic, and functional changes in humans with mild head injury.

Neuropsychological tests have shown impairment in sustained attention, delayed memory, and impaired ability to process multiple items of information simultaneously.[51,52] Such deficits usually clear over a 3-month period in patients without a history of previous head injury or drug abuse.[53]

These and other data indicate that the post-concussion syndrome cannot be explained solely on a psychological basis, as the result of emotional trauma, and a desire for legal compensation. The symptoms appear in the great majority of patients who have sustained mild head injuries. They occur frequently following sports-related injuries, in which case the motivation to return to athletic competition is high.[54] The symptoms of patients seeking legal redress may clear before settlement[55] and a lump sum award does not necessarily cure the condition.[56]

There are a number of reasons, however, why the symptoms cannot be accounted for on a traditional lesion deficit model, and why psychological and social factors are relevant. The severity of the brain injury as measured by the duration of the period of unconsciousness and the length of the post-traumatic amnesia does not correlate with the number and intensity of such symptoms as headaches, difficulty in concentration, irritability, noise sensitivity, and fatigue.[57] Even though test scores return to normal, and MRI abnormalities (if they have been present) clear, symptoms may persist.

The early symptoms that appear immediately or shortly after the injury, such as headache, dizziness, drowsiness, nausea, and blurred vision are thought to be a direct result of the brain injury. Later manifestations that come on a few weeks after injury include difficulties in memory (aside from the retrograde amnesia [RA] of which patients seldom complain) and concentration, fatigue, insomnia, irritability, noise sensitivity, and depression that can be regarded as responses to the stresses of the patient's cognitive and attentional deficits, and their anticipated consequences.

The persistence of headaches and dizziness or vertigo in the absence of signs of vestibular dysfunction indicates an association with anxiety or depression.

Despite the trauma, the patient is in some respects under less stress in the period immediately following the accident. He is likely to have been relieved that his injury was not serious, and to have been assured that he will recover completely. There is more stress when he returns to work and finds that his mental capabilities are reduced. The increased effort required causes fatigue, and he may become anxious and depressed. He may face the skepticism and disapproval of those who believe that he should have recovered from an apparently minor injury. These features are highly relevant to treatment.

The overall aim of treatment is the prevention of a secondary traumatic neurosis. If there is evidence of brain damage, the patient should be so informed. There is nothing more frustrating for the conscientious, intelligent patient than to be told that there is "nothing wrong" with him, a statement that suggests that he is malingering or not trying. Fatigue is the most troubling symptom interfering with return to work. The relationship of fatigue to diminished mental capacity and stress should be discussed with the patient and his supervisors. To control the situation, a graded work schedule should be instituted so that the patient can work within the limits imposed by his fatigue. Periodic neuropsychological testing may help to monitor progress.[58] A graded return to full workload over a period of 4 to 8 weeks is suggested.

MODERATE AND SEVERE HEAD INJURY

The severity of a head injury is evaluated by the findings on computed tomography (CT) and MRI scans, the depth of coma, the duration of the loss of consciousness, and the length of the anterograde amnesia (AA). Degrees of severity are differentiated as follows:

- Moderate and severe TBI lesions include contusions, hemorrhages, and hematomas, which are rare in mild head injury.
- Mild head injuries have scores of 13 to 15 on the Glasgow Coma Scale on which verbal, ocular, and motor responses are graded, while moderate head injuries score between 9 and 13, and severe head injuries place below 9.
- The loss of consciousness in moderate and severe TBIs is measured in hours and days, rather than in seconds and minutes as in mild head injuries.
- The AA in mild head injury is usually a matter of seconds or minutes, whereas in moderate and severe brain injuries there is an AA of days and weeks. Severe head injuries have an AA of 7 days or more. Whereas mild head injuries may have a momentary RA or none at all, more severe head injuries may have an RA of days, weeks, or months.

Patients recovering from more severe brain injuries with loss of consciousness usually go through several variable stages:

- A period of coma.
- A period of agitation, restlessness, overreaction to stimuli, combativeness, and rambling incoherent speech. Hallucinations may be present. This stage varies widely in incidence and intensity. It may not appear at all or may last up to several weeks.[59]
- A stage in which behavior is organized rather than random, and the patient is responsive to questions. There may be features of both the amnestic confabulatory state and the syndromes of denial, with anterograde and retrograde amnesia, confabulation, environmental and temporal disorientation, reduplicative misidentifications and delusions, and mood changes. Components vary in duration but may last for weeks and months and the patient later may be amnesic for much of the period. While there are deficits in memory and other forms of cognition, and in attention and perception, the behavior also has positive, symbolic, and adaptive aspects.

Post-Traumatic Amnesia

Anterograde amnesia (AA) is the period of time following the traumatic event or interruption of consciousness during which the patient is unable to retain new information and for which he later has no recall. Retrograde amnesia (RA) is the span of time prior to the injury that the patient does not recall. While post-traumatic amnesia (PTA) usually has anterograde and retrograde components, these may be dissociated and may have different mechanisms.[60,61] The length of the AA is a good indication of the severity of the brain injury but the extent of the RA is much more variable. A study of a group of soldiers with severe head injuries admitted to Walter Reed Army Medical Center showed that while some patients had extensive RA reaching back for years with no recollection of having served in the U.S. Army, others with comparable injuries had RA of days or weeks.[62] It is important to note that the events took place at a time when the patient's brain was functioning normally, while those of the AA occurred while he still had not attained full consciousness. The duration of the AA roughly corresponds to the period of time over which the patient was unconscious, confused, or disoriented. When interviewed later, patients are apt to estimate the length of the AA in terms of when they "woke up."

It may be difficult to precisely determine the duration of an RA from the patient's verbal report. For example, a patient may state that he remembers nothing since embarking on a trip days or weeks prior to his injury. On further questioning it turns out that he does not know the destination or purpose of the trip, even though it had long been planned. Some patients have a temporal gradient in accordance with Ribot's law, which states that memories more remote in time are spared. There are, however, many patients who do not show a temporal gradient.[61,63]

AA and RA differ in respects other than their temporal relationship to the traumatic event. Patients are likely to be unaware of an RA but may complain about their inability to retain information. The time span of the AA tends to remain fixed in terms of later recall, while the RA, on the other hand, shrinks in the course of clinical recovery so that eventually it covers only the seconds, minutes, or hours immediately preceding the traumatic event or loss of consciousness. While the moments preceding the loss of consciousness are irretrievable, earlier events may sometimes be recovered under hypnosis.[64] Interestingly, functional amnesias and fugue states not associated with brain damage are wholly retrograde.

RA involves more than memory loss per se in that it may be associated with feelings of unreality. Patients may not believe that they were actually in an accident, despite having been told about it many times, and despite the evidence of a cast on a leg or side rails on the bed. Some patients demand to see a photograph of the wrecked car, and even then may claim it is a different car. A soldier wounded in combat in Korea refused a Purple Heart, stating that if he had been wounded he would know it. Even after patients acknowledge that they have been injured, they may preface their answers to questions of what happened with "I don't know," "I don't remember," and "They say that..." There may be *jamais vu* experiences. A soldier returning home on leave said that he felt he had never been there before. Another complained that the old songs he knew were not familiar anymore.

Amnesic patients may have implicit knowledge of events that they cannot consciously recall. Performance may improve with successive trials on tasks that the patient may not recall having done previously. Soldiers who could not remember having been in the service retained knowledge of military protocol, and men who could not remember having been married could still recognize their wives. In one such case the patient commented that he knew his wife from their courtship days.

Amnesia can have positive as well as negative aspects in that the patient's last memory prior to "waking up" or "coming to himself" in the hospital may be a symbolic representation of current experiences and problems. Thus, the last memory of a patient with severe visual loss was of getting a new lens for his camera a few months before his injury. Such last memories may be veridical, actual events displaced in space and time, or confabulations. As new problems develop in the course of recovery, so may new last memories appear. A characteristic "last memory" occurs in patients who have been in an accident that resulted in fatalities. This has to do with sleep or other loss of consciousness; going to bed the night before, napping in the back seat of the car, or passing out at drill a few days previously. Over the period in which such memories are recalled, the patient usually expresses no conscious awareness that someone has been killed.[65]

Anosognosia

Anosognosia—literally lack of knowledge of disease—is closely related to amnesia as patients deny that they were injured or were in an accident. They may also disclaim such disabilities as hemiplegia, blindness, paraplegia, loss of a limb, facial disfigurement, and a craniotomy or tracheostomy. Patients may flatly deny that they are disabled in any way, or minimize impairment by attributing a paretic limb to a sprained ankle or "laziness." Some acknowledge the disability but regard it as outside of the self, referring to it as an animate or inanimate object or in the third syntactical person as "he," "she," or "it." They may claim that the accident happened to another person and do not get upset when their erroneous statements are challenged. Some claim that their disability was caused by rough handling by the hospital staff.[66] Many anosognosic patients, like amnesics, may appear quite normal on casual examination. Denial may also be expressed in the form of joking and punning and caricaturing disabilities.

As in amnesia, patients may indicate implicit knowledge of their problems and traumatic experiences, as in the case of a woman who denied that she had had a craniotomy but who complained of the "sawing and hammering" on her head. Selectiveness is another indication of awareness at a less-than-conscious level. Patients are not delusional or confabulatory about a part of the body that is not disabled in some fashion. Denial of physical disabilities usually clears within weeks, but denial of memory loss and other cognitive impairments may endure for months and years.

Laterality plays little role in the amnestic confabulatory state, which appears most prominently after bilateral orbitofrontal, anterior temporal, paralimbic, and diencephalic damage. Anosognosia occurs more frequently after right hemisphere lesions than after those of the left hemisphere. Such pathology is usually extensive and involves more than one lobe. In anosognosia for hemiplegia there is usually both frontal and parietal lobe damage. Patients with left hemisphere pathology may deny their aphasia, which is usually of a fluent type, often with jargon. Denial of memory loss is a feature of frontal and diencephalic amnesias in which the brain damage is bilateral.

Confabulation

Confabulations are defined as fictitious narratives without intent to deceive, or distorted versions of actual events. Some are spontaneous, fantastic, and unrelated to the person's experience, but most confabulations after brain injury are elicited in response to questions about the patient's disability and reason for coming to the hospital. A study of 100 moderately and severely head-injured patients seen at Walter Reed Army Medical Center found that 60 confabulated at some time during their hospital stay.[67] Initially confabulations tend to be brief, multiple, contradictory, and transient, but, after the stage of agitation, a patient may maintain a confabulation for weeks and months. Some, particularly early ones, are confabulations of exigency, as in the instance of a patient with his arms restrained who claimed that he had been shot in the hands. Others are amplifications of denial, as in the case of the man who explained his hemiparesis by stating he had sprained his ankle in a football game. Other confabulations are not associated with explicit denial, but are dramatizations, or allegorical or metaphorical representations of the patient's problems and disabilities. Although ostensibly referring to *past* events, they may symbolize the patient's *current* situation. The following is illustrative.

Case Study 1: Confabulation Following TBI

A 42-year-old field-grade supply officer sustained a head injury in Korea when his jeep overturned. He was left with slight weakness of his right upper extremity, and mild dysphasia, dyslexia, and dysgraphia. He was seen at Walter Reed Army Medical Center 4 months after his accident. When asked what had happened to him, he gave the following story, to be repeated on many occasions:

> I had a big job overseas. I was an intelligence officer for the Air Force. The man I replaced was a captain and his assistant a first lieutenant so that the two of them were working with me. I was sent to check on their security. They were just as Commie as if painted with a red brush. I had to write out everything I found so that it could be read in court in a court-martial for these men some day. I wrote it out and turned it into headquarters. I had enough written so that any jury in the right senses would give these guys 40 years in jail right away; they were just that Commie....[68(pp386–387)]

Comment: The repeated reference to reading, writing, and right senses and to intelligence indicate the patient's knowledge of his impairments, not otherwise expressed. The case also helps explain why patients may include apparently circumstantial and irrelevant details in their narratives and repeat them in each telling.

A new confabulation or a change in the content of an old one may indicate a new stressful experience. In the case just described, the patient was refused permission to visit his wife. He appeared angry but said nothing, but the next day he included a detail about threatening to shoot a man for giving food to Communists.

The content of confabulations is determined by several factors. One is the nature of the stress or disability. A second involves popular topics in the news such as Communism and space travel. A third factor concerns those themes that in the patient's past experience have been significant elements in patterns of social relatedness and important sources of identity. The Walter Reed study[67] showed that more than one half of the confabulators referred to family members, real or fictitious. They stated that a brother, child, or parent had been in the accident, often sustaining an injury identical with the patient's own. Confabulations about work and occupation were less frequent but were longer and more elaborate. Paratroopers injured in car accidents or fights were apt to confabulate that they had been hurt jumping and the inclusion of expressions like "had a Mae West" lent verisimilitude to the story. Confabulations about sports and minor illnesses were usually associated with denial of disability. Confabulations about great violence and death were associated with more disturbed behavior and somatic symptomatology.

As in amnesia and denial, patients may show implicit knowledge of the disability or traumatic event. This may appear in the content of the confabulation, as in the case of a soldier with a tracheostomy who confabulated that he had been a vocalist in a 17-piece band.[68]

In the course of clinical recovery, the content of an erstwhile confabulation may be represented in other forms of disturbed behavior. Following a head injury sustained in a car accident, a soldier confabulated about a girl passenger whom he said he had saved from injury by shielding her head at the moment of the impact. He was left with a left homonymous hemianopia, and on his first leave home, became extremely worried that a neighbor's child would go blind. He then became engaged to a 15-year-old retarded girl in the hope that U.S. Army doctors could operate and cure her.[67]

Environmental Disorientation

Disorientation for place or environmental disorientation takes on different forms depending on the stage of recovery. During the period of agitation, responses are random; the patient places himself at work, in combat, in a bar. As his behavior improves, disorientation may appear in successive patterns of misnaming, mislocation, condensation of time and distance, and the confabulated journey.[69,70] Patients usually say that they are in a hospital but they give it the name of another hospital, real or fictitious, or use euphemisms like "place for R and R," "repair shop," "retreat." In misnaming, the patient most often selects a hospital situated at his training base or in his home town. The patient may then name the hospital correctly but mislocate it in places associated with work or home. Or, a soldier may go on to name and locate the hospital accurately, but greatly condense the distance or travel time between the hospital and his home or base. After a patient appears to have established complete orientation, he may offer a confabulated journey as in the case of a soldier who stated that he had flown to Florida that morning.

Patients maintain their disorientation despite cues, clues, and corrections. Even with the name of the hospital in full view on bed linen, staff name tags, and desk plaques, and, despite having been told, patients refuse to accept the proper designation. The following case is illustrative.

Case Study 2: Environmental Disorientation Following TBI

A 21-year-old soldier was admitted to Walter Reed Army Medical Center after having sustained a head injury and a traumatic amputation of his left arm in an automobile accident. His home was in Massachusetts and he had been traveling to Washington from his station in Georgia. He denied that he had lost an arm and stated that he was in "Coolidge Memorial Hospital," which he located in Georgia. (It was later learned that the name was a condensation of Cooley-Dickerson Hospital and the Coolidge Memorial Bridge near his home.) Over the next 2 months, he successively located "Coolidge Memorial" in North Carolina, Virginia, and Washington. Then it became "Walter Reed Memorial Hospital." He gave up the disorientation with apparent reluctance, "they say it's Walter Reed or something," "it's supposed to be Walter Reed." At the same time he admitted the loss of his arm. Throughout the remainder of his 5-month hospital stay he was oriented, but expressed a "feeling that there must be a Coolidge Memorial Hospital somewhere."[66(pp46–47)]

Comment: Enduring environmental disorientation is not explicable in terms of confusion or overall memory loss, but has positive motivational aspects. Here the patient clung to his delusion in an apparent effort to maintain identity.

Temporal Disorientation

Disorientation for date and time of day are associated with environmental disorientation and RA. Patients displace backward in time and the greatest displacements occur in patients with amnesia of long duration.[71] In disorientation for time of day, the patient confuses morning and afternoon, and AM and PM. He appears to gauge the time in terms of his personal experiences and activities. No matter at what time of day he was examined, one man usually said it was 3 PM because that was when his wife visited. Disorientation for time is particularly striking after a patient has been sleeping or dozing. A man served with supper after awakening from an afternoon nap was indignant over having been given "spaghetti for breakfast." Such temporal disorientation occurs even with a large wall clock in full view, and when the patient is permitted to look at his watch. Nevertheless, such patients may be quite capable of drawing a clock and putting the hands at a designated time. Similarly, in disorientation for date, a patient may persist in his misdesignation even after being told or shown the correct date. Disorientation for person will be considered under the reduplicative disorders.

Reduplication

Reduplicative delusions and misidentifications occur in a number of modalities; those of place and person, time and event, objects, parts of the body, and the self. One form is usually associated with another. Like anosognosia and environmental disorientation, right hemisphere lesions are more common than those on the left even though both sides of the brain are usually involved.

Environmental reduplication or reduplication of place is the belief that there are two or more places of the same name although only one actually exists. The first case, in a woman with senile dementia, was described by Arnold Pick in 1903 under the designation, reduplicative paramnesia.[72] Henry Head[73] reported the case of a British soldier in World War I who, after sustaining a frontal missile wound, thought that there were two towns of Boulogne in France—one that he traversed on his way to the front, and the other through which he passed on his way home to England on leave. Head remarked that the man appeared rational in all other respects except that he wrote letters to his mother even though he knew that she had been dead for years.

Reduplication of person is the belief that a person has more than one identity. A soldier may believe that a corpsman is also a cook in his unit. In the syndrome of Capgras, which is not infrequent after head injuries,[74–77] the patient believes that a familiar person, usually a close relative, is an impostor. Another form of personal reduplication is the belief that one has an "extra" child.

Temporal reduplication is the belief that a current event has also occurred in the past, an enduring déjà vu experience. Patients hospitalized for a car accident state that they have been in several recent automobile accidents, or that they have previously been treated at the hospital for the same condition. It may be difficult to separate temporal from personal reduplication, as in an instance in which a patient claimed that a nurse was a high school classmate.

Patients may reduplicate both inanimate and animate objects, as in claims that personal possessions and domestic pets have been replaced by facsimiles. In reduplication of parts of the body, a patient believes that he has more than two arms, two legs, or one head. Reduplication of the self involves the belief that one's self is elsewhere or that one has a double.

The incidence of reduplicative phenomena in head injury varies with the method of study. Patients may not offer their beliefs unless specifically asked, and some do not volunteer them because they recognize their unusual nature. In the Walter Reed study[67] reduplication was found in 85% of patients, excluding those who were markedly aphasic or severely withdrawn. Reduplication is commonly associated with retrograde amnesia, confabulation, denial, and environmental and temporal disorientation, or it may first be noted after these conditions have improved or cleared. In one case a patient originally mislocated Walter Reed in Texas, his home state, then claimed that there were two Walter Reed hospitals, one in Texas, and one in Washington. Feelings of unreality and depersonalization often precede and are associated with reduplication. As noted, patients may not believe that they were really injured, or that people are who they say they are. In some instances, reduplication does not appear until weeks, months, and even years after the injury.

The two or more places, persons, events, objects, and parts of the body, although alike in many respects, are not identical. They differ in some way germane to the patient's experiences, feelings, and problems. For example, a patient admitted for multiple injuries thought that there were three Walter Reed Hospitals, one for head injuries, one for fractures, and one for plastic surgery. Aggrieved patients may believe that the nurses in the "other" hospital were kinder and more considerate. A patient with a draining suboccipital craniotomy wound complained of "bad drainage" from one of his heads, but claimed that his "other" heads were functioning well.[66] Alexander, Stuss, and Benson[75] studied a man who for several years after his head injury claimed that his family had been replaced by another almost identical one. The only difference was that the children of the "first" family were about a year younger than those of the "second" family. This difference appears to correspond with the period over which the patient estimated he had been disabled. The authors noted that the patient recognized the implausibility of his story while maintaining its correctness. He behaved in his usual manner toward his wife, showing neither anger nor distress at her putative desertion. With the breakdown in the unities of time and space, the "extra" person becomes a condensed symbolic representation, a reification or personification of the patient's own experience.

The delayed onset of reduplication and its relationship to depersonalization and derealization is well shown in a case reported by Staton, Brumback, and Wilson.[76] The patient had had a car accident at the age of 23 followed by a week of coma. He made what was apparently a good immediate recovery but several months later had episodes of irritability and complaints of memory difficulties. In the first few months after his accident he experienced feelings of unreality but did not report them until 4 years later. At that time he expressed the conviction that all of his current experiences had happened before. When examined by Staton et al 8 years after his accident, he described living in a world of fantasy in which his relatives were not the people he had known but were slightly different "look-alikes" or "doubles." The family farm was a false duplication because recent buildings looked like they should not have been built. Even his cat was not real because of a scar on its ear. He denied that he could be his real self because he was missing a tooth and wasn't working. He believed that the entire 8-year period of disability and unreality lived since the accident had occurred at some time in the past and resulted in complete recovery.

Reduplication and accompanying phenomena are adaptive in that patients expressing them are often less agitated and disturbed than they had been previously. Reduplication and confabulation combat feelings of unreality and nothingness, and the reification of an experience in terms of a place, person, or event may make it more "real" in the sense that metaphor may make reality more vivid. The validity of the denial and other symbolic representations of the patient's problem is reinforced by the way the content of the delusion identifies him with such significant values as home, family, work, health, and survival. Moreover, the delusion brings certainty, order, and unity to what would otherwise be masses of disparate, confusing, and contradictory data.

Mood Disorders

In general, the most conspicuous mood changes occur in patients in whom there is a relative paucity of verbal adaptive mechanisms. Patients with explicit denial tend to be bland and unconcerned, sometimes euphoric and witty. Those with partial denial might admit problems but attribute them to the inefficiency or malice of the staff. Patients without denial may be withdrawn and depressed, making references to being in a prison camp or cemetery, and such behavior may be punctuated by episodes of agitation. Others are hypomanic and ludic—a term introduced by Jean Piaget to describe the play and imitative aspects of the behavior of young children. These patients clown and joke, and caricature their disabilities. In their melodramatic presentations comic and tragic aspects are intermingled.[78] Altered sexual behavior is not uncommon, with lewd remarks, verbal and physical advances to staff, and confabulations of sexual activity. Aggressive and violent behavior may appear, often as a withdrawal manifestation, analogous to alcohol withdrawal, in patients who recover full consciousness rapidly and must face a new environment without going through a stage of denial and other adaptive coping mechanisms. As in anosognosia and reduplications, lesions are more likely to involve the right than the left hemisphere.

NEUROPSYCHOLOGICAL ASSESSMENT

Neuropsychological testing covers the areas of attention, memory, language, calculation, constructional and visuospatial skills, praxis, abstraction, and executive functions. It should be borne in mind that these categories are, in some degree, abstractions in the mind of the examiner rather than models of the organization of the brain. A single test may tap a number of functions. Clock drawing with the placing of the hands to a designated time, for example, requires attention, visuospatial, and constructional skills, and the ability to recognize that a 5 in one context means 25 minutes after the hour, and that in another it indicates the hour itself.

Formal neuropsychological testing is not performed during the first few weeks postinjury, because of impairments in attention, concentration, and inhibition, and because changes in the perception of reality do not lend themselves readily to tests for neural deficits. There are, however, a number of measures that can be used with the disoriented patient. The Galveston Orientation and Amnesia Test (GOAT) documents the disorientation, and estimates the duration and severity of the

PTA.[79] Patients are asked for the last event they remember before the injury, and for the first thing they can remember after it. Other tests that make minimal demands on the patient are tasks of reaction time, object naming, verbal fluency, and letter cancellation. The patient's ability to spell the word WORLD forward and backward and state how many nickels there are in a dollar and how many dollars there are in 60 nickels is a valuable index of cortical function. These measures can aid the investigator in establishing the recovery slope and determining when more extensive neuropsychological testing can be accomplished.

Attention

Two types of attention are recognized. A tonic form refers to the level of vigilance regulating overall information processing capacity. The second is a vector function, which regulates the direction and target of attention in any one behaviorally relevant area or space. Tonic attention is related to the activity of the reticular activating system. Directed, selective attention is associated more with neocortical activity. Marked disturbances of tonic attention are found in the acute confusional states in which the patient is highly distractible and cannot maintain vigilance, is unable to pursue coherent thought, and is unable to carry out a sequence of goal-directed movements. Impairment of focal directed attention is found in hemineglect in which a patient ignores or is unaware of one side of his body, or one half of circumambient space, or both. It occurs mainly with right hemisphere lesions involving the parietal and frontal multimodal association areas and their limbic, reticular, and sensorimotor connections.[80,81]

Overall attention can be tested by measuring digit span. The examiner orally presents a string of digits to the patient at a rate of one per second, and asks him to repeat the list forward and then backward. A normal digit span forward is five to seven items, and in reverse it is two digits less.[81,82] Sustained concentration can be evaluated by the "A" test in which the examiner reads aloud a list of 60 letters at a rate of one per second and the patient signs by raising his hand when he hears the letter "A." Normal persons perform error free while patients with deficits in attention tend to make errors of omission. The tendency of patients with impaired attention to have difficulty in inhibiting responses can be evaluated with a "go-no-go" paradigm. The patient is asked to raise his index finger when he hears a single tap and to make no response to two taps, which the examiner makes by hitting the undersurface of the table out of the patient's vision. In the Stroop interference procedure the patient is presented with color words, each printed in a color other than that spelled by the letters. The task is to give only the color and to inhibit the tendency to read the literal spelling.

Hemineglect has perceptual, motor, and motivational components. In drawing a clock the patient may omit the numbers on one side or in representing a daisy he may similarly leave off the petals on one side. Drawing of a human figure may show only one arm, leg, eye, and ear. The patient reads the word BRAKE as RAKE, or in the instance of right-sided hemineglect reads HERON as HERO. Writing may be confined to one side of a page. If the patient is asked to bisect a horizontal line he is likely to draw the vertical line on the side of the midline ipsilateral to the lesion. When both sides of the body are touched simultaneously the patient reports only the stimulus on the intact side, although a single stimulus on the affected side can be perceived, a phenomenon known as extinction. If the patient is asked to raise both arms aloft he may lift only one extremity, even though the other one is not weak and he uses it in other activities. On a letter cancellation task, performance in the detection of targets on the involved side may be improved by offering a reward.

Memory

There are various types and classifications of memory and memory loss. These include the amnesias; immediate, short-term and long-term memory; recent and remote memory; verbal and nonverbal memory; modality specific (visual, auditory, olfactory), episodic (autobiographical, specific events in time and space), semantic, and procedural (facts, procedures, skills) memory; and memory for geographical places, for people, and for animals. Testing therefore can be highly specialized.

Because of such specialization amnesics may do well on many recall tests, especially if they are allowed to rehearse silently. Rehearsal can be prevented by the Brown-Peterson interference technique, based on the known sensitivity of patients with AA to distraction. The patient is presented with trigrams or groups of 3 words over varying intervals, and asked to count backward aloud during the intervals. Performance is far inferior to that which would be accomplished had rehearsal been permitted. The Famous Faces test in RA is based on the concept of a temporal gradient. The patient is asked to recognize the faces of people prominent in the news over periods in the past, and scores for different decades compared. However, because autobiographical memory can be profoundly impaired while knowledge of famous people and events is spared[83] and a considerable number of patients do not manifest temporal gradients, the test is of limited clinical value.

Story recall is routinely used. The patient is asked to recall a 6-item passage such as "St Joseph's School burned down and 3 firemen were overcome by smoke" immediately and after an interval of 5 minutes. Nonverbal memory can be evaluated by having the patient watch the examiner conceal several of his personal possessions, and find them 5 to 10 minutes later. A more complex evaluation of verbal memory can be done through the Rey Auditory Verbal Learning Test. The Rey-Osterrieth Figure Test provides a quantitative measure of nonverbal learning and memory.[84]

Language

Evaluation of language functions mainly concerns aphasia. Patients are tested from the standpoints of fluency of conversational speech, comprehension, repetition, reading and writing, object naming, and word-word relationships. Note should also be taken of handedness.

Nonfluent aphasia is characterized by sparse verbal output (less than 50 words/min), effortful speech, short phrase length, sometimes a single word, poor articulation of speech sounds, and dysprosody, the loss of melodic quality.[85] Agrammatism, the omitting of function words such as "and" and "to," and of syntactic indicators such as verb tenses and plurals, may be a feature. Fluent aphasia, on the other hand, involves a normal or excessive production of words, normal phrase length, and intact articulation and prosody. There may be paraphasic word errors, and jargon, the use of neologisms or standard English words given in meaningless or inappropriate contexts. Nonfluent aphasias occur with lesions of the anterior dominant, usually the left, hemisphere while fluent aphasias are found with more posterior lesions.

Comprehension is tested by having the patient follow commands: Point to the window, Clap and clasp hands, Stand up and walk to the door. If severely impaired or apraxic he can be asked questions such as, "How many wheels are there on a bicycle?" or asked to give yes or no answers to questions such as, "Are the lights on in this room?" or "Did George Washington have a beard?" The patient may be asked to decipher passive sentence structures such as "The lion was killed by the tiger; which animal is dead?" Comprehension can be impaired by lesions of both anterior and posterior parts of the left hemisphere.

Repetition can be tested by having the patient repeat words, phrases, and sentences. Aphasic patients generally have more difficulty in repeating passages with function words such as "no ifs, ands, or buts" than they do with phrases containing content words such as "correspondents write frequently." Failure of repetition is a cardinal feature of conduction aphasia produced by lesions of the perisylvian area.

Reading should be assessed both by reading aloud and testing comprehension. While alexia without agraphia is a reliable sign of a posterior left hemisphere lesion, alexia and agraphia may occur with lesions at various points in the hemisphere.

Writing can be evaluated by asking the patient to write his name, and take down a dictated sentence. Note is made of word accuracy, spelling, and calligraphy. Disorders of writing are common in confusional states and are of limited value in localization.

The patient is asked to name common objects and movements or pictures of them, along with colors. Items that are most apt to yield errors are those that are parts of wholes, such as a button hole, cuff, or lapel, or have compound names such as doorknob or coathanger. Color anomia may occur in association with alexia without agraphia. Generally, aphasic naming errors are not of value in localization. Nonaphasic naming errors may also occur with lesions of the right hemisphere and with bilateral damage. These are apt to involve items connected with the patient's disability or that have other personal significance for him, as in referring to a wheelchair as "a director's chair" or a plastic drinking straw as a "cigarette."[86]

Calculation

In testing a patient's ability to add, subtract, multiply, and divide it must first be determined that he can comprehend the concept of an arithmetical operation, and that he is attentive to the task. Serial subtractions of 7s is a useful test that depends not only on calculation skills but on attention. Normal persons may make errors in the unit column, so that the significant mistakes are in the tens column such as "93, 76 ..." or "93, 86, 79, 82." Tests of addition and subtraction should involve carrying, and in evaluating multiplication, rote tables should be avoided. The finding of dyscalculia is not of great localizing value but the combination with agraphia, difficulty in identifying and naming fingers, and left right disorientation is highly suggestive of a lesion in the left parietal lobe.

Constructional and Visuospatial Skills

These are tested by drawing and making designs. The patient is asked to draw a clock, house, or cube, or copy a complex design like the Rey-Osterrieth Figure. In the block design subtest of the Wechsler Adult Intelligence Scale, the patient arranges a group of colored blocks in a design shown on a card. Impairment occurs with lesions of either hemisphere. Evidence of hemineglect may also be found in the drawings of patients with right hemisphere lesions. Topographical orientation and memory can be tested by having the patient draw a map of his quarters or describe a familiar route. Impairment occurs with both bilateral and unilateral posterior brain lesions, the latter located more frequently in the right hemisphere.

Praxis

Apraxia is the inability to carry out a skilled movement on command or in imitation even though the person understands the task and there is no primary motor disability. Ideomotor apraxia is the inability to perform an act, such as a salute, although the patient can do it spontaneously. Ideational apraxia refers to the failure to carry out a sequence of actions, such as folding a letter, putting it in an envelope, and sealing it. The ability to pantomime may also be tested by asking the patient to pretend to comb his hair, brush his teeth, cut with scissors, and fire a pistol. An apraxic patient is apt to substitute a body part for the object. He may run his fingers through his hair, rub his index finger against his teeth, use his index and middle fingers as scissor blades, and point his index finger and say "boom, boom." Serial hand movements can be tested by having the patient assume three consecutive hand postures, first in a fist position with the knuckle downward, then with hand open and palm down, and then with hand open and edge down while saying the positions aloud, "fist, slap, cut." Ideomotor apraxia is often associated with aphasia, but other forms are difficult to localize. Interestingly, apraxic patients rarely complain of any difficulty.

Dressing apraxia is the failure of a person to put on a coat or a pair of trousers after the garments are handed to him. He may get the sleeves reversed or even try to put both legs into the same trouser. It is considered to be a constructional difficulty rather than a true apraxia. It may occur with right parietal lesions along with topographical disorientation and hemineglect, and is common in dementia and confusional states.

Abstraction

Abstraction is the derivation of a common principle or category from diverse elements. In the Similarities subtest of the Wechsler Adult Intelligence Scale, the patient is asked how such items as a chair and a table, or a cup and a saucer are alike. Aphasic difficulties and loss of inhibition may contribute to failures as in the statement that "You drink from a cup." Proverb interpretation is commonly used, but has the disadvantage that most proverbs are overlearned and do not require abstract thinking. Nonverbal categories can be tested by asking the patient to sort out stimuli on the basis of color, shape, or size. Impaired abstraction is traditionally associated with frontal lobe lesions, but may be a feature of more widespread brain involvement.

Executive Functions

Defects in executive functions are characterized by inability to plan and organize behavior and set priorities among competing tasks. Such a patient may do well on a large battery of neuropsychological tests including those of memory, abstraction, and reasoning.[87–89] He might answer a test question of what he would do if he found a stamped and addressed envelope on the street, but act quite differently. Testing should approximate real life situations. Loss of executive functions with preservation of other faculties is a reliable indicator of focal frontal lobe damage.

LONG-TERM SEQUELAE

The long-term sequelae of TBI cover a broad range of cognitive, affective, and personality changes. While some patients show striking changes in language, perception, and visuospatial processing, the more typical picture emphasizes disturbances in memory, attention, personality, and the cognitive and affective aspects of social behavior.

Cognitive Changes

Memory problems include a deficit in the explicit retrieval of new information (AA), and a much more modest and variable RA. Immediate recall and older memories are generally intact as are implicit memory processes. The deficit thus appears to be primarily in the consolidation of new episodic memory. These memory problems may be accompanied by slowed reaction times and reduced information processing skills, attentional deficits, and impaired ability to divide cognitive resources. Related to this may be a deficit in concept formation with difficulty in changing set, manifested by perseveration on such tasks as the Wisconsin Card Sort Test.

The follow-up study of head-injured Vietnam veterans showed that damage to the basal forebrain (BFB) in the proximal orbitofrontal lobe made a large contribution to the episodic memory loss as well as to the slowed reaction time and attentional deficits. BFB-injured men differed from their non-BFB-injured matches only in having a longer loss of consciousness postinjury, more episodic memory deficits and poorer performance in the Wisconsin Card Sort Test.[90,91] The basal forebrain lesions alone, however, were not sufficient to produce dementia as suggested by studies of Alzheimer's disease.

In addition to residuals of aphasia, there are nonaphasic disturbances of language that are more difficult to classify. These include tangential and fragmented speech, loose connections between words and ideas, cryptic expressions, and a tendency for the patient to refer to himself and his experiences in the third person. Thus, he may describe his injuries as if they had happened to someone else.[62,92,93] These nonaphasic language disorders are mentioned not because they appear in a majority of patients but because they may be mistaken for schizophrenic phenomena.

Affective Disorders

These depend only partly on the severity of the brain injury and the location of the lesion. The disorders are also influenced by associated verbal behavior, premorbid experience, and by environmental events. Efforts to localize individual mood states have led to variable, sometimes contradictory, results.

Anxiety

Anxiety has traditionally been regarded as a reflection of the patient's efforts to cope with his deficits and the social limitations imposed by them. Extreme degrees of anxiety are expressed in the catastrophic reaction, a term introduced by Kurt Goldstein[94] to describe the behavior of brain-injured German veterans of World War I. It consisted of outbursts of frustration and emotional distress experienced by the patient confronted by a task or situation beyond his capabilities. Catastrophic reactions occur predominantly in patients with left hemisphere lesions, especially those situated anteriorly, and associated with nonfluent aphasia. A study of Vietnam veterans seen 15 years after injury showed, however, that feelings of anxiety and "edginess" were experienced most frequently by men with right orbitofrontal damage, while feelings of anger/hostility were most frequent after left dorsofrontal lesions. Generally, patients with orbitofrontal lesions appeared more affectively blunted and hostile than any other lesion group or controls.[2] The study also showed that cognitive deficits played a lesser role in right hemisphere mood change than they did in left hemisphere lesions.

Some forms of anxiety disorder have been related to serotonin excess[95] or excessive noradrenergic activity.[96] Other neurotransmitter systems including γ-aminobutyric acid (GABA) have also been implicated in anxiety disorders.[96]

Denial or Unawareness

While anosognosia for physical defects such as hemiplegia usually clears within 2 or 3 months, denial or unawareness of cognitive and other behavioral disabilities may persist much longer. The so-called anosognosic attitude, while it combats anxiety and depression, may lead to a number of undesirable consequences. The patient may blame his problems in social relationships on weakness or an unsteady gait. He may have unrealistic work expectations, and be unwilling to accept a job that he feels is beneath his capabilities. He may see no need for training or rehabilitation.

In the early stages when the anosognosia is complete and has the supporting cognitive framework of confabulations and delusions, the patient is usually serene, but as brain function improves, he may become anxious and depressed. He may develop headaches and other somatic complaints. He may become obsessively concerned with his own health and that of others. He may express concern about minor facial blemishes or his teeth, and express fears of falling or getting a haircut. Some patients become preoccupied with God and sin and leading a better life. Paradoxically, the patient becomes more emotionally disturbed at a time when his brain function is recovering.

Dealing with denial and the catastrophic reaction is a major task of neuropsychological rehabilitation, and unless these phenomena are dealt with, improvement in psychosocial adjustment is much less likely to occur.[93] Awareness allows the patient to experience a normal grief reaction and adjust to lost skills and loss of status. On the other hand, other patients with severe brain injuries remain aware of their problems. A soldier who had returned to duty complained on follow-up that it was difficult for him to make new friends because he could not stop himself from talking so much.

Depression

Depression in the form of feelings of helplessness, unworthiness, guilt, reduced self-esteem, loss of interest and initiative, and diminished libido is a common later sequel and can appear at any time postinjury. Depression is not directly related to the severity of the brain injury or the degree of neuropsychological impairment.[93,97] The depression may not be a classical one, worse in the morning, and associated with weight loss and psychomotor agitation or retardation;[98] however, the classical symptom of insomnia is common. Social withdrawal may be a feature of depression, but in other instances it may be simply the avoidance of coping with a stressful situation.[93] Decreased sexual drive and diminished erectile function may or may not be associated with depression.[99] While reduced sexual drive along with cognitive loss, and physical complaints like headache and fatigue are factors in troubled domestic relationships, increased sexual drive may also be a problem.

Location of the lesion is another determinant. Major depressions are more common after left than right hemisphere lesions, with the greatest frequency following left frontal damage.[100,101] Depression, however, is also common with right hemisphere pathology, especially in patients without denial and the associated phenomena that have been described.[93,102] The hemispheric asymmetry has been attributed to differences in cognitive capacities of the hemispheres, to the adaptive role of denial, confabulation, and reduplication, and to direct biochemical effects. Some forms of depression appear to be related to depletion of brain serotonin,[103] and it has been shown that after brain injury there is increased serotonin receptor binding in intact areas of the right hemisphere suggesting better biological adaptation.[104]

Premorbid experience and the quality of psychosocial functioning also play a role in depression following brain injury, and in later-onset depression these factors are of greater importance than lesion location.[105] A recent civilian study of acute and late-onset depression after closed-head injuries found that patients in both groups had more psychiatric disorders and poorer social functioning than controls; but, while acute onset depression was significantly related to left anterior frontal lobe localization, late onset depression was not related to the site of brain damage.[105]

Secondary mania after TBI is far less common than depression as a long-term sequelae. Case reports indicate onsets of from weeks to years postinjury with involvement of orbitofrontal and basal temporal regions and other subcortical structures, and greater on the right side of the brain.[106–108]

Aggressive and Paranoid Behavior

Aggressive behavior may appear at any time after a brain injury. Outbursts of temper with verbal and physical aggression may be a response to frustration, and be triggered by small amounts of alcohol or other drugs. Violence in the sense of directed physical force against persons or property may occur when the patient feels that he is being threatened or persecuted or will be harmed, and also in the absence of paranoid delusions. Paranoid attitudes may be expressed in justification of acts of violence. When episodes of explosive rage are out of proportion to any precipitating stimulus and especially when they are followed by amnesia, they raise the question of temporal lobe epilepsy. It is likely, however, that the incidence of both post-traumatic temporal lobe epilepsy and directed assaultive destructive behavior in epilepsy has been exaggerated.[109–112] More relevant considerations are a history of severe combat stress, violence in civilian life, and the immediate environmental situation. While a history of head injury is very common among patients who come to medical attention because of violence, the incidence of violence in controlled follow-up studies of patients with head injuries is far lower. A 5-year follow-up study of 1,830 Finnish veterans of World War II, 32 to 37 years after the end of the war, who had sustained penetrating brain injuries did not show a higher frequency of violent crime than did nonwounded veterans. Nor was there more violent crime in men with frontal or temporal lobe lesions.[113]

The Overt Aggression Scale[114] grades a spectrum of aggressive and violent behavior ranging from verbal threats, curses, and insults to physically destructive acts against objects, to physical harm to the self, to physical aggression against other persons.

Psychoses

Psychosis can be a late sequel of combat-incurred brain injury recognized months, years, or decades after the trauma. A review of the German literature of the Franco-Prussian War of 1870 to 1871 by Adolf Meyer[115] noted that less than 1% of soldiers with serious brain damage became insane, but the belief that dementia praecox, catatonic psychoses, and schizophrenia could be caused by brain trauma was prevalent during and following World War I. Long-term follow-ups of American casualties of World War II are not available, but a Soviet investigation of 1,168 brain injured veterans reported a 9.8% incidence of schizophrenia mainly of the depressive-paranoid and depressive types.[116] It can be pointed out that many diagnoses of schizophrenia were made before standard classifications were established and before the delusional misidentification reduplicative syndromes of organic origin and the metabolic dementias were well known.

More recent studies, notably those of Finnish veterans of the 1939 to 1944 wars with the Soviet Union, have shown that brain trauma is not a significant cause of schizophrenia. In the Finnish series, schizophrenic psychoses appeared more frequently in men who had had mild head injuries and had not lost consciousness than in the more severely injured, and there was a larger proportion of patients under the age of 20 at the time of the wounding than there was in the 20- to 34-year-old group.[117] A British study[118] found that while the number of schizophrenic-like states following brain damage exceeded that expected by chance, schizophreniform reactions were more frequent than process schizophrenia, and there was no increase in genetic loading.

The most extensive and detailed investigations of psychoses following combat-incurred brain injuries have been carried out at the Kauniala Hospital for Disabled War Veterans in Finland where the treatment and rehabilitation of all brain injuries from World War II are centralized. Investigators there have found a rising incidence of psychoses over the past 40 years; rates of 4.4% in 1951, 8.9% in 1969, and 12% in 1993.[117,119,120] A control group of pneumonia patients in the most recent study had an incidence of psychosis of 3.3%. The most frequent diagnoses were paranoid delusional state, major depression, epileptic psychoses consisting of confusional states after seizures, and organic psychosis (dementia). Delusional psychoses lasted less than a year in 28% of cases, and more than 5 years in 40%. Jealousy and the fear of being sexually betrayed constituted the most prominent delusional content.

The delayed onset of psychosis requires explanation. One aspect is that with the passage of time the risk factors for further brain damage, such as the use of alcohol and other drugs including anticonvulsive medication, additional injuries, cerebral vascular impairment, and systemic disease, increase. Second, the damaged brain is more sensitive to the effects of the stresses of living associated with the person's diminished capacities. Another issue concerns the time that a psychotic reaction becomes overt. As in the case reported by Staton et al,[75] feelings of unreality and reduplicative phenomena may long antedate the florid manifestations. Other studies have linked late onset psychoses with epilepsy, even though only a minority of psychotic episodes are associated with seizures.[121]

TREATMENT

One of the most encouraging aspects of TBI rehabilitation is the amazing ability of the young adult brain to compensate for many aspects of injury naturally. Over the past 2 decades, however, it has become apparent that most TBI patients will benefit from some level of TBI-specific rehabilitation. The field of TBI rehabilitation has grown exponentially over this time, but the exact form and intensity of rehabilitation indicated for a given patient remains debatable.

Multiple therapeutic strategies, including coma stimulation, reality orientation, cognitive therapy, speech therapy, occupational therapy, recreation therapy, and music therapy, have been applied to the TBI patient. While selected elements of many of these will undoubtedly prove useful in the

TBI setting, there has been a paucity of scientific validation for these often expensive interventions (including comparison with minimal care, supportive models).

If progress is to be made in this area, rehabilitation modalities must be subject to the same scrutiny for indications, dose, duration of treatment, and efficacy as are other medical treatments, including drugs. The ultimate goal of therapy should be the independence and community reintegration of the patient within his or her limits, rather than the specialized treatment of specific deficits simply because "they are there."

All too often, scarce resources available to the patient are used up in the early acute and postacute phases on evaluation and therapy of deficits that will improve anyway or that are relatively unimportant to the ultimate goal of independence. Some programs may be actually counterproductive by fostering continued dependence. Relatively cost-effective interventions such as training in specific community reintegration skills (eg, decision making) and certain forms of behavioral modification may end up being omitted because the limited funds available were used up in earlier, less relevant therapies.

Although cognitive rehabilitation has yet to fulfill its promise by submission to careful group and case-series analyses, the reality is that most TBI patients will receive some form of cognitive rehabilitation during their postinjury course. In fact, some drug therapies may potentially be most effective when used in conjunction with cognitive remediation programs. Thus, the possibility of rehabilitation-drug interactions when evaluating drug effects on independent variables must be addressed in pharmacological studies by, at a minimum, categorizing the type, frequency, and duration of remediation. More sophisticated studies can adapt both therapy and agent as dependent factors.

Behavioral Management

The treatment of the behavioral consequences of serious brain injuries varies with the stage of clinical recovery. During the initial acute stage of agitation, aiding orientation and cutting down on environmental diversity may be useful. After the initial phase, it should be recognized that denial, amnesia, confabulation, and reduplicative misidentifications are "normal" phenomena and do not have the same ominous significance of delusions in nontraumatic mental illnesses. Barring abnormal neurological signs and impairments from other injuries, patients are usually discharged from the hospital after they become oriented and able to retain new information. They are then reevaluated after a 6-month period over which the greatest part of improvement in cognitive functions occurs.

Caution should be exercised in sending patients with a great deal of denial back to duty or accepting their statements about their condition at face value. Patients about to be discharged from the hospital or allowed leave should be warned about the effects of alcohol, indulgence in which is particularly apt to occur after weeks of confinement. An apparently recovered patient may become disoriented and disturbed after relatively small amounts of alcohol. In anticipating such situations, the Amytal Test described in Chapter 15, Conversion Disorders, is useful. If a patient becomes disoriented or confabulatory under the effects of barbiturates, then alcohol is apt to produce a similar reaction.

While the major recovery of cognitive functions takes place in the first 6 months, patients may continue to make progress in adapting to their deficits. It is doubtful if cognitive retraining is of value in that the damaged brain can relearn lost function, but rehabilitative measures may improve behavior and social skills. The aims of such therapy are to provide the patient with the conceptual or analogical model of what has happened to him, help him to recognize both his defects and remaining strengths, train him in alternate strategies, and teach him how to behave in social situations.[92]

Pharmacological Management

While behavioral rehabilitative measures are the cornerstone of therapy, psychopharmacology has a role in the management of symptoms. Drugs may be indicated for the treatment of depression, agitation, violence, and psychoses, and for the control of pain and seizures. Accounts of anticonvulsant therapy are available in standard neurological texts, and this section focuses on the treatment of disturbances of mood and behavior and of pain in the brain-injured patient.

It must be pointed out that the use of drugs in the control of behavioral changes, particularly agitation and aggression, is controversial and in some situations such control is best achieved by nonpharmacological intervention. Drugs may have undesirable effects, and brain-damaged persons are not only more sensitive to the actions of alcohol and barbiturates but to those of other drugs as well. Antidepressants, for example, have more sedative, disorienting, hypotensive, and anticholinergic effects than in non-brain-injured patients. Neuroleptics such as the phenothiazines and the butyrophenones may be helpful in diminishing strong emotional outbursts, but they also produce affective and cognitive deficits, lower seizure thresholds, and may actually exacerbate aggressive behavior. These medications may also increase the risk of abnormal involuntary movements and parkinsonism acutely, and tardive dyskinesia, tardive dystonia, and tardive akathisia with chronic use.

In theory, cholinergic, noradrenergic, and dopaminergic drugs tend to activate or increase aggression in TBI patients, while serotonergic (fluoxetine, trazodone) and GABA-ergic (benzodiazepines, valproate) drugs tend to decrease it. In practice, however, pharmacological management of symptoms in a given individual remains largely empirical. The choice of drug is also determined by the postinjury stage. Whereas a neuroleptic like haloperidol may be indicated for acute initial violent behavior, it is contraindicated for later episodes of aggression in a neurologically stable patient.

Pharmacotherapy of Pain

Pain as a direct result of brain tissue damage is uncommon, but headaches are a complaint, and pain may be a feature of associated injuries involving the spinal cord and peripheral nerves. Narcotic analgesics are generally contraindicated in the treatment of chronic pain especially in patients with impaired brain function, and combinations of nonsteroidal antiinflammatory drugs (NSAIDs) and antidepressants are preferred.

Headaches are more apt to be a problem in later stages when patients must face the stress of diminished capability and altered life style. Treatment is much like that of non–brain-injured patients. In headaches of a vascular type β-adrenergic blockers and antidepressants are often effective. Antidepressants have also been of benefit in headaches caused by muscle contraction. Interestingly, depression rating scales may show little change in the level of depression despite marked improvement in headache control.

Antidepressants probably should be given a different name because they are useful in treating a variety of other conditions including anxiety disorders, panic disorders, PTSD, obsessive-compulsive disorders, bulimia and anorexia, phobic disorders, personality disorders, mitral valve prolapse, peptic ulcers (doxepin is a stronger histamine-2 blocker than cimetidine), and some chronic pain disorders.[122]

The antidepressants of choice for chronic pain appear to be those that affect noradrenergic neurotransmission (imipramine, amitriptyline, desipramine, doxepin, etc.) rather than those affecting serotonergic neurotransmission (fluoxetine, sertraline, fluvoxamine, paroxetine, etc.). An exception to this generalization is fibromyalgia, which appears to respond better to serotonergic drugs. Because the tricyclic antidepressants (including those affecting noradrenergic neurotransmission given above) can lower seizure threshold, patients with head injuries must be carefully assessed. Furthermore, anticonvulsants (most notably carbamazepine and phenytoin) can cause induction of enzymes in the liver that rapidly detoxify tricyclic antidepressants (TCAs), making it difficult to achieve therapeutic blood levels. Some patients respond at dosages of TCAs that would be subtherapeutic for depression; however, many cases require higher dosages. Despite prescribing difficulties, TCAs can give dramatic pain relief.

A report of cases of causalgia resulting from missile and fragment wounds sustained in the fighting in Lebanon from 1975 to 1981 indicated marked relief of pain with phenoxybenzamine, an α-1,2-noradrenergic antagonist.[123] The drug, however, may be contraindicated in head injuries, as it has been found experimentally to retard recovery following brain damage in animals.[124]

Pharmacotherapy of Mood and Behavior Disorders

Standard antidepressant and anxiolytic medications are usually efficacious for these conditions. Anxiolytics, preferably less sedating ones, should be used cautiously and usually briefly because of their euphoriant and addictive potential. Because the antidepressants, particularly those affecting serotonergic neurotransmission, are effective anxiolytics in chronic usage, a useful approach is to start an antidepressant and anxiolytic together for rapid control of anxiety then discontinue the anxiolytic in a few weeks, after the latency period of the antidepressant has ended.

Electroconvulsive therapy is particularly benign compared to drug therapy for patients with various medical conditions, and this applies as well to those with TBI. Due to legal considerations, electroconvulsive therapy is often reserved for patients unresponsive to antidepressant therapy; however, this legal artifact should not prevent its use in cases likely to respond.

If mania occurs, mood stabilizers such as lithium, carbamazepine, or valproic acid may be used. Obviously, in mixed conditions (seizures plus mania, depression plus anxiety, depression plus pain) a single agent efficacious for both conditions may be selected.

PTSD is a common sequela not only of psychological trauma but also of physical trauma. Its treatment is described in Chapter 16, Chronic Post-Traumatic Stress Disorders. In terms of the brain-injured patient with PTSD, nonsedating agents are preferred and if a seizure disorder coexists, anticonvulsants (carbamazepine, clonazepam) should be tried first. Because clonazepam has serotonergic activity, it may be helpful through a dual mechanism.

Alcoholism, which is often associated with PTSD, poses particular problems in patients with TBI because of the intermittent withdrawal from alcohol, which is sometimes complicated by seizures. Fortunately, benzodiazepines used for withdrawal are effective anticonvulsants.

Inasmuch as aggressive behavior may be modulated through changes in a number of neuroanatomic sites and many neurotransmitter systems, including serotonin, norepinephrine, dopamine, acetylcholine, GABA and the opioids,[125] a variety of medications including neuroleptics, anticonvulsants, β-adrenergic blockers, benzodiazepines, and serotonergic agents (including lithium) may be useful in chronic aggression.[126] When aggression is severe or dangerous, neuroleptics (phenothiazines, butyrophenones, etc.) may be initially required to gain control. Neuroleptics may be helpful but the complications have been noted. Attempts should be made to replace them with more benign and often more efficacious medications such as mood stabilizers (lithium, carbamazepine, valproic acid, clonazepam, and occasionally calcium channel blockers).

β-adrenergic blocking agents (propranolol, metoprolol, etc.) have been used for decreasing aggression, particularly in patients with organic brain syndromes[127] and α-adrenergic blocking agents (clonidine) for reducing disinhibited behaviors such as sexual exposure, lewd remarks, etc. Serotonergic agents (trazodone) and benzodiazepines (lorazepam, clonazepam) have been found useful in some patients with chronic aggression.[126] Usually, treatment requires experimentation with a variety of medications until one that is efficacious is found.

Silver, Yudofsky, and Hales[128] recommend the use of propranolol in the management of the violent patient, beginning with a 20 mg thrice daily schedule and increasing it by 60 mg/d every 3 days, while monitoring blood pressure. They note that daily doses above 800 mg are not usually required and recommend that the patient should be maintained for at least 8 weeks before concluding that the medication is ineffective. In heavy smokers, atenolol may be preferable because it tends to spare the lungs; however, its latency period is longer than propranolol.

Because of success in the treatment of attention deficit and hyperactivity disorders, the use of psychostimulant drugs such as methylphenidate and amphetamine has been suggested for the management of the behavioral sequelae of TBI. Animal studies have also indicated a possible role. Dopamine agonists have been found to attenuate or abolish the septal rage syndrome, which follows lesions of the septal nuclei in rats.[129] A single dose of d-amphetamine given 24 hours after injury has been reported as accelerating recovery of motor function after unilateral sensorimotor and bilateral frontal cortex ablation in rats and cats, an effect blocked by haloperidol given 24 hours after surgery or by restraining the animals.[130] These remarkable findings in different functional areas offered hope that stimulation of catecholaminergic systems might facilitate processes of cognitive and other behavioral recovery in TBI. To date, however, there is insufficient evidence that psychostimulants can improve brain function.

Individual case reports and anecdotal observations[131–133] have indicated that psychostimulant drugs may relieve tiredness, improve initiative and concentration, promote feelings of well-being, and result in better performance on some tests of memory and attention. The one controlled study of a case series, however, has yielded disappointing results.[134] Methylphenidate was superior to placebo but there was a marked discrepancy between subjective report and performance. Only a few objective measures showed clear stimulant effects, and there was no coherent pattern to the measures that were responsive to the drug. Patients with mild and moderate head injuries with symptoms of impulsiveness, hyperactivity, distractibility, and emotional lability may be given a trial of psychostimulants under close supervision, with consideration of the dangers of abuse, increased risk of seizures, withdrawal manifestations on cessation, and a psychotic reaction.[135]

OUTCOME

A surprisingly good overall outcome can be seen in many young, moderately severely to severely injured patients, a finding that probably reflects compensation for lost functions more than recovery of the injured tissue itself. Thus, "floating" or dynamic endpoints can be identified in the post-TBI course: recovery from coma, return of orientation, resolution of post-traumatic amnesia, shrinking of retrograde amnesia, number of significant deficits identified on initial neuropsychological testing, number of significant deficits identified on the last neuropsychological evaluation, and the steepness of the recovery slopes. Nevertheless, an important milestone yet to be reached in the TBI field is the development of reproducible, universally accepted measures of function and long-term outcome with which to compare the value of various interventions.[1]

Final outcome is a composite of a number of elements, including preinjury, neurologic, cognitive, behavioral, and psychosocial function, all of which may interact differently in each individual patient. When evaluating efficacy of a given therapy it is necessary to study all of these elements in the context of outcome as a whole; any evaluation battery should thus include at least some measure of each. It is misleading, for example, to use improvement in a particular overlearned memory task as a measure of outcome. While there may not be any ideal surrogate or summary measure for outcome, return to gainful employment may be a useful one in most TBI populations.

The second author has had the opportunity to study the disabilities that affect return to work in a large cohort (N=520) of head-injured Vietnam veterans participating in the Vietnam Head Injury Study. A 1-week, standardized, multi-disciplinary outcome evaluation was completed on each of them. Some 15 years postinjury, 56% of these men were gainfully employed, compared to 82% of an uninjured Vietnam veteran control group.[136] The occupational distribution of those who were working was essentially no different from that of normal uninjured young American males.[137] After exclusion of severe aphasic and triplegic patients, none of whom worked, a multistage statistical analysis of this data, including factor and multiple logistic regression analyses, identified seven specifically defined disabilities that had a significant impact on return to work: post-traumatic epilepsy, hemiparesis, visual field loss, verbal memory loss, visual memory loss, psychological problems, and violent behavior. Interestingly, these seven items were found to be relatively equipotent, so that a simple sum of any of them could yield a "disability score," which predicted return to work.

Patients were able to compensate relatively well for up to any three impairments, but beyond that there was a sharp drop in work rates. Other factors contributing significantly to return to work included preinjury intelligence, total brain volume loss on CT scan, and education postinjury. This experience is a further reminder of the importance of considering outcome from TBI as dependent on a set of functional skills, rather than identifying one or two disabilities as its principal determinant.

PREDICTABILITY AND PREDISPOSITION

It is difficult to predict the long-term social outcome of individual brain injuries even though the location and extent of the lesions are known. There are, however, a number of useful observations. Men whose injuries were sustained under particularly severe combat conditions, and those who have had a prior head injury or a history of combat-induced stress reactions, are apt to have more severe behavioral consequences. Injuries to other parts of the body are a factor. A follow-up study of military personnel treated at Walter Reed Army Medical Center for mainly closed-head injuries showed that patients who were violent in the acute stage and who used language of violence with references to death, blood, and mangling went on to have higher problem ratings on a scale based on employment record, social sexual adjustment, somatic symptoms, and emotional state than did men with less disturbed initial behavior.[138] Similar findings in civilian patients are reported.[139] Alcohol consumption at the time of injury is said to increase the severity and duration of initial agitation and the amount of later memory loss.[140,141] Also, premorbid personality factors may play a role. The following case is illustrative.

Case Study 3: Disastrous Social Consequences of a Brain Injury

A 44-year-old infantry commanding officer sustained a head injury and a fractured femur in a car accident while on a training exercise. His wife, who was driving, and his five children were also injured. On admission to the hospital he responded only to painful stimuli, and, because of extreme agitation, was restrained over the next 10 days. After transfer to Walter Reed Army Medical Center 6 weeks after injury, he was restless, overtalkative, tangential, and suspicious. He spoke incessantly of his children, and believed that one of them had been killed in the accident. He accused the hospital of running a dope ring and demanded an investigation.

In the first formal interview on the psychiatric ward he appeared hypomanic. He was unsure of the date, mistaken about his age (giving his wife's), and did not know the name of the hospital beyond calling it "the best hospital in the world." When asked about his accident he went into a lurid account of the consequences of nuclear and biological warfare (the subject of his course) and talked at length about his children. The RA was estimated at one half hour and the AA later determined as having endured for 7 to 10 days. His "last memory" was of scolding his wife for not having arrived to pick him up in the car. There was temporal reduplication; he stated that the examiner had given him a mental examination at Fort Benning, where the accident occurred. He admitted having suffered a head injury and a broken leg, but denied any memory loss or mental problems. He agreed that he was emotionally overstimulated and attributed this to his eagerness to see his family. He complained of blurred vision on reading, and neurological examination disclosed a partial internuclear ophthalmoplegia.

Orientation cleared over the next few days but the temporal reduplication persisted. Following a carotid angiogram, performed with some difficulty, he confabulated the next day that he had acted as defense counsel for several soldiers convicted of rape and attempted murder. He claimed that one of the men had been hanged and described in vivid detail, indicating on himself, how the man's neck had been stretched at least 18 inches. He also believed that he had been given electroconvulsive therapy (ECT).

At the time of discharge from the hospital, 4 months after his injury, the patient's mood was subdued but he would become overexuberant during testing and interviews. He was no longer confabulatory but believed that a steel plate had been placed in his head. (A pin had been inserted in his femur.) He also became preoccupied with repairing the leaky roof of the buildings on his farm. He had considered having this done prior to his injury, but had given up the idea because of the great expense. Now, however, he was determined to proceed regardless of cost. Despite the recommendation that he not resume his occupation as an agricultural administrator for several months, he insisted on returning to work immediately.

Follow-up over a 5-year period revealed a pattern of domestic and emotional difficulties. He became increasingly critical of his children and demanded perfection from them. He also projected his concerns with his own health upon them. He forbade them to watch television as it was bad for their eyes (he had some residual blurred vision), and would not allow his daughter to ride her horse for fear of a head injury. He was sexually demanding, insisting on intercourse several times a day, without any display of affection. After his wife had a hysterectomy following a hemorrhage, he accused her of evading her conjugal duties. After one of his sons drank poison in a suicidal gesture, he considered shooting himself in the head for having failed as a parent. He was technically competent on his job, but was overbearing with subordinates and charged that his secretary was talking about him behind his back. After 3 years his wife obtained a separation, and he went to live with his widowed mother and to work for his brother.

Some of the behavior was an exaggeration of premorbid personality traits. The patient had grown up in a prosperous Calvinistic work ethic family, in which the rod was not spared. His mother recalled him as a quiet, timid child who might be punished by his father for showing fear. His wife described him as a driving—and driven—perfectionistic, stubborn person, proud of his success in his several businesses and his military activities. He was the dominant member of his family, very attentive to his children and intent on making them responsible and achieving. His wife noted that he never played with them. He took pride in his good health, and regarded illness as a sign of weakness of character. He was intolerant of the ills of others, except in the case of his children, about whose even minor ailments he would become excessively worried; he was particularly unsympathetic with mental illness. He had been sexually active, and had taken any refusal by his wife as a personal rejection. Overall, he had been concerned with the physical aspects of relationships and situations with strong views of race and blood lines, looks, smells, diet, and nutrition.

Comment: The following features are noteworthy.

- Preservation of technical competence with marked disturbances in social and emotional behavior.
- Association of a long initial period of violence with an unfavorable outcome.
- Confabulation about the hanging of a deserter as a symbolic representation of the patient's traumatic carotid angiogram.
- The "last memory" prior to the injury of scolding his wife as symbolic of the patient's habitual hypercritical attitude toward her.
- The replacement of the patient's initial preoccupations and delusions about his children with a projection onto them of his own physical problems.
- A premorbid predisposition to denial and the role of denial in the patient's premature return to work.
- A possible connection between the patient's premorbid emphasis on the physical aspects of personal relationships with later paranoid attitudes, including these expressed through sex.

The mechanisms by which premorbid experience interacts with alterations in brain function following TBI are poorly understood. Most clinicians are aware of a relationship but the lack of a method of study has hampered research in the field. There are so many theories of personality that selection of measuring instruments appropriate for brain injuries is a problem.[142] Patients are often not good informants, and interviews carried out with relatives are of necessity retrospective. Another difficulty is that the life experience of a 17- or 18-year-old youth is so limited that his character cannot be fully evaluated. Some writers believe that behavioral traits such as disorderliness, argumentiveness, suspiciousness, and anxiousness become more pronounced and that extroverted patients become more boisterous.[97] However, disorderly patients may previously have been orderly, and patients with frontal lobe lesions may have deficits in executive functions and the social proprieties regardless of premorbid personality.

Another approach has been based on the idea that premorbid experience influences the positive, adaptive—or maladaptive—aspects of behavior following brain injury, as opposed to such negative symptoms as lack of empathy, loss of initiative, impaired emotional recognition, and diminished impulse control. Denial and some other delusions and confabulations are adaptive in the sense that they are attempts by the patient to cope with and interpret what has happened to him, make sense of his environment, and gain a *feeling* of reality. Interviews with relatives are directed toward learning how the patient has reacted to stress in the past, and toward determining the values through which he has structured his social environment. These values include attitudes toward health and illness, work and efficiency, physical appearance, family, sex, violence, religion, and ethnicity. Patients with marked and enduring delusional denial have been described variously as dogmatic and inflexible, highly work-oriented with emphasis on self-sufficiency, reserved with their feelings, and as regarding incapacity or illness as a personal failure.[66,143,144] Patients who had been more emotional and open with their feelings, and in whom these were expressed as "physical" symbols such as those relating to the body, looks, food, and sexual activity, were more likely to have paranoid forms of denial. Patients with violent backgrounds have been found to be predisposed to violence after brain injury.[126] As in the case described, patients who identified strongly with children and whose lives were structured in terms of a parent-child relationship may have delusions and preoccupations about children.[145] Patients who made inappropriate sexual remarks and gestures, who had delusions about sex, and who structured their problems in sexual language often had a history of hypersensitivity to the implications of sex in personal relationships and of highly stereotyped views of the roles of men and women.[146] It should be noted that these personality factors contribute to the behaviors described only after particular types of brain damage, but it is also noteworthy that patients with comparable lesions may exhibit marked differences in the cognitive and affective aspects of social behavior.

In recent years more attention has been paid to genetic and early acquired genetic factors, child abuse and possible brain damage, mental illness and alcoholism in close relatives, attention deficit and hyperactivity, and other learning disorders. Although interest in personality factors has declined, a knowledge of the premorbid personality characteristics of the brain-injured subject is of great importance in rehabilitation.[93] Discussion with a patient may help to show him how his own personality may be contributing to his failure in adaptation or conversely be helping him to adapt.

SUMMARY AND CONCLUSION

These are exciting times for the field of TBI. The understanding of the complex pathogenesis of acute TBI has grown exponentially over the past few decades with the delineation of focal injury, diffuse axonal injury (DAI), hypoxia and ischemia, and diffuse microvascular injury with loss of autoregulation. With the possible exception of DAI in penetrating brain wounds, these processes occur in both closed and penetrating head injuries. This initial brain damage is followed by secondary tissue injury at the cellular level, involving particularly oxygen free radicals, which affects otherwise viable tissue, so that much of the loss of function after TBI is not due to the injury itself but to a vicious cycle of subsequent biochemical events. Treatment, along with conventional measures to control shock and intracranial pressure and to evacuate hematomas, is aimed at the prevention and correction of secondary tissue damage. Among the more promising medical therapies now entering clinical trials are the inhibiting of lipid peroxidation with 21-amino steroids, and the control of oxygen free radicals with superoxide dismutase and catalase.

DAI has been demonstrated even after minor head injury, and occurs in the absence of morphopathological change in any other vascular, glial, or neural element. The finding establishes a possible organic base for "postconcussion syndrome," once thought to be of psychological origin.

While penetrating and closed-head injuries (CHI) share a number of pathological features, there are clinical differences. Patients with an acceleration/deceleration CHI are by definition unconscious, while those with penetrating head wounds frequently do not lose consciousness or have amnesia. Penetrating head wounds have a much higher incidence of subsequent seizures. The neurological deficits following penetrating wounds are more focal and include aphasia, lateralized motor and somatosensory loss, and visual field defects. Patients with CHI have predominant damage to frontal and temporal limbic structures and are more apt to develop impairments of memory and attention, in the perception of reality, and in social and emotional behavior. These differences are not absolute: penetrating injuries of basilar and other deep brain structures can result in prolonged unconsciousness and memory loss.

In recovery from severe head injuries, coma may be followed by a period of restlessness and agitation, and by a stage of altered interaction in the environment with features of the amnestic confabulatory state and the denial syndromes, that may endure for months. This latter stage involves not only deficits in cognition, the perception of reality and affective control, but modes of adaptation to the stresses of reduced capacity.

While long-term cognitive loss depends mainly on the location of the lesion, notably damage to the basal forebrain, changes in social and emotional behavior, such as depression and other mood changes, and aggressive acts and attitudes derive not only from lesion location, but from premorbid experience and environmental events. Return to work after penetrating wounds sustained in Vietnam was unfavorably affected by post-traumatic epilepsy, hemiparesis and visual field loss, verbal and visual memory impairment, psychological problems, and violent behavior. Changes in personality and affective relationships are less predictable.

It is doubtful if cognitive retraining can enable the damaged brain to regain lost skills. Rehabilitative measures, however, can provide the patient with a conceptual or analogical model of what has happened to him, help him to overcome denial and recognize both his deficits and remaining strengths, train him in alternate strategies, and teach him how to behave in social situations. Drugs have an important role in symptom management, in the control of disturbances of mood and behavior, in seizures, and in pain resulting from associated injuries.

REFERENCES

1. Department of Health and Human Services. *Interagency Head Injury Task Force Report.* Washington, DC; 1989.

2. Grafman J, Vance SC, Weingartner H, Salazar AM, Amin D. The effects of lateralized frontal lesion on mood regulation. *Brain.* 1986;109:1127–1148.

3. Hume Adams J, Graham DI, Gennarelli TA. Contemporary neuropathological considerations regarding brain damage in head injury. In: Becker DP, Povlishock JT, eds. *Central Nervous System Trauma Status Report.* Bethesda, Md: National Institute of Neurological and Communicative Disorders and Stroke, NIH; 1985: 65–77.

4. Gennarelli T, Thibault LE. Biological models of head injury. In: Becker DP, Povlishock JT, eds. *Central Nervous System Trauma Status Report.* Bethesda, Md: National Institute of Neurological and Communicative Disorders and Stroke, NIH; 1985: 391–404.

5. Marshall LF, Toole BM, Bowers S. The National Traumatic Coma Data Bank, Part II: Patients who talk and deteriorate: Implications for treatment. *J Neurosurg.* 1983;59:285–288.

6. Gennarelli TA, Thibault LE, Adams JH, Graham DI, Thompson CJ, Marcincin R. Diffuse axonal injury and traumatic coma in the primate. *Ann Neurol.* 1982;12:564–574.

7. Strich S. The pathology of brain damage due to blunt head injuries. In: Walker AE, Caveness WF, Critchley M, eds. *The Late Effects of Head Injury.* Springfield, Ill: Charles C Thomas; 1969: 501–526.

8. Povlishock JT. The morphopathologic responses to head injuries of varying severity. In: Becker DP, Povlishock JT, eds. *Central Nervous System Trauma Status Report*. Bethesda, Md: National Institute of Neurological and Communicative Disorders and Stroke, NIH; 1985: 443–452.

9. Povlishock JT, Coburn TH. Morphopathological change associated with mild head injury. In: Levin HS, Eisenberg HM, Benton AL, eds. *Mild Head Injury*. New York: Oxford University Press; 1989: 37–53.

10. Oppenheimer DR. Microscopic lesions in the brain following head injury. *J Neurol Neurosurg Psychiatry*. 1968; 31:299–306.

11. Gajdusek DC. Hypothesis: Interference with axonal transport of neurofilament as a common pathogenetic mechanism in certain diseases of the central nervous system. *N Engl J Med*. 1985;312:714–719.

12. Clinton J, Ambler MW, Roberts GW. Post-traumatic Alzheimer's disease: Preponderance of a single plaque type. *Neuropath Appl Neurobiol*. 1991;17(1):69–74.

13. Roberts GW, Allsop D, Burton C. The occult aftermath of boxing. *J Neurol Neurosurg Psychiatry*. 1990; 53(5):373–378.

14. Roberts GW, Gentleman SM, Lynch A, Graham DI. Beta A4 amyloid protein deposition in brain after head trauma. *Lancet*. 1991;338:1422–1423.

15. Ishige N, Pitts LH, Hashimoto T, Nishimura BS, Bartkowski HM. Effect of hypoxia on traumatic brain injury in rats: Part 1. Changes in neurological function, electroencephalograms, and histopathology. *Neurosurgery*. 1987; 20(6):848–853.

16. Kontos HA, Wei EP. Superoxide production in experimental brain injury. *J Neurosurg*. 1986;64(5):803–807.

17. Proctor HJ, Palladdino GW, Fillipo D. Failure of autoregulation after closed head injury: An experimental model. *J Trauma*. 1988;28(3):347–352.

18. Muizelaar JP, Marmarou A, Ward JD, et al. Adverse effects of prolonged hyperventilation in patients with severe head injury: A randomized clinical trial. *J Neurosurg*. 1991;75:731–739.

19. Allen IV, Kirk J, Maynard RL, Cooper GK, Scott R, Crockard A. An ultrastructural study of experimental high velocity penetrating head injury. *Acta Neuropathol (Berl)*. 1983;59:277–282.

20. Maxwell WL, Irvine A, Adams JH, Graham DL, Gennarelli TA. Response of cerebral microvasculature to brain injury. *J Pathol*. 1988;155:327–335.

21. Povlishock JT. Experimental studies of head injury. In: Becker DP, Gudeman SK, eds. *Textbook of Head Injury*. Philadelphia, Pa: WB Saunders; 1989: 437–450.

22. Carey, ME, Sarna GG, Farrell JB. The effect of an experimental missile wound to the brain on brain electrolytes, regional cerebral blood flow and blood brain barrier permeability. US Army Medical R & D Command, 1987. Annual report DAMD17-83-C-3145.

23. Palmer RMJ, Ferige AG, Moncada S. Nitric oxide release accounts for the biological activity of endothelium-derived relaxing factor. *Nature*. 1987;327:524–526.

24. Lawson DL, Mehta JL, Nichols WW, Mehta P, Donnelly WH. Superoxide radical-mediated endothelial injury and vasoconstriction of rat thoracic aortic rings. *J Lab Clin Med*. 1990;115(5):541–548.

25. Ward PH, Maldonado M, Moreno M, Gunther B, Vivaldi E. Oxygen derived free radicals mediate the cutaneous necrotizing vasculitis induced by epinephrine in endotoxin primed rabbits. *J Infect Dis*. 1990;161:1020–1022.

26. Lamb FS, King CM, Harrell K, Burkel W, Webb RC. Free radical mediated endothelial damage in blood vessels after electrical stimulation. *Am J Physiol*. 1987;252(5 pt 2):H1041–1046.

27. Wei EP, Kontos HA, Dietrich WD, Povlishock JT, Ellis EF. Inhibition by free radical scavengers and by cyclooxygenase inhibitors of pial arteriolar abnormalities from concussive brain injury in cats. *Circ Res*. 1981; 48(1):95–103.

28. Ellis EF, Wright KF, Wei EP. Cyclooxygenase products of arachidonic acid metabolism in cat cerebral cortex after experimental concussive brain injury. *J Neurochem*. 1981;37:892–896.

29. Faden AI. Neuropeptides and CNS Injury. *Arch Neurol*. 1986;43(5):501–504.

30. McIntosh TK, Faden AI, Yamakami I, Vink R. Magnesium deficiency exacerbates and pretreatment improves outcome following traumatic brain injury in rats. *J Neurotrauma*. 1988;5(1):17–31.

31. Faden AI, Demediuk P, Panter SS, Vink R. The role of excitatory amino acids and NMDA receptors in traumatic brain injury. *Science*. 1989;244:798–800.

32. Hayes RL, Pechura CM, Katayama Y, Povlishock JT, Giebel ML, Becker DP. Activation of pontine cholinergic sites implicated in unconsciousness following cerebral concussion in the cat. *Science*. 1984;233:301–303.

33. Suguru I, Marmarou A, Clarke GD, Andersen BJ, Fatouros PP, Young HF. Production and clearance of lactate from brain tissue, CSF, and serum following experimental brain injury. *J Neurosurg*. 1988;69:736–744.

34. Giulian D, Chen J, Ingeman JE, George JK, Noponen M. The role of mononuclear phagocytes in wound healing after traumatic injury to adult mammalian brain. *J Neurosci*. 1989;12(9):4416–4429.

35. Demopoulos HB, Flamm E, Seligman M, Pietronigro DD. Oxygen free radical in central nervous system ischemia and trauma. In: Autor AP, ed. *Pathology of Oxygen*. New York: Academic Press; 1982: 127–155.

36. Ikeda Y, Long DM. The molecular basis of brain injury and brain edema: The role of oxygen free radicals. *J Neurosurg*. 1990;27(1):1–11.

37. Bochicchio M, Latronico N, Zani DG, et al. Free radical induced lipoperoxidation and severe head injury: A clinical study. *Intensive Care Med*. 1990;16(7):444–447.

38. Hall ED, Yonkers PA, McCall JM, Braughler JM. Effects of the 21-aminosteroid U74006F on experimental head injury in mice. *J Neurosurg*. 1988;68(3):456–461.

39. Hall ED. Intensive antioxidant pre-treatment retards motor nerve degeneration. *Brain Res*. 1987;413:175–178.

40. Yoshida S. Brain injury after ischemia and trauma: The role of vitamin E. *Ann N Y Acad Sci*. 1989;570:219–235.

41. Manning AS, Coltart DJ, Hearse DJ. Ischemia and reperfusion-induced arrhythmias in the rat: Effect of xanthine oxidase inhibition with allopurinol. *Circ Res*. 1984;55(4):545–548.

42. Taylor MD, Palmer GC, Callahan AS. Protective action by methylprednisolone, allopurinol and indomethacin against stroke-induce damage to adenylate cyclase in gerbil cerebral cortex. *Stroke*. 1984;15(2):329–335.

43. Willmore LJ, Hiramatsu M, Kochi H, Mori A. Formation of superoxide radicals after FeC_{13} injection into rat isocortex. *Brain Res*. 1983;277(2):393–396.

44. Schettini A, Lippman HR, Walsh EK. Attenuation of decompressive hypoperfusion and cerebral edema by superoxide dismutase. *J Neurosurg*. 1989;71:578–587.

45. Muizelaar JP, Marmarou A, Young HF, et al. Improving the outcome of severe head injury with the oxygen radical scavenger polyethylene glycol-conjugated superoxide dismutase: A Phase II trial. *J Neurosurg*. 1993;78:375–382.

46. Salazar AM, Brown HR, Schwab K, Grafman J. The Vietnam Head Injury Study: Background and overview of results. In: Dagi TF, George ED, eds. *Penetrating Head Injury*. Boston: Little Brown; in press.

47. Salazar AM, Grafman JH, Vance SC, Weingartner H, Dillon JD, Ludlow C. Consciousness and amnesia after penetrating head injury: Neurology and anatomy. *Neurology*. 1986;36:178–187.

48. Wolfe J, Wine P, Grafman J, Salazar AM. Brain-behavior interaction in assessment of posttraumatic stress disorder (PTSD) in veterans with penetrating head injuries. International Neuropsychological Society, Orlando, Florida, February, 1990.

49. Keane TM, Malloy PF, Jackson JA. Empirical development of an MMPI subscale for the assessment of combat-related posttraumatic stress disorder. *J Consult Clin Psychol*. 1984;52:888–891.

50. Rutherford WH. Post concussion syndrome: Relationship to acute neurological indices, individual differences, and circumstances of injury. In: Levin HS, Eisenberg HM, Benton AL, eds. *Mild Head Injury*. New York: Oxford University Press; 1989: 217–228.

51. Gronwall D, Wrightson P. Delayed recovery after minor head injury. *Lancet*. 1974;2:605–609.

52. Stuss DT, Ely P, Hugenholtz H, et al. Subtle neuropsychological deficits in patients with good recovery after closed head injury. *Neurosurgery*. 1985;17(1):41–47.

53. Levin HS, Mattis S, Ruff RM, et al. Neurobehavioral outcome following minor head injury: A three-center study. *J Neurosurg*. 1987;66:234–243.

54. Barth JT, Alves WM, Ryan TV, et al. Mild head injury in sports: Neuropsychological sequelae and recovery of function. In: Levin HS, Eisenberg HM, Benton AG, eds. *Mild Head Injury*. New York: Oxford University Press; 1989: 257–275.

55. Kelly R, Smith BN. Post-traumatic syndrome; another myth discredited. *J R Soc Med*. 1981;74(4):275–277.

56. Miller H. Accident neurosis. *Br Med J*. 1961;April 1:919–925, 992–998.

57. Dikmen SS, Temkin N, Armsden G. Neuropsychological recovery: Relationship to psychosocial functioning and post concussional complaints. In: Levin HS, Eisenberg HM, Benton AL, eds. *Mild Head Injury*. New York: Oxford University Press; 1989: 229–241.

58. Wrightson P. Management of disability and rehabilitation services after mild head injury. In: Levin HS, Eisenberg HM, Benton AL, eds. *Mild Head Injury*. New York: Oxford University Press; 1989: 245–256.

59. Brooke MM, Questad KA, Patterson DR, Bashok KS. Agitation and restlessness after closed head injury: A prospective study of 100 consecutive admissions. *Arch Phys Med Rehabil*. 1992;73:320–323.

60. Goldberg E, Antin SP, Gerstman LS, Hughes JEO, Mattis S. Retrograde amnesia: Possible role of mesencephalic reticular activation in long-term memory. *Science*. 1981;213:1392–1394.

61. Kapur N, Ellison D, Smith MP, McLellan DL, Burrows EH. Focal retrograde amnesia following bilateral temporal lobe pathology. *Brain*. 1992;115:73–85.

62. Weinstein EA, Marvin SL, Keller NAJK. Amnesia as a language pattern. *Arch Gen Psychiatry*. 1962;6:259–270.

63. Sanders HI, Warrington EK. Retrograde amnesia in organic amnesic patients. *Cortex*. 1975;11:397–400.

64. Spiegel H, Spiegel D. *Trance and Treatment*. New York: Basic Books; 1978: 297.

65. Weinstein EA. Linguistic aspects of amnesia and confabulation. *J Psychiatr Res*. 1971;8:439–444.

66. Weinstein EA, Kahn RL. *Denial of Illness: Symbolic and Physiological Aspects*. Springfield, Ill: Charles C Thomas; 1955.

67. Weinstein EA, Lyerly OG. Confabulation following brain injury: It's analogues and sequelae. *Arch Gen Psychiatry*. 1968;18:348–354.

68. Weinstein EA, Kahn RL, Malitz S. Confabulation as a social process. *Psychiatry*. 1956;19:383–396.

69. Paterson A, Zangwill OL. Recovery of spatial orientation in the post-traumatic confusional state. *Brain*. 1944;67:54–68.

70. Weinstein EA, Kahn RL. Patterns of disorientation in organic brain disease. *J Neuropathol Clin Neurol*. 1951;1(3):214–225.

71. Levin AS, O'Donnel VM, Grossman RG. The Galveston Orientation and Amnesia Test: A practical scale to assess cognition after head injury. *J Nerv Ment Dis*. 1979;167:675–684.

72. Pick A. Clinical studies:III. On reduplicative paramnesia. *Brain*. 1903;26:260–267.

73. Head H. *Aphasia and Kindred Disorders*. Cambridge, England: Cambridge University Press; 1926.

74. Weston MS, Whitlock FA. The Capgras Syndrome following head injury. *Br J Psychiatry*. 1971;119:25–31.

75. Alexander MP, Stuss DT, Benson DF. Capgras Syndrome: A reduplicative phenomenon. *Neurology*. 1979;29:334–339.

76. Staton RD, Brumback RA, Wilson H. Reduplicative paramnesia: A disconnection syndrome of memory. *Cortex*. 1982;18:23–35.

77. Weinstein EA, Burnham DL. Reduplication and the Syndrome of Capgras. *Psychiatry*. 1991;54:78–88.

78. Weinstein EA, Kahn RL, Sugarman LA. Ludic behavior in patients with brain disease. *J Hillside Hosp* 1954;3:98–106.

79. Levin HS, Goldstein FC. Neurobehavioral aspects of traumatic brain injury. In: Bach-y-Rita, ed. *Traumatic Brain Injury*. New York: Demos; 1989.

80. Mesulam MM. A cortical network for directed attention and unilateral neglect. *Ann Neurol*. 1981;10:309–325.

81. Mesulam MM. *Principles of Behavioral Neurology*. Philadelphia, Pa: FA Davis; 1985.

82. Spitz HH. Note on immediate memory for digits: Invariance over the years. *Psychol Bull*. 1972;78:183–185.

83. Hodges JR, McCarthy RA. Autobiographical amnesia resulting from bilateral paramedian thalamic infarction. *Brain*. 1993;116:921–940.

84. Rey A. *L'examen Clinique en Psychologie*. Paris, France: Presses Universitaires de France; 1970.

85. Goodglass H, Quadfasel F, Timberlake W. Phrase length and the type and severity of aphasia. *Cortex*. 1964;1:133–153.

86. Weinstein EA, Kahn RL. Nonaphasic misnaming (paraphasia) in organic brain disease. *AMA Arch Neurol Psychiatry* [superseded in part by *Arch Neurol* and *Arch Gen Psychiatry*]. 1952;67:72–79.

87. Eslinger PJ, Damasio AR. Severe disturbance of higher cognition after bilateral frontal lobe ablation. *Neurology*. 1985;35:1731–1741.

88. Stuss DT, Benson DF. *The Frontal Lobes*. New York: Raven Press; 1986.

89. Shallice T, Burgess PW. Deficits in strategy application following frontal lobe damage in man. *Brain*. 1991;114:727–741.

90. Salazar AM. Penetrating war injuries of the basal forebrain: Neurology and cognition. *Neurology*. 1986;36(4):459–465.

91. Salazar AM, Grafman JH, Vance SC, Weingartner H, Dillon JD, Ludlow C. Unconsciousness and amnesia following penetrating head injury: Neurology and anatomy. *Neurology*. 1986;36:178–187.

92. Levin HS, Grossman RG, Rose JE, Teasdale G. Long-term neuropsychological outcome of closed head injury. *J Neurosurg*. 1979;50:412–422.

93. Prigitano GP. *Neuropsychological Rehabilitation after Brain Injury*. Baltimore, Md: The Johns Hopkins Press; 1986:19–22, 36–38, 41, 71, 109.

94. Goldstein K. *Aftereffects of Brain Injury in War*. New York: Grune and Stratton; 1942: 255.

95. Meltzer H. Multiple roles and actions of serotonin systems. *J Clin Psychiatry*. 1991;52(12)(supplement):3.

96. Dubovsky SL. Generalized anxiety disorder: New concepts and psychopharmacologic therapies. *J Clin Psychiatry*. 1990;51(1)(supplement):3–10.

97. Lishman WA. *Organic Psychiatry*. Oxford, England: Blackwell Scientific Publications; 1987.

98. Saran AS. Depression after minor closed head injury: Role of dexamethasone suppression test and antidepressants. *J Clin Psychiatry*. 1985;46:335–338.

99. Kreutzer JS, Zasler ND. Psychosexual consequences of traumatic brain injury: Methodology and preliminary findings. *Brain Inj*. 1989;3(2):177–186.

100. Robinson RG, Kubos KL, Starr LB, Rao K, Price TR. Mood disorders in stroke patients. *Brain*. 1984;107:81–93.

101. Sinyor D, Jacques P, Kaloupek DG, Becker R, Goldenberg M, Coopersmith H. Poststroke depression and lesion localization. *Brain*. 1986;109:537–546.

102. Gainotti G. Emotional behavior and hemispheric side of lesion. *Cortex*. 1972;8:41–55.

103. Coccaro EF, Sieve LJ, Klar HM, et al. Serotonergic studies in patients with affective and personality disorders. *Arch Gen Psychiatry*. 1989;46:587–599.

104. Mayberg HS, Robinson RG, Wong DF, et al. PET imaging of cortical S2 serotonin receptors after stroke: Lateralized changes and relation to depression. *Am J Psychiatry*. 1988;145:937–943.

105. Jorge RE, Robinson RG, Arndt SV, Forrester AW, Geisler F, Starkstein SE. Comparison between acute- and delayed-onset depression following traumatic brain injury. *J Neuropsychiatry Clin Neurosci*. 1993;5(1):43–49.

106. Shukla S, Cook BL, Sukdeb M, Godwin C, Miller MG. Mania following head trauma. *Am J Psychiatry*. 1987;144:93–96.

107. Starkstein SE, Boston JD, Robinson RG. Mechanisms of mania after brain injury: 12 case reports and review of literature. *J Nerv Ment Dis*. 1988;176:87–100.

108. Starkstein SE, Mayberg HS, Berthier ML, et al. Mania after brain injury: Neuroradiological and metabolic findings. *Ann Neurol*. 1990;27:652–659.

109. Rodin EA. Psychomotor epilepsy and aggressive behavior. *Arch Gen Psychiatry*. 1973;28:210–213.

110. Mathiesen G. Pathology of temporal lobe foci. In: Penry JK, Daly DD, eds. *Complex Partial Seizures and Their Treatment*. New York: Raven Press; 1975: 163–181.

111. Delgado-Escueta AV, Mattson RH, King L, et al. The nature of aggression during epileptic seizures. *N Engl J Med*. 1981;305:711–716.

112. Hauser WA, Hesdorffer DC. *Epilepsy: Frequency, Causes and Consequences*. New York: Demos Publications; 1990: 253–255.

113. Virkkunen M, Nuutila A, Huusko S. Brain injury and criminality: A retrospective study. *Dis Nerv Syst*. 1977;38(11):907–908.

114. Yudofsky SC, Silver JM, Jackson MD, Endicott J, Williams D. The Overt Aggression Scale for the objective rating of verbal and physical aggression. *Am J Psychiatry*. 1986;143:35–39.

115. Meyer A. The anatomical facts and clinical varieties of traumatic insanity. *Am J Insanity* [now *Am J Psychiatry*]. 1903;60:373–441.

116. Lobova LP. The role of trauma in the evolution of schizophrenia. *Zh Nevropatol Psikhiatr*. 1960;60:1187–1192.

117. Achté KA, Hillbom E, Aalberg V. Psychoses following war brain injuries. *Acta Psychiatr Scand*. 1969;45:1–18.

118. Dawson K, Bagley CR. Schizophrenia-like psychosis associated with organic disorders of the central nervous system. In: Herrington RN, ed. Current Problems in Neuropsychiatry. *Br J Psychiatry*. 1969;Special Publication:113–184.

119. Hillbom E. Schizophrenia-like psychoses after brain trauma. *Acta Psychiatr Scand*. 1951;Suppl. 60:36–47.

120. Achté K, Jarho L, Kyykka T, Vesterinen E. Paranoid disorders following war brain damage. *Psychopathology*. 1991;24:309–315.

121. Levine DN, Finklestein S. Delayed psychoses after right temporoparietal stroke or trauma: Relation to epilepsy. *Neurology*. 1982;32:267–273.

122. Jones FD. Newer uses of psychotropic drugs. *Med Bull US Army Europe*. 1986;43(4):3–8.

123. Ghostine SY, Comair YG, Turner DM, Kassell NF, Azar CG. Phenoxybenzamine in the treatment of causalgia: Report of 40 cases. *J Neurosurg*. 1984;60:1263–1268.

124. Feeney DM, Sutton RL. Catecholamines and recovery of function after brain damage. In: Stein DG, Sabel BA, eds. *Pharmacological Approaches to the Treatment of Central Nervous System Injury*. New York: Plenum Press; 1988: 121–142.

125. Eichelman B. Aggressive behavior: From laboratory to clinic—Quo Vadis? *Arch Gen Psychiatry*. 1992;49:488–492.

126. Tardiff K. The current state of psychiatry in the treatment of violent patients. *Arch Gen Psychiatry*. 1992;49:493–499.

127. Yudofsky S, Williams D, Gorman J. Propranolol in the treatment of rage and violent behavior in patients with chronic brain syndromes. *Am J Psychiatry*. 1981;138:218–220.

128. Silver M, Yudofsky SC, Hales RE. Neuropsychiatric aspects of traumatic brain injury. In: Hales RE, Yudofsky SC, eds. *Textbook of Neuropsychiatry*. Washington, DC: APA; 1987:179–187.

129. Marotta RF, Logan N, Potegal M, Glusman N, Gardner EL. Dopamine agonists induce recovery from surgically-induced septal rage. *Nature*. 1977;269:513–515.

130. Feeney DM, Gonzalez A, Law WA. Amphetamine, Haloperidol and experience interact to affect rate of recovery after motor cortex injury. *Science*. 1982;217:855–857.

131. Stern SM. Cranio-cerebral injured patients: A psychiatric clinical description. *Scand J Rehabil Med*. 1978;10:7–10.

132. Haas JF, Cope N. Neuropharmacologic management of behavioral sequelae in head injury. A case report. *Arch Phys Med Rehabil*. 1985;66:472–474.

133. Evans RW, Gualtieri CT, Patterson D. Treatment of chronic closed head injury with psychostimulant drugs-a controlled case study and an appropriate evaluation procedure. *J Nerv Ment Dis*. 1987;175(2):106–110.

134. Gualtieri CT, Evans RW. Stimulant treatment for the neurobehavioral sequelae of traumatic brain injury. *Brain Inj*. 1988;2:273–290.

135. Lipper S, Tuckman MM. Treatment of chronic post-traumatic organic brain syndrome with dextroamphetamine. *J Nerv Ment Dis*. 1976;162:366–371.

136. Schwab K, Grafman J, Salazar AM, Kraft JK. Residual impairments and work status 15 years after head injury: Report from the Vietnam Head Injury Study. *Neurology*. 1993;43:95–103.

137. Kraft J, Schwab K, Salazar AM, Brown HR. Occupational and educational achievements of head injured Vietnam veterans at 15-year follow-up. *Arch Phys Med Rehabil*. 1993;74:596–601.

138. Weinstein EA, Lyerly OG. Language behavior during recovery from brain injury as predictive of later adjustment. *Trans Am Neurol Assoc*. 1968;93:292–294.

139. Levin HS, Grossman RG. Behavioral sequelae of closed head injury: A quantitative study. *Arch Neurol*. 1978;35:720–777.

140. Brooks N, Symington C, Beattie A, Campsie L, Bryden J, McKinlay W. Alcohol and other predictors of cognitive recovery after severe head injury. *Brain Inj*. 1989;3(3):235–246.

141. Sparadeo FR, Gill D. Effects of prior alcohol use on head injury recovery. *J Head Trauma Rehabil* 1989;4(1):75–82.

142. Brooks DN, McKinlay W. Behavioural change after severe blunt head injury—a relative's view. *J Neurol Neurosurg Psychiatry*. 1983;46:336–344.

143. Gainotti G. Confabulation of denial in senile dementia: An experimental study. *Psychiatr Clin (Basel)*. 1975; 8(3):99–108.

144. Levine DN, Calvanio R, Rinn WE. The pathogenesis of anosognosia for hemiplegia. *Neurology*. 1991;41:1770–1781.

145. Weinstein EA, Kahn RL, Morris GO. Delusions about children following brain injury. *J Hillside Hosp*. 1956;5:290–300.

146. Weinstein EA, Kahn RL. Patterns of sexual behavior following brain injury. *Psychiatry*. 1961;24:60–78.

Chapter 14

DISABLING AND DISFIGURING INJURIES

EDWIN A.WEINSTEIN, M.D.*

**Consultant in Neurology, National Naval Medical Center, Bethesda, Maryland; Consultant in Psychiatry, Walter Reed Army Medical Center, Washington, D.C.; and Formerly Chief, Fifth Army Neuropsychiatric Center (World War II)*

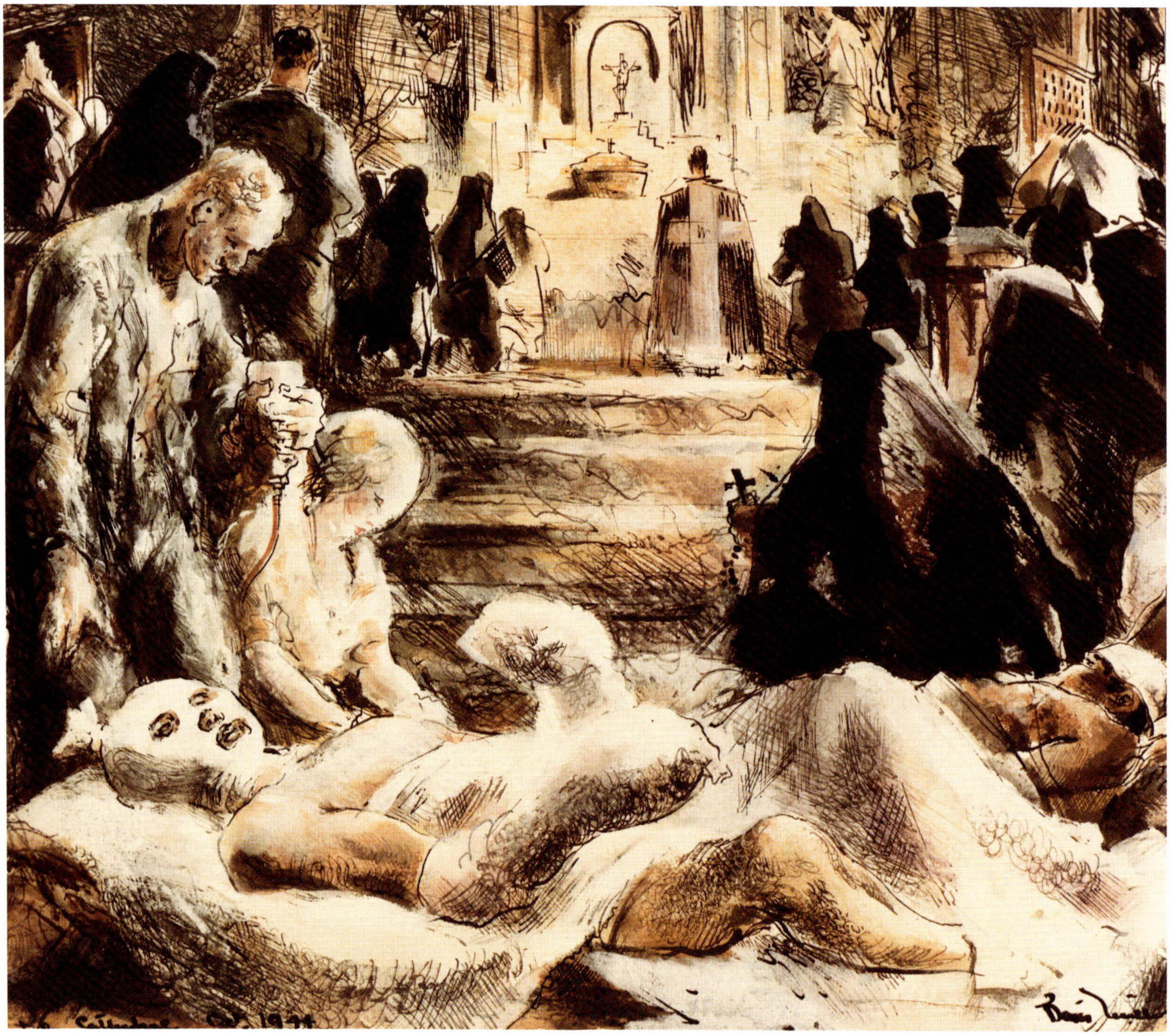

Barse Miller *Requiem Mass* 1944

Barse Miller was an artist for Life Magazine before he enlisted in the U.S. Army in 1943. He served with the Corps of Engineers before becoming the War Art Leader of the Combat Art Section. In this watercolor, Miller portrays the interior of a church in World War II that has been converted to a makeshift hospital to care for combat-injured soldiers. The man in the foreground has sustained wounds to his hands and face, the two areas most associated with visible expression of emotions. These are among the injuries that soldiers fear the most—those that leave them permanently disfigured or disabled or both.

Art: Courtesy of US Center of Military History, Washington, DC.

INTRODUCTION

This chapter takes up the neurological and physiological disturbances and the behavioral changes that follow major amputations, spinal cord injury with paralysis, facial disfigurement from missile wounds and burns, blindness, and mutilating and castrating wounds of the external male genitalia. Changing conditions of warfare and the greater explosive power of weapons have raised the proportion of some types of wounds, and increased the incidence of multiple injuries. Improved methods of evacuation and the development of new surgical techniques have resulted in the survival of many men who previously would have died. Whereas the combat zone hospital mortality rate in World War II was 3.3%, the rate in Korea was 2.4%, and that in Vietnam 1.8%.[1] The changing nature of future combat actions, to include nation assistance, foreign internal defense, and operations other than war (OOTW), broadens the range of patients that may be seen.

Survivors of disabling and disfiguring injuries share a number of problems. Along with their physical limitations, they experience an altered body image, lowered self-esteem, and changes in their personal relationships. Some bear the social stigma associated with crippling and deformity. It is only since World War II that these features have been recognized and specialized programs set up for amputees, paraplegics, and the burned and the blind. Sustaining a combat wound does not preclude the development of post-traumatic stress disorder (PTSD), and depression, denial, and drug abuse pose major problems in therapy. While the management of each type of disability will be considered separately, overall principles of management are presented.

AMPUTATION

Amputation of a limb as a result of an injury in combat has profound and special behavioral consequences. These are the emotional reactions to the initial trauma, the problems of coping with the motor disability, the alterations of body image caused by the loss of a previously healthy arm or leg, and the neurophysiological and psychological aspects of phantom limb phenomena.

Lower-limb amputations are much more common than amputations of the upper extremity; in Vietnam these wounds were caused predominantly by antipersonnel land mines and booby traps, and might extend to involve the scrotum, buttocks, and abdomen. The limbs might be severed by the injury, or a surgical amputation was carried out, usually within hours of the initial trauma. In cases in which attempts were made to preserve a shredded limb the amputation might not be performed until days or weeks later.

Behavioral Effects

Behavioral disturbances are not usually a problem in the early postoperative period over which the combating of infection, the maintenance of metabolic balance, and the management of other injuries are the paramount considerations. Also, newly wounded soldiers are apt to be euphoric, glad to be alive, and thankful that their injuries were not more severe. Even at this early stage, however, what the emergency room, surgical, and ward staff say to the patient (or to each other within hearing distance) is important even if they think the patient is unconscious. Depression may follow elation, but it is mainly when the patient encounters the stresses of further treatment and recovery, and begins to realize the extent of his physical and social limitations, that emotional problems arise. The physical stresses include surgical revisions of an infected, often painful, stump, learning to use a temporary prosthesis, and experiencing the fatigue caused by alterations in posture, balance, and locomotion. Patients worry how they will be accepted by their family and community, and whether they will be able to make a living and lead a normal life. They are concerned with physical attractiveness and sexual ability.

Anxiety and Depression

Anxiety and depression are the most common forms of emotional distress. These states are experienced as feelings of tension, sleep disturbances, somatic complaints, phobias such as fears of falling or otherwise injuring the amputation stump, irritability, outbursts of anger, and feelings of worthlessness and social withdrawal. The circumstances of the initial injury are a factor in that soldiers who have undergone a particularly traumatic experience involving the death or mutilation of others are more severely stressed.

Case Study 1: Lord Nelson at Tenerife

Admiral Lord Nelson, England's greatest naval hero, had his right arm amputated above the elbow following a wound sustained in an attack on the Spanish fortress of Tenerife in 1797. The assault failed with heavy British casualties, largely because of Nelson's overconfidence induced by his contempt for the Spaniards, his faith in Providence, and his belief in his own magical qualities of leadership. He was initially elated but several days later he wrote in left-handed script to his superior, Lord St. Vincent, "I am become a burden to my friends and useless to my country. When I leave your command I become dead to the world; I go hence and am no more seen. I hope you will give me a frigate to convey the remains of my carcass to England."[2(p145)] The wound healed but Nelson continued to experience phantom pain for the rest of his life.[3]

Comment: Lord Nelson believed that the phantom fingers of his amputated arm provided a direct proof of the existence of the soul.

In World War II it was observed that amputees who had been injured through their own negligence, or while they were absent without leave (AWOL), were more apt to be depressed and have disciplinary problems.[4] Some patients deal with the stresses and boredom of hospitalization by resort to alcohol or other drugs.

Denial

Denial is the most prominent defense mechanism. Patients do not deny the actual loss of a limb unless there is brain dysfunction such as might result from an associated head injury, or a toxic or metabolic encephalopathy. Amputees may deny phantom sensations for fear of being thought mentally abnormal. Denial may be expressed in dreams in which the patient sees himself with his limbs intact or as having sustained some lesser damage such as a fracture. An occasional patient expresses the idea that his limb will grow back or that he can get a transplant. Some have the unrealistic expectation that an artificial limb will allow them to function as well as they did before they were injured. Most commonly, patients deny concern, depression, and other negative feelings. Some have a paranoid reaction and blame the staff and hospital equipment for their less than satisfactory progress. Amputees may manifest denial by not recognizing the need for rehabilitative procedures. Others offer a show of bravado, and boast of their physical and sexual prowess. They may engage in reckless behavior such as racing wheelchairs down hospital corridors.[5] Preoccupation with religion may become a form of denial as patients avoid discussion of their problems by engaging in theological speculations.[4,6]

Denial appears on both conscious and unconscious levels. It may function temporarily as an adaptive mechanism but, if continued over time, poses barriers to treatment. It keeps the soldier from coming to terms with his loss and prevents the development of close personal relationships with other patients and staff; it is often followed by depression.

Phantom Limb

Phenomenology

The phantom limb, the experience of sensation in the severed extremity, is virtually universal. The phantom may be so mild that the amputee is aware of it only when his attention is directed toward it; in other cases it is more vivid. The phantom may originally duplicate the normal limb, but over time differs in size, sensation, shape, position, and completeness—in the case of an amputation at the shoulder, there may be a gap between the shoulder stump and the phantom elbow. The foot and hand are felt most prominently. Sensations range from a not unpleasant tingling and feelings of warmth, cold, and heaviness, to cramping, twisting, burning, or lancinating pain. The phantom usually appears immediately after amputation, so that patients on awakening from anesthesia do not believe that the limb has been removed, but it occasionally comes on later. Most phantoms begin to fade within weeks, with sporadic later occurrences over a period of years.[7,8] Fading of the phantom, which is felt more vividly in the upper extremity, may be associated with telescoping, the sensation that the fingers or toes, or hand or foot are attached directly to the stump. Chronically painful phantoms, however, do not telescope.

Pain occurs in both the stump and the phantom. Stump pain is almost always present. It is usually severe immediately after the operation and subsides in a few days. If it persists, then there is likely a problem with the stump, such as infection or poor blood supply. Recurrence may often be traced to local abnormalities such as bone spurs, deficient soft tissue padding, difficulties with the prosthesis, and alterations in gait and posture.[9] Phantom pain is much more variable. Whereas the phantom itself appears immediately, the pain may not come on for months or years after the amputation, with disagreeable feelings replacing the original benign sensations.[8] Phantom pain is more likely to be present in persons who have had pain prior to operation.[10] The pain may be described as similar in type and location to that previously experienced, with even the limb in the same distorted position.[11,12]

Somatosensory memories, most of which are painful, may be multimodal involving not only pain, but tactile, visual, motor, and even olfactory components. Riddoch[7] described the case of a soldier whose arm was blown off by the premature explosion of a bomb that he was holding. In the painful phantom, his hand was still grasping the bomb. A phantom reported by Henderson and Smythe[8] included the sensation of blood trickling down the limb. A soldier whose leg was amputated in the Italian campaign of World War II could still feel and visualize the fragments of his shattered bones. Some somatosensory memories are benign as in the instance of the man who reexperienced the sensation of a bandage being applied to his wounds, but most are associated with high levels of anxiety and emotion.[12]

Phantoms, painful and nonpainful, may appear without apparent cause, or they may be brought on by a wide variety of perceptual, cognitive, or affective experiences. Sensory stimulation of the stump and elsewhere on the body or face can produce or accentuate a phantom, as may pain from an arthritic shoulder or an anginal attack. Visual experiences can elicit a phantom, as in a case described by Varna, Lai, and Mukherjee,[13] in which a man, after an upper-limb amputation, would feel his ring on an absent finger when he saw someone wearing a ring on the corresponding digit. Micturition, defecation, yawning, and sexual activity may occasionally elicit phantom sensations and images. A phantom may be evoked by thinking of it, and a sense of movement created by willing it. Bailey and Moersch[11] reported a patient who related that while his amputated arm was being burned at his request, he had felt the ashes gradually dropping from the phantom. Riddoch[7] described an amputee in whom pleasant excitement caused his phantom to tingle along with the rest of his body. When, however, his mind was fully occupied, he was as unaware of the phantom as he was of the rest of the body. Episodes of phantom pain can be precipitated or intensified by emotional stress.

Neurophysiological Aspects

Observations that could not be explained by current neurophysiological concepts, and the failure of surgery to help phantom pain more than temporarily, led to the belief that phantom limb phenomena were of psychological origin, and various theories were advanced. One view was that the symptoms were caused by the amputee's narcissistic reluctance to accept the reality of his physical mutilation—in essence a denial. Another was that the phantom represented mourning for the lost limb.[15] A number of the patients studied by Kolb[16] had had a close emotional attachment to another amputee, and pain was thought to express the patient's feelings of hostility and guilt toward persons with whom he identified as mutilated or mutilating, and on whom he was dependent. It was also believed that amputees who developed phantom pain had a high incidence of premorbid psychopathology.[16–18]

Psychological, cultural, and emotional factors enter into the perception of pain, but recent psychological and neurophysiological investigations have not yielded evidence that phantom phenomena are psychogenic. Pain is often precipitated by stress and associated with anxiety and depression; and, patients with adjustment problems are apt to focus on pain as the source of their discontents. In World War II, amputees referred to a psychiatrist for disturbances in behavior or disciplinary infractions were more likely to complain of pain than those who sought help voluntarily.[19] Such observations, however, do not mean that pain, per se, is necessarily of psychogenic origin. Patients with chronic pain, however, whether of organic or functional origin, have high scores for "neuroticism" on the Eysenck Personality Inventory, and are notoriously difficult to treat.[20]

Older neurophysiological theories of phantom limb involved the action of afferent fibers from the stump on spinal and supraspinal cells and the sending of abnormal impulses to cortical sensory areas. Most hypotheses focused on pain rather than other sensory disturbances and, in particular, did not offer an explanation of telescoping. More recent formulations have utilized the evidence of brain plasticity, that is, the manner in which the brain can modify its connections in response to experience, and the way in which it can reorganize function after damage.

In World War II, a study of amputees showed that the thresholds for two-point discrimination on the skin of a stump were consistently lower than those in the homologous area of the sound limb. This suggested that there had been a central cortical reorganization of function, in which the stump had taken on features of the amputated hand or foot.[21] Subsequent studies also showed lower thresholds (ie, finer discrimination for light, touch, and point localization). Furthermore, accuracy in point localization was significantly influenced by telescoping, in that it was most efficient in above elbow amputees who perceived their phantom to be within the stump.[22]

The work of Merzenich and his associates[23–25] has established a basis for the understanding of the mechanism of cortical reorganization after peripheral trauma. It was found that after amputation of a finger in the adult monkey, the cortical area that had been deprived of its original input could be activated by touching the adjacent fingers, and even by stimulation of other points on the body and face, in the way a phantom in man can be elicited by a stimulus on the stump and elsewhere. The perceived length, size, and shape of the phantom may thus be a peripheral marker of the extent to which input from the stump and other regions has taken over cortical areas originally driven by input from the amputated limb. Plasticity of cortical reorganization is also determined by the use of the digit, paralleling the observation in man that the length and shape of the phantom changes after extensive use of the stump. If a stump is surgically cleft and the two parts used as a forceps, patients may report a cleft phantom hand.[26] Severe pain prevents the use of a prosthesis, and may contribute to the failure of telescoping to develop in such patients.

Phantom-limb phenomena also have a temporal dimension in that preamputation sensations, particularly painful ones, may be reproduced in vivid detail. Katz and Melzack[12] emphasize that the patient not only remembers that he had pain but has the direct experience of pain. Pain, or stress, or both appear to be crucial for the development of somatosensory memories because most of them are painful. The authors suggest that sensitized cells in the spinal cord activate the structures in the brain which subserve sensory memories, a process resembling the flashbacks of PTSD. The highly emotionally laden features of multimodal phantom representations may relate to the fact that multimodal association areas, rather than the primary unimodal cortical sensory areas, are interconnected with the paralimbic regions concerned with the affective coloring of experience.

Treatment

There has been an apparent decline in the incidence of severe and enduring phantom pain since World War II. Prior literature and reports of observations early in the war described suffering so intense as to lead to serious depression, morphine addiction, and suicide. A noted neurosurgeon, James C. White, recommended surgical intervention in amputees with severe phantom pain of more than 6 months duration before psychic changes became irreversible.[27] Unfortunately, procedures such as sympathetic block, chordotomy, tractotomy at medullary and midbrain levels, and cortical parietal ablation failed to provide lasting relief. Revisions of the stump for ulceration, necrosis, and neuromas might relieve local stump pain but did not, as a rule, help phantom pain.

More recent studies present a more favorable picture. A 1955 review of 400 amputees treated at the U.S. Navy Amputee Rehabilitation Center in Oakland, California, the majority of whom were battle casualties, found that 94% were employed and wearing their prostheses.[28] Painful phantoms were rare among British amputee prisoners of war (POWs) in Germany in World War II.[8] A long-term follow-up of Finnish amputee veterans of the wars with the Soviet Union (1939–1946) showed persisting debilitating pain in only 2% of subjects.[29] No painful phantoms were encountered among Vietnam amputees treated at Valley Forge General Hospital in Pennsylvania.[6] Two thirds of Israeli amputees of the Yom Kippur War of 1973 had phantom pain, but in the great majority of cases it decreased in intensity and disappeared after a few weeks or months.[30]

The method of study influences the evaluation of phantom pain. A 1979 poll of U.S. medical schools, Veterans Administration (VA) hospitals, pain clinics, and pain specialists found that 58% of respondents who had treated amputees reported no experience with phantom pain.[31] A mailed questionnaire, however, sent by the same investigators to 5,000 U.S. veteran amputees yielded an incidence of pain in 78%, and 85% of subjects who reported pain experienced it for 6 or more hours a day. However, 90% of the respondents were able to use their prostheses more than 8 hours a day.[32,33]

The decline in the frequency of severe chronic pain may be attributed to a number of advances in medicine stemming from World War II. These include the shortening of the period between wounding and hospitalization, better surgical techniques, a broader spectrum of antibiotics and analgesics, recognition of the special behavioral problems of amputees with the setting up of amputee centers, and changes in the attitudes of society toward the handicapped.

The treatment of an amputee begins prior to surgery. It is important to control pain and avoid unnatural positions of the injured limb, and to operate as soon as feasible to diminish the likelihood of painful somatosensory memories. The patient should be told what to expect in the way of phantom phenomena. If there is pain after surgery, its relationship to tension and stress should be discussed with the patient. Maximum use of his prothesis should be encouraged. He should be urged to keep a log, so that any correlation with weather, diet, alcohol, smoking, or a particular type of stress can be noted. Sources of referred pain into the phantom—from pathology in the stump, a faulty prosthesis, an arthritic joint or an intervertebral disc abnormality—should be identified.

In the absence of specific precipitating factors, treatment of phantom pain can be very difficult, and none of the numerous methods that have been employed have been consistently efficacious. In World War II, Russell[34] reported that percussion or vibration of the stump alleviated pain. Measures that reduce tension and interrupt the pain-anxiety cycle, such as biofeedback and relaxation training, have been suggested.[35] An occasional patient benefits from self-hypnosis. Transcutaneous electrical nerve stimulation (TENS), a procedure based on a reported concordance between points of tenderness and skin conductance on the outer ear and pain in an extremity, is said to have resulted in a moderate reduction of phantom pain.[36]

Many medications have been used, and relief has been reported with the anticonvulsant, carbamazepine,[37] antidepressants used alone or in combination with other drugs,[38,39] phenothiazines,[40] and propranolol, a beta-blocker.[41,42] Such studies, however, have been poorly controlled with insufficient data for critical evaluation. Narcotic analgesics usually result in increasing dosage and drug dependence with poorer and poorer pain control and depression. Sedatives and hypnotics are not only ineffective in relieving phantom pain, but tend to be habit-forming and increase depression.[39]

The treatment of the amputee goes beyond the control of pain and extends into the broader behavioral area. In former years the emphasis was on the promotion of denial as amputees were encouraged to be optimistic and not give into their fears and doubts in the interest of maintaining good ward morale. Frank[6] noted that the objective of the hospital staff was to keep the patient so busy with activities that he did not have time to dwell on his problems. Staff also tended to give an overly rosy picture of what the prosthesis could accomplish. Interest by psychiatrists was discouraged on the grounds that it would stir up new problems or reactivate old ones.

Currently, there is more cooperation among surgeons, psychiatrists, nurses, and rehabilitation personnel. The amputee is given a realistic account of the difficulties he will encounter and asked to participate in his own treatment, as in the care of his stump. He is allowed to speak openly of his feelings, whether of powerlessness, shame, anger, or self-blame, and pass through the period of mourning for the dismembered part of his body, which is essential for the eventual acceptance of loss. Efforts are made to help the soldier incorporate the prosthesis into his body image, for example, by doing his exercises in front of a mirror rather than regarding it as a foreign object.

The amputee must acquire a new identity. This involves not only in some cases training for a new occupation, but new ways of thinking, feeling, acting, and relating to others. Actions that were once carried out automatically now require focused attention. The amputee must reevaluate himself and, if necessary, change old attitudes, notably those concerning physical attractiveness, masculinity or femininity, and self-sufficiency. If he persists in the belief that a physically handicapped person is also psychologically and socially inferior he is likely to perceive these attitudes in others.[43] The successful amputee must have qualities of concentration, flexibility, and sensitivity.

SPINAL CORD INJURIES

The systematic study of the behavioral aspects of spinal cord injuries (SCI) did not begin until World War II, as in World War I 80% of men with SCI died within a few weeks of injury.[44] Even with the advances in surgery, antibiotics, and methods of evacuation in World War II, the majority of patients arrived at hospitals in the United States suffering from decubitus ulcers, urinary tract infections, and malnutrition. It was largely through the work of Donald Munro and Ernest Bors in America and Sir Ludwig Guttmann in Great Britain that the humanitarian needs of paraplegics and quadriplegics were recognized and comprehensive spinal cord injury centers were established.

Neurological Aspects

Spinal cord transections vary in completeness and are classified according to the level of the lesion into cervical, thoracolumbar, and cauda equina types. The wounds are most often caused by shell fragments or bullets with the foreign bodies piercing the cord directly, or driving bone into the spinal canal. Blast injuries may produce intramedullary hemorrhages. Falls and vehicle accidents are other sources of injury. Alcohol exacerbates the neurochemical and behavioral effects of spinal cord trauma.[45] SCIs are commonly associated with abdominal and chest injuries, and with brain damage, especially with high cervical cord lesions. Shock, loss of blood, sepsis, stress hormonal responses, anoxia from respiratory embarrassment, and the administration of morphine for pain also contribute to impairment of brain function. Opioids apparently decrease spinal cord perfusion, and opioid receptor antagonists can reduce tissue damage following central nervous system trauma.[46]

There is no immediate intrinsic phenomenological awareness of disability and many patients sustaining acute SCIs initially deny or are unaware of their paralyses and sensory loss. Such anosognosia may persist for days or weeks. Heilporn and Noel[47] found that only 4 of 40 paraplegics were immediately and spontaneously aware of their deficits. Others realized that their legs were paralyzed and had lost feeling when they tried to move them, and some recognized their disabilities after they were demonstrated on a neurological examination. Anosognosia is more marked and more enduring in patients who have been unconscious and who have gone through a period of amnesia and disorientation. Quadriplegics show more denial/unawareness because of the more frequent association with brain damage. Another factor in early unawareness of paralysis is that patients may be confused by phantom sensations. Paraplegics who have had an initial loss of consciousness may have the illusion that the lower part of their bodies have been amputated.[48]

As in the experience of amputees, phantom phenomena are common. Bors[49] found them in all of the 50 paraplegic veterans of World War II whom he studied. The most frequent abnormal sensations were paresthesias in the anesthetic limbs, and feelings that the legs were floating upward from the bed or frame, extended at the knees or ankles, and slightly flexed at the hips.[50] Other phantoms are more bizarre. Patients may feel that their legs have been cut off, and one described the feeling that blood was oozing from the stumps.[51] Another paraplegic felt as if he had an extra pair of legs that, at times, were tied up in knots.[52] If there is associated brain damage, the patient may have the persistent delusion that he has another pair of arms or legs.[53,54] In the absence of significant brain injury, phantoms usually disappear in a few weeks, except those resulting from cauda equina lesions. Unlike amputees, however, SCI patients do not experience telescoping, possibly because of inability to move their legs.

Toxic psychosis caused by sepsis from urinary tract infections and deep decubitus ulcers are rare when adequate treatment facilities are available.[55] However, brief episodes of delirium and agitated behavior may be associated with fever or occur after general anesthesia for operative procedures in the first few months after injury. Hypoxic episodes occurring during sleep in patients with high cervical cord lesions may contribute to cognitive impairment.[56]

Patients with high cervical cord lesions necessitating traction with tongs and neck and head immobilization may show manifestations of sensory deprivation.[57] They are lethargic, with little interest in food or surroundings, and in interviews they keep their eyes closed. They comprehend and retain orientation, but respond slowly. Alertness and eye contact can be restored by a tactile stimulus to the neck, but they may revert to the previous state until stimulated again. Hallucinations may occur. This condition usually disappears when the restraint is removed and the patient is helped to sit upright. Loss of spinal cord function produces many physical problems in addition to the paralysis. Laminectomy and surgical stabilization of the spine may be necessary followed by immobilization in a prone position on a Stryker frame for several weeks to avoid pressure sores. A study by Jacobson and Bors[58] found decubiti in almost half of men sustaining SCI in combat in Vietnam. There is impairment of bowel and bladder function, pain, leg spasms that may be very painful, and defective autonomic reflexes with reduced capacity for blood pressure regulation. Genitourinary complications include irritation from catheters, infection, calculosis, hydronephrosis, and epididymitis. Complete spinal cord transection may require an orchiectomy adding to the sense of emasculation. Insomnia may be a problem because of frequent turning on a frame and the diminished amount of REM (rapid eye movement) and deep sleep associated with cervical cord lesions.[56]

Behavioral Effects

Patients respond to the loss of control over their bodies and the overwhelming sense of helplessness and dependence in a number of ways. Some become childish and demanding while others withdraw and show little emotion. Some are hostile, others are anxious or depressed. Many express denial. Several models of the behavioral course of SCI patients have been offered. Guttmann[55] described a first stage of anxiety and regression, sometimes associated with negativistic behavior and provocative attitudes, followed by denial, and then by adjustment. Another proposed sequence is one of initial denial, succeeded by depression with grief and mourning, with eventual acceptance of disability.[59,60] However, not all patients get depressed. Others become depressed in response to some disappointment such as the failure of a laminectomy to clear up the paralysis. Patients may or may not express hostility or denial. Behavioral manifestations such as withdrawal and indifference can be interpreted as either depression or denial.

Depression

Estimates of the incidence and significance of depression vary. Some authors believe that it is normal for a severely disabled person to become depressed.[61] It has been stated that when a newly paralyzed person does not appear to be depressed he is denying his loss of function and its social implications.[60] Other observers have not found depression to be inevitable, and believe that the incidence has been exaggerated through the expectations of the hospital staff.[62] A prospective study[63] of 71 civilian patients followed through the acute and rehabilitative stages found that 14 fulfilled the criteria of the Diagnostic and Statistical Manual, 3rd edition, of the American Psychiatric Association (DSM-III)[64] for major depressive disorder, and that another 13 had transient periods of depressive mood. The time of onset of depression was from 3 to 40 weeks after injury. Remarkably, depressive disorders appeared with comparable frequency in paraplegics (17%) and quadriplegics (23%). Similarly, Lawson[65] showed that the level of cervical cord injury was not a factor in the incidence or severity of depression. These observations were made in civilian hospitals but there is no reason to believe that there would be different findings in military personnel. Thom and Von Salzen[66] noted no difference in the incidence or severity of depression in World War II veterans who sustained SCIs in combat and in those hurt in accidents.

While a period of grief and mourning is helpful in allowing the patient to work through his feelings of loss on the way to acceptance, prolonged depression has disastrous effects. Self-neglect is a frequent feature of depression. Such patients present with either angry, rebellious attitudes, or are withdrawn, indifferent, and overtly self-destructive.[67] They do not cooperate with the hospital staff, may refuse medication or other treatment, refuse to eat or maintain fluid intake or breathe deeply, and fail to attend to skin care or manage their catheters. They may demand unnecessary surgery and have alcohol or other drug problems.

Suicidal ideation is very common in the first days after injury but it rarely materializes.[55] Suicide, however, may be a problem later on and Hohmann[60] warns that it is a great mistake to assume that because a patient is disabled his incapacity will physically preclude his trying to kill himself. Suicidal intent should be suspected in patients with self-neglect who deny having ever having harbored thoughts of ending their lives.[56] A 20-year follow-up of veterans of World War II with traumatic myelopathies revealed suicide to be the third most common cause of death, ranking behind only renal failure and secondary amyloidosis.[68] The figure does not include other deaths involving self-destructive behavior such as alcoholism, smoking, and motor vehicle accidents.

Denial

Unless there is associated brain dysfunction, SCI does not result in classical anosognosia in the sense that the patient explicitly denies or is unaware of his paralysis, forgets that he cannot walk, or represents the disability in delusional fashion. Brain damage is produced by the injury, or by a toxic or metabolic encephalopathy. An investigation of fatal craniocerebral injuries, principally from motor vehicle crashes, noted that 46% of victims with spinal cord damage also had brain pathology.[69] Wilmot, Cope, Hall and Acker[70] identified four risk factors for brain dysfunction: (1) quadriplegia following a high deceleration accident, (2) loss of consciousness, (3) cortical or brain stem neurological signs, and (4) required respiratory support at the time of injury. Of patients with one or more risk factors, 64%

showed impairment on neuropsychological testing a median 48 days after injury.

Apart from classical anosognosia, denial is expressed in a number of ways. Unlike the amputee whose loss is visible, the SCI patient may cling to the hope that he will regain the function of his limbs through some new medicine or operation. A form of denial encountered by Guttmann[55] in young soldiers wounded in World War II was a defiant "we can take it" mentality, with rejection of advice and instruction by the hospital staff. Some patients are highly euphoric and joke about their problems. As amputees do, some engage in reckless behavior such as the wheelchair racing portrayed in the Marlon Brando movie, *The Men*. Others are indifferent and are not motivated to participate in self-care or rehabilitation. Denial of loss of sexual function may be shown in inappropriate boasting of sexual prowess and excessive interest in pornography.[71] Paranoid forms of denial are shown by patients who charge that newly discovered treatments are not being made available to them, or who blame paralysis on being kept on a Stryker frame.

It may be difficult to separate denial from hope and faith, and in the earliest stages it can be a help in survival. Denial, while it may make a patient more comfortable and provide a temporary solution to his problems, is ultimately maladaptive. It deprives him of the opportunity to grieve, prevents the formation of intimate relationships, and blocks rehabilitative efforts. Moreover, the collapse of a denial system is apt to be followed by depression.

Personality Factors

While no type of premorbid personality has been found to be predictive of adaptation to SCI, previous experience is significant. Social background, academic and vocational achievement, quality of interpersonal relationships, habitual modes of coping with stress, and the values that determine the meaning of the incapacity are all relevant.

Civilian patients with histories of sociopathic behavior, poor school and job records, drug abuse, and painful punishment in childhood were found to adjust poorly after SCI, with more depression and disruptive behavior.[59,72] Similarly, soldiers who have had problems with authority may find it difficult to establish a trusting relationship with the professional staff. Patients who have been well educated and have developed skills are better able to occupy themselves productively and plan for the future than those whose vocational abilities are limited and involve physical work. A study of the individual beliefs of SCI patients showed that those who believe that they exercised control over their lives and health were less depressed than those who thought that rewards and punishments resulted from chance, luck, fate, or the actions of powerful others.[73]

The meaning of the disability in terms of the person's value systems is highly significant. Some patients with pain are mainly concerned with what the pain means in regard to their health and prognosis, and are apt to refuse medication unless it serves some therapeutic purpose. Others react in terms of their current suffering and want relief. Patients who have needed physical activity, such as jogging, to ease tension, are apt to find the limitation of mobility particularly difficult to accept. Some feel that the disability means loss of manhood, and a loss of sexual attractiveness. Or, they may equate the incapacity with inferior status as a person, and a loss of love and respect. A soldier who has had an authoritarian religious upbringing may perceive in this injury a manifestation of God's will, and a punishment for sin.

Roberts,[74] from his experience in a rehabilitative facility, regards spontaneity, ability to show emotional experience, the holding of conventional but not fundamentalist or dogmatic religious beliefs, good contact with reality, and feelings of personal adequacy as predictive of good adjustment.

Treatment

The aims of treatment are: (*a*) managing of the initial state of impaired awareness, (*b*) motivating the patient to participate in self-care and rehabilitation, (*c*) addressing denial, and (*d*) dealing with the problems of pain, depression, and sexual dysfunction.

It is useful to point out to the patient that phantom sensations are normal and do not mean that he is losing his mind. The staff should avoid fostering denial unwittingly. A corpsman who might feel sorry for a soldier should not try to cheer him up by telling him that he will recover the use of his limbs. Similarly, a physician may believe that if the patient is given the facts of his situation, hope will be destroyed and that he will have no motive to work in therapy. Roberts[74] is of the opinion that loss of motivation, over time, is more often due to the patient's failure to achieve unrealistic goals based on misleading information. When should a patient be told of his prognosis? It should not be in the acute stage when he may have impaired brain function, or when he is too sick or uncomfortable for the information to matter. He should be told at the point at which he is able to retain information and participate in treatment. He should receive an explanation of SCI, and be told the reasons why procedures are being carried out and why it is important for him to attend to skin care, breathe deeply, and maintain fluid intake and nutrition.

Pain following SCI is of different types and degrees of severity. Pain in the area of the wound usually clears in a few weeks. Pain in the shoulders, elbows, and fingers of paraplegics may be due to tendinous and articular contracture, often caused by faulty positioning of the upper limbs following injury.[55] Radicular pain, along with hyperesthesia, results when damaged nerve roots are encased in an adhesive arachnoiditis, and is particularly severe, with a causalgic quality, in cauda equina lesions. Flexor leg spasms can be painful. Visceral pain that may be referred to anesthetic areas can occur because of distension or reflex activity of the bladder, colon, uterus, or ureter. Syringomyelic pain may develop in chronic cases as a consequence of cavitation in the spinal cord above the level of the lesion.[75]

Phantom sensations are not usually painful, but tingling, pressure, and burning sensations in areas below the level of the lesion are common and may be perceived as painful. The dysesthesias recede in most cases, but they can be long-lasting. While such central pain is not psychogenic, it is affected by emotional and attentional factors. It is also influenced by fatigue, weather, alcohol excess and other drug abuse, smoking, and pressure sores.[52,76] It is unlikely that a pressure sore causes pain by direct neural transmission, but the need to lie in a bed or on a frame for long periods contributes to depression. Moreover, depression may have led to self-neglect and the development of a bed sore.

Drugs can create problems in a number of ways. Patients may resort to marihuana and alcohol to relieve pain and boredom. The cord injury may exacerbate preexisting drug dependency. Insomnia may lead to excessive use of hypnotics, especially benzodiazepines.

Local pain responds to nonnarcotic analgesics, but radicular pain and central pain are much more difficult to treat. Some patients with radicular pain are helped by carbamazepine (Tegretol) or phenytoin (Dilantin) but in most chronic cases not even chordotomy gives permanent relief.[52] One must rely on directing the patient's attention away from his symptoms into other activities such as prevocational training and sports. If possible, the patient should be taught relaxation techniques and self-hypnosis. Anxiolytic or antidepressant drugs may be given if there is evidence that anxiety or depression is present.

Antidepressant drugs should be used when appropriate with great caution. Depression should be distinguished from sorrow, despair, and grief. It should also be differentiated from states of conservation-withdrawal in which patients weakened by long bed rest, intercurrent infections, and nutritional depletion are apathetic.[77] Drugs with anticholinergic effects can compromise the function of a neurogenic bladder, and those with alpha-adrenergic blocking can induce dangerous hypotension. Tricyclic antidepressants, and especially the nontricyclic, bupropion, can lower seizure threshold, a significant factor for patients with brain damage. Levin, Burtt, Levin, and Ginsberg[78] reported ventricular fibrillation in quadriplegic patients on therapeutic levels of imipramine. Of tricyclic antidepressants, desipramine and nortriptyline have the least alpha-blocking actions and relatively few anticholinergic effects. However, newer generations of antidepressants (fluoxetine, paroxetine, sertraline, bupropion) are virtually free of alpha-blocking, anticholinergic, and antihistamine effects. In treating psychotic states, haloperidol and piperazine have the fewest anticholinergic effects. They may, however, require the addition of anticholinergic agents (preferably amantadine) to prevent extrapyramidal syndromes, such as dystonia, pseudoparkinsonism, and akathisia. Stewart[57] notes that it is important to avoid drugs such as trazodone (Desyrel) which have soporific side effects, as vigilance is necessary for self-care. Electroconvulsive therapy should be considered in severe depression when rapid action is required. With anesthesia, muscle relaxants, and oxygenation, the risk of fracture or further cord damage is low.

The effects of spinal cord damage on sexual functions is a serious concern of the recovering patient. While sexual competence is impaired in ways that depend on the completeness and level of the lesion, patients have normal desires, fantasies, and erotic dreams. The issue should be addressed, and a physician should overcome whatever inhibitions he or she may have in the matter. It can be pointed out that marriage is feasible, that a majority of males have erections, and that some can consummate intercourse. The therapist can indicate that other methods of gaining sexual satisfaction are not necessarily perversions, and that stimulation of erotic areas other than the anesthetic parts of the body can be enjoyable. Above all, the need of a loving relationship to accommodate mechanical handicaps should be emphasized.

DISFIGUREMENT

Major disfigurement, involving the face and hands, occurs mainly as the result of burns, and of blast and missile wounds. Thermal injuries include exposure to flames, flash burns from gas explosions, the effects of chemical and high-voltage electrical agents, and smoke and carbon monoxide inhalation. Burns occur principally in tank warfare, and after vehicle explosions including airplane crashes and ship sinkings. Burns accounted for 4.6% of all casualties in Vietnam, for 12.5% in the 1973 Yom Kippur War, and for 18% of British casualties in the 1982 Falkland Islands War. It is estimated that 9% of the casualties in the 1991 Persian Gulf War had burn injuries.[79] Facial injuries are produced by bullet wounds, and by blast from mortars, mines, and other explosive devices, which commonly cause other disabilities such as blindness. Survivors of high-velocity missile wounds are more apt to have had maxillofacial and mandibular fractures than penetrating orbital injuries, which are often fatal.

This section focuses on burns because they are more likely to involve other organs including the brain, pose the most difficult problems in cosmetic surgery, and have the most severe and lasting behavioral consequences. The survival rate following even severe burns is high: more than 50% of patients 15- to 40-years-old with burns covering 75% of total body surface (TBS) live.[79] Life-threatening complications, however, are frequent with burns involving more than 30% of TBS. These involve the hormonal and cell immune systems, heart, lungs, liver, adrenals, kidneys, gastrointestinal tract, hematopoietic and blood clotting systems, and central nervous system and peripheral nerves.

Brain Syndromes

Delirium

Burn encephalopathies, which develop in the majority of patients with burns involving 30% or more TBS, have a number of etiologies. These include hypoxia, hypovolemia, electrolyte imbalance, notably hyponatremia resulting in seizures, acidosis, and sepsis. Patients may be awake, alert, and well-oriented on admission to the hospital, but within hours or days may become restless, agitated, disoriented, with fluctuating levels of consciousness, memory lapses, hallucinations, and paranoid ideation. Fear, pain, terror, and immobilization contribute, but the more massive the burn, the more likely the patient is to develop delirium, which is almost always associated with an abnormal electroencephalogram (EEG).[80] Some patients are only mildly disoriented, a condition that may be overlooked. Delirium usually clears in a few weeks but abnormal behavior may persist for weeks or months.[81]

Delayed Manifestations

There are also delayed complications, appearing weeks or months after the burn and usually associated with sepsis or fluid or electrolyte imbalance. These include focal neurological manifestations such as seizures, cranial motor nerve palsies, hemipareses,[82] spinal cord and peripheral nerve disabilities,[83] behavioral disorders including paranoid disorders, hallucinations,[84] psychoses,[82,85] and somatic delusional states, notably anosognosia and reduplicative misidentification syndromes.

Anosognosia and Reduplication

Patients deny or appear unaware of the somatic manifestations and obvious consequences of their injuries. If a burned limb has been amputated, its loss may be denied or represented in delusional fashion. Thus a patient in danger of losing a severely burned hand developed the idea that the doctors had removed the hand and was angry at their delay in putting it back.[81] Damage to the body can be selectively ignored, as in the case of a man who failed to notice the silver-nitrate–blackened skin of fellow patients in the burn unit.[81] Reduplication of the self was noted in a case described by Steiner and Clark.[86] In an apparently lucid period in which the patient expressed concern for her status, she told the staff to debride the sick woman in bed with her while she and her husband went to have a cup of coffee in the cafeteria.

Some anosognosic patients are bland and unconcerned, others paranoid or euphoric. A paranoid form of implicit denial was noted in a man with burns over 60% of his body. Despite being so weak that he was unable to raise his head from the pillow, he threatened to punch his physician in the nose.[87] A state of blissful euphoria associated with anosognosia was described by Hamburg, Hamburg, and de Goza.[88] The patient was a woman with extremely severe burns necessitating maintenance on a Stryker frame. She had initially thought that she would die, following which she claimed that she had recovered and would be able to go home in a few days and care for herself and her children. She died 2 weeks later. The experience at the A.V. Vishnevskii Institute of Surgery in Moscow is that euphoria succeeding depression is a grave prognostic sign.[82]

Neuropathology

Examination of the brains of persons who have died of burns and their complications has shown very little. In the great majority of instances no pathology has been found, although in a few cases cerebral edema, small infarcts and hemorrhages, and neuronal degeneration have been noted.[89,90] The cause of the delayed onset of symptoms referable to the central nervous system is unclear beyond that which can be attributed to sepsis or fluid or electrolyte imbalance, or a vascular complication. It is likely that burn encephalopathy is relatively common with many manifestations and few deaths.[90]

Stresses of Recovery

The surviving patient is subject to a broad range of stresses throughout the process of recovery. Pain is exacerbated by debridement, dressing changes, skin grafts and other plastic surgery, and the need to exercise burned limbs to avoid contractures. Gastric stress ulcers are another source of pain. The patient may have to be isolated until the danger of infection has passed, and extensive bandaging further reduces environmental contact. A tracheostomy may interfere with communication. In the patient's state of relative sensory isolation all fears are magnified. If he has facial burns and edema of the eyelids he worries that he will be blind, and burns in the genital area cause concern about sexual function. Insomnia can be a problem. When he is with other patients, the sight of charred bodies and the odor of wounds and dressings are distressing. The patient's first look at himself in the mirror can be a shocking experience and should be managed sensitively.

After survival is assured and the patient is no longer preoccupied with the issue of life and death new problems arise. As he is now able to participate in his own care, he needs less attention from nurses and other staff members to whom he may have become attached, and may thus feel betrayed and abandoned. Although his wounds have healed or been covered by grafts, he must face the fact of disfigurement and wonder if he will be socially rejected or unable to work. Burns of the exposed parts of the body, the face and the hands, have the most serious social consequences. The burned soldier must anticipate the reactions of people who may be horrified, curious, hostile, or pitying. Eventually he must come to recognize that burned faces may all look much the same, without individuality, and that his capacity to smile or use other muscles of expression to convey emotion may be reduced. If his hands have been severely burned, he is handicapped in using them in gesture. Moreover, posture, which reflects so much of personality and attitudes, may become rigid and distorted by contractures about joints.[91]

Coping Mechanisms

Patients react to disfigurement in various ways. Some accept their misfortune and cooperate in treatment. Most are depressed and anxious in some degree. There may be post-traumatic stress disorder with agitation, tremulousness and startle responses, nightmares or flashbacks concerning the circumstances of the injury, and difficulty in concentrating. Depression is usually self-limiting. It may come on at any time—on emergence from delirium, or weeks or even months later. It may be precipitated by the discovery that grafted skin does not look quite normal. Serious depression is manifested in feelings of hopelessness and thoughts of suicide, insomnia, lethargy, and poor cooperation as in refusal to eat. Suicidal ideation and gestures are rare during initial hospitalization, but they may occur following discharge. Some patients react with anger and bitterness, directing their resentment against the hospital staff. Others show what has been called regressive behavior, because it suggests a return to childhood attitudes. Such patients are excessively dependent, demanding, and demonstrative. They are apt to complain a great deal, and feel neglected or mistreated.

Denial in patients without impaired brain function usually does not involve somatic delusions, but takes other forms that may be adaptive or maladaptive. It helps the person combat anxiety and depression and may give him hope for the future. On the other hand, it leads to lack of concern about problems, unrealistic expectations of the future, and, at best, passive participation in therapy. Many patients seek religious meaning as they struggle to come to terms with their suffering.[92] These have positive and negative aspects. A person may feel sustained by God's presence or by the idea that he has been purified by fire. Others may see the injury as a punishment for sin or misconduct, or as some other manifestation of divine will.

Adaptive—and maladaptive—mechanisms have been usually formulated in psychodynamic terms, but organic neurological features must be considered in patients who have severe burns. One of the effects of such brain damage is a lowered threshold for the effects of acute environmental stress and the action of drugs. One of the survivors of the Coconut Grove fire disaster in Boston of November 1942 was a woman who showed no evidence of impairment of brain function until she received the news that her husband and son had died. She responded to the news with a state of excitement and paranoid suspicions that the doctors and nurses considered her to be a sinful, immoral person.[93] A U.S. Army sergeant, burned in a fire in his apartment, was ordinarily quiet and cooperative. He would, however, become extremely demanding, critical, and combative following the recovery of consciousness after the administering of a general anesthetic for dressing changes and skin grafting.[88] Similarly, burn patients may be sensitive to drugs used to control pain, anxiety, and depression.

Treatment

The aims of therapy are the management of delirium, the control of pain, anxiety, and depression, and the establishing of a social milieu in which the patient can come to terms with his disability and participate in his care.

Pharmacotherapy

Treatment of delirium involves the correction of disturbances of fluid and electrolyte balance, providing orientation cues such as keeping lights on at night, and protection of patients from self-injury. Neuroleptics are the drugs of choice, given orally if possible, with checking for hypotension. High-potency neuroleptics with minimal anticholinergic effects and alpha-adrenergic blocking are preferred.

Pain is especially severe in the first few weeks. If necessary, morphine or meperidine is indicated as the danger of addiction is slight. Respiratory depression may be more of a problem. For the control of acute anxiety provoked by the anticipation of pain, oral diazepam given one hour prior to the treatment has been effective, with intravenous (IV) administration of diazepam or chlordiazepoxide in more severe cases.[94] These drugs can impair cognition and are long-acting. Chronic use can cause depression. Intramuscular use is contraindicated because of poor absorption by that route. If major depression or chronic anxiety states supervene, antidepressants should be used, as they are effective for both the depression and the anxiety. Doxepin may be particularly useful for depressed or anxious patients who also have peptic (stress) ulcers because it is one of the most potent histamine-2 receptor blocking agents, more potent than cimetidine (Tagamet) in reducing gastric acid secretion. It is primarily a noradrenergic modifying antidepressant, hence useful in chronic pain disorders as well. Its anticholinergic and antihistamine effects can, of course, be detrimental for alertness, bladder function, and vascular reflexes.

Behavioral Management

As soon as the patient's medical condition permits and he is able to retain information, he should be given a statement of the extent of his injuries, the type of and rationales for the treatment that will be required, and the anticipated length of his hospital stay. As noted by Kjaer,[95] the often heard phrase, "You're lucky to be alive," is rarely helpful. In the absence of information, rumors and irrational fears flourish, and it is important for physicians and nurses to maintain communication with patients other than that which involves a dressing change or some other painful procedure.

The belief that the soldier has some control over his destiny should be fostered. The first self-feeding or unassisted bath should be met with expressions of approval. If possible patients should be taught self-hypnosis or other relaxation techniques. These are not only helpful in the relief of pain, nausea, anorexia, and tension, but provide a sense of mastery and raise self-esteem. Group therapy allows for the ventilation of feelings, mutual support, and the building of a common identity. If there are multiple survivors of the same event, critical event debriefing may be helpful. Chapter 11, Debriefing Following Combat, discusses several methods available.

The management of demanding and dependent patients is difficult, in part because such behavior brings out resentment in the staff. It is important to keep in mind that the behavior has an adaptive function in that many of these patients are dramatizing their problems by taking the role of a child. Limits should be set, with some choices left to the patient to enable him to keep some sense of autonomy.

Physical and adjustment problems may persist after the soldier has left the hospital. He may need further surgery to correct scars and contractures. While such reconstruction is helpful, the patient should be cautioned that scarring may never be entirely eradicated, or a burned face restored completely. Patients who have been disappointed with the results of surgery may demand further operations that are not medically indicated. Some may use relatively minor disfigurement as a focus for their discontents, and blame job failures, inability to make friends, or domestic difficulties on others' reaction to their appearance.

Case Study 2: Fall of a Hero

A 24-year-old decorated combat infantry officer sustained fractures of the left zygoma and mandible, multiple facial lacerations, injury to the left ear canal, and a left facial nerve palsy in an airplane crash. He was comatose on admission to the hospital and over the next 2 to 3 weeks he was restless, combative, and feared that he would be killed. In this state, he reenacted scenes of battle in Korea. After recovering orientation he complained a great deal of pain in his jaw. Following each of two corrective surgical procedures he became confused and hostile. Routine mental status, however, was normal and he returned to duty 5 months after his injury.

In Korea, he experienced dizziness, diplopia and unsteadiness of gait, was depressed, had nightmares and flashbacks, and found that he was intolerant of the noise of grenade and rifle fire. He did not seek medical aid for these complaints, but rather focused on his disfigurement. He had several scar revisions and was noted as being unusually sensitive about his appearance. Following a complaint of pain and photophobia in his left eye, a blepharoplasty was performed. A small foreign body was found and it was suspected that he had inserted it himself.

Four years after his initial injury he was referred by his commanding officer for psychiatric observation because of disrespectful behavior and for having made allegations, out of channels, of inefficiency and security violations. This conduct contrasted with his previously excellent efficiency reports and his reputation for bravery in combat. Examination showed no evidence of organic brain damage, neurosis, or psychosis and he was discharged to duty. His full scale intelligence quotient (IQ) of 115, however, was considered to represent a fall from his premorbid level.

Following his resignation from the service, the patient continued to have difficulties. He attributed his employment and marital problems to his facial disfigurement and was preoccupied with violence. He carried pictures of his men who had been killed in combat and made several suicidal gestures. Following the assassination of President Kennedy, he claimed that he had known Lee Harvey Oswald, that he had had foreknowledge of the assassination, and feared that he would be set up by the same conspirators who had murdered Oswald.

Comment: This case illustrates the association of traumatic facial disfigurement with a brain injury (the severity of which was not recognized), PTSD, and a paranoid delusional state.

BLINDNESS

Loss of vision is a catastrophic event that thrusts a soldier into an unfamiliar world, profoundly alters his perception of reality, robs him of mobility, and ends a way of life. Changing conditions of warfare have markedly increased the incidence of eye injuries. In the Civil War ocular wounds made up 0.5% of surviving casualties. The figure rose to 2.14 % in World War I.[96] In Korea the rate was 8.1%,[97] and in Vietnam 9% of surviving combat casualties had ocular injuries.[98,99] In Vietnam the great majority of wounds were generated by fragments from explosive projectile shells, rockets and bombs, grenades, booby traps, and land mines. Tank warfare, which requires commanders to expose their upper bodies for better vision, produces many eye injuries, totalling 25% of all Israeli casualties in the 1967 Arab-Israeli War.[100] Most casualties sustain other wounds as well. In Vietnam, it was not uncommon for a man to be blinded by the same explosion that caused multiple facial fractures, and blew off a leg. Chemical agents may result in blindness as occurred with mustard gas in World War I. Ocular trauma from high-velocity fragments is frequently accompanied by brain injury, and blindness of central origin results from intracranial wounds involving the visual pathways.

The current battlefield laser rangefinders and designators produce multiple pinpoint burns on the retina, where the beam has been focused by the lens of the eye. This can occur at distances of several kilometers if the source of the laser is viewed with the naked eye, and out to many kilometers if viewed through binoculars, gunsights, or other optics. The tiny burns are quickly surrounded by edema. While loss of peripheral vision may go unnoticed, burns in the fovea produce sudden impairment of vision. Depending on size and location of the retinal burns, recovery of vision may take days, and can leave visual field defects.

Cerebral Blindness

Cerebral or cortical blindness is usually the result of bilateral occipital lobe lesions involving the striate cortex. It is characterized by failure to see light or movement, even though the pupils are dilated and react to light, and in attempted convergence. Blindness may not be total, but as most patients have mental changes it is sometimes difficult to be certain of the degree of visual loss. Binocular blindness may also be caused by lesions of the optic chiasm, and by anoxia, such as that resulting from carbon monoxide poisoning. Anoxia may also result in selective visual impairments such as achromatopsia, and loss of perception of form and motion in which the patient tries to identify an object by color alone.[101] Lesions of the visual pathways cause hemianopias in both the vertical and horizontal planes.

Anosognosia for Blindness

The most striking behavioral abnormality associated with cerebral blindness is anosognosia for visual loss, known as Anton's syndrome, in which patients deny or appear unaware of their blindness. Even though they appear to be totally blind, they confabulate descriptions of the examiner and their surroundings. Denial may be incomplete in that a patient may complain of dim vision, but attribute it to the darkness of the room, or being kept in a dungeon. Some patients are cheerful and unconcerned about their deficits; others become angry and hostile when their claims to vision are challenged.[102] Patients may behave in ludic fashion, joking and clowning. Such apparent emotional indifference or inappropriateness could contribute to a mistaken diagnosis of conversion disorder. Patients are usually disoriented for place and time, and may have visual hallucinations. They are amnesic, particularly when the injury has resulted in loss of consciousness, and they confabulate about their activities and reason for coming to the hospital.

The pathology is bilateral and extensive. When the occipital lobes are involved, the lesions usually extend from the ventromedial portions into the temporal lobes. When blindness is caused by damage to the optic chiasm at the base of the brain there are commonly lesions of the frontal lobe. Anton's syndrome also appears with blindness of peripheral origin provided there is additional cerebral damage. Recovery from cortical blindness caused by occipito-temporal lesions may go through various stages of visual agnosias and homonymous scotomata.[103]

Case Study 3: Denial of Blindness

A 21-year-old paratrooper, while on maneuvers in Germany, was thrown from a moving vehicle sustaining a basilar skull fracture and bleeding from his right ear canal. He lapsed into unconsciousness, and a subdural hematoma and necrotic brain tissue was removed from the right parietal-temporal region. Papilledema developed, followed by optic atrophy and bilateral loss of vision.

On arrival at Walter Reed Army Medical Center in Washington, D.C. 6 weeks after his injury, the right pupil was fixed to light and the left reacted sluggishly. Visual acuity in the better eye was 20/200. The patient was disoriented for place and date, was amnestic for his injury, and did not remember that he was married. He denied anything was wrong with his vision, even though he identified objects mainly by feeling them. He was cheerful and uncomplaining; at times he stated that his vision was dim because the ward was so dark, and that maybe he should get goggles. There were many references to vision in colloquial speech, as in reporting on his first leave. "Well, I got home and *seen* my uncle, and *seen* nearly everybody. I went and got baptized. I went to *see* everybody. I *seen* my aunt and grandmother and everyone else. *Seen* people I hadn't *seen* for a long time." Denial of blindness lasted for 3 to 4 weeks by the end of which period he was completely oriented. He then developed a hysterical tremor of his head.

Comment: The case is of particular interest because it demonstrates that patients with anosognosia can have unconscious awareness of their deficits, and that a conversion reaction can be a late consequence of brain injury.

Anosognosia for Hemianopia

Whereas patients with Anton's syndrome have other disorders of consciousness, patients with a homonymous hemianopia from a head injury may be unaware of their visual loss even though their mental faculties are intact. Such patients do not see only one half of space. Because of the phenomenon of completion, they "fill in" the part of the image falling in the hemianoptic field, and report a complete circle when a semicircle is presented. Such patients may not complain of visual loss or they may have noticed only a slight difficulty in picking up a line in reading. Although such soldiers might function well in ordinary surroundings, they are at serious risk if exposed in a combat situation.

Visual Phenomenology

Visual hallucinations, as distinguished from mental imagery, may occur during a period of delirium, but are rare in traumatic blindness of peripheral origin unless it is associated with brain damage, drug effects, or extended sleep deprivation. Transient episodes of phantom vision comparable to phantom limb sensations have been described in Vietnam combat veterans following enucleation of one or both eyes.[102] Some had had brain injuries but all were aware of their blindness. As in cases of extremity phantoms, the men were reluctant to report their experiences of seeing out of an empty socket out of fear of being thought mentally unbalanced. Patients stated that they had seen clouds, flashing lights, and movement—in one case the man's mother—even though they knew that there was nothing there. The visions appeared under a variety of circumstances, often while the patient was relaxed. Phantom vision should be differentiated from the pseudo-hallucinations of the Charles Bonnet syndrome. These are well-formed, often of marching soldiers, and are common after cataract extraction in the aged, but rare after trauma in the young.[104] Visual phantoms should be discussed with patients, not only to allay fears of being mentally disturbed, but to remove false hopes that they are a sign of recovery of vision.

There may be a cessation of dreaming for a period after brain injury, but most recently blinded persons have an active dream life. Many report that their dreams are more vivid and the colors more intense since the loss of sight.[105] Soldiers in the early stages are apt to reenact battle experiences or other trauma, but as nightmares recede, dreams become more varied. Men may dream that they can see, while knowing that they are blind. One man would dream that he could see but not reach the object. Wittkower and Davenport[106] described the case of a soldier at St. Dunstan's who dreamed that he could see his empty sockets in a mirror. When disturbing dreams do occur, the dreamer, rather than being a victim, may be a detached spectator of some trauma.

Early Reactions

Soldiers who have been blinded in combat are not usually unconscious unless they have sustained a brain injury but, as in paraplegia, they may not be immediately aware of their visual loss. When they find they cannot see they react in various ways. In some cases, they go into in a state of emotional and cognitive withdrawal. They may believe that the visual loss is only temporary, and that they will see when the swelling subsides or the bandages are removed. Some are in a state of despair, talk of suicide, and express regret that they were not killed outright. Some do commit suicide "accidentally" in such mishaps as falling out of a window.[107] Others are relieved and thankful that they were not injured more seriously.

Stresses and Coping Mechanisms

As a patient's condition stabilizes he encounters the consequences of his blindness—the sensory isolation, the loss of autonomy, and the impairment of communication. He must attend to countless actions that formerly were carried out unconsciously. He must learn how to walk again, to wash, bathe, dress, and feed himself. He must rely to a much greater degree on the senses of hearing, touch, proprioception, and smell and be able to visualize the information. He must depend more on his memory. He must acquire the ability to form visual and affective images of people he knows only by their voices, and overcome the handicap of not being able to see their facial expressions and gestures. If there is the additional loss of hearing, this interferes with his ability to judge depth and distance of objects. If he is also disfigured, the inability to observe the reactions of people whom he meets may be especially troubling. He must learn to use the aids that will enable him to be literate again, and acquire new work skills and modes of recreation. If he has lost a limb or sustained hearing loss or brain damage these tasks are more difficult. He must accustom himself to the fact that he will never drive a car again, play or watch a baseball game, or see the faces of his children.

Blindness imposes a loss of status and self-esteem. Many soldiers feel deprived of their manhood and dignity. In the hospital some are too ashamed or embarrassed to tell people at home what has happened to them. They are concerned with whether they can function as a husband or father and associate with people. As one man noted, "It's hard to make friends with people you can't see." They worry about making a living, and being dependent on the charity or pity of others. Many feel inferior to and are resentful of the sighted. Patients respond to these stresses with varying degrees of denial and depression, frustration, anger, and anxiety and resort to alcohol or other drugs. Moreover, blindness exacerbates previous emotional and social problems.

Denial and Nonacceptance

Patients do not continue to deny or appear unaware of their blindness unless they have severe brain damage, as in Anton's syndrome, but manifest denial in other ways. They may cling to the hope that sight will be restored by a transplant or some miracle. Denial may be expressed by inappropriate cheerfulness and unrealistic plans for the future. Nonacceptance is indicated by such statements that if the surgeons had performed the right operation the patient would be able to see. Denial is also shown in patients' refusal to use the Hoover light cane as an aid to spatial orientation and mobility and participate in other training exercises.

Patients who have light perception and some useful vision within the definition of blindness as central visual acuity of 20/200 or less in the better eye, or central visual acuity of more than 20/200 if there is a peripheral visual field subtending an angular distance no greater than 20 degrees in the better eye, have some advantage over the completely blind. They, however, on the whole are less accepting of their disability and make a poorer adjustment.[106,108,109] The minimally sighted are more reluctant to enter into rehabilitation training, and continue to rely on their residual sight which may provide erroneous information. Whereas the completely blinded have come to terms, once and for all, with the fact that they will never see, the partially blinded often retain false hopes and are beset by fears that they will lose their remaining vision. The earlier the person accepts his blindness, the more favorable the behavioral outcome.[110] Some patients show "blindisms," (ie, vacant stare, grimacing, overloud voice and failure to look at the person with whom they are conversing). It has been noted that men with the grossest "blindisms" are particularly apt to resist training.[111]

Denial may be unwittingly reinforced by the attitudes of caretakers. A staff member may give a patient an assurance that his sight will return in a well-meant effort to keep up his morale. Physicians may contribute to denial by their reluctance or inability to give the patient a definitive evaluation. Statements such as "one chance in a million" and "perhaps a miracle will happen" should be avoided.[108] Soldiers are apt to remember such phrases to the exclusion of everything else they have been told and become bitter over what they consider to have been a deception.

Depression

The majority of men blinded in combat are depressed to some degree and feelings of hopelessness and suicidal ideation are common during hospitalization. The experience at St. Dunstan's, the training center for British soldiers blinded in World War II, was that 29% of patients were depressed, although very few were "grossly and patently" so.[106] Mainly, they were withdrawn and moody and dwelled on the past. Feelings of guilt and self-blame are more likely to be expressed by soldiers blinded by disease or in accidents than those wounded in combat.[108] Depressed patients regard training as another stress to be avoided rather than an opportunity to overcome some of their handicaps.

An initial period of depression has been considered to be a mourning process through which the person grieves for the death of the sighted self in order to be reborn as a blind man. Cholden[112] believed that such depression was necessary before the patient could accept his loss and that it diminished with time. A blinded veteran recalled:

> I think it must have been or was a lot like dying. Anyway I know I went through all the stages of "dying" that some one who is terminally ill goes through when he's told he's dying. I remember how strenuously I demanded that the doctors do everything to restore my vision, even though it was hopeless. I called them "idiots" and "fools" for not knowing what to do to help me. I prayed and made promises to God. But I was blind and no amount of denial of the fact could change it. I was angry and resentful for a long time, and I remember how often I asked, "Why me?" I went through a stage where I cried a lot and was really depressed. I still feel that way sometimes but I've learned to accept my blindness the best I can. I came to a point where I started having some good days. Now most of them are okay.[113(p35)]

Other observers, however, have not found this sequence to be necessary or inevitable.[114] Some men are briefly devastated by the news that they will not see again, but then work vigorously on a rehabilitation program.[109,115] Depression may not come on until after the patient has left the hospital, and some men are chronically depressed. In the St. Dunstan's study, 50% of the patients followed for periods of from 1 to 4 years were depressed, resentful, or showed other psychiatric abnormalities.[106] If depression is severe or enduring, it should be actively treated. Along with denial, prolonged depression poses the greatest barrier to successful adaptation.

Anxiety is manifested in fears of falling, and in suspicions of being watched by sighted people. Insomnia may occur, due in part to the absence of the light-dark cycle, and some patients develop a fear of the dark. There may be accompanying PTSD and psychosomatic complaints include headache, dizziness, gastrointestinal discomfort, and eye strain. Blind men may complain of eye strain after Braille reading even after both eyes have been enucleated.[106]

Adaptation to blindness is determined by the extent of other injuries, personality and social factors, and the quality of the training program. Patients with concomitant brain damage and deficits in memory and attention, and those with amputations, marked facial scarring, and hearing loss are at a disadvantage. Certain premorbid personality features favor the development of denial. Such patients are described as having been compulsive and perfectionistic, as reluctant to share their feelings, and as priding themselves on their self-sufficiency. They had regarded disability as a personal failure or disgrace.[116,117] Patients with a history of dependency, on the other hand, may find it all too easy to accept any assistance that is offered and be reluctant to work on their own.[109] Levels of education and degree of family support correlate positively with successful adjustment.[118] According to one combat-blinded veteran (known to the author), who was active in rehabilitation, macho types see in blindness a loss of masculinity and have particular difficulty in enduring the limitations of physical activity.

Treatment

Modern treatment of blindness resulting from combat began during World War II and is based on the principles of orientation and mobilization (O & M), acceptance of blindness, and the forming of a group esprit. Despite the experience of World War I, the U.S. armed services were not fully prepared for the care of the 1,400 men blinded in World War II. Soldiers were evacuated to Dibble General Hospital in Menlo Park, California or Valley Forge General Hospital in Phoenixville, Pennsylvania. U.S. Navy and Marine Corps personnel were sent to the Philadelphia Naval Hospital in Pennsylvania, but the first center devoted exclusively to the rehabilitation of the blind was not set up until June 1944 at Avon Old Farms, Connecticut. Treatment had consisted of instruction in self-care, posture, and facial expression; physical exercise and sports activities; social recreation; and industrial, vocational, and academic classes. Morale was not good, and over 40% of the men at Dibble General Hospital were considered by a psychiatrist to be maladjusted.[108]

The prevailing philosophy at Avon Old Farms was that the blind could be taught to "see" through "facial vision." This was the idea that the person could perceive obstacles in front of him by changes in the sensations of touch, pressure, and temperature emanating from the object. The method had had rare success with the congenitally blind but was ineffective for the war-wounded. Locomotion was aided by an ordinary wooden walking cane.

What came to be known as the Hoover light cane was introduced at Valley Forge by Sergeant Richard E. "Dick" Hoover[119] (who completed medical school after World War II), and the O & M technique was to be developed with the collaboration of Russell C. Williams who had been blinded in the Normandy campaign, and C. Warren Bledsoe, who had been a teacher of the blind. Hoover found the conventional cane to be too cumbersome, and devised a lightweight longer one made of steel—subsequently aluminum or fiberglass—that the patient swung in an arc in front of his trailing foot. This extension of the patient's arm enabled him to "feel" objects and gain an appreciation of their qualities through the transmitted vibrations. The metallic body was a good sound conductor that gave information about the presence of walls, open spaces, or changes in terrain. The cane tip also gave auditory information. Even some bilateral upper limb amputees could use the cane which was more of a wand and light enough to be attached to a stump. Hoover and his associates trained many instructors, and the technique has spread around the world. The shift to O & M occurred in the context of a change in social attitudes toward the blind. An original objection to O & M was that the Hoover cane made the user conspicuous while "facial vision" disguised the blind so that they would not upset or offend the sighted.

A follow-up study (1952–1953) of 1,949 veterans blinded in World War II and the Korean conflict[118] showed a high level of adjustment, considering that so many men had other disabilities. Of these blinded veterans, 50% were employed and 82% of these expressed satisfaction with their jobs. A much higher employment rate was found in men who had completed rehabilitation training. Nine of 10 were reported as coping well with community attitudes and relating well in their families. The same number expressed themselves fluently, and appeared orderly in their thinking processes. Eight of 10 did not appear nervous or depressed during interviews, and 8 of 10 did not show "blindisms." As for manifestations of denial, 30% had unrealistic plans for the future, 15% were reported as using cheerfulness to mask other feelings, and 32% had retained hopes of seeing for 10 or more months after their injuries.[118] No comparable study of Vietnam veterans has been published.

The following do's and don'ts in dealing with a blind patient have been suggested:

1. Address him directly rather than his escort.
2. Do not shout unless the patient has a hearing loss.
3. Do not avoid the words "look" and "see" for fear of embarrassing the blind person.
4. Do not hesitate to ask the person how much sight he has.
5. Announce when you are entering or leaving his room.
6. Give specific directions on location of objects rather than using the vaguer term, "over there."
7. Ask the patient to take your arm rather than taking his and propelling him.
8. Tell a patient you have not guided before when coming to steps.
9. Walk in line with the patient but in going up and down stairs keep one step in front of him.
10. Do not feel offended if the blind person refuses help.

CASTRATION AND GENITAL MUTILATION

Wounds of the external genitalia are the most feared combat injuries. Soldiers in foxholes have been observed to place their helmets over their genitalia, and airmen noted to reinforce their seats with life jackets. While the incidence is low as compared to other wounds, it has risen over the years with the change from the static trench warfare of World War I to more mobile modern tactics. Wounds of the penis, scrotum, and testicles made up 2% to 3% of American casualties in Vietnam,[120] and comprised from 40% to 67% of all genitourinary injuries.[121–124] The rate was higher before the 1968 Tet offensive because there were more below-the-waist explosions from mines and booby traps than after Tet when there was a higher proportion of shell-fragment wounds.[122,123] Burns are another source of genital injuries.

The great majority of genital wounds are associated with other organ damage—to the extremities, other parts of the genitourinary tract, the abdomen, and chest—and the greater explosive power of weapons over the years has increased the incidence of such injuries. Spinal cord damage, amputations, and even blindness may result. Such extensive injuries differ strikingly from the castrating and mutilating genital wounds of civilian life. The latter are caused mainly by low-velocity bullets, now commonly used in drug wars, and by knives, razors, and scissors wielded by vengeful lovers or rivals. Self-castrations are performed by mentally disturbed persons. Such wounds do not produce the massive tissue destruction and the extensive contamination that result from the impact of the high-velocity particles of combat.

Patients are usually admitted to the hospital in shock and early attention is directed to life-threatening problems, so that definitive treatment is delayed until their condition has stabilized. Complete loss of external genitalia was reported as a common occurrence in the Soviet Army in World War II[125] but penile amputation has been encountered much less frequently by American surgeons.[124,126–128] Superficial penile injuries involving the skin and glans or subcutaneous tissues or both, are much less likely to be accompanied by other genital wounds and generally heal without major complications.[122] Severe penile wounds with injury to the corpora cavernosa are apt to be associated with urethral and testicular damage but partly severed penises can be reconstituted provided sufficient corpus cavernosum is retained. Later complications include penile pain and fibrosis, and chordee interfering with erection.

Scrotal-testicular wounds are the most common external genital injuries. They made up 32.8% of all genitourinary wounds in a series of 124 patients evacuated from Vietnam to Japan. It was usually possible to preserve at least part of a testicle. Orchiectomy or partial orchiectomy was performed in 77 of 98 men with unilateral testis injury, and total bilateral orchiectomy was done in only 5 of 28 patients with damage to both testicles.[124] Loss of one testicle does not interfere with potency or cause sterility, and does not contraindicate return to duty. After bilateral orchiectomy, hormone replacement with depo-testosterone maintains potency and bone density. The course and disposition depends not only on the severity of the genital wounds but on the extent of other injuries.

Behavior

There are no published studies of the behavioral sequelae of combat-incurred genital mutilations. One reason is that such wounds are relatively uncommon. Another is that because of the frequently associated injuries, patients with genital wounds, unlike amputees and those with spinal cord damage or blindness, do not form a distinct group with a training program from which data can be derived.

As noted, it may be some time before the wounded soldier becomes aware of the extent of his injuries. The first sight of a mutilating genital wound may be so distressing that some surgeons perform the first procedures with the patient under anesthesia.[124] While some men react with equanimity, depression ensues in the great majority of cases. It usually improves over time but may persist, especially if the patient is septic or in pain. Patients experience the emotional problems of the disabled and disfigured, along with those specifically related to sexual functions. The incidence of impotence associated with persisting penile deformity is not known, but the sensitivity to the cosmetic aspects is an important psychological factor. For some, disfigurement of sexual organs is equivalent to the loss of all manly qualities. Adding to the sense of alienation in some cases is the lack of a reference group such as those with which the amputee, the paraplegic, and the blind can identify and gain support.

The major behavioral disorders in the chronic stages are depression, social withdrawal, and substance abuse. Statistical data are lacking so it is not known if the association of genital wounds with amputations, spinal cord injuries, and blindness or facial disfigurement or both adds to the suicide rate or increases the incidence of behavioral disturbances. Phantoms of the genitals may occur but have not been reported in the literature of recent wars. Patients with relatively minor genital injuries may also have psychiatric problems. A man with a slight penile deformity may believe he is physically repulsive and make it the focus of all his personal problems. A patient with loss of one testicle may be beset by fears that the other will be damaged or he may engage in compulsive sexual activity to prove his potency.

Treatment

Treatment depends on the extent of genital loss and the nature and severity of other injuries that determine the patient's ability to participate in a rehabilitation program. Unfortunately a man with a genital injury cannot improve his performance the way a blind man can become proficient in orientation and mobilization techniques. There should, in any case, be a doctor-patient relationship in which feelings of despair, loneliness, anger, and shame can be expressed. The patient must be assured that loss of physical capacity does not mean loss of personal integrity and that all that can be done for him is being done. Some of the more successful outcomes have been associated with the initiative and resourcefulness of surgeons who have followed their patients over the years and the personal qualities of the patients themselves.

The following cases are illustrative of some of the features that have been presented.

Case Study 4: Of Arms and the Man

On Friday, 13 October 1967, a 17-year-old machine-gunner in Vietnam was struck by a high-velocity missile that pierced his left flank and exited from the right, destroyed his left kidney and one half of his right one, damaged extensive areas of bowel and penetrated the cauda equina. At an evacuation hospital where he arrived within 15 minutes of his injury, a surgical team performed a left nephrectomy, a right heminephrectomy, multiple bowel anastomoses and a colostomy, and inserted drains in the pelvic area. In Japan, the patient was noted to be paraplegic and underwent a lumbar laminectomy after which he developed a bloody pleural effusion and contracted a severe urinary tract infection. At a hospital in the United States to which he was admitted 1 month after his injury he was still paraplegic, had large decubiti over the sacrum and other pressure points, and had osteomyelitis of the lumbar vertebrae and pelvic bones. To protect what was left of his remaining kidney from infection, an ileal conduit was constructed. The patient was confused and lethargic as a result of his sepsis, was in constant pain, became addicted to several drugs, and was deeply depressed. He tolerated food poorly and his weight had dropped to 57 pounds.

At this point his physician, recognizing the noxious effects of his pain-racked, functionless, septic lower body, conceived of a translumbar hemicorporectomy, an operation that had been performed on patients with advanced cancer of the bladder and pelvis. Following the procedure, the patient's condition improved remarkably. He was free of pain, came off drugs, and was no longer depressed. He entered a rehabilitation program, developed great arm strength, and was able to use and transfer himself from a wheelchair. One year after his injury he was discharged to his home and, with the support of his family and the community, has led an active life. He operates a small-engine repair shop, drives a number of vehicles, and serves as a member of a radio emergency-action communication team. He collects guns, target shoots, hunts with a rifle and crossbow, and fishes. He was fitted with a prosthetic trunk and legs but has discarded these, as he finds it easier to ambulate on his hands which he does without embarrassment. He cares for his personal hygiene and handles his colostomy and ileal bags successfully.[129]

In a 1993 interview, the veteran reported that he had had no emotional problems. For several years after his return home from the hospital he drank heavily but stopped after he put on a great deal of weight. He has not been depressed and never thought of suicide. He recalled that he had been immediately aware of his paralysis after being wounded in Vietnam, and that in the hospital there he had been terrified during shelling because of his immobility. He since has had no symptoms of PTSD. He has experienced a phantom of his right lower extremity with a sensation of dull pain from his knee upward, but no genital phantoms. He has had no sexual sensations, desires or imagery, and no erotic dreams. When asked how he sees himself in dreams, he replied that he does not visualize himself, only others. He states that he does not regret not having gotten married and having children, and that he regards his nephews as his sons. He is not bitter over his war experience, but rather, he is proud of having served his country as his father and brother have, and is grateful to the doctors for saving his life.

Comment: One can only marvel at the superb medical care he received and the patient's survival skills.

Case Study 5: Against All Odds

An 18-year-old combat engineer was injured in Vietnam in 1968 when his helicopter was struck by rocket fire and crashed into a mountain. Both legs were sheared off above the knees on impact, his right little finger was amputated, there were fractures of both arms, and he had facial and genital wounds. There was penetration of the left orbit into the frontal lobe necessitating enucleation of the left eye and injury to the right eye left only light perception. The right eye was subsequently enucleated. The genital wounds consisted of penile lacerations closed by primary repair, and a damaged right testicle requiring orchiectomy. He later had a craniotomy for an infected frontal sinus, reparative upper-limb procedures, a number of revisions of his amputation stumps, and in 1972 exenteration of his right hip joint for osteomyelitis.

The veteran was interviewed 20 years after his injury when he was located by his surgeon, Dr. Kenneth Swan. He recalled that he had been unconscious only briefly, but that it was not until several days later, and then only after he had been told by a fellow soldier, that he discovered he could not see, and that he had lost his legs. He stated that he was not depressed or concerned over his condition while in Vietnam. He thought that he would be able to get along fine with wooden legs, and that his remaining vision would suffice. Following a craniotomy in Japan, he had an episode of delirium lasting 4 months, over which time he was agitated and hallucinatory, reexperiencing combat. This was followed by long periods of lethargy and depression that improved after the removal of his infected hip joint. Subsequent depressive episodes associated with aggressive behavior have appeared mainly in response to frustration. He recalled that the first time he struck his wife was when he was having difficulties with college courses. He also has had problems of drug abuse, but gave up drinking after a grand mal seizure. Symptoms of PTSD appeared in 1972, 4 years after his injury, and anniversaries of traumatic experiences such as the 1968 Tet offensive have been associated with emotional distress.

He had been told during his last military hospitalization that he would be sterile; subsequently he engaged in excessive sexual activity after discharge. He later married and fathered two children. He is potent except for brief periods when he is under stress. He remains totally blind and navigates from a wheelchair with the aid of a sonar path sounder. He has experienced phantoms of both lower extremities with sharp pains that may last up to 24 hours. He has not had phantoms of the missing testicle or little finger. Since enucleation of the right eye, there has been phantom vision in which he "sees" bright lights.

In the late 1980s, the veteran's wife suffered a nervous breakdown, an episode of depression brought on by his social withdrawal, his abusive behavior, and her inability to cope with the management of the household. The couple went into counseling and the veteran feels he has been able to resolve his feelings about the war and his own experiences as an abused child. Although he states that he is making a better adjustment at home, he still finds it difficult to be comfortable with people in public.

Comment: One factor contributing to the worse adaptation of the this second patient is the brain injury that he suffered.

SUMMARY

Amputation, spinal cord injury, facial disfigurement from wounds and burns, blindness, and mutilating and castrating genital injuries have a number of features in common. Each involves the loss of a major function of the body that is largely irreparable. The injuries are frequently associated in that a mine explosion may blow off one or more limbs, damage a testicle, and blind a soldier. Following the initial shock and the undertaking of life-saving measures, most patients must endure a long hospitalization, often with complications necessitating arduous and painful surgical procedures. Psychologically, there is a profound alteration of body image, a loss of self-esteem and, for many, the end of a way of life. Injuries may be associated with PTSD, depression, and denial as prominent behavioral features, and brain dysfunction is common.

Brain dysfunction occurs in a number of ways. It may result from direct impact as in spinal cord injuries, notably cervical cord lesions, and from penetrating head wounds in blinded patients. Brain abnormalities can also be caused by anoxia, sepsis, and metabolic abnormalities. Sensory isolation consequent to head immobilization for cervical cord injuries may bring on behavioral disturbances. Phantom-limb manifestations were once regarded as psychogenic, but current findings suggest that the phenomena are the result of reorganization of denervated cortical sensory areas. Burn encephalopathies are manifested in initial delirium and occasionally in delayed focal neurological signs and psychotic reactions. Among the organic mental syndromes subsequent to severe burns that have been reported are depressive-withdrawn and paranoid-aggressive states, anosognosia in which the patient denies or appears unaware of his bodily deformities, and delusional misidentifications. In patients without overt behavioral disorders, brain damage lowers thresholds for stress and increases the complications of drug therapy. Psychoses in the absence of evidence of brain dysfunction are rare.

A wounded soldier may not be spontaneously and immediately aware of the loss of a limb or of paralysis, blindness, or disfigurement. The duration of such anosognosia depends on the state of brain function and the degree of interaction in the environment. Later manifestations of denial include unrealistic expectations of the future, faith in a miracle cure, and a defiant "we can take it" attitude. Blind patients may persist on relying on an inadequate fragment of remaining vision and refuse training to help them compensate for the loss of sight. Denial may take a paranoid form in which a patient may angrily blame his incapacity on improper treatment. In the early stages denial may detach a patient from the catastrophic reality and help him preserve a sense of identity, but it is ultimately maladaptive. It deprives the patient of the opportunity to grieve, hinders the development of group relationships, and blocks rehabilitative efforts.

Depression at some stage is almost universal. While a period of grief and mourning is helpful in allowing a patient to come to terms with his loss, prolonged depression with dwelling on the past has disastrous effects. It leads to noncooperation in treatment and to self-neglect. Suicide is a danger even in severely incapacitated patients, especially those with self-neglect who deny ever having harbored thoughts of ending their lives.

Although disabling and disfiguring injuries present a variety of problems, there are some common principles of treatment. The staff should avoid statements and attitudes that reinforce denial. Patients should be told of their prognoses and given the rationale for their treatment as early as they can retain and evaluate information and cooperate in self-care. The development of a new identity should be facilitated by acceptance of a handicapped status and by participation in a rehabilitative training program. Feelings about disability should be shared in group sessions and the patient should be helped to understand how his feelings about himself affect his perceptions of the attitudes of others. Depression, aggression, and pain should be managed with both behavioral and pharmacological measures.

ACKNOWLEDGEMENT

The author is pleased to acknowledge the assistance of the following people:
C. Warren Bledsoe, formerly Chief Blind Rehabilitation, Physical Medicine and Rehabilitation Service, Veterans Administration; Don Garner, Director Blind Rehabilitation Service, Department of Veterans Affairs; Frank La Piana, M.D. Col M.C., Chief Ophthalmology Service, Walter Reed Army Medical Center; David G. Mc Leod, M.D. Col M.C., Chief Urology Service, Walter Reed Army Medical Center; Thomas H. Miller, Director of Governmental and Community Affairs, Blind Veterans Association; Basil A. Pruitt Jr., M.D. Col M.C., Commander and Director U.S. Army Institute of Surgical Research, Brooke Army Medical Center, Fort Sam Houston, TX; Stuart M. Selikowitz, M.D., Section of Urology, Department of Surgery, Department of Veterans Affairs, White River Junction, Vermont; Kenneth Swan, M.D., Professor of Surgery, University of Medicine and Dentistry of New Jersey, New Jersey Medical School; Paul F. Vinger, M.D., Associate Professor of Ophthalmology, Tufts University Medical School; John N. Wettlaufer, M.D. Col M.C., Department of Urology, Madigan Army Medical Center, Tacoma, WA; and Russell C. Williams, formerly Chief Blind Rehabilitation, Veterans Administration.

REFERENCES

1. Hardaway RM III. Vietnam wound analysis. *J Trauma*. 1978;18(9):635–643.

2. Pocock T. *Horatio Nelson*. New York: Alfred A Knopf; 1988.

3. Pugh RDG. *Nelson and His Surgeons*. Edinburgh, Scotland: E. & S. Livingstone; 1968.

4. Randall GC, Ewalt JR, Blair H. Psychiatric reactions to amputation. *JAMA*. 1945;128:645–652.

5. Noble D, Price DB, Gilder R Jr. Psychiatric disturbances following amputation. *Am J Psychiatry*. 1954;110:609–613.

6. Frank JL. The amputee war casualty in a military hospital: Observations on psychological management. *Int J Psychiatry Med*. 1973;4(1):1–16.

7. Riddoch G. Phantom limbs and body shape. *Brain*. 1941;64:197–222.

8. Henderson WR, Smythe GE. Phantom limbs. *J Neurol Neurosurg Psychiatry*. 1948;11:88–112.

9. Sherman RA. Stump and phantom limb pain. *Neurol Clin*. 1989;7(2):249–264.

10. Jensen TS, Krebs B, Nielsen J, Rasmussen P. Immediate and long-term phantom limb pain in amputees: Incidence, clinical characteristics and relationship to pre-amputation limb pain. *Pain*. 1985;21:267–278.

11. Appenzeller O, Bicknell JM. Effects of nervous system lesions on phantom experience in amputees. *Neurology*. 1969;19:141–146.

12. Katz J, Melzack R. Pain "memories" in phantom limbs: Review and clinical observations. *Pain*. 1990;43:319–336.

13. Varna SK, Lai SK, Mukherjee A. A study of phantom experience in amputees. *Indian J Med Sci*. 1972;26:185–188.

14. Bailey AA, Moersch FP. Phantom limb. *Can Med Assoc J*. 1941;45:37–42.

15. Szasz T. *Pain and Pleasure*. New York: Basic Books; 1975.

16. Kolb L. *The Painful Phantom*. Springfield, Ill: Charles C Thomas; 1954.

17. Hoffman J. Phantom limb syndrome. *J Nerv Ment Dis*. 1954;119:261–270.

18. Miles JE. Psychosis with phantom limb treated by chlorpromazine. *Am J Psychiatry*. 1956;112:1027–1028.

19. Ewalt JR, Randall GC, Morris H. The phantom limb. *Psychosom Med*. 1947;9:118–123.

20. Merskey H. Psychological aspects of pain. *Postgrad Med J*. 1968;44:297–306.

21. Teuber HL, Krieger HP, Bender MB. Reorganization of sensory function in amputation stumps: Two-point discrimination. *Federation Proceedings* [now *FASEB J*]. 1949;8:156.

22. Haber WB. Effects of loss of a limb on sensory functions. *J Comp Neurol*. 1955;40:115–123.

23. Merzenich MM, Kaas JH, Wall JT, Sur M, Felleman J. Progression of change following median nerve section in the cortical representation of the hand in areas 3b and 1 in adult owl and squirrel monkeys. *Neuroscience*. 1983;10:639–665.

24. Merzenich MM, Nelson RJ, Stryker MP. Somatosensory cortical map changes following digit amputation in adult monkeys. *J Comp Neurol*. 1984;224:591–605.

25. Jenkins WM, Merzenich MM, Ochs MT, Allard T, Guic-Robles E. Functional reorganization of primary somatosensory cortex in adult owl monkeys after behaviorally controlled tactile stimulation. *J Neurophysiol.* 1990;63(1):82–104.

26. Kallio KE. Phantom limb of forearm stump cleft by kineplastic surgery. *Acta Chir Scand.* 1950;99:121–132.

27. White JC. Pain after amputation: Its treatment. *JAMA.* 1944;124:1030–1040.

28. Canty TJ, Bleck EE. Amputation stump pain. *US Armed Forces Med J.* 1955;9:635–647.

29. Solonen KA. The phantom phenomenon in amputated Finnish war veterans. *Acta Orthop Scand.* 1962; Supplementeum no. 54:1–119.

30. Carlen PL, Wall PD, Nadvorna H, Steinbach T. Phantom limbs and related phenomena in recent traumatic amputations. *Neurology.* 1978;28:211–217.

31. Sherman RA, Sherman CJ, Galt NG. A survey of current phantom limb pain treatment in the United States. *Pain.* 1980;8:85–99.

32. Sherman RA, Sherman CJ. Prevalence and characteristics of chronic phantom limb pain among American veterans. *Am J Phys Med* [now *Am J Phys Med Rehabil*]. 1983;62(5):227–238.

33. Sherman RA, Sherman CJ, Parker L. Chronic phantom and stump pain among American veterans: Results of a survey. *Pain.* 1984;18:83–95.

34. Russell W. Painful amputation stumps and phantom limb treated by repeated percussion to stump neuroma. *Br Med J.* 1947;1:1024–1026.

35. Sherman RA, Galt N, Gormly J. Treatment of phantom limb pain with muscular relaxation training to disrupt the pain-anxiety cycle. *Pain.* 1979;6:47–55.

36. Katz J, Melzack R. Auricular transcutaneous electrical nerve stimulation (TENS) reduces phantom limb pain. *J Pain Symptom Manage.* 1991;6(2):73–83.

37. Elliott F, Little A, Milbrandt W. Carbamazepine for phantom-limb phenomena [letter]. *N Engl J Med.* 1976;295:678.

38. Urban BJ, France RD, Steinberger EK, Scott DL, Maltbie AA. Long-term use of narcotic/antidepressant medication in the management of phantom pain. *Pain.* 1986;24:191–196.

39. Loeser JD. Pain after amputation: Phantom limb and stump pain. In: Bonica JJ, ed. *The Management of Pain.* Philadelphia, Pa: Lea and Febiger; 1990.

40. Logan TP. Persistent phantom pain: Dramatic response to chlorpromazine. *South Med J.* 1983;76:1585.

41. Ahmad S. Phantom limb pain and propranolol [letter]. *Br Med J.* 1979;1(6160):415.

42. Marsland A, Weekes JW, Atkinson RL, Leong MG. Phantom limb pain: A case for beta blockers. *Pain.* 1982; 12:295–297.

43. Dembo T, Leviton LL, Wright BA. Adjustment to misfortune: A problem of social-psychological rehabilitation. *Artificial Limbs.* 1956;3:4–62.

44. Cushing H. Organization and activities of the Neurological Service, American Expeditionary Forces. In: Weed FW, McAfee L, eds. *Surgery: Part 1.* Vol 11. In: *The Medical Department of the United States Army in the World War.* Washington, DC; Office of The Surgeon General, US Army; 1927: 749–758.

45. Halt PS, Swanson RA, Faden AI. Alcohol exacerbates behavioral and neurochemical effects of rat spinal cord trauma. *Arch Neurol.* 1992;49:1178–1184.

46. Faden AI, Salzman S. Pharmacological strategies in CNS trauma. *Trends Pharmacol Sci.* 1992;13(1):29–35.

47. Heilporn A, Noel G. Reflections on the consciousness of disability and somatognosis in cases of acute spinal injuries. *Paraplegia*. 1968;6:121–127.

48. Ettlin TM, Seiler W, Kaeser HE. Phantom and amputation illusions in paraplegic patients. *Eur Neurol.* 1980; 19:12–19.

49. Bors E. Phantom limbs of patients with spinal cord injuries. *Arch Neurol Psychiatry* [superseded in part by *Arch Neurol* and *Arch Gen Psychiatry*]. 1951;66:610–631.

50. Conomy JP. Disorders of body image after spinal cord injury. *Neurology*. 1973;23:842–850.

51. Wittkower ED, Gingras C, Mergler L, Wigdor B, Lepine A. A combined psychosocial study of spinal cord lesions. *Can Med Assoc J*. 1954;71:109–115.

52. Davis R. Pain and suffering following spinal cord injury. *Clin Orthop*. 1975;112:76–80.

53. Weinstein EA, Kahn RL, Malitz S, Rozanski J. Delusional reduplications of parts of the body. *Brain*. 1954;77:45–60.

54. Ohry A, Gur M, Zeilig G. "Duplicate limbs" sensation in acute traumatic quadriplegia. *Paraplegia*. 1989; 27:257–260.

55. Guttmann L. *Spinal Cord Injuries. Comprehensive Management and Research*, 2nd Edition. Oxford, England: Blackwell Scientific Publications; 1976: 280, 506–511.

56. Adey W, Bors E, Porter R. EEG sleep patterns after high cervical lesions. *Arch Neurol*. 1968;19:377–383.

57. Stewart TD. Psychiatric diagnosis and treatment following spinal cord injury. *Psychosomatics*. 1988;29:214–220.

58. Jacobson SA, Bors E. Spinal cord injury in Vietnamese combat. *Paraplegia*. 1970;7:263–281.

59. Kerr WG, Thompson MA. Acceptance of disability of sudden onset in paraplegia. *Paraplegia*. 1972;10:94–102.

60. Hohmann GW. Psychological aspects of treatment and rehabilitation of the spinal cord injured patient. *Clin Orthop*. 1975;112:81–88.

61. Bracken MB, Shephard MJ. Coping and adaptation following acute spinal cord injury. *Paraplegia*. 1980;18:74–85.

62. Frank RG, Wonderlich SA, Umlauf RL, Ashkanazi GS, Buckelew SP, Elliot TR. Differences in coping style among persons with spinal cord injury: A cluster analysis approach. *J Consult Clin Psychol*. 1987;55:727–773.

63. Judd FK, Stone J, Webber JE, Brown DJ, Burrows D. Depression following spinal cord injury: A prospective in-patient study. *Br J Psychiatry*. 1989;154:668–671.

64. American Psychiatric Association. *Diagnostic and Statistical Manual of Mental Disorders, Third Edition (DSM III)*, Washington, DC: APA; 1980.

65. Lawson N. Significant events in the rehabilitation process: The spinal cord patient's point of view. *Arch Phys Med Rehabil*. 1978;59:573–577.

66. Thom A, Von Salzen CF. Psychological aspects of the paraplegic patient. *Med Clin North Am*. 1946;30:473–480.

67. Macleod AD. Self-neglect of spinal injured patients. *Paraplegia*. 1988;26:340–349.

68. Nyquist R, Bors E. Mortality and survival in traumatic myelopathy during 19 years from 1946 to 1965. *Paraplegia*. 1967;5:22–48.

69. Davis D, Bohlman H, Walker AE, Fisher R, Robinson R. The pathological findings in fatal craniospinal injuries. *J Neurosurg*. 1971;34:603–613.

70. Wilmot CB, Cope DN, Hall KM, Acker M. Occult head injury: Its incidence in spinal cord injury. *Arch Phys Med Rehabil*. 1985;66:227–231.

71. Petrus J, Balaban AB. Special psychiatric problems of the paraplegic. *Am J Psychiatry*. 1953;109:693–695.

72. Katz V, Gordon R, Iversen D, Myers SJ. Past history and degree of depression in paraplegic individuals. *Paraplegia*. 1978;16:8–14.

73. Frank RG, Elliott TR. Spinal cord injury and health locus of control beliefs. *Paraplegia*. 1989;27:250–256.

74. Roberts A. Spinal cord injury: Some psychological considerations. *Minn Med*. 1972;55:1115–1117.

75. Frisbie JH, Aguilera EJ. Chronic pain after spinal cord injury: An expedient diagnostic approach. *Paraplegia*. 1990;28:460–465.

76. Burke DC. Pain and paraplegia. *Paraplegia*. 1973;10:297–313.

77. Weiner MF, Lovitt R. Conservation-withdrawal versus depression. *Gen Hosp Psychiatry*. 1979;1:347–349.

78. Levin R, Burtt DM, Levin WA, Ginsberg MG. Ventricular fibrillation in a tetraplegic patient who had a therapeutic level of a tricyclic antidepressant. *Paraplegia*. 1985;23:354–357.

79. Pruitt BA Jr. Personal Communication, 1993.

80. Andreasen NJC, Hartford CE, Knott JR, Canter A. EEG changes associated with burn delirium. *Dis Nerv Syst*. 1977;38:27–31.

81. Noyes R, Andreasen NJC, Hartford CE. The psychological reaction to severe burns. *Psychosomatics*. 1971;12(6): 416–422.

82. Gelfand VB, Nikolajev GV. The burn encephalopathy: Its origin, clinical picture and treatment. *Acta Chir Plast*. 1986;28(2):103–110.

83. Levine NS, Atkins A, McKeel DW Jr, Peck SD, Pruitt BA Jr. Spinal cord injury following electrical accidents: Case reports. *J Trauma*. 1975;15:459–463.

84. Antoon AY, Volpe JJ, Crawford JD. Burn encephalopathy in children. *Pediatrics*. 1972;50(4):609–616.

85. Quindlen EA, Abram HS. Psychosis in the burned patient: A neglected area of research. *South Med J*. 1969; 62:1463–1466.

86. Steiner H, Clark WR. Psychiatric complications of burned adults: A classification. *J Trauma*. 1977;17:134–143.

87. Andreasen NJC, Noyes R, Hartford CE, Brodland G, Proctor S. Management of emotional reactions in severely burned patients. *N Engl J Med*. 1972;286:265–269.

88. Hamburg DA, Hamburg B, de Goza S. Adaptive problems and mechanisms in severely burned patients. *Psychiatry*. 1953;16:1–20.

89. Pruitt BA Jr. Other complications of burn injury. In: Artz CP, Moncrief JA, Pruitt BA Jr, eds. *Burns: A Team Approach*. Philadelphia, Pa: WB Saunders Company; 1979: 523.

90. Sevitt S. A review of the complications of burns, their origin and importance for illness and death. *J Trauma*. 1979;19:358–369.

91. Avni J. The severe burns. *Adv Psychosom Med*. 1980;10:57–77.

92. Sherrill KA, Larson DB. Adult burn patients: The role of religion in recovery. *South Med J*. 1988;81:821–825.

93. Cobb S, Lindemann E. Symposium on management of Coconut Grove burns at Massachusetts General Hospital. *Ann Surg*. 1943;117:814–824.

94. Watkins PN, Cook EL, May SR, Ehleben CM. Psychological stages in adaptation following burn injury. *J Burn Care Rehabil*. 1988;9:376–384.

95. Kjaer GC. Psychiatric aspects of thermal burns. *Northwest Med*. 1969;68:537–541.

96. Duke-Elder PM, McFaul S. *System of Ophthalmology*, Volume 14. St Louis, Mo: CV Mosby; 1972: 51–56.

97. Lowrey A, Shaffer F. Eye, ear, nose and throat injuries sustained in the Korean theatre. *Trans Pac Coast Oto-Ophthalmol Soc*. 1954;35:39–44.

98. Hoefle FB. Initial treatment of eye injuries. *Arch Ophthalmol*. 1968;79:33–35.

99. LaPiana FG. Unpublished analysis prepared for the Center of Military History, US Department of the Army, Washington, DC, 1985.

100. Treister G. Ocular casualties in the Six-Day War. *Am J Ophthalmol*. 1969;68:669–675.

101. Zeki S. The visual image in mind and brain. *Sci Am*. 1992;267:68–76.

102. Cohn R. Phantom vision. *Arch Neurol*. 1971;25:468–471.

103. Bender MB. Disorders in visual perception. In: Halpern L, ed. *Problems in Dynamic Neurology*. Jerusalem, Israel: Hebrew University Hadassah Medical School; 1963: 356–358.

104. Damas-Mora J, Skelton-Robinson M, Jenner FA. The Charles Bonnet syndrome in perspective. *Psychol Med*. 1982;12:251–261.

105. Fitzgerald RG. Visual phenomenology in recently blinded adults. *Am J Psychiatry*. 1971;127:1533–1539.

106. Wittkower E, Davenport RC. The war blinded. *Psychosom Med*. 1946;8:121–137.

107. Vinger PF. Personal Communication, 1993.

108. Diamond BL, Ross A. Emotional adjustment of newly blinded soldiers. *Am J Psychiatry*. 1945;102:367–371.

109. Williams RC. Personal Communication, 1993.

110. Keegan DL, Ash DG, Greenough T. Blindness: Some psychological and social implications. *Can Psychiatr Assoc J* [now *Can J Psychiatry*]. 1976;21:333–340.

111. Carroll TJ. *Blindness: What It Is, What It Does, How To Deal With It*. Boston, Mass: Little Brown; 1961: 73.

112. Cholden L. Some psychiatric problems in the rehabilitation of the blind. *Bull Menninger Clin*. 1954;18:107–112.

113. Brown R, Schutte H. *Our Fight: A Battle Against Darkness*. Washington, DC: Blinded Veterans Association; 1991.

114. Fitzgerald RG, Ebert JN, Chambers M. Reaction to blindness: A four year follow-up study. *Percept Mot Skill*. 1987;64:363–378.

115. Hoehn-Saric R, Frank E, Hirst LW, Seltser CG. Coping with sudden blindness. *J Nerv Ment Dis.* 1981;169:662–665.

116. Weinstein EA, Kahn RL. *Denial of Illness: Symbolic and Physiological Factors.* Springfield, Ill: Charles C Thomas; 1955.

117. Adams GL, Pearlman JT, Sloan HS. Guidelines for the psychiatric referral of visually handicapped patients. In: Adams GL, Pearlman JT, Sloan SH, eds. *Psychiatric Problems in Ophthalmology.* Springfield, Ill: Charles C Thomas; 1977: 142–151.

118. Bledsoe CW. *War Blinded Veterans in a Postwar Setting.* Washington, DC: Veterans Administration; 1958.

119. Greear JN. The rehabilitation of blinded casualties. In: Coates JB Jr, ed. *Ophthalmology and Otolaryngology.* In: *Surgery in World War II.* Washington, DC: Office of The Surgeon General, US Army; 1957 (reprint 1986): 147–209.

120. Aaby G. USARV [US Army Vietnam] Surgery Consultant's Report, July 1967–June 1968. 35–40.

121. Busch FM, Chenault OW, Zinner NR, Clarke BG. Urological aspects of Vietnam war injuries. *J Urol.* 1967;97:763–765.

122. Selikowitz SM. Penetrating high-velocity genitourinary injuries. Part I: Statistics, mechanisms, and renal wounds. *Urology.* 1977;9(5):371–376.

123. Selikowitz SM. Penetrating high-velocity genitourinary injuries. Part II: Ureteral, lower tract, and genital wounds. *Urology.* 1977;9(5):493–499.

124. Wettlaufer JN. Personal Communication, 1993.

125. Frumkin AP. Reconstruction of the male genitalia. *Am Rev Sov Med.* 1944;2:14–21.

126. Marshall DF. Urogenital wounds in an evacuation hospital. *J Urol.* 1946;55:119–132.

127. Umhey CE. Experiences with genital wounds in Vietnam: A report of 25 cases. *J Urol.* 1968;99:660–661.

128. Selikowitz SM. Personal Communication, 1993.

129. Margolis G, Selikowitz SM. A soldier and a physician: Two decisions for life. *Dartmouth Med Sch Alum J.* 1980;Fall Issue:24–26.

Chapter 15

CONVERSION DISORDERS

EDWIN A. WEINSTEIN, M.D.*

*Consultant in Neurology, National Naval Medical Center, Bethesda, Maryland; Consultant in Psychiatry, Walter Reed Army Medical Center, Washington, D.C.; and Formerly Chief, Fifth Army Neuropsychiatric Center (World War II)

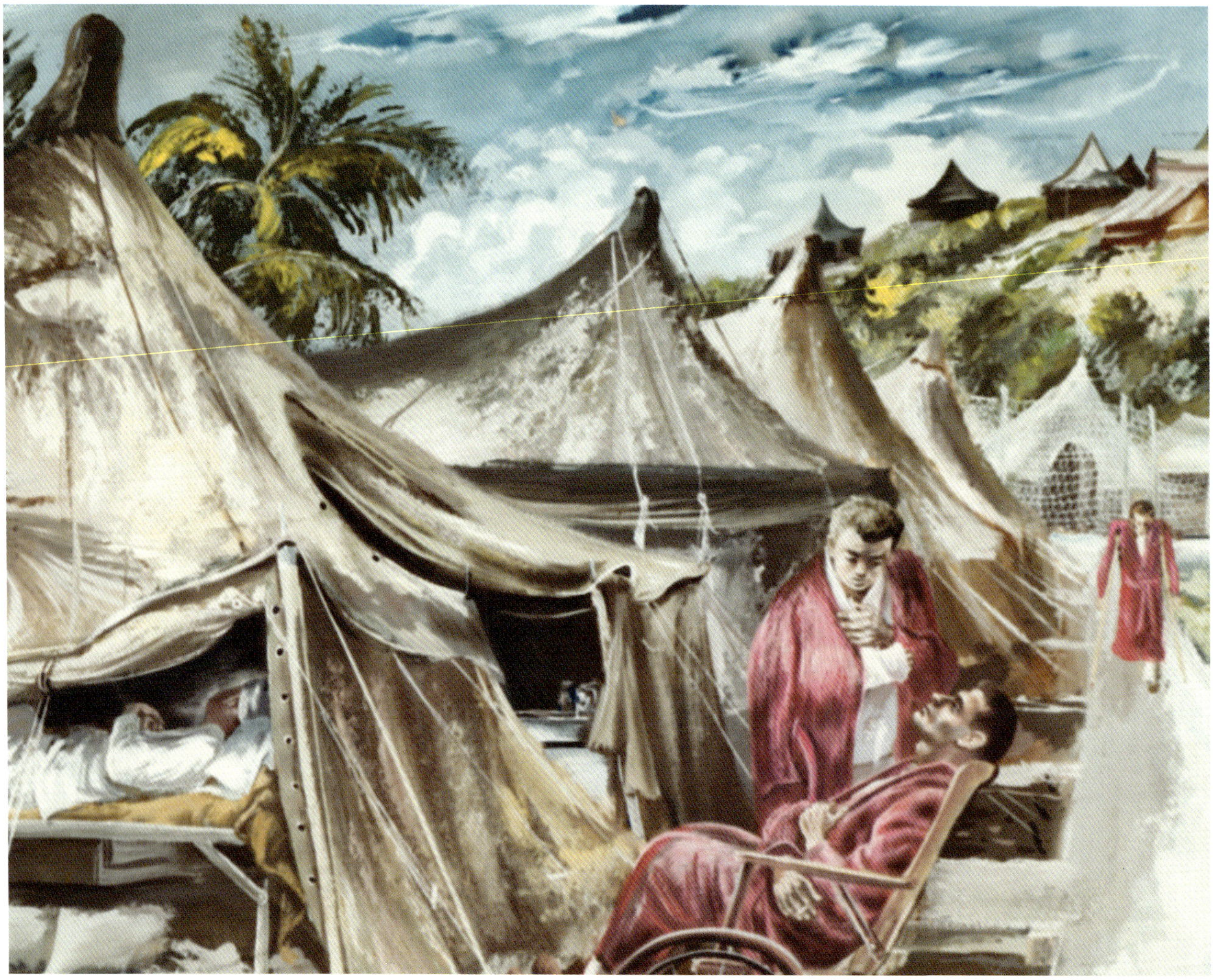

Aaron Bohrod *Tent Hospital* 1943

Aaron Bohrod was engaged as an artist by the War Department Artist's Advisory Committee and was in the South Pacific, England, and France during World War II. In this painting, he captures the variety of patients seen in a field hospital. Of particular interest is the patient in the wheelchair—slumped down, arms completely limp, head back, vacant stare—a soldier who has seen too much and cannot even move himself into an upright seated position. He presents as a classic conversion disorder with the obvious conflict between his desire to serve and his invalidism which prevents it.

Art: Courtesy of US Center of Military History, Washington, DC.

INTRODUCTION

Although ideas of hysteria and conversion disorders have changed radically over the centuries, almost all have emphasized emotional and physical traumas and their effects on the brain or mind. While the incidence of conversion reactions has declined in developed countries, the occurrence of the condition in association with violence and stress makes it particularly relevant to military medicine. Military approaches have been shaped by concepts derived from civilian practice, and, in turn, wartime experiences have contributed greatly to current theoretical formulations. This chapter provides a historical review of conversion disorders in wartime, considers epidemiological and demographic aspects, examines psychological, symbolic and neural factors, and takes up problems of differential diagnosis and treatment.

A conversion disorder, as defined by the Diagnostic and Statistical Manual, 3rd edition, of the American Psychiatric Association (DSM-III),[1] is a loss or alteration of physical functioning suggestive of physical disease but expressing a psychological conflict or need in a nonvoluntary fashion. In practice, the term is limited to findings on neurological examination that imitate neurological disease, but do not conform to anatomical or physiological patterns. It includes paralysis, somatic and special sensory disturbances, involuntary movements, pseudoseizures, speech, gait, and memory disorders, and excludes symptoms referable to the gastrointestinal, cardiorespiratory, and genitourinary systems. Broadly, the symptom can be seen as the symbolic representation of some problem or disability. Conversion disorders are differentiated from hysterical personality, somatization disorder, hypochondriasis, and psychogenic pain. Pain, however, is commonly associated. The terms conversion disorder and hysteria will be used interchangeably here depending on contemporary reference.

HISTORY

The Civil War

By the middle of the 19th century it had been recognized that hysteria was a disease of the mind and the brain, but it was still considered a female malady. The gender difference was variously attributed to reflex irritation from the uterus and ovary, to women's greater sensitivity, emotionality, and impressionability, which made them more sensitive to the effects of fear, excitement, grief and jealousy, and to sexual repressions and frustrations. Both abstinence and overindulgence were invoked as causes. Hysteria was known in men, but only in those who were effeminate or homosexual. Authors also emphasized heredity, citing mental illness and diseases such as epilepsy and syphilis.

Against this background, it is not surprising that cases of hysteria were not recorded in the Civil War, in which the major neuropsychiatric disabilities were nostalgia, soldier's heart, and insanity. A review, however, of individual cases in the medical journals of the day suggests that a considerable number of the 28.3% of discharges for epilepsy, and of the 20.8% for paralysis involved conversion disorders.[2] One such case was that of a 28-year-old recruit who, after an altercation with an officer while seeking to desert, became unable to move any of his limbs. Subsequently, he developed violent tremors of his head and upper extremities. Pressure on the soles of his feet produced saltatory arching of his back. On attempting to walk he would take a few powerful and ungoverned steps and then throw himself on a bed. He was discharged from service with a diagnosis of choreic convulsion, and, 2 months later was reported to be completely recovered.[3]

Further evidence for the existence of conversion disorders in the Civil War comes from the records of the military hospital set up at Turner's Lane in Philadelphia by William A. Hammond, Surgeon-General of the Union Army, for the study and treatment of wounds and other injuries of the nervous system. There, Silas Weir Mitchell and his colleagues, George D. Morehouse and William W. Keen,[4] described seven cases of "reflex paralysis" which were almost certainly conversion reactions. In these patients a missile wound of an extremity which had not damaged a major nerve resulted in a transient paralysis of all four limbs or an enduring weakness and sensory loss in several extremities. In one instance, a man who had been shot through the right thigh developed a loss of sensation over the entire right half of his body. Patients responded to faradic stimulation but only up to a point short of complete recovery. Mitchell had studied in Paris, then the leading center of neurology in the world, and was familiar with the manifestations of hysteria. He may have considered the diagnosis as he mentioned the case of an officer in the Mexican War who had become "almost hysterical" after having been shot through the heel. The officer, however, had a reputation for courage under fire and it was an article of faith that hysteria did not occur in strong men not weakened by indulgence in sex, alcohol, or tobacco.[4]

After the Civil War

The decades following the Civil War may be regarded as the golden age of hysteria. The condition was romanticized in Victorian novels, and provided the central theme for the concepts of mental illness put forward by Paul Briquet, Jean-Martin Charcot, Pierre Janet, and Sigmund Freud.

Briquet[5] found that hysteria occurred predominantly in lower-class women who led lives of hardships and poverty, rather than among the privileged groups of society. Taking up the role of sexuality, he compared the incidence of hysteria—as diagnosed by the standards of the time—in chaste nuns, female domestic servants (who might supplement their incomes through sexual accommodations), and professional Parisian prostitutes. He discovered the highest rate in prostitutes and the lowest in nuns, with servants in between. Briquet concluded that the significant agent was not sexual indulgence per se but the distressing conditions under which the activity was carried out. He thought that emotions such as fear and grief affected the part of the brain which was the seat of feelings and that this in turn produced the hysterical symptom.

Jean-Martin Charcot[6] believed that a past psychological trauma could affect the function of the cerebral cortex, and produce such hysterical disorders as aphonia, hemiplegia, and seizures. He showed that symptoms could be both produced and removed by suggestion, and regarded susceptibility to suggestion and hypnosis as evidence of hereditary weakness of the nervous system. Charcot thought that a volitional element might be present and emphasized the need for discipline in treatment. He urged that patients be isolated from their families and from others with hysteria to provide a better moral environment. Charcot and his followers, known as the school of La Salpetriere, stressed the so-called stigmata of hysteria, such as ovarian tenderness, pharyngeal and corneal anesthesia, and concentric constriction of the visual fields. Joseph Babinski, one of Charcot's pupils, believed that hysterical hemianesthesias, and other manifestations were artifacts of the neurological examination produced by unconscious suggestion by the physician.

Pierre Janet,[7] another of Charcot's disciples, believed that the traumatic event occurred in a setting of altered consciousness or trance state, and was not integrated into conscious awareness. The dissociated ideas and affects produced the hysterical symptoms. Janet thought that chronic disease, organic affections of the nervous system, psychic weakness, and a succession of cumulative emotional effects made the individual more vulnerable to dissociation.

John Russell Reynolds[8] in London proposed that a hysterical paralysis was caused by the *idea* of a paralysis and the emotion associated with it and by a loss of the will to move the limb(s), and that treatment depended on the removal of that idea. Reynolds noted that in men the hysterical manifestations frequently came on after a fall from a horse or other accident, and that in women idleness, preoccupation with domestic matters, and frigidity were the principal factors. He also remarked on the association with organic brain disease and physical illness.

Joseph Breuer and Sigmund Freud[9] in 1895 cited such emotional traumas as guilt over a father's illness, unrequited love, and remorse over the wish to marry a dying sister's husband. They found that hysterical symptoms brought on by even minor upsets or injuries could be traced back to traumas early in life for which the memory and associated affect had been repressed. After Freud gave up the seduction theory—the idea that the origin of hysteria lay in the sexual abuse of children—he held that the original trauma involved emotions connected with the child's own sexual and aggressive drives. These affects and memories were converted into somatic symptoms in order to maintain a constant level of energy in the nervous system. The hysterical manifestation, in Freud's view, was the expression of sexual gratification along with efforts to suppress it, although he agreed that nonsexual impulses might be involved.[9] He later was to attribute the traumatic neurosis of World War I to the narcissistic attachment of the libido to the ego, engendered not only by fear of battle but by reactivation of the castration complex. Freud, like others, believed in a hereditary factor, noting that one half of his patients with hysteria and psychasthenia (ie, obsessions and phobias) had a syphilitic father.

Briquet, Charcot, and Freud had all described hysteria in female patients. It was, however, not until the rapid industrial growth following the Civil War, particularly the expansion of the railroads and the advent of compensation legislation and litigation, that the existence of male hysteria in the form of the traumatic neurosis was generally recognized.

A man who had been shaken up or bruised in a fall or a railway accident would complain of pain and inability to move his legs, and examination would show tenderness over the spine, and apparent paralysis and anesthesia below the waist. At first these findings were attributed to injury of the spinal column, or to concussion or anemia of the spinal cord, but the observations of Herbert Page, surgeon to the London and Northwest Railway, and James J. Putnam of Boston established the functional nature of the condition. By 1895, James Hendrie Lloyd, writing in Francis X. Dercum's authoritative textbook on nervous disease, could state that next to heredity, trauma was the most important cause of hysteria and that some of the worst cases occurred in men. Others thought that patients with railway spine were malingerers and, like Weir Mitchell, did not accept the existence of male hysteria until World War I.

World War I

Conversion disorders, along with neurasthenia (ie, anxiety and exhaustion), were the leading categories of neuropsychiatric breakdown in both combat and noncombat situations in World War I. There were 6,250 cases, representing an incidence of 1.53/1,000/y of total strength, admitted to U.S. military hospitals from 1 April 1917 to 31 December 1918.[10] Although Congress declared war in April 1917, it was more than a year before U.S. troops engaged in significant combat, and the data are derived mainly from British, French, and German sources.

In the early years of the war, ideas of hereditary and acquired predisposition to the effects of shell shock provided explanations of conversion disorder and neurasthenia. Frederic W. Mott, a British medical officer in charge of a large hospital in London, was the leading advocate of the view that the concussive action of the shell explosions caused minute brain hemorrhages, and that the large majority of men who broke down after such an experience had inborn neuropathic or psychopathic tendencies, a family history of alcoholism, insanity, or epilepsy, or a timorous disposition.[11,12] The French differentiated the contusional effects of shell explosions with focal neurological signs and bloody or xanthochromic spinal fluid, from the commotional or concussional effects, and from the emotional sequelae.

It was soon evident that conversion reactions occurred in men who had not been in the immediate proximity of an exploding shell. They appeared in soldiers who had undergone terrifying and life-threatening experiences, such as witnessing scenes of death and mutilation or undergoing torpedoing at sea. They were more apt to appear in places of relative security before the opening of a barrage, or after a man had reached a clearing station rather than in the midst of combat. Conversion reactions also occurred after relatively minor trauma—a slight wound, bruises, or burns. It was not uncommon for the conversion symptom to come on days, weeks, or even months after the reported trauma, after what Charcot had referred to as a *phase de meditation*. There was a very low incidence of traumatic neurosis in prisoners of war.[13]

British, French, and German observers noted that conversion reactions were more common at base installations than in forward or combat support areas. Eder[14] found that 77% of patients at a British hospital in Malta were so classified. U.S. experience was similar in that there was a higher rate of hospital admissions for conversion disorders in men who had never left the continental United States than in those who had served overseas.[10] Among patients in General Hospital No. 3 set up in Plattsburg, New York for the treatment of war neuroses, conversion disorders outnumbered other categories combined.

The significance of preexisting constitutional factors was a controversial issue in the German as well as the Allied armies. At the German Neurological Congress held in Munich in September 1916, R. Gaupp presented the case for predisposition, while M. Nonne was the leading advocate of the view that the cause of the war neuroses lay less in the personal constitution than in the nature of the trauma. Working in hospitals in Hamburg and Schleswig Holstein, Nonne found that the "hysterical character" was lacking in the majority of his cases.[15] Hurst[16] found many cases of gross hysterical symptoms in British soldiers who had no family or personal history of neurosis and who were perfectly fit up to the time of the traumatic incident. It should be noted that the original British Army in France was made up largely of volunteers. Even Mott stated later in the war that premorbid factors were important only in neurasthenia.[11] Rather than occurring in men with timorous dispositions, many conversion disorders were observed in noncommissioned officers and enlisted men with good combat records, and in daredevil types who had volunteered for hazardous assignments such as dispatch rider, stretcher bearer, or sniper.

Both British and American data indicated a marked difference in the incidence of conversion disorders in commissioned officers and enlisted men. The British found that the symptoms displayed by officers were predominantly of the neurasthenic type, while enlisted men had mainly hysterical manifestations. In the British Army, rank was an indicator of social class, and it was believed that the forces of education, tradition, and example in the officer groups made for greater self-control and better ability to resist a sudden breaking emotion or trauma.[17] In the U.S. Army, disability discharges for hysteria in officers were four times less frequent than those for neurasthenia, whereas in enlisted personnel the ratio was approximately equal.[10]

Conversion symptoms included mutism and stammering, deafness, gross tremor and other involuntary movements, paralysis and anesthesia, abnormal postures and contractures, astasia (an inability to maintain stance), abasia (an inability to coordinate movements in walking), and other gait disturbances, seizures, amnesia, and fugue states. In the French Army paraplegia and monoplegia were the most frequent forms of paralysis.[18] Blindness was less common than blurring of vision and blepharospasm. It was usual for soldiers to report having been blown up or buried after a shell explosion, and then having no memory of events prior to arriving at the clearing station. There were episodes of excitement and delirium for which the soldier would later be amnesic, and periods of stupor often preceded muteness, deafness, and paralysis. The type and location of the conversion manifestation was frequently determined by the character of the trauma. Astasia-abasia, the most common conversion manifestation of the war, occurred frequently in men who had been thrown violently to the ground and who had rolled into a trench or hollow and had been able to get to an aid station by laboriously walking or crawling.[18] Hemiparesis might be preceded by an injury to that side of the body. Paralysis or contracture of a limb might follow a local wound, or might come on after a period of immobilization in a splint, sling, or cast.

A large number of cases, sometimes in epidemic proportions, followed gas attacks. Chlorine and mustard gas caused conjunctivitis making it painful for the man to close his lids, produced irritation of the throat, larynx, and bronchial tree, and resulted in gastritis from swallowed saliva. These symptoms usually cleared within 2 to 3 weeks, but some soldiers developed hysterical blindness, ptosis, aphonia, vomiting, and respiratory difficulty. (Adolf Hitler became blind and mute for several weeks after having been exposed to mustard gas in the last days of the war, and may well have had a hysterical disorder.) Gas neurosis epidemics also occurred after desultory gas shelling or even after an alarm had been erroneously sounded, even without evidence of inhalation or vesicant action.

Problems in diagnosis arose. Prior to the war most physicians who had been engaged in private practice or administrative work were not familiar with the traumatic neuroses. Early in the war, cases of conversion disorder were considered to have organic disease and were evacuated to the neurological centers in base areas where they might be treated with rest, hydrotherapy, and other measures which perpetuated the symptoms. It was also shown that patients with evidence of brain damage could have conversion manifestations.[16,19] Moreover, such stigmata as hysterogenic zones (ie, areas of anesthesia or tenderness on the back or abdomen, concentric constriction of the visual fields, and corneal and pharyngeal anesthesia) proved to be unreliable indicators.[15,16] As Babinski had found, narrowing and spiraling of the visual fields were frequently an artifact of the examination of the perimeter of men who had no visual symptoms. Similarly the classical *la belle indifference* (being indifferent to the situation) might not be present.

Treatment included suggestion, persuasion, explanation, reeducation, hypnosis, and more physical measures such as isolation and deprivation, faradization (stimulation by electrical current), and sedation. Hypnosis was used with suggestion, and also in attempts to recover repressed feelings and memories. Psychotherapy strove to encourage catharsis, and deal with feelings of grief, shame, fear, anger, and guilt. The overall experience was that the efficacy of whatever treatment was employed increased with proximity to the front and the promptness with which it was applied. While hysterical manifestations might be removed at a base hospital, the majority of such cases did not return to successful combat duty. The soldier might develop headaches and other manifestations of anxiety or depression, or his conversion symptom might return during some frightening situation, such as a London air-raid.[17,19] The British found that amnesia, mutism, and paralysis responded readily as did gas hysteria, while deafness was the most intractable.[20] The American experience was that symptoms which occurred in conditions in which there had been a definite trauma or acute emotional insult succeeded by a stage of amnesia or dissociation had the best outcome.[10]

The French, in the tradition of Charcot and Babinski, regarded conversion disorders not as diseases but as failures of will or attitude. Conditions such as mutism, trembling, and paralysis were treated first by persuasion and encouragement, and if these measures were inadequate, by isolation and bed rest without permission to read, write, or smoke. If cure still had not resulted, painful faradic stimulation, *torpillage* (*torpille* = torpedo [numb fish]) was applied. Inveterate hysterics were regarded as malingerers and might be subject to court-martial.[18] The French were the first to treat such "emotional" cases in forward areas, a policy not adopted in the British Army until the winter of 1916 to 1917.

There were also cases in which conversion symptoms cleared after some emotional shock as in the instance of a man with hysterical blindness following torpedoing whose sight returned after he was thrown into the sea. Another man suddenly regained speech during a bombing raid by Zeppelins.[17]

The observations of conversion disorders in World War I can be summarized as follows:

1. The conversion symptom was often a reenactment or symbolic representation of recent traumatic experience.
2. Trauma was a necessary but not sufficient agent in that the incidence did not depend on the severity of the injury or emotional insult.
3. Symptoms might come on at a considerable interval following trauma and persist in chronic form.
4. Social class and education were significant factors in that the incidence was greater in enlisted men than in commissioned officers.
5. Individual predisposition was not a factor in the sense that men who developed conversion disorders had had more mental illness or were of a more timid, nervous temperament.
6. Many forms of therapy were effective provided that they were administered promptly and in close proximity to the soldier's unit.

World War II

There was little academic interest in conversion disorders in the decades following World War I. The condition was thought to be disappearing because of greater sophistication and sexual liberation—actually a decline in incidence and less dramatic presentation had been noted at the turn of the century—but other factors were involved. Nineteenth century physicians had focused on the physical stigmata of mental illness, whereas later ones were more concerned with psychological mechanisms. New neurological procedures such as the introduction of the Babinski sign and the delineation of the functions of the parietal lobe led to better diagnosis. A number of the manifestations of conversion disorders were placed in the growing category of psychosomatic disease. Patients with conversion symptoms, who tended to be less educated and more apt to come from rural areas, were not considered good candidates for psychoanalytically oriented therapy, and were likely to be treated by local practitioners or referred to public clinics.[21,22] Compensation traumatic neuroses were not considered worthy of scientific study.

Theoretical formulations, despite the experience of the war, were for the most part reiterations of Freudian concepts. These emphasized intrapsychic struggle and regression to earlier stages of psychosexual development. Little attention was given to current trauma which was regarded mainly as a trigger of hitherto repressed drives and conflicts. Hypnosis fell into disuse, as it was felt that symptom removal did not touch the deeper problems. It was also believed that conversion symptoms might serve as a defense against a psychosis.[23] Nonanalytically oriented psychiatrists saw the issue as a conflict between the instinct of self-preservation and the demands of society without regard for situational factors and group interactive processes.

Conversion disorders were much less common in World War II than they had been in World War I, but they made up a significant proportion of neuropsychiatric casualties. Comparisons are difficult because revision of nomenclature had removed the somatic manifestations of anxiety and cardiorespiratory, gastrointestinal, and genitourinary symptoms from the conversion reactions. The rates as a consequence of combat varied with the intensity of the fighting, the location and expertise of the medical facility, and the conditions of evacuation. Reports from combat support areas in Italy[24] and

Normandy and Germany[25,26] showed an incidence of about 5% of neuropsychiatric casualties. The incidence among men evacuated to one hospital in the South Pacific 4 to 6 weeks after the onset of symptoms was 17%.[27] A British report of neuropsychiatric casualties admitted to a rear-area installation during the retreat to El Alamein and the advance into Tripolitania gave an incidence of 26%.[28] After a study of documents and interviews with former Wehrmacht psychiatrists, Schneider[29] concluded that conversion manifestations such as trembling and paralysis were common in the German Army.

The conversion manifestations matched those of World War I with paralysis of limbs, bizarre postures and gaits, involuntary movements and seizures, muteness and stammering, hearing and visual loss, and amnesia. There were also the stupors and other acute dissociative reactions, referred to as pseudopsychoses in which men experienced episodes of agitation, hallucinations and paranoid ideation, and performed such stereotypic activities as digging foxholes with their fingers, and taking shelter under cots at any sudden sound. These reactions occurred predominantly in young soldiers new to their units. Swank,[26] on the basis of his experience in Normandy and Germany, noted that hysterical paralyses and anesthesias occurred more frequently in airborne troops with good combat records than in other U.S. Army personnel and that the manifestations were almost always superimposed on a wound, injury, or surgical procedure. Swank found that all of his cases showed emotional tension rather than the traditional *la belle indifference*.

Symptoms were also occupationally determined. Anderson[30] noted that airmen developed complaints which did not totally incapacitate them, but which did not allow them to carry out certain types of operations. The symptoms included reduced visual acuity, impaired depth perception, diminished night vision, and altered hearing. These caused minimal discomfort, but disqualified the man from formation and night flying and from use of the intercommunication system. In many instances flyers could hear everything perfectly well with the sole exception of the radio beam. Blindness and concentric visual field constrictions were rare. The disability might be stated in terms of performance rather than symptoms as a patient might complain of difficulties in gauging distances when flying in formation.[31] Similarly, hysterical amblyopia was observed to appear suddenly in soldiers in whom the eye was particularly important in fighting, such as sharpshooters.[32] The following is an account of an acute combat conversion reaction.

Case Study 1: One More Shot

A 23-year-old infantry staff sergeant was admitted on a litter to the 601st Clearing Company in June 1944 during the fighting about Grossetto, Italy. His right arm was paralyzed below the elbow with a corresponding anesthesia. He stammered and said he could not see objects on his left side, and could not recall the first three digits of his serial number. He could recall nothing since being blown up and buried in a shell explosion. He expressed great fear that he would be killed. After examination which did not show a hemianopia or organic weakness or sensory loss, and assurances that he would recover, he was placed in isolation. When interviewed 8 hours later he was markedly improved. He could move his arm, talk clearly, and walk without assistance. He told the following story.

"First day of battle I shot a dago eight times because he shot at me. I guess I must have just lost my head. We dug in and went to bed. I was with the Armd. Div. [Armored Division] riding tanks—three of my men got killed by shells then just this side of Rome. We took Grossetto—took a hill, man hit me with a rifle butt [scar in left supraorbit] that scared me—I killed him with a bayonet—that bothered me, my father taught me never to kill—he's an invalid; he's a Christian man too....[W]alked some more, kept going north into the mountains. Got pinned down, shelled for 2 hours, killed two of my men and a lieutenant. Got to a little town; Battalion Commander lost his head, ordered four men in; he got nicked then ordered us to withdraw. Then went on tanks that shelled us [weeps], killed my lieutenant ...[m]y platoon leader was hit, I was in charge. I ordered my men out. I stopped to take one more shot. I heard the Germans holler FIRE in English and that's all I remember until they picked me up in a jeep. My gas mask and shoulder straps had been shot off. Then I went to sleep and don't remember anything until this morning. The gun was blown out of my hand, all that was left was the trigger part. I guess the flash must have blinded me."[24(p135)]

Comment: The case illustrates a number of features:

1. The manner in which the symptom is a condensed symbolic representation of current experience rather than a revival of some childhood conflict.
2. The relationship of the site of the conversion manifestation to the type of physical injury.
3. The amnesia in which soldiers commonly reported that they remembered nothing from the time they were "blown up" in a shell explosion and "buried." As noted in World War I, actual burial incidents were infrequent although soldiers might be covered with debris. Rather the "burial" symbolized fear and feelings about death.
4. The coincidental occurrence of recovery and a dramatic account of traumatic experience.

5. The association of a conversion reaction with a high degree of anxiety.

As in this patient, some men with conversion reactions responded to suggestion and a period of sleep and isolation. In others hypnosis and the techniques of narcoanalysis[33] or narcosynthesis[34] were used. Each aimed at restoring the memory of the combat experience and allowing the ventilation of the affect. If the patient was amnesic it was suggested after the injection intravenously of sodium pentothol or Sodium Amytal that he go over the events immediately preceding the period for which he had no recall. If there was no amnesia he was asked to revisualize the scene just prior to the onset of his symptoms.

The recall or revisualization was usually associated with marked emotion and excitement. Events would be reenacted vividly: patients would yell, cower in fear, or strike at an examiner who was apparently mistaken for an enemy or a hated officer. In the method of narcosynthesis described by Grinker and Spiegel the examiner would simulate the sounds of combat, mimicking the antiaircraft fire and the shouts of the bomber crew. Or if it was known that the soldier was in a tank unit he would be warned that his tank was on fire and he had to climb out. Even though the patient might recall events for which he had been amnesic, the therapeutic effects seemed to depend on the degree of emotion displayed.

It was noted that patients might abreact with the introduction of the drug even though no suggestion that he recall the trauma was made. Also, the events that were reproduced were not necessarily those that preceded the onset of amnesia or other conversion manifestations. Recollections might be highly melodramatic with a mixture of fact and fantasy.[24,35,36] In a case treated by the author at the U.S. Army's 601st Clearing Company in Italy, the patient who had become dramatically blind "recalled" how he had been searching for his brother among the dead and wounded. He later admitted that his actual brother was safe in the United States.

As in World War I, once patients had been evacuated from their units, removal of a major conversion symptom by any method did not in most instances result in a successful return to combat duty even though in some cases soldiers asked to go back. It did, however, diminish the need for further hospitalization, and the majority of such soldiers could be released for noncombat service. By the end of the Italian campaign, the use of barbiturates at the U.S. Army level had been reduced. If symptoms persisted, despite attempts at abreaction, the patient was placed in an isolation tent with minimal privileges and told when his nervous condition cleared up he would be assigned to less hazardous duty. If these measures failed, the man was evacuated to a base section installation, where electroconvulsive treatment was effective in treating amnesias, mutism, seizures, astasia-abasias, deafness, and hyperkinesias.[37]

The experience of the Holocaust emphasizes the importance of motivation and secondary gain. Despite the terror, the gruesome conditions, and the appalling amount of physical injury, conversion reactions in the concentration camps were almost unknown. Eitinger, a Norwegian psychiatrist, who was a prisoner himself, commented on their rarity in Auschwitz where the appearance of a symptom meant instant death.[38] Kral[39] noted a few cases in Terezin that occurred while prisoners were awaiting transportation to extermination camps further eastward. Later studies of survivors showed a high incidence of brain damage and post-traumatic stress disorder.[40]

Korea and Vietnam

Rates of conversion disorders along with those for other psychiatric casualties were lower in Korea and Vietnam than they had been in World War II. In Vietnam, character and behavior disorders and substance abuse predominated, and the incidence of conversion reactions appeared to vary with proximity to combat. Jones,[41] who served with an infantry division and field hospital in Vietnam, remarked on the rarity of both combat fatigue and conversion reactions, while a higher rate was suggested by Carden and Schramel[42] who saw their 12 patients after they had been evacuated to the Philippines. In a temporal frame, while the overall combat casualty rate reached its peak in 1968 and 1969, the incidence of conversion disorders continued to increase, reaching a 1975 high of 95/100,000/y in patients in U.S. Army medical facilities worldwide, followed by a steady decline.[43]

A prior wound was an important risk factor both for conversion reactions and other psychiatric disorders among U.S. Marines.[44] In U.S. Army personnel, Jones noted, similarly, that *conversion manifestations were apt to appear when a wounded hospitalized soldier was about to return to duty.*

DEVELOPMENTS AFTER WORLD WAR II

Whereas the combat experience of World War I had little impact on psychiatric thought, that of World War II profoundly affected developments in areas relevant to conversion disorders. These concerned the:

1. Psychological and physiological effects of stress and violence associated with traumatic life events in persons without prior personality disorders or unusual emotional problems. These include assaults and injuries, rape, medical and surgical illnesses, natural catastrophes, political terrorism, family violence, and death of a loved one.
2. Concept of denial as a coping mechanism during and following trauma. Prior to the war and the Holocaust, psychoanalysis had focused on the denial or repression of unacceptable inner drives. Denial of external reality was considered to be indicative of severe psychopathology or a weak ego. The war experience showed that denial could be used by normal persons in adaptive—or maladaptive—fashion. The soldier who was well-integrated into his unit perceived the hostile environment as less life-threatening than the man who had little confidence in his leaders, and was otherwise not identified with the values of his group. When, however, denial of danger was expressed in a failure to follow safety procedures, it became highly maladaptive. In concentration camps it was observed that prisoners who could deny the inevitability of death by selective inattention and emotional numbing, and carry on by helping others, were most likely to survive. Those who expressed denial by escape into day dreaming and by not accepting the grim realities soon perished.[38]
3. Dissociative states such as feelings of depersonalization, derealization and detachment from one's body, and amnesia and fugues, which, like denial, are commonly associated with trauma. Patients with multiple personality have a high incidence of conversion disorders.[45]
4. Development of procedures and methods of study which established the organic nature of conditions once thought to be of hysterical origin, such as the focal dystonias, reflex sympathetic dystrophy and transient global amnesia.
5. Investigation of the roles of brain damage and cerebral hemisphere asymmetry in the incidence of and lateralization of symptoms in conversion disorders.
6. Sociocultural and epidemiological aspects of mental illness.

Role of Violence

The relationship of violence to conversion disorders was studied in a series of investigations at the Veterans Administration Hospital in Salem, Virginia and the Walter Reed Army Medical Center in Washington, D.C.[46–48] A majority, 70%, of patients, including men and women, attributed their symptoms to an injury, or placed the onset in a traumatic setting, even though the trauma may have been minor and occurred months or years previously. Reports included falls, wounds, blows, vehicle accidents, surgical operations, a dental novocaine injection, family quarrels, witnessing an act of violence, and, in one instance, a voodoo spell. Women were more apt to cite sexual violence, such as an attempted rape or seduction or a Lesbian solicitation. In contrast, control subjects with organic impairments comparable to the conversion symptom did not invoke trauma unless the disability had actually been caused by an injury. Similarly, none of a group of patients with anxiety states that served as another control attributed his illness to injury.

A content analysis of verbal language showed that conversion subjects also used more words of violence to describe their symptoms and experiences. Patients with hemisensory syndromes spoke of a side as "dead," and as feeling as if they had been "cut in half." Men who had been in vehicle accidents used more expressions such as, "smashed," "mashed," and "killed" than controls who had sustained comparable accidents and injuries. A soldier who developed a functional paralysis of his right arm after bayonet practice characterized the exercise as "kill or be killed." Violence was the metaphor through which the patient organized his experience, and his idea of what happened to him was, in terms of the response of his nervous system, as important as what actually happened. A decorated veteran of the Korean conflict, the sole survivor of an airplane crash in which 20 people had died, described the screams of the dying and the smell of the flesh of burning bodies, even though he had been unconscious at the time.

The following case illustrates how the recall of traumatic events and the idiom of violence may serve as symbolic or metaphorical representations of current problems, and how the intensity of such recollections may vary with changes in the person's present circumstances. The case also indicates the association of a conversion disorder and features of a post-traumatic stress disorder.

Case Study 2: Forgetting Remembrance of Things Past

A 44-year-old dairy farmer was admitted to the Salem Virginia VA Hospital in 1963 with complaints of nervousness, blackouts, dizziness, headaches, and loss of feeling and weakness over the left side of his body. He stated initially that the left-sided symptoms had come on during World War II service in Italy after a shrapnel injury to his left sciatic nerve.

On examination, there were mild residuals of sciatic nerve involvement, along with marked weakness and sensory loss of a functional type over the entire left side of his body, reduced vision in the left eye, and diminished hearing in the left ear. When asked how his symptoms had begun, the patient gave a dramatic account of the death of his commanding officer, and the loss of most of the men in his company. He went on to tell how he had been ordered to target a church in which German soldiers were thought to be hiding. After the church had been demolished, it was found to have been filled with women and children. He had been continually troubled by recollections of the event and when he entered any church became disturbed by the thought of the massacre.

The patient improved over the course of hospitalization, and at follow-up a year later he reported that he had done well except for some irritability and nervousness. He no longer complained of the loss of feeling over his left side, and examination showed only a faint diminution of sensation. He now attributed his nervousness to overwork, business problems, and difficulties with a brother-in-law on whom he had depended. He thought that his left-sided symptoms had come on several years earlier after he had done some heavy lifting on the farm. When asked about his wartime experiences, he said he could remember little or nothing about them.

Comment: In one situation a conversion symptom may be associated with traumatic events; after the patient has recovered he may have an amnesia for the traumatic experience.

Denial

Patients denied concern over the emotional, social, and occupational problems that appeared connected with the conversion symptom. They might deny fear of combat, job dissatisfaction, and feelings of incompetence. Some tended to resent psychiatric investigation and statements by examiners that they did not have an organic condition. They also showed no appreciation of the consequences of the putative organic disease. The following cases indicate how the traditional *la belle indifference* may be regarded as a form of denial.

Case Study 3: Movements that Prevented A Move

A 41-year-old infantry platoon sergeant with 12 years of active duty was hospitalized at Walter Reed Army Medical Center in July 1991 because of bizarre involuntary movements that had come on in January after his unit had been notified that they had been ordered from Germany to the Persian Gulf. He also complained of numbness and weakness of his left side since a head injury in 1984. Neurological examination revealed a staggering, saltatory gait, and a left hemisensory syndrome with jerking of his left limbs. A work-up including magnetic resonance imaging (MRI) yielded no evidence of organic involvement. During a Sodium Amytal interview, the patient walked normally, but his symptoms soon recurred and he refused another session. He had a cheerful, unworried demeanor despite his objection to being on a psychiatric floor and his demand to be seen by an expert in Huntington's disease, a condition that had been diagnosed by a German civilian neurologist.

The soldier had grown up in the rural South and had less than a high school education. He gave a dramatic family history of poverty, violence, and serious illnesses. His father was described as having a bad temper that led him into frequent fights and, when enraged, he had fits in which he trembled all over. Mother did the whipping and was very religious. Siblings were said to have illnesses that included schizophrenia, a cerebral hemorrhage, and neuritis with difficulty in walking.

Comment: The denial was shown in several ways. The patient maintained a cheerful manner and lack of concern for both his own and his family's disabilities. The spectacular gait and bizarre involuntary movements may also be seen in terms of adaptation, as a tragi-comic caricature or parody of disease. While such extreme melodramatic behavior is uncommon, many patients appeared unruffled by their situation. Some may be unconcerned with the conversion manifestation itself but are tense, withdrawn, and even hostile.

Case Study 4: Denial by Bravado

A 27-year-old female U.S. Marine was admitted to the hospital 2 weeks after she had passed out on a run at boot camp. She complained of numbness of her left ankle and toes and received a negative work-up for reflex sympathetic dystrophy. She developed weakness in her legs and impaired walking and was diagnosed as Achilles tendonitis. Examination showed functional weakness of both lower extremities and hyperesthesia with no evidence of spinal cord, root, or peripheral nerve disease. She had difficulty in standing and could only walk on crutches. Despite her condition, she was eager to return to duty saying in rather belligerent fashion that she was too tough to be laid up by a sprained ankle. She wanted to serve in the U.S. Marines to fight terrorists, then join the FBI [Federal Bureau of Investigation] to fight crime, and then use the GI bill to become a coroner.

Comment: The case illustrates how an obviously incapacitated conversion patient may insist on returning to duty, often with boasts of prowess and intent to wreak mayhem on the enemy.

Dissociation

Conversion disorders have dissociative aspects in that somatic and cognitive experiences may occur out of the sphere of conscious awareness. As in the two cases cited above, patients may regard the affected part of the body as outside and emotionally irrelevant to the self. The following excerpt illustrates an acute dissociative reaction in the form of a functional amnesia.

Case Study 5: A Fall From Battle

A 25-year-old U.S. Marine was evacuated from the fighting in Panama after a fall on his head. For a period of a week he did not know his name or anything of his past life. He spoke with a Latin accent that he had not had prior to his injury, and did not recognize his wife. There was no anterograde amnesia; he watched television and was able to remember what he had seen. He knew of Mohammed Ali and Babe Ruth because he had seen them on television since coming to the hospital. Neurological study found no evidence of brain damage and his memory suddenly returned.

Comment: More often the amnesia does not involve such a profound loss of the data of personal identity, and a patient may report no memory of an experience or limited span of time. Commonly, the person states that he will find himself in a certain place, and will have no recollection of going there. Functional amnesia may follow a fugue state, the essential feature of which is the assumption of a new identity without awareness of the previous identity. In the classical form the person is not aware of his memory loss, and the condition often involves travel away from his base.

Organicity

Estimates in the literature of central nervous system pathology in conversion disorders vary widely depending on symptomatology, type of medical facility, methods of investigation, and criteria of organicity. The highest incidence of 62.5% is reported by Whitlock[49] whose 56 patients were studied, in most instances retrospectively, on inpatient psychiatric services in England and Australia. The major categories of organicity were a concussive head injury during the preceding 6 months and a history of epilepsy. A similar study in Canada by Roy[50] yielded evidence of neural pathology in only 16% of cases. At the other extreme, is the report of about 1% of conversion disorders in neurological patients admitted over 3 decades to the National Hospital for Nervous Diseases, Queen Square, London.[51] Brandt[52] found an incidence of 9% among over 4,000 neurological patients admitted to a general hospital in Munich. Pain and dizziness were among the most common symptoms and this may account for the difference from the Queen Square findings. Weinstein[53] reported functional paralysis, sensory loss, and involuntary movements in 16 of 200 soldiers hospitalized for closed-head injuries with documented periods of unconsciousness followed by disorientation, amnesia, and confabulation. Conversion manifestations appeared after these disturbances of consciousness had cleared, at intervals up to 8 months.[46]

The author's ongoing study of 90 patients with conversion disorders admitted to the neurological and psychiatric services of the National Naval Medical Center and Walter Reed Army Medical Center (both in Washington, D.C.) has yielded evidence of neural pathology in 20 cases. The criteria are objective clinical signs of brain damage confirmed by laboratory findings, a head injury or anoxic episode with loss of consciousness within the previous 6 months, or a documented history of brain disease. Five patients had clear cut neurological conditions; two had multiple sclerosis, two had cerebral vascular involvement (one with collagen disease), and another patient had progressive supranuclear palsy with dementia. Eleven patients had had head injuries with loss of consciousness or anoxic episodes, that were momentary in most instances. Four of the 11 had computed tomography (CT), magnetic resonance imaging (MRI), or electroencephalogram (EEG) abnormalities. Two patients had had a bona fide seizure prior to developing psuedoseizures. One had a dural sinus thrombosis with a persisting abnormal MRI. A patient with pseudoseizures and a functional left hemisensory syndrome had an Arnold-Chiari malformation, and one soldier had a history of childhood hyperactivity/attention-deficit disorder.

These data may be interpreted in a number of ways. One is that organic neurological disease may be misdiagnosed. Another is that there may be functional elaboration of deficits caused by the brain lesion. Third, brain injury may facilitate the dissociative process and lower the threshold for conversion disorders. On the other hand, there is no correlation between the severity of brain damage and the occurrence of conversion reactions. The high proportion of head injuries reported may be a reflection of the tendency of patients with conversion disorders to focus their problems on trauma. Head injuries or other brain disease including seizures in childhood may contribute to less education and lower socioeconomic status, both risk factors for conversion disorders.

Laterality

Almost all 19th and early 20th century neurologists believed that hysterical phenomena occurred predominantly on the left side of the body, and a number of modern studies[51,54,55] have confirmed an asymmetry. Handedness was shown not to be a factor.[55] Several explanations, some based on investigations of hemisphere specialization in neurological conditions, have been offered. One is that the right brain is specialized for the monitoring of somatic states and the mediation of negative emotional processes. A recent literature review[56] of the thalamic pain syndrome of Dejerine-Roussy showed a significant predominance of right thalamic lesions in cases with lateralized pain. In contrast, the incidence of the other components of the syndrome—hemiparesis, sensory impairment, ataxia, and choreoathetosis—did not differ significantly in the left and right groups.

Another approach draws on the analogies of hysterical hemisensorimotor syndromes with anosognosia and hemineglect, both of which occur mainly as a result of right brain lesions. In the various forms of anosognosia, the patient denies, caricatures, or appears indifferent to his deficits, and may even feel that the affected parts of the body do not belong to him. In hemineglect, he ignores stimuli and events on the impaired side of his body and in circumambient hemispace. Patients with hemineglect following strokes, brain traumas, or mass lesions may show a midline split to all sensory modalities, including vibration, and a disinclination to use the impaired extremities or look to the affected side even though such movements can be elicited in other contexts.[57–59]

One may speculate that patients with functional hemisensorimotor syndromes show the affective, subjective aspects of anosognosia and hemineglect. They may feel that the affected side of the body is dead, insensitive, or detached from the self. From the standpoint of diagnosis, however, such patients do not have tactile or visual extinction. Nor do they bisect a line or draw a clock or human figure in asymmetrical fashion, or show the eye shift to the unaffected side on visual confrontation characteristic of organic visual neglect.

Epidemiology

Major conversion disorders occur predominantly in the lower social classes, among the poor and less educated,[22,60–62] and in certain cultural groups. They are also common in societies in which violence is an important source of identity and mode of social relatedness.[47,63] The Salem, Virginia Veterans Administration Hospital was chosen for study because of its high rate of conversion disorders. Over a 4-year period in the 1960s, 25% to 30% of all patients admitted showed conversion manifestations at some time during hospitalization.

The patients were drawn mainly from the Appalachian counties of Virginia and West Virginia. The region was rural but nonfarming, and had an ethnically homogenous (mostly old, Anglo-Saxon, white, and Protestant) population. The decline of the extractive industries of mining and logging had led to economic depression. Educational facilities were limited, and the average school attainment at the time of the study was eighth grade.

Since the days of the Hatfields and the McCoys down through the mine union wars, Appalachia has had a tradition of violence. While the blood feuds have ended, a high rate of murder and nonnegligent homicide has persisted. Violence was a form of communication, occurring principally among relatives, friends, and acquaintances. Ownership of guns was universal and hunting and automobile racing the most popular sports. Violence in the form of physical beatings and the instillation of fears of ghosts and graveyards was a prominent instrument of child raising. The theme of violence pervaded religious beliefs—mainly of the Fundamentalist type. These emphasize divine punishment and forgiveness of sin, salvation and the next world, and saw in physical catastrophes evidence of the power of the Lord.

Attitudes toward health and illness were tied to the idea of a dangerous environment. As the economy dictated hazardous jobs, and safety standards were low, there was a high accident rate, and men worked until they were disabled or laid off. The manifestations of disability were a badge that indicated that the person had worked and suffered, and many people grew up in a home with a disabled or crippled relative who was receiving compensation. These conditions, along with the military tradition of the region, produced a high rate of enlistment in the armed forces, particularly the combat branches, and the role of wounded or disabled veteran was a familiar, sanctioned, and rewarding one.

These features are present in some Latin American societies with their high homicide rates, male macho roles, and violent, bloody religious imagery. The so called *ataque* was not uncommon among Puerto Rican troops, usually in noncombat situations. It was characterized by the sudden onset of violent behavior, thrashing about, striking out and pseudoseizures, with homicidal and suicidal ideation, and, in some cases, belief of being affected by spirits of the dead. The attack lasted from a few minutes to one half hour and was followed by amnesia. It was brought on by feelings of rage, frustration, and disappointment, and usually cleared when the man was placed in isolation.[64] Compton and Jones[65] showed that the syndrome (sometimes called the Puerto Rican Syndrome) occurred in all Hispanic military populations and appeared to be culturally determined.

A major reason why conversion disorders have occurred more commonly in women is that, historically, except in wars, women have been subjected to more physical and sexual violence—much of it institutionalized—than men. Currently in the armed forces conversion disorders occur with equal frequency in men and women.

DIFFERENTIAL DIAGNOSIS

The diagnosis of a conversion disorder depends primarily on the neurological examination in which the findings symbolize some traumatic experience or conception by the patient of a loss of function, but do not conform to a neuroanatomical or neurophysiological pattern. The existence of an emotional conflict may not be helpful as anyone in a stressful situation may have problems. Similarly, determination of secondary gain is difficult to evaluate as soldiers with a variety of ailments may be seen as deriving some benefit from them.

Motor Disorders

Loss of motor power appears as weakness or paralysis of single limbs, paraplegia or paraparesis, hemiparesis or hemiplegia. Quadriplegia as a conversion disorder is almost unknown. While the patient cannot move a limb voluntarily, or fails to exert sustained power on effort—so-called give-away weakness—there are no postures indicative of weakness. In the supine position, the leg on the putatively hemiplegic side is not more externally rotated nor is the foot more dropped than its fellow, and when the upper limb is extended in pronation, the thumb does not droop. There is likely to be a Hoover sign in hemiplegia. When the supine putatively hemiparetic patient is asked to raise a leg alternatively or sit up, he does not press down harder with the heel of the good leg, as one would expect if the weakness were of organic origin. There is not the motor gradient characteristic of a cerebral lesion in which the greatest weakness is in the most distal muscles. In a hysterical hemiplegia the facial and tongue muscles are spared. Also, a patient with a hemiplegia may exhibit diminished power in turning his head to that side even though the action is performed by the contralateral sternomastoid muscle. He is apt to drag the leg or walk with a limp rather than with the circumduction of an organic hemiparesis. In hysterical monoplegia all movements about a joint are equally affected whereas in peripheral nerve or radicular lesions there is a segmental distribution.

Disorders of Stance, Gait, and Balance

The classical astasia-abasia refers to the person's inability to stand (astasia) or walk (abasia) even though other actions of the legs can be performed. In the Romberg position, there is an increasing amplitude of sway after a latency of a few seconds, and the patient avoids falling by grasping the examiner or staggering across the room to gain support from a wall. In walking there are exaggerated efforts to maintain balance by using the arms as if the patient were on a tightrope, or by flexing hips and knees to gain a lower center of gravity. There may be a fluctuation in performance, and the patient may walk as well in tandem or on his toes as in more conventional forms of locomotion. Gait may be very slow and hesitant with short steps and apparent sticking of the feet to the ground. Unlike the situation in Parkinson's disease, the inhibition is not overcome after the first few steps. Sudden buckling of the knees may occur, usually but not always, without falling. Other conversion manifestations (sensorimotor, visual, oculomotor, speech, or pseudoseizures) may be associated. Chorea and dystonia are the neurological conditions most likely to be misdiagnosed. Also disturbances of gait and balance can be caused by drugs, anticonvulsants, antidepressants, alcohol, sedatives, and tranquilizers.

Vertigo, the sensation of the apparent movement of one's body or of an object in one's line of vision, may accompany astasia-abasia, but as a presenting symptom it is only rarely of hysterical origin. It is much more common in anxiety, panic and phobic states, and depression. Psychogenic vertigo is differentiated from disease of the vestibular system by the absence of nausea and vomiting and of rotational vertigo with direction-specific falling. If a complaint is of a rotational component, the absence of concurrent spontaneous nystagmus under Frenzel's glasses, which suppress nystagmus by fixation, suggests a functional etiology.[52,66]

Involuntary Movements

Tremor and myoclonus are the most common of the involuntary movements of psychological origin. Tremor consists of oscillatory movements produced by contractions of reciprocally innervated antagonistic muscles. Myoclonus is a quick involuntary jerk. These disorders usually have an abrupt onset following a head or back injury, a car accident, a surgical procedure, or some emotional upset. Psychogenic tremor generally combines resting, postural, and kinetic components, and varies in amplitude, frequency, and time of appearance. Both tremor and myoclonus may be relieved by placebos, reduced when the patient is distracted, increased by attention, and associated with other conversion manifestations such as sensory loss and giveaway weakness in the affected limbs, speech and gait disorders.[67,68]

Camptocormia is a postural disorder in which a soldier presents with severe forward flexion of the spine, often along with flexion at the knees and dangling of the arms. The position persists in walking but disappears when the man lies down. He complains of pain that he attributes to a back injury, and there is often a family history of back disability. A herniated disc or spinal stenosis is occasionally found but these are not causes of the deformity[69,70] although they determine its site.

Dystonia was formerly thought to be of psychological origin but studies in recent decades have established it as a neurological entity. It is a syndrome dominated by muscle contractions frequently causing twisting and repetitive movements, or abnormal postures that may be sustained or intermittent.[71] It can be focal or generalized and includes torticollis, involuntary movements of the thumb and limbs, orofacial and mandibular dystonia, blepharospasm, and dysphonia. Focal dystonia also includes writer's and piano and violin player's cramp and other specific task or instrument conditions. Electromyography reveals that reciprocal muscle inhibition is impaired so that there is cocontraction of agonists and antagonists.

The clinical picture may be bizarre—in dystonia involving the legs the patient may be able to walk forward but not backward. About 9% of cases are preceded by trauma and remissions occur in 12% of cases of torticollis.[72] However, dystonic movements and postures of psychogenic origin are rare.[73] In such cases the dystonic manifestations are apt to be associated with peculiarities of gait and functional types of sensory and motor loss. The following case excerpt illustrates some of the diagnostic pitfalls that may be encountered.

Case Study 6: The Wry Neck Recidivist

The patient was a 45-year-old field grade officer who was referred to a base section hospital in North Africa with a diagnosis of hysterical torticollis. The involuntary turning movements of his head to the left had come on while he was awaiting a court-martial for alleged black market dealings. The movements were interpreted as symbolic of his unconscious wish to turn away from the problems. Subsequent investigation, however, established a neurological diagnosis of torsion dystonia.

Comment: Stressful events may coincide with the onset of an organic neurological condition.

Sensory Disorders

Loss of sensation in conversion reactions involves a diminution or absence of feeling over one side of the body or in one or more limbs resulting in glove and gauntlet, and sock and stocking distributions. In hemisensory syndromes all or several modalities are involved without the dissociation usually found in cerebral lesions in which stereognosis, 2-point discrimination, graphesthesia, and position sense are more impaired than pain, temperature, touch, and vibration. During testing for astereognosis, the patient may manipulate the test object skillfully in his fingers indicating intact proprioception but still fail to identify it. There is commonly a midline demarcation in which the patient feels all stimuli less intensely on one complete half of the body, perceiving the tuning fork differently on either side of the sternum and forehead, even though vibration is transmitted through the bone. A midline split on sensory examination is not necessarily present even though patients complain of a loss of feeling over the entire half of the body. The special senses are also involved: on being tested the patient reports poorer vision in one eye, reduced hearing in the corresponding ear, and even less smell in one nostril and less taste on one side of the tongue.

The phenomenon of extinction elicited by the method of double simultaneous stimulation is useful in distinguishing a hemisensory deficit of hysterical origin from one caused by structural brain damage. Patients with pathology in one hemisphere may have normal or slightly reduced responses to touch and pinprick with a single stimulus to the side opposite the brain lesion, but when bilateral simultaneous stimuli are applied sensation is extinguished or further reduced on the side contralateral to the lesion. The responses of patients with a conversion disorder, however, are not affected by the method of testing.

In conversion disorders involving single limbs there is a loss of a sensory gradient. If impaired sensation in the lower extremities is caused by a spinal cord lesion, then vibratory sensation is most impaired in the toes and less affected over the more proximal areas. In conversion reactions, on the other hand, the vibratory sensation may be not only absent in the toes but over the ankles and knees. The examiner should avoid suggesting to the patient that his sensation is impaired; hemisensory syndromes can be created iatrogenically.

Visual Disorders

In no area of neurological examination is the physician–patient interaction more likely to affect results than in the plotting of the visual fields. Fatigue, inattention, or suggestibility on the part of the patient and overzealousness and impatience of an examiner can produce abnormal visual fields even in people who have no visual complaints, and the findings may differ on successive examinations. Functional visual field loss takes the forms of constricted or tubular fields in which the size of the field does not vary with distance of the target, spiral fields that progressively diminish during testing so that only central fields remain, and focal field defects that do not follow an anatomical or physiological pattern. Tunnel fields may occasionally be found in patients with frontal lobe tumors.

Functional blindness can be detected by normal pupillary light reactions (impaired in blindness of organic neurological origin except in cortical blindness due to bilateral occipital lobe lesions), by producing a blink response to visual threat, by eliciting eye movements with an optokinetic tape or drum, and by moving a large mirror to and fro and up and down in front of the patient while observing eye movements corresponding to the movement of the mirror.[74] The red glass test is particularly useful in monocular blindness. The patient is asked to read a line of alternating black and red letters with a red glass placed over the good eye. Any reading of the red letters must accordingly be done by the supposedly bad eye. Patients with functional reductions of visual acuity can be shown to have normal vision by retesting, encouragement, or subterfuges designed to identify normal acuity.[75]

Hearing Loss

Functional hearing loss is indicated when the behavioral response is inconsistent with auditory findings on examination. Psychogenic deafness is initially suggested if the patient speaks in a loud voice and refuses to communicate except in writing. Eye blink in response to a loud noise, or awakening from sleep after a loud sound indicates that hearing is present. More sophisticated procedures include delayed auditory feedback which normally disrupts performance on reading aloud. In unilateral hearing loss a tuning fork placed over the mastoid on the affected side should produce hearing, via the good ear through bone conduction, so the patient's report that he hears nothing indicates psychogenicity. The Stenger test makes use of the observation in normal persons that if identical signals differing in intensity by more than 20 decibels are presented to each ear, the sound appears to come from the ear in which the intensity was greater. If a high-intensity signal is put into the supposedly impaired ear at the same time that a low-intensity stimulus is delivered to the good ear, a failure of the good ear to hear indicates that there is auditory function in the involved ear.[76]

Speech Disorders

Stuttering is the most common hysterical speech disorder. It frequently occurs after trauma, and may be preceded by a period of mutism. It contrasts with conventional stuttering which begins in early childhood and starts only rarely in adults. Conventional stuttering is variable, occurs in different situations, with different words, typically involves the initial sound of a word, and does not occur in singing or more automatic speech like greeting and counting. Conventional stutterers adapt with avoidant measures such as the use of a substitute word when they anticipate difficulty. Conversion subjects are rigid and unvarying, stuttering in all situations, and there may be associated jaw, face, tongue, and vocal cord tremors. Other functional disturbances include slow, labored, staccato, and syllabic deliveries.

Pseudoseizures

The differentiation of pseudoseizures (also known as psychogenic seizures) from bona fide epileptic fits depends on a number of criteria, no one of which is sufficient for an unequivocal diagnosis.[77] Moreover, pseudoseizures may coexist with true seizures (Table 15-1).

TABLE 15-1

CRITERIA FOR DIAGNOSIS OF EPILEPTIC AND PSYCHOGENIC SEIZURES

Characteristics	Generalized Tonic Clonic Seizures	Complex Partial Seizures	Psychogenic Seizures
Onset	Usually paroxysmal; may be preceded by seizures of different muscles or auras	Usually paroxysmal; may be preceded by aura of only few seconds	Often gradual; prolonged, nonspecific warning may occur
Postictal confusion	Prominent	Almost always present	Often conspicuously absent; patient may be normal immediately after attack
Recollection of events	None	Usually scant and most often none	Sometimes detailed
Suggestibility	None	Rare	Occasionally
Violent behavior	None	Rare; virtually always in response to restraint and not highly directed	Rare; but may be highly directed
Weeping*	None	Very rare	Common
Comparison with known seizure types	Relatively little variation in events	Wide range of events, but most common are well described	Extremely wide range of events with bizarre and unusual behavior
EEG during seizure	Abnormal and changed from preictal	Frequently abnormal and changed from preictal	Usually normal and unchanged from preictal
EEG immediately after seizures	Almost always abnormal and changed from preictal	Frequently abnormal and changed from preictal	Usually normal and unchanged from preictal
Abnormal neurological signs during seizure	May be present (example: Todd's paralysis)	May be present	None
Relation of attacks to medical regimen	Prominent, especially in severely affected patients	Usually related	Usually unrelated but anticonvulsive medication may increase frequency of seizures
Nocturnal occurrence	Common	May occur	Rare

*Source: Bergen D, Ristanovic R. Weeping as a common element of pseudoseizures. *Arch Neurol.* 1993;50:1059–1060.
Adapted from Desai BT, Porter RJ, Penry JK. Psychogenic Seizures: A study of 42 attacks in six patients, with intensive monitoring. *Arch Neurol.* 1982;39:207-208.

More recent studies have shown that frontal lobe seizures from mesial and orbital foci in which vocal profanities and obscenities, rocking, and pelvic thrusting are apt to occur and seizures arising from the supplementary motor area with thrashing movements and tonic posturing are particularly apt to be mistaken for psychogenic seizures. They are distinguished from the latter principally by short duration (usually less than a minute), stereotypy and nocturnal occurrence, as well as EEG and MRI findings.[78–80]

Amnesia

Amnesia is a loss of memory for periods of time and personal experiences, rather than inability to remember facts and procedures. Amnesia may occur on an organic or functional basis, and usually follows some interruption of consciousness or emotional trauma. Anterograde amnesia (AA) refers to the period of time following the acute event over which the patient is unable to retain new information, and for which he later has no memory. Retrograde amnesia (RA) refers to the period prior to the acute episode for which the person reports no memory. Following loss of consciousness from a concussion or other brain injury there is both an AA and an RA, even though the RA may be very brief, and the patient may remember everything up to a few seconds before impact. One does not remember the blow or other agent causing loss of consciousness. If, however, the patient recalls and describes the crash of the car or the bursting of a shell, the inference is that he did not lose consciousness, and even though he may state that he does not then remember anything until he found himself in a clearing station or hospital, unable to walk or talk, it is likely that the amnesia is not directly caused by brain injury.

The profound amnesias of dissociated and fugue states such as that described in Case Study 5 are differentiated from the amnesias of brain injury by the loss of data of personal identity and the exclusively retrograde character of the memory loss. Even when the RA following brain damage is extensive, the person knows his name, address, occupation, religion, and other autobiographical information. He may not remember his actual marriage ceremony, but he knows he is married and recognizes his wife. He may not remember actually enlisting, but he knows he is in the U.S. Army. Also most organic amnesias show a temporal gradient in that more remote events are recalled better.

Amnesia resulting from alcoholic intoxication usually covers only the period of intoxication and prolongation beyond that period suggests functional elaboration. Transient global amnesia (TGA) should be considered in cases of sudden onset in persons over the age of 40. TGA involves the sudden occurrence of a marked anterograde and variable retrograde amnesia, typically accompanied by bewilderment and agitation, with the patient repeatedly asking the same questions. Data of personal identity are retained, and immediate recall is preserved. The condition clears within hours. The cause is unknown, but a migrainous etiology is likely.[81]

Simulated Amnesia

Patients may simulate, exaggerate, or dramatize memory loss. Useful but not infallible aids in distinguishing such states are:

1. Absence of a gradient of difficulty in that subject may do as poorly on a difficult task as an easier one.
2. Responses may be very slow.
3. Recognition is not better than recall.
4. Immediate recall, which is intact in most organic conditions, is involved.
5. Performance is not improved with cues and clues.
6. Elements of a Ganser syndrome may be present.

Ganser Syndrome or Pseudodementia

In 1898, Sigbert J. Ganser, a German psychiatrist, described four prisoners with episodes of clouding of consciousness, disorientation, hysterical conversion symptoms, hallucinations, a recent history of head injury or typhus, and *vorbeireden*.[82] The last feature consists of "talking past the point," in which the patient gives approximate answers such as stating that 2 plus 2 are 5, and calling a blue object pink. The behavior was of short duration and subjects were later amnesic. The syndrome has occurred not only in prisoners but in persons awaiting trial, in military personnel facing disciplinary action or being otherwise embittered with military life. The complete syndrome is only rarely present but fragments, particularly *vorbeireden*, are common. Patients state that the capital of France is Marseilles or may draw a clock with the numbers reversed. Responses may be very slow. Violence and suicidal gestures may occur. Malingering is often suspected, as patients seem to be simulating insanity, or exaggerating a psychotic experience. In recent years, cases with Ganser features have been reported following not only head injury, but also strokes, brain tumors, and acute psychosis, and have occurred in women as well as men.[83,84]

TREATMENT

In the treatment of conversion disorders, the major emphasis should be placed on removal of symptoms. If these are not cleared, they take on a life of their own, and persist even after the underlying emotional problems are no longer relevant. These emotional problems are rarely "deep" in the sense that they represent repressed unconscious conflicts, but are usually situational. In general, the most effective treatments are those that emphasize affect and relatedness rather than insight. These involve the induction of a state of mind or milieu of brain function in which affect is released and the person can reformulate stressful experiences in symbols and imagery. This may come about in the context of a rapport with the therapist, via the product of trance state by hypnosis, and through the alteration of brain function provided by such drugs as Sodium Amytal. The following three cases are illustrative.

Case Study 7: Abreaction through Confession

A 20-year-old combat infantry private first class (PFC) was seen in April 1969 at Phuoc Vinh, Vietnam by Captain [later Major General] James H. Rumbaugh because of a complete paralysis and loss of feeling in his left upper extremity. He reported that he had tripped over a tree trunk and landed on his left shoulder. Because of soreness and some deviation of his head to the left he was taken to a hospital, put in head traction, and given a soft collar. On the night following his discharge his unit was mortared. He rolled out of his bunk, fell on his arm, and "tore it up so bad" that he had to go back to the hospital. Neurological examination now showed a functional paralysis of the entire left arm and a sensory loss for all modalities which included the shoulder area. There were two circumscribed burns on the left forearm where the soldier had not felt a lit cigarette. Medical history disclosed that after lifting paper at a factory, a year prior to enlistment, he had "messed up" his back and had been unable to move his legs or walk for several weeks.

The patient stated that he had been in service for 9 months and had gone to jump school at Fort Benning. When asked why he had gone he said that it was to do something outstanding for the glory of it. He had been born in rural Tennessee and had graduated from high school in Michigan where his father had become an automobile worker. He had gotten along well with his parents, but described his father as having a high temper. He and his brothers would get beaten with a switch or a strap, particularly when his father had been drinking. He was devoted to his mother whom he depicted as suffering from "heart spells" and as very religious.

A few hours after the initial interview, the soldier approached Captain Rumbaugh to say that there was something on his conscience. With considerable emotion he confessed that the jump wings he was wearing were not his own, but had been given to him by a boy whom he had met on the plane. He was told he could still be an outstanding soldier, and Captain Rumbaugh assured him that very soon feeling and then motor function would return. The next day he had pins and needles sensations in his fingers, followed by twitches in his thumb. At the end of a 2-week period he had completely recovered. Follow-up from brigade surgeons indicated a successful return to duty.

Comment: In this case the development of the conversion symptom may have been facilitated by the hospitalization and the orthopedic procedures.

Hypnosis and abreaction through the intravenous administration of barbiturates are indicated when the patient has not responded to suggestion and encouragement. Hypnosis is indicated especially in subjects with a high-induction profile (HIP).[85] The HIP is an indicator of hypnotizability consisting of a biological component, the ability to maintain upward gaze during slow lid closure, and a psychophysiological one, the capacity for arm levitation. According to Spiegel and Spiegel,[85] the highly hypnotizable individual has a reliance on feeling rather than reasoning, a tendency to live in the present, and a capacity for intense focal concentration. These features are enhanced in combat.

Case Study 8: Revisualization of Trauma

A medic, seen by Captain Herbert Spiegel during World War II, was returned from a battlefield in Tunisia with inability to use his legs, despite the absence of organic findings. He and his unit had come under heavy fire, and, after the sergeant ordered retreat, the soldier heard the cry of a friend for help, and saw the foot of someone who might have been the friend lying behind a rock. However, he obeyed the order and retreated and his friend never returned. He was overwhelmed with remorse at not having tried to rescue him. The man was highly hypnotizable and was able to readily regress to the past. He was instructed to revisualize the scene of leaving the battlefield with one modification, that the foot he had seen was facing downward, with the implication that the man was already dead. The soldier came out of the trance with an exhilarating sense of "discovery" that his friend could not have been saved. Within a few days he regained his ability to walk and returned to active duty.[85(p140)]

Comment: In combat areas where alertness and mobility are important, hypnosis is in some ways preferable to techniques involving barbiturates. Hypnosis does not require venipuncture or sterile procedures and precautions against respiratory and circulatory depression, and is not followed by drowsiness and ataxia. An occasional subject becomes agitated and violent with barbiturate administration, while in hypnosis the degree of abreaction can be controlled. Also, posthypnotic suggestions may be made for the handling of anticipated symptoms.[86,87]

The Amytal interview is indicated in situations in which the patient is not communicative and related, especially in cases of stupor, muteness, and deafness. It is also preferable to hypnosis when there is lack of motivation, and where there is an inability or unwillingness to focus attention.

Case Study 9: Abreaction in Dramatic Metaphor

An 18-year-old radio operator with 6 months service was evacuated to Walter Reed Army Medical Center from Germany because of difficulty in articulation. He spoke in garbled fashion clicking his tongue against the roof of his mouth. The symptom had come on the day after receiving a painful novocaine dental injection and had gotten worse over the next 2 months. The soldier was from a rural Southern area and had had 4 years of high school.

Under Sodium Amytal he became very drowsy but recovered to speak understandably. He told of his dissatisfaction with his job, the shock of seeing black men with white women. He described how upset he was when he found that the dentist was a black woman. He went on to say how worried he was about his mother, who had no one to take care of her. She had told him that she, too, had a burning in her mouth after dental work. He was vague about his father who, he said, had been killed by the Mafia. He, himself, had almost been killed in an accident but had been saved by a miracle. The patient spoke normally but the following day had relapsed halfway. Following a leave home, he talked normally. A psychiatric evaluation noted dependent and avoidant personality traits and he was not returned to overseas duty.

Comment: The case illustrates how, under the conditions of brain function supplied by a barbiturate, the soldier could restructure the problems of job inadequacy and homesickness in metaphors of race, violence, and filial devotion.

The Amytal procedure is helpful in the detection of volitional elements and malingering. Such patients may become excessively drowsy even before there is a sufficient amount of the drug to have any physiological effect. The subject may keep his eyes tightly closed when the examiner is eliciting eye movements and may not answer questions or may respond in inaudible fashion.

The Amytal Test[88,89] also serves in the diagnosis of brain disease. Prior to injection the patient is asked a series of questions dealing with orientation and awareness of impairment, and answers are recorded. (If the patient is already disoriented this is indicative of brain dysfunction and the procedure is not indicated.) The drug is then introduced intravenously at a rate of 50 mg/min until errors in counting backward, slurring of speech, mood change (usually euphoria), and nystagmus are observed. The questions are then repeated. One or more persisting errors constitute a positive result indicative of organic brain dysfunction. Patients without brain damage remain oriented and aware of impairment throughout with only occasional transient self-corrected errors.

Case Study 10: Misdiagnosis Revealed by the Amytal Test

A 44-year-old naval petty officer jet mechanic with 19 years active duty had a 10-year history of reduced color vision that came on while he was on sea duty off Vietnam. It became difficult for him to work with color-coded wires, and subsequently he became unable to move his eyes. Most recently he had complained of difficulty in remembering names and telephone numbers. Routine mental status was within normal limits and on neuro-ophthalmological examination he could not move his eyes laterally or vertically on voluntary effort, but some movement was noted when he was distracted. Optokinetic nystagmus was obtained and the vestibular ocular reflex was normal. A diagnosis of conversion disorder was made.

He was given the Amytal Test at the National Naval Medical Center in Bethesda. He answered the preinjection questions accurately, and these were repeated after the administration of 300 mg of the drug. He became disoriented for place, stated repeatedly that he was in Pensacola, a former duty station, and was also disoriented for month and year. Subsequent MRI showed evidence of bilateral occipital lobe lesions, and he went on to develop a frank dementia.

Comment: This case illustrates the value of the Amytal Test in detecting neural pathology in cases in which routine examination and laboratory tests have been normal.

When soldiers do not respond to therapy there arise questions of associated brain damage, depression, or mechanisms beyond the original dissociative process that are not entirely out of conscious control. It is uncommon for a patient to manufacture symptoms out of whole cloth, but the idea of incapacity has been implanted by the initial injury, real or fancied, and after separation from his or her group, the conversion symptoms symbolize and maintain a new identity as a disabled soldier. This role is reinforced by each neurological or orthopedic examination, and by the prospect of secondary gain.

After a conversion symptom has been present for weeks and the soldier has been evacuated, it is unlikely that he will return to combat. The emphasis should now be on the avoidance of procedures that support the idea of physical disease or increase secondary gain. Hospital privileges should be made dependent on clinical improvement, and the prospect of another assignment or a favorable discharge held out. Certain hysterical conditions such as camptocormia are notoriously resistant to treatment and such patients should generally be promptly separated from the service.

SUMMARY AND CONCLUSION

Conversion disorders have historically been associated with violence. They have been attributed to the malign influence of devils and witches, to divine wrath, to the sexual abuse and forcible subjugation of women, to industrial trauma, and to shell shock in war.

Patients with conversion reactions describe their symptoms in idioms of violence, ascribe them to an injury, and depict their onset in a violent setting, even though the traumas may have been relatively minor and removed in time. The conversion symptom is a symbolic representation of a felt disability or a traumatic experience. The language, verbal and gestural, imparts meaning and a *feeling* of reality not only by reason of the trauma itself, but because violence and the anticipation of violence have been such important elements in patterns of social relatedness. There is predisposition not in the sense of mental illness or personality disorder—although these are often deduced after the fact—but because of lower class status, limited education, cultural tradition, family violence or physical disability, previous conversion episodes, and, more immediately, a recent wound or injury requiring hospitalization.

Conversion disorders are not disease entities but signs and symptoms. Their character and incidence have varied over the centuries with the forms of trauma, cultural change, and the degree to which the behavior is reinforced by society. One no longer sees the stigmata of the Crucifixion, or the *attitudes passionelles* of Charcot's day. Conversion hysteria was the hallmark of World War I, exhaustion featured World War II, and post-traumatic stress disorder came out of Vietnam. Conversion reactions occur in the course of a number of conditions: post-traumatic stress disorder (PTSD), adjustment disorders, depression, multiple personality, Axis II disorders, and brain damage. The roles of brain dysfunction and hemisphere specialization, and the physiological mechanisms of dissociation are as yet not well understood; but, depending on the circumstances under which people are exposed to threats of death and mutilation and loss of personal integrity, then dissociative processes in the form of conversion disorders, PTSD, or some clinical syndrome yet to be described will appear.

REFERENCES

1. American Psychiatric Association. *Diagnostic and Statistical Manual of Mental Disorders, Third Edition (DSM III)*, Washington, DC: APA; 1980.

2. Barnes JK. *The Medical and Surgical History of the War of the Rebellion*. Prepared under the direction of Surgeon General Joseph K. Barnes, United States Army. Washington, DC: GPO, 1870–1888.

3. Porter IG. Case report. *Am J Med Sci*. 1864;134–137.

4. Mitchell SW, Morehouse GD, Keen WW. Reflex Paralysis, Article 6. Washington, DC: The Office of the Surgeon General; 1864.

5. Briquet P. *Traité de l'Hystérie*. Paris, France: JB Ballière et fils; 1859.

6. Charcot JM. Discussed in: Ellenberger HF. *The Discovery of the Unconscious: The History and Evolution of Dynamic Psychiatry.* New York: Basic Books; 1970.

7. Janet P. Discussed in: Ellenberger HF. *The Discovery of the Unconscious: The History and Evolution of Dynamic Psychiatry.* New York: Basic Books; 1970.

8. Reynolds JR. Remarks on paralysis, and other disorders of motion and sensation. *Br Med J* [now *Br Med J (Clin Res)*]. 1869;6:483–485.

9. Breuer J, Freud S. Studies on hysteria. In: Strachey J, Freud A, eds; Strachey J, trans-ed. *The Standard Edition of the Complete Psychological Works of Sigmund Freud*, Vol 2. London, England: Hogarth; 1953.

10. Bailey P, Haber R. Occurrence of neuropsychiatric diseases in the Army. In: Bailey P, Williams FE, Komora PO, eds. *Neuropsychiatry.* Vol 10. In: *The Medical Department of the United States Army in the World War.* Washington, DC: Office of The Surgeon General, US Army; 1929: 154.

11. Mott SW. War psycho-neurosis. *Lancet.* 1918;Jan 26:127–129, Feb 2:169–172.

12. Wolfsohn JM. The predisposing factors of war psycho-neuroses. *Lancet.* 1918;Feb 2:177–180.

13. Farrar CB. War and neurosis. *Am J Insanity* [now *Am J Psychiatry*]. 1917;73(12).

14. Eder MD. *War Shock.* London, England: Heinemann; 1917.

15. Nonne M. Hypnotism in war hysteria. (Berlin Letter. Dec 14, 1915) *JAMA.* 1916;66:440–441.

16. Hurst AF. Hysteria. *Lancet.* 1919;Nov 1:771–779.

17. Myers CS. *Shell Shock in France 1914–1918.* Cambridge, England: Cambridge University Press; 1940.

18. Roussy G, Lhermitte J. *The Psychoneuroses of War.* Paris, France: Masson et cie; 1918.

19. Ross TA. The prevention of relapse of hysterical manifestations. *Lancet.* 1918;Oct 19:516–517.

20. Hurst AF, Peters EA. The pathology, diagnosis and treatment of absolute hysterical deafness in soldiers. *Lancet.* 1917;Oct 6:517–519.

21. Chodoff P. A re-examination of some aspects of conversion hysteria. *Psychiatry.* 1954;17:75–81.

22. Ziegler FS, Imboden JB, Meyer E. Contemporary conversion reactions. *Am J Psychiatry.* 1959;116:901–910.

23. Noble D. Hysterical manifestations in schizophrenic illness. *Psychiatry.* 1951;14:153–160.

24. Weinstein EA. The Fifth Army Neuropsychiatric Center—"601st". In: Glass AJ, ed. *Overseas Theaters.* Vol 2. In: *Neuropsychiatry in World War II.* Washington, DC: Office of The Surgeon General, US Army; 1973: 127–141.

25. Wagner PS. Psychiatric activities during the Normandy Offensive: June 20–August 20, 1944. *Psychiatry.* 1946;9:341–364.

26. Swank R. Combat exhaustion. *J Nerv Ment Dis.* 1949;109:475–508.

27. Fisher ED. Psychoneurosis in the armed forces. *Bull US Army Med Dept.* 1947;7:939–947.

28. Torrie A. Psychosomatic casualties in the Middle East. *Lancet.* 1944;Jan 29:139–143.

29. Schneider RJ. Stress breakdown in the Wehrmacht: Implications for today's Army. In: Belenky G, ed. *Contemporary Studies in Combat Psychiatry.* New York: Greenwood Press; 1987: 87–101.

30. Anderson RC. Neuropsychiatric problems of the flier. In: Glass AJ, ed. *Overseas Theaters*. Vol 2. In: *Neuropsychiatry in World War II*. Washington, DC: Office of The Surgeon General, US Army; 1973: 881–891.

31. Ironside R, Batchelor IRC. The ocular manifestations of hysteria in relation to flying. *Br J Ophthalmol*. 1945;29:88–98.

32. Kardiner A, Spiegel H. *War Stress and Neurotic Illness*. New York: Paul B. Hoeber; 1947.

33. Horsley JS. *Narco-analysis*. London, England: Oxford; 1943.

34. Grinker RR, Spiegel JP. *Men Under Stress*. Philadelphia, Pa: Blakiston; 1945.

35. Sargant W, Slater E. Amnesic soldiers in war. *Proc R Soc Med* [now *J R Soc Med*].1941;35:757–760.

36. Parfitt DN, Gale CMC. Psychogenic amnesia: The refusal to remember. *J Ment Sci*. 1944;XC:33–41.

37. Boshes B, Roberts LP, Tureen LL. Base section psychiatry. In: Glass AJ, ed. *Overseas Theaters*. Vol 2. In: *Neuropsychiatry in World War II*. Washington, DC: Office of The Surgeon General, US Army; 1973: 148–185.

38. Eitinger L. Denial in concentration camps: Some personal observations on the positive and negative aspects of denial in extreme life situations. In: Breznitz S, ed. *The Denial of Stress*. New York: International Universities Press; 1983: 199–212.

39. Kral VA. Psychiatric observations under severe chronic stress. *Am J Psychiatry*. 1951;108:185–192.

40. Eitinger L. Pathology of the concentration camp syndrome. *Arch Gen Psychiatry*. 1961;5:371–379.

41. Jones FD. Experiences of a division psychiatrist in Viet Nam. *Milit Med*. 1967;1:1003–1008.

42. Carden NL, Schramel DJ. Observations of conversion reactions seen in troops involved in the Viet Nam Conflict. *Am J Psychiatry*. 1966;123:21–31.

43. Personal Communication. Statistical data provided by US Patient Administration Systems and Biostatistics Activity, Department of the Army, 1991.

44. Palinkas LA, Coben P. Psychiatric disorder among United States Marines wounded in action in Viet Nam. *J Nerv Ment Dis*. 1987;175(5):291–300.

45. Putnam FW. The scientific investigation of multiple personality disorder. In: Quen JM, ed. *Split Minds Split Brains: Historical and Current Perspectives*. New York: New York University Press; 1986: 109–125.

46. Weinstein EA, Lyerly OG. Conversion hysteria following brain injury. *Arch Neurol*. 1966;15:545–548.

47. Weinstein EA, Eck RA, Lyerly OG. Conversion hysteria in Appalachia. *Psychiatry*. 1969;32: 334–341.

48. Weinstein EA, Lyerly OG, Rumbaugh JH. Conversion reactions in military personnel. Read at Seminar of Department of Military Psychiatry. Walter Reed Army Institute of Research. 25 March 1989.

49. Whitlock FA. The aetiology of hysteria. *Acta Psychiatr Scand*. 1967;43:144–162.

50. Roy A. Hysteria: A case note study. *Can J Psychiatry*. 1979;24:157–161.

51. Trimble MR. *Neuropsychiatry*. New York: John Wiley; 1981.

52. Brandt T. *Vertigo: Its Multisensory Syndromes*. London, England: Springer Verlag; 1991.

53. Weinstein EA. Conversion hysteria after brain injury. *Trans Am Neurol Assoc*. 1966;91:361–362.

54. Galin D, Diamond R, Braff D. Lateralization of conversion symptoms: More frequent on the left. *Am J Psychiatry*. 1977;134(5):578–580.

55. Stern DB. Handedness and the lateral distribution of conversion reactions. *J Nerv Ment Dis*. 1977;164(2):122–128.

56. Saver JL. Right diencephalic lesions predominate in thalamic pain. *Neurology*. 1992;42(Suppl. 3):162.

57. Weinstein EA, Kahn RL. *Denial of Illness: Symbolic and Physiological Aspects*. Springfield, Ill: Charles C Thomas; 1955.

58. Weinstein EA, Kahn RL, Slote WH. Withdrawal, inattention and pain asymbolia. *Arch Neurol Psychiatr*. 1955;74:235–248.

59. Weinstein EA, Kahn RL, Sugarman LA. Ludic behavior in patients with brain disease. *J Hillside Hosp*. 1954;3:98–106.

60. Ljungberg L. Hysteria: A clinical prognostic and genetic study. *Acta Psychiatr Scand*. 1957;Supplement 112.

61. Guze SB, Woodruff RA, Clayton PS. A study of conversion symptoms in psychiatric outpatients. *Am J Psychiatr*. 1971;128:643–646.

62. Steffanson JA, Messina JA, Meyerowitz S. Hysterical neurosis, conversion type: Clinical and epidemiological considerations. *Acta Psychiatr Scand*. 1976;53:119–138.

63. Wiesel C, Arny M. Psychiatric study of coal miners in eastern Kentucky area. *Am J Psychiatry*. 1952;108(8):617–624.

64. Kepecs SG. Psychiatric disorders in Puerto Rican troops. *War Med*. 1945;8:244–249.

65. Compton A, Jones FD. Clinical features of young adult Hispanic psychiatric in-patients: The so-called Puerto Rican Syndrome. *Milit Med*. 1991;156(7):351–354.

66. Lempert T, Brandt T, Dietrich M, Huppert D. Psychogenic disorders of stance and gait in neurology. In: Brandt T, ed. *Disorders of Posture and Gait*. Stuttgart, Germany: G. Thieme Verlag; 1990.

67. Koller W, Lang A, Vetere-Overfield RN, Findley L, Cleever L, Factor S, Weiner W. Psychogenic tremor. *Neurology*. 1989;39:1094–1099.

68. Monday K, Jankovic J. Psychogenic myoclonus. *Neurology*. 1993;43(2):349–352.

69. Sandler SA. Camptocormia: A functional condition of the back in neurotic soldiers. *War Med*. 1945;8:26–45.

70. Miller RW, Forbes JF. Camptocormia. *Milit Med*. 1990;155(11):561–565.

71. Fahn S, Marsden CD, Calne DB. Classifications and investigations of dystonia. In: *Movement Disorders*. London, England: Butterworths; 1987.

72. Chan J, Brin MF, Fahn S. Idiopathic cervical dystonia: Clinical characteristics. *Mov Disord*. 1991;6(2):119–126.

73. Fahn S, Williams DT. Psychogenic dystonia. *Adv Neurol*. 1988;50:431–455.

74. Kramer KK, LaPiana FG, Appleton B. Ocular malingering and hysteria: Diagnosis and management. *Surv Ophthalmol*. 1979;24(2):89–96.

75. Kathol RG, Cox TA, Corbett JJ, Clancy J. Functional visual loss: A true psychiatric disorder? *Psychol Med*. 1983;13:307–314.

76. Cooper JC, Meyerhoff WL. Functional hearing loss. In: Paparella MM, Shumrick DA, Gluckman JL, Meyerhoff WL, eds. *Otolaryngology*. Philadelphia, Pa: WB Saunders Co; 1991: 1161–1165.

77. Desai BT, Porter RS, Penry JK. Psychogenic seizures: A study of 42 attacks in six patients. *Arch Neurol.* 1982;39:202–209.

78. Williamson PO, Spencer D, Spencer SS, Novelly RA, Mattson RH. Complex partial seizures of frontal lobe origin. *Ann Neurol.* 1985;18:497–504.

79. Kanner AM, Morris HH, Luders H, Dinner DS, Wyllie E, Mendendorp SV, Rowan AJ. Supplementary motor seizures mimicking pseudoseizures. *Neurology.* 1990;40:1404–1407.

80. Saygi S, Katz A, Marks DA, Spencer SS. Frontal lobe partial seizures and psychogenic seizures. *Neurology.* 1992;42:1274–1277.

81. Hodges JR, Warlow CP. The aetiology of transient global amnesia. *Brain.* 1990;113:639–657.

82. Ganser SJ. Uber einen eigenarten hysterische Dammerzustand. *Arch fur Psychiatrie Berlin.* 1898;30:633–640.

83. Whitlock FA. The Ganser Syndrome. *Br J Psychiatry.* 1967;103:19–29.

84. Latcham R, White A, Sims A. Ganser syndrome: The aetiological argument. *J Neurol Neurosurg Psychiatry.* 1978;41(9):851–854.

85. Spiegel H, Spiegel D. *Trance and Treatment: Clinical Uses of Hypnosis.* New York: Basic Books; 1978.

86. Spiegel H. The grade 5 syndrome: The highly hypnotizable person. *Int J Clin Exp Hypn.* 1974;22(4):303–319.

87. Kartchner FD, Korner IN. The use of hypnosis in the treatment of acute combat reactions. *Am J Psychiatry.* 1947;103:630–636.

88. Weinstein EA, Kahn RL, Sugarman LA, Linn L. Diagnostic use of amobarbitol sodium ("Amytal sodium"). *Am J Psychiatry.* 1953;109:889–894.

89. Weinstein EA, Kahn RL, Sugarman LA, Malitz S. Serial administration of the "Amytal test" for brain disease. *AMA Arch Neurol* [now *Arch Neurol*].1954;71:217–226.

Chapter 16

CHRONIC POST-TRAUMATIC STRESS DISORDERS

FRANKLIN D. JONES, M.D., F.A.P.A.*

*Colonel (ret), Medical Corps, U.S. Army; Clinical Professor, Uniformed Services University of the Health Sciences, Bethesda, Maryland; Past President and Secretary and currently Honorary President of the Military Section, World Psychiatric Association; formerly Psychiatry and Neurology Consultant, Office of The Surgeon General, U.S. Army

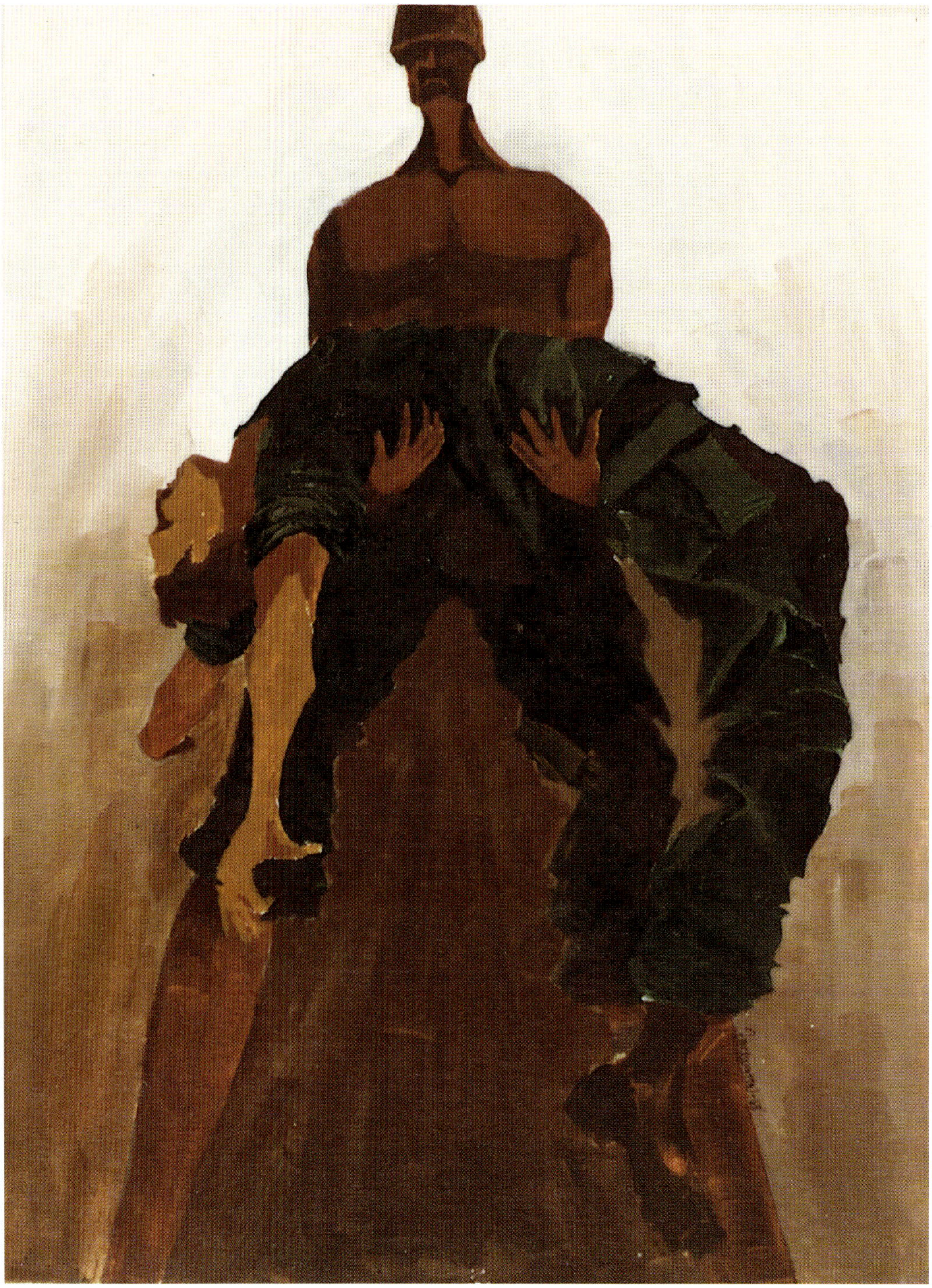

David N. Fairrington *Long Binh* 1968

David N. Fairrington was a member of the U.S. Army Artist Team #6 and was in Vietnam from February through June of 1968. In this striking visual presentation from that conflict, Fairrington captures the essence of every soldier's worst nightmare—carrying the body of his dead buddy and fearing that he himself may be the body being carried. Post-traumatic stress disorder is a complex of symptoms most often predominated by flashbacks and repetitive nightmares of this nature.

Art: Courtesy of US Center of Military History, Washington, DC.

INTRODUCTION

Post-traumatic stress disorders (PTSDs) comprise the majority of stress disorders associated with the trauma of combat, either of the acute, chronic, or delayed type. Combat fatigue may be considered a form of acute PTSD in its original understanding. Chapter 1, Psychiatric Lessons of War, describes this in greater detail. The chronic and delayed forms of PTSD have assumed considerable importance as sequelae of combat in Vietnam and in the 1982 Lebanon War.[1] The specific criteria for a diagnosis of PTSD, as delineated by the American Psychiatric Association's descriptive and nontheoretical *Diagnostic and Statistical Manual*, Fourth Edition (DSM-IV),[2] are presented in Exhibit 16-1.

History

Modern theories of PTSD begin with the 19th century concept of traumatic neurosis. Railway accidents from the middle of the century had seen the development of increasing litigation by injured persons suffering from pain and paralysis. The new specialty of neurology initially attributed these apparent neurological deficits to spinal cord injury; however, clinical and autopsy evidence began to accumulate, revealing little correspondence between tissue destruction (usually absent) and degree of disability. It was recognized that "railway spine" was a functional disorder. Charcot's[3] demonstrations of the production of paralysis and other symptoms in "hysterical" women suggested to Freud in 1893 a psychological etiology of hysteria. Charcot retained his belief in a neurological cause of hysteria and its manifestations. This was the prevailing idea. In 1889 Charcot's student, Oppenheim,[4] coined the term "traumatic neurosis" to describe what he thought was a "molecular derangement" of nerve tissue. Initially Freud accepted this idea, postulating with Breuer in their classic work, *Studies in Hysteria*,[5] an organic "hypnoid state" that made one vulnerable to hysterical symptoms when stimulated by a traumatic event. Freud believed that the traumatic event in hysteria was sexual. Later, when evidence accumulated that cast doubt on the presence of actual sexual trauma, he postulated that a fantasized sexual trauma could produce hysteria.[6] Later Freud attributed war neuroses to conflicts in ego structures (ego, id, superego) and instinctual drives (libido, destrudo).[7]

The idea that psychological trauma could produce apparent physical disabilities became generally recognized, especially with the appearance of numerous "shell shock" casualties of World War I. The pendulum swung from considering those with traumatic neuroses as neurological cases to considering them to be of purely psychological causation. Eventually traumatic neurosis was mostly subsumed under conversion or somatoform disorders but a large group, whose symptoms took the form of mood and behavioral disturbances, did not fit this categorization.

The first edition of the American Psychiatric Association Diagnostic and Statistical Manual of Mental Disorders published in 1952 (DSM-I)[8] included combat reactions under Gross Stress Reaction that corresponded in the *International Statistical Classification*[9] 1948 revision to Acute Situational Maladjustment. In DSM-I Gross Stress Reaction was to be reserved for "conditions of great or unusual stress" in which "a normal personality may utilize established patterns of reaction to deal with overwhelming fear."[8(p40)] These were differentiated from neurosis and psychosis on the basis of "clinical history, reversibility of reaction, and its transient character."[8(p40)] In terms of prognosis the following was stated: "When promptly and adequately treated, the condition may clear rapidly. It is also possible that the reaction may progress to one of the neurotic reactions. If the reaction persists, this term is to be regarded as a temporary diagnosis to be used only until a more definitive diagnosis is established."[8(p40)] The diagnosis was stated to be "justified only in situations in which the individual has been exposed to severe physical demands or extreme emotional stress, such as in combat or in civilian catastrophe (fire, earthquake, explosion, etc.)."[8(p40)] In many instances this diagnosis applied to previously more or less "normal persons who have experienced intolerable stress."[8(p40)]

The second edition of the Diagnostic and Statistical Manual (DSM-II, 1968)[10] substituted the term Adjustment Reaction of Adult Life for Gross Stress Reaction. This was in the general category of Transient Situational Disturbances, which were defined as follows:

> This major category is reserved for more or less transient disorders of any severity (including those

EXHIBIT 16-1

APA DIAGNOSTIC CRITERIA FOR DSM-IV 309.81 POST-TRAUMATIC STRESS DISORDER

A. The person has been exposed to a traumatic event in which both of the following were present:
   (1) the person experienced, witnessed, or was confronted with an event or events that involved actual or threatened death or serious injury, or a threat to the physical integrity of self or others
   (2) the person's response involved intense fear, helplessness, or horror. **Note:** In children, this may be expressed instead by disorganized or agitated behavior

B. The traumatic event is persistently reexperienced in one (or more) of the following ways:
   (1) recurrent and intrusive distressing recollections of the event, including images, thoughts, or perceptions. **Note:** In young children, repetitive play may occur in which themes or aspects of the trauma are expressed.
   (2) recurrent distressing dreams of the event. **Note:** In children, there may be frightening dreams without recognizable content.
   (3) acting or feeling as if the traumatic event were recurring (includes a sense of reliving the experience, illusions, hallucinations, and dissociative flashback episodes, including those that occur on awakening or when intoxicated). **Note:** In young children, trauma-specific reenactment may occur.
   (4) intense psychological distress at exposure to internal or external cues that symbolize or resemble an aspect of the traumatic event
   (5) physiological reactivity on exposure to internal or external cues that symbolize or resemble an aspect of the traumatic event

C. Persistent avoidance of stimuli associated with the trauma and numbing of general responsiveness (not present before the trauma), as indicated by three (or more) of the following:
   (1) efforts to avoid thoughts, feelings, or conversations associated with the trauma
   (2) efforts to avoid activities, places, or people that arouse recollections of the trauma
   (3) inability to recall an important aspect of the trauma
   (4) markedly diminished interest or participation in significant activities
   (5) feeling of detachment or estrangement from others
   (6) restricted range of affect (eg, unable to have loving feelings)
   (7) sense of a foreshortened future (eg, does not expect to have a career, marriage, children, or a normal life span)

D. Persistent symptoms of increased arousal (not present before the trauma), as indicated by two (or more) of the following:
   (1) difficulty falling or staying asleep
   (2) irritability or outbursts of anger
   (3) difficulty concentrating
   (4) hypervigilance
   (5) exaggerated startle response

E. Duration of the disturbance (symptoms in Criteria B, C, and D) is more than 1 month.

F. The disturbance causes clinically significant distress or impairment in social, occupational, or other important areas of functioning.

Specify if:

Acute: if duration of symptoms is less than 3 months

Chronic: if duration of symptoms is 3 months or more

Specify if:

With Delayed Onset: if onset of symptoms is at least 6 months after the stressor

Reprinted with permission from American Psychiatric Association. *Diagnostic and Statistical Manual of Mental Disorders,* 4th ed. (DSM-IV). Washington, DC: APA; 1994: 427–429.

of psychotic proportions) that occur in individuals without any apparent underlying mental disorders and that represent an acute reaction from overwhelming environmental stress.[10(pp48–49)]

It is further stated in terms of prognosis that, *"If the patient has good adaptive capacity, his symptoms usually recede as the stress diminishes"* (author's emphasis). If, however, the symptoms persist after the stress is removed, the diagnosis of another mental disorder is indicated."[10(p49)]

This is a most unfortunate change because one gains the impression that therapy should be aimed at removing the individual from the stressful environment; in fact, a brief respite from the stressors is needed, but removal too far produces chronic symptoms, and the object of treatment is rapid return to the high-stress environment. Furthermore, it implies that outcome is dependent only on the individual's innate adaptive capacity rather than requiring therapeutic interventions to permit that adaptive capacity to recover. Contrast this impression with that given in DSM-I: "When promptly and adequately treated, the condition may clear rapidly."[8(p40)]

In the third edition of the Diagnostic and Statistical Manual (DSM-III),[11] published in 1980, the clinician may place the combat stress reaction in the Adjustment Disorder category specifying the presentation (depressed mood, anxious mood, etc.) or may choose the Post-Traumatic Stress Disorder category. In the former, outcome as in DSM-II is stated to be dependent on removing the stressor: "It is assumed that the disturbance will eventually remit after the stressor ceases."[11(p299)]

Post-Traumatic Stress Disorder, among other criteria, lists "a recognizable stressor that would evoke significant symptoms of distress in almost everyone."[11(p238)] By dividing these disorders into acute (duration of symptoms or onset of symptoms, less than 6 mo following the onset of the traumatic event), chronic (duration of symptoms 6 mo or more) and delayed (onset at least 6 mo after the traumatic event), the impression is given that one is dealing with a lengthy disturbance due to psychological trauma.

In DSM III-R,[12] the 1987 revision of DSM-III, and DSM-IV,[2] the 1994 edition, there is a requirement for symptoms to last longer than a month. Presumably this was intended to make a distinction from transient adjustment disorders; however, this requirement introduces an unnecessary disjunction to the clinical and theoretical understanding of PTSD as an exaggeration of normal responses to psychic trauma. It does underscore the fact that the eventuation of chronic symptoms suggests perhaps persistent biological changes.

DSM-IV adds a new category, Acute Stress Disorder, for similar symptoms that occur during or soon after the trauma, last for at least 2 days, and cause clinically significant distress or impairment. If this persists beyond 4 weeks, it becomes Acute PTSD. This category corresponds reasonably well to those stress (battle fatigue) casualties who require "restoration" at medical holding facilities (clearing stations) for 2 to 3 days. It also covers those who require "reconditioning" for 7 to 14 days (or up to 4 wks) further to the rear. The DSM-IV also notes that "some symptomatology following exposure to extreme stress is ubiquitous and often does not require any diagnosis." This could apply to those battle fatigued service members who can remain in their own small unit or be given 1 to 2 days of rest in a nonmedical support element, or who recover and return to duty with only 24 to 36 hours of treatment at a forward medical (clearing) company. The DSM-IV has also shortened the onset time of chronic PTSD to 3 months post-trauma, although "delayed onset" is still after 6 months.

In summary, DSM-I, having been published shortly after the Korean conflict and based in large part on the U.S. Army nomenclature growing out of World War II experience, retained the correct concept for battle fatigue, which was placed under Gross Stress Reaction. In fact, the description of Gross Stress Reaction was almost an exact reiteration of that for Combat Exhaustion given in TB Med 203, the War Department Technical Bulletin, Nomenclature and Method of Recording Diagnoses, published 19 October 1945.[13] DSM-I was heavily influenced by the psychobiology of Adolf Meyer and the experiences of World War II psychiatrists.[14] DSM-II, however, was published in 1967, over 15 years after the end of the Korean conflict, the last conflict in which large numbers of battle fatigue casualties were seen. The Vietnam conflict was in its early stages; however, very few battle fatigue cases were produced primarily because of the low-intensity nature of combat and other factors.[15,16] Consequently the treatment lessons implicit in labeling did not have an urgent, emotional reality to the authors of DSM-II.

The authors of DSM-III were well aware of the effect of labeling as can be seen in the use of "schizophreniform" instead of "schizophrenia" but lack of familiarity with battle fatigue cases again led to a failure to understand the treatment implications of the labels involved.

Some of the thought involved might have been due in part to the need to view Vietnam veterans as having been damaged by their experiences in Vietnam and as appropriate recipients of psychiatric care. Such concern might have led to the acceptance of post-traumatic stress disorder (PTSD) and delayed post-traumatic stress disorder (DPTSD) for a larger cohort of behaviors (such as addictive and aggressive acts) than had previously been considered as sequelae of psychological trauma. Unfortunately, such labels hold potential untoward consequences for the perception, diagnosis, and treatment of the varied stress disorders that can be generated in combat and that are amenable to rapid intervention, very brief therapy, and quick restoration to duty. DPTSD must be seen as a special case that undoubtedly involves more complex historical factors both pre- and post-combat than the usual stress responses to the trauma of combat.

The DSM-IV category of Acute Stress Disorder helps to restore a distinction between the transitory reactions to extreme stress and more persistent symptoms, "Acute" may also have fewer negative connotations than DSM-I's use of "Gross," although "gross" does imply more than a trivial stressor.

Proposed Nomenclature for the Military

The following guidance was given when the author was Psychiatry and Neurology Consultant to the U.S. Army Surgeon General. It encapsulates ideas on proper nomenclature for combat psychiatric casualties, drawing from the *Manual of International Statistical Classification of Diseases, Injuries and Causes of Death*[9] (also known as ICD-9):

> Psychiatric combat casualties consist of a unique group of military patients for whom the diagnosis has strong possibilities for adversely affecting recovery. The term "battle fatigue" is ideal in that it suggests a nearly normal response, is relatively nonspecific in allowing for labeling of the great variety of symptom syndromes known to occur, and most importantly conveys an expectancy of rapid resolution. The disadvantage is that many psychiatric casualties occur so soon in combat that fatigue cannot reasonably be presumed to be a factor. Policy will be that patients in whom fatigue can reasonably be considered a factor will continue to be diagnosed as battle fatigue while those in whom fatigue cannot be so considered will be diagnosed transient battle reaction. Both terms should be considered roughly equivalent, should be treated similarly and will be coded with ICD-9 number 308.4 (mixed disorders as reaction to stress). Avoidance of technical terms that could be regarded as diagnoses (eg, "anxiety," "conversion," "paralysis") is desirable. Two examples follow:
>
> 1. Unwounded soldier presenting with tremor, tachycardia, sweating, paralysis of right arm, and glove anesthesia of right hand ten minutes after observing a friend killed in the first hour of battle:
> *(Axis I) 308.4 Transient battle reaction* manifested by numbness and weakness of right arm and hand, sweating, and rapid pulse.
> 2. Unwounded soldier developing fatigue, tremor, tachycardia, sweating, paralysis of right arm, and glove anesthesia of right hand following 36 hours of sustained combat exposure:
> *(Axis I) 308.4 Battle fatigue* manifested by fatigue, numbness and weakness of right arm and hand, sweating, and rapid pulse.

Subsequently, in current doctrine, the distinction between battle fatigue and transient battle reaction was abandoned. The rationale is that fatigue, by definition, is impaired performance due to doing something too long *or* too hard. As S.L.A. Marshall observed, fatigue or exhaustion can be brought on very rapidly by extreme fear. Anticipatory anxiety, as well as physiologic strain can bring on battle fatigue even before the battle starts. Therefore, the one term, battle fatigue, suffices. As operations other than war, such as disaster relief or peacekeeping in high stress conditions have increased while combat has decreased, the terms "contingency fatigue" and "conflict fatigue" have also been proposed.

ETIOLOGY

Psychiatric theories of etiology generally derive from the cultural or scientific zeitgeist. Ancient Egyptian healers, noting almost exclusive incidence of hysteria in women and being well-versed in anatomy, assumed that the multiple somatic symptoms of hysteria were due to migration of the uterus, a theory that held sway until the medieval Catholic Church, emphasizing the conflict between Satan and God, attributed hysteria to possession by evil spirits. After Isaac Newton revolutionized science with his theory of universal gravitation, Anton Mesmer began treating hysteria with magnets thought to have effects similar to planetary bodies. In a contest with the renowned exorcist Father Gassner, Mesmer demonstrated the superiority of his "scientific" approach over the older theory of possession.[17]

Likewise, in an era in which the intelligentsia accepted Charles Darwin's concepts of the evolution of increasingly complex structure and behavior based on the survival of animals with the best instincts, Freud saw various neuroses as resulting from instinctual drives clashing with reality. Thus, those with hysteria suffered from unfulfilled sexual wishes and those with obsessions and compulsions suffered from expressions of or defenses against anal eroticism and aggression. In this view, psychological trauma could cause anxiety symptoms due to the activation of unacceptable sexual and aggressive wishes. While temperament varied, the psychological conflict was considered paramount. Until the late 1970s psychological explanations of PTSD etiology, usually based on psychoanalytic or learning theories, predominated.

Gradually, perhaps presaged by the Watson-Crick discovery of the molecular structure of DNA, biological explanations of causality in mental disorders have gained hegemony. The concept of hysteria has almost disappeared except as a cluster of personality traits; and obsessive-compulsive disorders are viewed by many as the survival in some persons of instinctual grooming and other social behaviors of our mammalian ancestors, often best treated with medications.[18] Concerning PTSD, this biological supremacy has emphasized the physiological and neural aspects.

Biological Models of PTSD

Patients with chronic PTSD present with "positive" symptoms such as anxiety, tachycardia, muscle tension, shortness of breath, insomnia, irritability, and exaggerated startle response, which have been postulated as arising from conditioned autonomic activation to innocuous stimuli.[19–23] PTSD is also characterized by "negative" symptoms such as diminished interest in formerly significant activities, interpersonal detachment, restricted affective range, and a feeling of foreshortened future. These symptoms have been likened to the animal model of learned helplessness.[24]

Biological models of PTSD have emphasized the role of noradrenergic systems in the brain (primarily the locus ceruleus and its projections), which are activated by situations of alarm or trauma, the fight-flight reaction of Cannon.[25] Such "trauma centers" in the brain could be conditioned by threatening environmental events or stimuli associated with threat (conditioned fear stimuli) to respond to innocuous situations with PTSD symptoms.[26]

Drugs that inhibit noradrenergic brain systems have been used to treat stress symptoms including those of PTSD. These include clonidine, β-adrenergic blocking agents (propranolol), antidepressants (which downregulate β-adrenergic receptors), and benzodiazepines (GABA facilitators).[26] Many substances abused by persons with PTSD may be attempts at self-treatment because they share the ability to inhibit noradrenergic systems, at least temporarily. These include alcohol, benzodiazepines, barbiturates, and opiates.[26] The effectiveness of serotonergic attenuating agents (such as buspirone, a partial mixed serotonin 1A/1B receptor agonist) in treating anxiety disorders suggests serotonergic excess theories of anxiety as well.

Stress-mediated changes in neuronal structures of lower animals suggest that PTSD could be associated with fundamental and long-lasting modifications, including alterations in neuronal structure and gene expression.[26] Treatment, therefore, must often be intensive and prolonged and preventive measures should be the first approach.

While traumas cannot be prevented in conflicts, it is noteworthy that not all those exposed to severe traumas develop PTSD. In animal experiments of inescapable shock or stress (ie, the learned helplessness model of PTSD and depression)[27] those animals that could gain control over stress presentation and the severity, duration, and repetition of the aversive stimulus did not develop learned helplessness. The presence of a supportive peer and previous escape experience have protective effects in animals though biological and social vulnerabilities are factors.[26]

Studies also revealed that animals given antidepressants, clonidine, and benzodiazepines did not develop learned helplessness when exposed to inescapable stress.[27] Substances often abused by PTSD sufferers (stimulants, barbiturates, ethanol, and chronic use of benzodiazepines) were ineffective in reversing learned helplessness once it developed; however, antidepressants, clonidine, and buspirone, had a normalizing effect in animal studies.[26]

In summary, while older theories emphasized psychological trauma or conflict and conditioning aspects of PTSD etiology, more recent investigators have emphasized lasting neuronal changes and behavior in traumatized animals, postulating a hyperadrenergic state with hypercortisolism and physiological arousal to innocuous stimuli that resemble the original stressor. Others[28,29] have pointed out the aspect of repetition of the trauma manifested by intrusive thoughts, nightmares, and even hallucinations, thus implicating memory systems as paramount. The author has emphasized a multifactorial etiology or biopsychosocial model of chronic PTSD.[30]

A Biopsychosocial Model of Etiology

Chronic PTSD symptoms develop in those with social and biological predispositions in whom the stressor is meaningful when social supports are inadequate and the symptoms are maintained because of subsequent inadvertent reinforcement of the maladaptive behaviors.

Following both World War I and World War II, large numbers of combat veterans were treated in Veterans Administration hospitals for chronic "war neuroses." Many of these former soldiers had broken in combat and had been evacuated, never to rejoin their comrades. In many such soldiers a dynamic was set up that produced increasing disability. The dynamic developed as follows: (*a*) the soldier was conflicted over almost instinctual urgings to leave the combat arena to secure personal survival, battling with his own concepts of duty, honor, and responsibility to his comrades requiring him to remain in combat, (*b*) medical symptoms developed offering an honorable route out of combat, (*c*) the symptoms were accepted as a legitimate reason for leaving and the soldier was evacuated, (*d*) the soldier experienced guilt for abandoning his comrades because at some level he did not accept the legitimacy of his symptoms, (*e*) the symptoms became strengthened and exaggerated because of the soldier's need to prove to others and himself that he was really disabled and legitimately left combat, and finally, (*f*) any reproach either from internal guilt or from external doubt as to the medical necessity for his symptoms resulted in further strengthening of the symptoms.

Such a dynamic would explain the development, progression, and persistence of symptoms in the improperly treated acute post-traumatic stress casualty who becomes chronically disabled; but how can one explain the development of delayed PTSD symptoms, often occurring years after combat exposure? Such cases suggest that the dynamic described may represent only a special case of a more pervasive condition. Based on his study of psychiatric casualties in the 1973 Yom Kippur War and the 1982 Israel-Lebanon War, Belenky[31] has postulated that psychiatric casualties form a spectrum ranging from immediate ("battle shock") through acute ("combat fatigue") to late (chronic and delayed PTSD) combat stress reactions. In each case the etiopathogenic element is combat stress. The distinctions are based on certain intrinsic (personality, prior adjustment) and extrinsic (degree and quality of trauma, presence of ameliorating influences) factors. This conceptualization complements Marlowe's battle ecologies scheme, with the latter focusing on environmental factors (combat intensity).[32]

In Belenky's conceptualization, delayed PTSD results from the traumatic process itself, depending on degree of trauma, and develops somewhat independently of subsequent events. The author's view of the development of delayed PTSD is slightly different. While he agrees that a psychologically traumatic event will result in PTSD symptomatology, he would emphasize the contingent nature of the maintenance of, or delayed appearance of, disabling symptoms. As with the dynamic described earlier, *acute* post-traumatic symptoms are maintained and become chronic by their reinforcing value in preventing guilt or admonishment for the soldier's evasion of combat responsibilities. This has sometimes occurred because of improper or absent treatment.

The *delayed* PTSD syndrome, however, has a slightly different history. In these cases the soldier has experienced a traumatic event with variable degrees of subsequent symptoms that eventually disappear and may not even be remembered. Often, these soldiers performed without obvious impairment at the time, perhaps by denying fear or grief. After a symptom-free interval, the former combatant again experiences environmental stress. Such stress may or may not resemble the stress of combat; however, it evokes anxiety symptoms that usually are similar to those of combat. This similarity evokes memories of combat trauma and even produces in some instances reaction patterns similar to combat. These symptoms are reinforced in a variety of ways, including the concern of friends, justification for acting out otherwise unacceptable feelings, sustaining the patients' indignation over being abused by society, and monetary reinforcement (Veterans Administration [VA] pension).

Within the past decade the belief has developed that delayed and chronic PTSD are more common following unpopular conflicts. This belief is based on experience with U.S. veterans of the Vietnam conflict and more recently with Israeli veterans of the 1982 Lebanon War. In the Vietnam instance, estimates as high as 700,000 or 25% of Vietnam veterans were given as suffering from chronic

PTSD.[33,34] Other estimates as high as 60% of combat veterans have been given.[35] A more accurate figure for Vietnam appears to be 17%,[36] less than the 25% psychiatric disabilities given for World War II veterans. In the Lebanon instance studies[37] have revealed that two thirds of Israeli psychiatric casualties have been of the chronic or delayed PTSD type. This is exaggerated because all Lebanon War veterans reporting to a mental health facility were labeled as suffering from PTSD even though they had prior psychiatric diagnoses including manic-depressive disorder.[38]

Despite the possible exaggeration of PTSD prevalence, some relationship between unpopular wars and chronic and delayed PTSD seems to exist. Goodwin[33] has identified the following variables as producing chronic PTSD in Vietnam veterans: it was a teenage war (average age 20 for combatants); there was a fixed tour (unrealistic expectations after return to the states); the ideological basis of the war was unclear (saving the corrupt South Vietnamese "democracy" from the North Vietnamese, not Soviet or Chinese Communists); the enemy was hard to identify (sometimes the enemy appeared to be civilians—including women and children); there was widespread use of illicit drugs (especially heroin and cannabis); tranquilizing drugs were first used in combat (may have suppressed symptoms of stress); administrative discharges were frequent (often for drug abuse) and were only temporary solutions to stress; and the rapid return to the United States did not allow for decompression, with the returnee often being met with a hostile or indifferent homecoming. This may be a reflection of the lack of societal support for wars of this type. They are frequently ambiguous with a large percentage of the population indifferent or hostile to the war. Such wars are usually prolonged beyond the expectations of the initiators of combat and the patience of the populations, and they often include actions against civilians.

PTSD can be conceptualized as a special case of a broader mechanism by which the mental apparatus handles aversive stimuli. Freud's postulate, described shortly after World War I, of a repetition compulsion in which the organism replays the psychic trauma in an attempt to gain mastery, may play a role, especially with the early symptoms.[7] This replaying may take the form of dreams or nightmares, recurrent memories, or even hallucinatory "flashbacks" of the traumatic event. The sufferer may be preoccupied with "if only I had (or hadn't...)" thoughts. Other mechanisms such as positive reinforcement (secondary gain in Freud's model) seem more important in the chronic maintenance of symptoms. The emergence of delayed symptoms may be explained on the basis of an association between the current situation and an aspect of the traumatic situation. Ullmann and Krasner[39] have used the term "redintegration" for such evocation of behavior more appropriate to an earlier life event. Whatever the theory of causation, PTSD symptoms appear to be relatively universal given a severe enough stressor; however, it is not the presence of symptoms but the psychological purposes they serve that determines the degree of disability.

PTSD PRESENTATIONS

Diagnosis, treatment, and prevention of PTSD will be considered in the context of the following cases, which illustrate some of the features of chronic and delayed PTSD. Diagnosis, treatment, and prevention of *acute* PTSD have already been described in Chapter 1, Psychiatric Lessons of War, and Chapter 2, Traditional Warfare Combat Stress Casualties, in terms of combat fatigue or combat stress reactions. The following two cases, known to the author, illustrate some of the features of *chronic* and *delayed* post-traumatic stress, ranging from normal memories which are not a disorder to disabling PTSD.

Case Study 1: Just Bad Dreams

June K., now 60 years old, has never sought mental health care despite mild, chronic post-traumatic stress symptoms. Typically she develops nightmares after seeing a war movie or when undergoing unusual psychological stress such as the death of a family member. The nightmares awaken her and her husband who reassures her; then she falls asleep without further incident.

The psychic trauma that she experienced occurred at the age of 18 when she was captured by the North Koreans when they invaded Seoul in 1951. From a prominent South Korean family, she and her parents and siblings had been targeted for capture, torture, and death. Knowing this, the family had dispersed throughout Seoul. June K., the oldest child, had found work under an assumed name in order to buy food for her family (forced rationing and use of North Korean money prevented purchase of food with family resources). She was turned in to the North Koreans by a collaborator who had recognized her from newspaper photographs. After several days' captivity, which included occasional beatings, she escaped when the compound was bombed by U.S. planes.

She hid for several weeks until Seoul was recaptured by UN forces.

June K. served as a laboratory technician with U.S. forces until the war ended; then she came to the United States on a Fulbright Scholarship. Other than rare nightmares about her war experiences, there are no other symptoms and no apparent secondary gains.

Comment: This person exhibits typical mild chronic post-traumatic stress symptoms that do not appear to serve any adaptive role in her current functioning. Her symptoms are evoked by associations with the traumatic event.

Case Study 2: The Assassination Witness

While the author was consulting in the psychiatric unit of a military hospital in an Arabic country in 1985, he interviewed a 54-year-old army major, formerly a Warrant Officer, with 32 years of active duty. The major was married with five children. He dated the onset of his symptoms to an incident several years earlier when he was present at the assassination of the leader of his government, having been invited by his oldest son to see him march in the parade.

Sitting near the leader, he initially thought that the firing of weapons was part of the normal demonstration of support for him. When he recognized the hostile nature of the firing, which killed the head of state, the patient ran in a panic about 3 miles, collapsing at the gate to his military unit. He stated that ever since that time he has had headaches, nightmares, and giddiness. Physical exams and neurological studies revealed no apparent physical basis for his symptoms.

The symptoms persisted roughly a year at which time he was admitted to a hospital where he remained for another year. In the hospital he was found to be severely depressed but not suicidal. He also had severe anxiety, trembling, elevated heart rate, complaints of irritability, and dreams of airplanes bombing. He had also become angry with his oldest son, who had urged him to attend the ceremony. On one occasion he had even started choking him. Psychometrics revealed that he had average intelligence and neurotic symptoms, primarily a depressive disorder with hysterical personality. He was treated with thioridazine, lorazepam, and psychotherapy. His request for a medical separation from the military was denied.

Past history revealed that he had similar symptoms in the 1956 Arab-Israeli War when, as an officer candidate at the military academy, he was in a building that was bombed, causing it to collapse. He remained terrified underneath his bed for hours until he was dug out. Shortly thereafter, a bullet from a second air raid narrowly missed him. Afterwards he collected bullets as souvenirs. He had a period of nightmares and anxiety following these episodes, but this did not persist beyond a few weeks.

A decade later he was an advisor to the Yemen Army during their civil war. He stated that for a period of about 6 months he was constantly panicked. Several of his fellow soldiers were ambushed and their bodies mutilated; however, he did not witness these episodes. He felt isolated, alone among foreigners. A psychiatrist who served at about the same time verified that such incidents did occur but that the biggest problem was material deprivation in an inhospitable climate. Following that tour he again developed symptoms of anxiety and nightmares that lasted for several months, but then they dissipated and he experienced no particular problems until the assassination.

Currently, the patient appeared as a middle-aged man with gray hair who was anxious and sweating profusely while recounting his symptomatology. He presented my fellow psychiatrists, some of whom had treated him, with a letter that detailed his current complaints. He could not tell us why he had persistent symptoms after the assassination, but did not after the barracks bombings in 1956 and after his Yemen tour. He did not participate in the 1967 or the 1973 wars with Israel.

The following were the patient's complaints: giddiness, especially when walking, with a tendency to be worse on the right side; tinnitus leading to irritability and sometimes violent actions toward his wife or children; numbness or tingling in his scalp, "like I had a helmet on"; general paresthesias all over the body; sleep disturbances (early morning awakening, fatigue after having nightmares, and frightening awakenings). During the day he often felt tense as if his "head were full of blood" and as if the blood in his head were "boiling." He stated that he would become irritable if in crowds or if he heard loud noises, especially shooting. He also stated that he had profuse sweating of the right hand. He described sexual difficulties (impotence for the past 3 years); pessimistic outlook (that he hadn't achieved anything in his life); withdrawal and suspiciousness of other people; impulsiveness, depression, and sadness (in contrast to formerly being friendly and energetic); anorexia with mild weight loss; and smelling something burning. (The author's colleagues pointed out that this is a common symptom among PTSD sufferers who were exposed to napalm or burning flesh in various wars; however, this patient was not exposed to those conditions, so the etiology of this symptom is obscure. Perhaps it may have been modeled after the symptoms of other PTSD patients on the wards; such "contagion" of symptoms among suggestible battle fatigue cases is common.)

During the interview the patient was very energetic and animated, sweating profusely at times when recalling his symptoms; but, at the same time he seemed to derive some relief or even pleasure from sharing those symptoms and his suffering. His physician said that this patient, despite the diagnosis on psychological testing of a hysterical personality, actually had many features of an obsessive-compulsive personality (having been meticulously clean, very organized, very attentive to details, and somewhat rigid in interpersonal relationships).

Etiologically, this patient appeared to have all of the elements of a post-traumatic stress disorder: a severe stressor (the assassination in which he could have been killed) and recreation of this and earlier traumas in nightmares and perhaps the smelling of something burning (which could have been reminiscent of the gun powder at the time of the assassination—an intrusion of the trauma into the present). He also displayed the explosive irritability and aggressiveness as well as the withdrawal from social contact that are often found in PTSD. The irritability in the presence of loud noises, particularly the firing of weapons, has some components of a startle reaction.

In terms of treatment, group psychotherapy should be considered in this case although the lack of patients with PTSD symptoms from the assassination episode would weaken this approach. Usually group therapy works best when all group members have been exposed to a similar stressful situation.

Past individual psychotherapy apparently had focused on ventilation and supportive treatment. It had also emphasized work because he was denied compensation and a medical separation. Such an emphasis on "here and now" issues is desirable.

Comment: This patient exhibited a plethora of symptoms that, while typical of chronic PTSD, are seldom all found in one person. His symptoms appear to serve a current adaptive role in his functioning in making him a focus of attention and sympathy and excusing him from some military duties. Pharmacotherapy in such cases is often quite rewarding. The patient had received some anxiety relief from the thioridazine and lorazepam; however, he continued to be troubled by a multiplicity of symptoms. Recent studies have shown that the use of benzodiazepines beyond a few months may actually be countertherapeutic due to the development of tolerance effects.[40] He had not yet been treated with antidepressants, particularly monoamine oxidase inhibitors (MAOI) or the tricyclics. Although the mechanism of action of these agents is unknown (their effectiveness might be related to suppression of dreaming or REM (rapid eye movement) sleep (and thus nightmares), due to a general antidepressant effect or due to a specific anxiolytic action related to downregulation of β-adrenergic or serotonin 1-A receptors), these antidepressants often produce dramatic relief of symptoms. The author recommended a trial of phenelzine (a hydralazine-type MAOI—Nardil) in a dose of up to 90 mg per day. If there were problems with his use of MAOI, perhaps dietary restrictions not being enforceable, or other problems such as hypotension, then a trial with a tricyclic, probably imipramine, was recommended. At the time, selective serotonin reuptake inhibitors (SSRI) were not available. Currently, a trial of an SSRI might be helpful.

The following case, provided by Dean A. Inouye, M.D., reveals an aspect of personality, alexithymia, that may play a role in chronic PTSD. Alexithymia (literally "inability to read emotions") was described as a characteristic of some patients who appear unable to properly interpret emotions in themselves and others.[41]

Case Study 3: Chronic PTSD and Alexithymia

First sergeant (1SG) MC is a 43-year-old married white male with 22 years of service, self-referred for feelings of distress following his involvement in a shooting incident. In July 1991, 1SG MC and a security officer had attempted to evict an occupant from the company barracks. The occupant produced a gun and, without warning, shot 1SG MC in the chest and killed the security officer. The patient underwent surgery, which revealed no injury to vital structures. His post-operative course was unremarkable.

Past medical history revealed that the patient experienced three injuries during his two tours as a medic in the Republic of Vietnam: 1969, gunshot wound to right thigh; 1970, fragment wounds to right leg and head; 1971, burns to right hand and head. He had no other significant past medical history or current medications. He rarely used alcohol and denied use of tobacco or caffeine. He had no known drug allergies.

Social history revealed that he was adopted in infancy with a fraternal twin brother into an upper middle class family. He was close to both parents, did well in school, graduating from high school. He had no behavior problems and joined the Army at age 20 after 2 years of business college, "because I always wanted to." His military history was exemplary with many awards and citations.

Course: The patient first presented to outpatient psychiatry 1 month after his injury, complaining of rumination about the shooting incident, decreased appetite, and early insomnia with multiple awakenings, which he stated was "no different than when I was shot in Vietnam." He appeared anxious but his mental status exam was otherwise unremarkable. He was given a diagnosis of adjustment disorder with mixed emotional features. He was briefly tried on lorazepam (Ativan) 1 to 2 mg at bedtime to improve the insomnia. The medication was discontinued when the patient terminated treatment after three visits.

The patient returned to psychiatry 6 months after his injury complaining of rumination with depressed mood, pan-insomnia, increased appetite with 22 lb weight gain, lack of energy and initiative, pervasive anxiety, sudden crying spells and angry outbursts, decreased self-esteem and social withdrawal, and a feeling of loss of control of his emotions.

He had experienced the death of friends during the war but denied survivor guilt. After returning from Vietnam he had complained of prominent generalized anxiety; pronounced startle reaction without hypervigilance; pan-insomnia with multiple awakenings; nightmares of battle scenes and ambush; difficulty concentrating; angry outbursts; fear of flying in helicopters but no vivid recollections while awake. He received no specific treatment for his symptoms except diazepam (Valium). His symptoms gradually abated after a few years although he continued to have occasional nightmares. He believed that his present PTSD symptoms were worse than those after the Vietnam conflict. He was anxious and tearful during his exam. He was given a provisional diagnosis of post-traumatic stress disorder. He was started on doxepin

(Sinequon) 25 mg at bedtime to improve his anxiety and insomnia. Six weeks later, his treatment was terminated due to his unwillingness to attend his appointments.

The patient returned to psychiatry a year after his injury, 3 weeks before the anniversary date of the shooting incident. He complained of vivid recollections and nightmares of the shooting event, hypervigilance and easy startle, fear of situations similar to the shooting event, difficulty falling and remaining asleep with multiple awakenings, generalized irritability with occasional explosive anger, decreased concentration, and thoughts of death. He denied feelings of guilt over his survival. He expressed ambivalence about "coming for help" and fear of becoming a patient in the hospital. On exam, he was restless, with labile affect, and was frequently tearful. During all interviews he was remarkably without insight and unable to verbalize his feelings. His diagnosis of post-traumatic stress disorder was confirmed. He was given an additional diagnosis of alexithymia. He was started on fluoxetine (Prozac) 20 mg tablets once a day and clonazepam (Klonopin) 0.5 mg tablets three times a day to improve his anxiety and insomnia. The patient was placed on buspirone (BuSpar) 15mg per day, later increased to 30 mg per day.

He experienced a marked increase in his symptoms during the anniversary week of the shooting. After that, his anxiety decreased slightly and he experienced occasional nights of improved sleep, with fewer awakenings. He complained of mild daytime sedation and the buspirone was discontinued. His PTSD symptoms, in general, remained unchanged. In October 1992, buspirone 5 mg tablets three times a day was reintroduced to improve anxiety, with the goal to discontinue clonazepam and morning drowsiness. He reported gradually decreasing anxiety and improved sleep. However, his anxiety was often markedly worse on weekends and he continued to have two to three awakenings per night.

The patient continued on the above medications with clonazepam reduced to 0.5 mg at bedtime. After 2 months on the medication regimen, the patient reported significantly decreased anxiety, improved feeling of control, and improved sleep quality with fewer awakenings. On exam, his restlessness and lability of affect were improved. His other PTSD symptoms were unchanged and he could not do his work satisfactorily. He was therefore presented to a medical evaluation board (MEB) for separation from the military.

Comment: This soldier had continued to experience difficulties at work and he anticipated difficulties working in a foreign country after impending retirement. The symptoms may have represented an attempt to delay retirement and hold on to his U.S. Army identity. They may also have been an attempt to convey his feelings of disability for compensation purposes.

These case studies suggest that varying degrees of symptoms will follow a traumatic event. Whether they become disabling depends on the use to which they are put. In some circumstances, they can be highly adaptive. The Arabian major, for instance, trapped for 6 more years in a job that he did not enjoy with little chance of promotion, would have gained not only an exit from the army but also additional money for a disability separation. Furthermore, his possible envy and anger toward his upwardly mobile officer son could be justified by making him responsible for the major's current distress. June K., however, does not utilize her symptoms for current conflicts, having other adaptive mechanisms.

1SG MC functioned adequately until the time approached for his retirement from the military with the turmoil and uncertainties of a civilian life in a foreign country. The symptoms kept him his military identity and allowed him to express his distress in an acceptable manner, a common finding in alexithymic persons who cannot express feelings directly but do so with symptoms, usually physical.

One of the main methods of preventing chronic PTSD is by preventing (or properly treating) acute post-traumatic stress symptoms.[42,43] An important element in preventing acute post-traumatic stress (combat breakdown) is the presence of cohesive units or social support *during* the stressful event. Stretch[44] has shown that social support *following* the stressful event is also important in preventing or attenuating symptoms of chronic or delayed PTSD. He found, for example, that soldiers who remained in the U.S. Army (which is socially supportive of the combat role) following combat in Vietnam had significantly less symptomatology than controls who left the military following assignment in Vietnam. It is possible, of course, that self-selection accounted for some differences (with those more prone to PTSD disaffiliating themselves from the military); however, other studies[45] reinforce the importance of social support in the prevention of PTSD.

TREATMENT

The treatment of chronic PTSD, like its etiology, involves multiple modalities including emotional conditioning, cognitive restructuring, and pharmacological interventions.[46]

Psychotherapy

Individual therapy is often too intense for both patient and therapist, and group therapy with peers is usually preferable. While some "debriefing" (abreaction and ventilation) of the original traumatic events must be expected, it is important to prevent these sessions from becoming "stuck in the past," endlessly reiterating old guilts and grudges and trying to outdo others' stories. Here, and in individual therapy if it is undertaken, the focus is on current issues as in Glasser's reality therapy approach.[47] It is usually clear to an objective observer what reinforcements are maintaining the symptoms. To help clarify this area and intervene in diminishing this reinforcement, family and other interested parties may need to be interviewed individually and conjointly. This may also reveal that the patient has minimized significant alcohol or other substance abuse. When substance dependency is clearly established, an intervention and referral for detoxification and rehabilitation in a specialized program is indicated. Self-help groups such as Alcoholics Anonymous (AA), Narcotics Anonymous (NA), and Cocaine Anonymous (CA) should play a prominent part in the treatment.

Deconditioning by teaching the evocation of the relaxation response[48] can help alleviate not only the heightened tension of the hyperadrenergic state but also the tendency to use substances for relaxation. Exercise programs can also be beneficial in this respect.

Pharmacotherapy

Since the early descriptions of barbiturate treatment of combat stress casualties of World War II,[49] a variety of medications have been used to treat acute and chronic PTSD symptoms. The first relatively effective use was reported in an uncontrolled study of five war veterans utilizing phenelzine.[50] Subsequent studies have validated the usefulness of MAOIs and tricyclic antidepressants (TCAs) in the treatment of some PTSD patients, particularly when complemented with psychosocial therapies.[51–54] More recently, the SSRIs may be useful for some of these patients.

Most reports have emphasized the presence of concurrent disorders with PTSD, particularly substance abuse, depressive disorders, and personality disorders.[52,54] These concurrent disorders often require different approaches and may prevent effective pharmacotherapy of PTSD symptoms.

For the different PTSD symptoms themselves, different medications may vary in efficacy. Antidepressants appear to improve intrusive symptoms (such as recurrent intrusive recollections, nightmares, and panic episodes) but may be less effective with avoidant symptoms (such as withdrawal, emotional numbing).[54] Intrusive symptoms as well as hostility and feelings of violence were improved by the tricyclic anticonvulsant carbamazepine (Tegretol) in 70% of Vietnam veteran inpatients in a study by Lipper and others.[55] Again, improvement in the avoidant symptoms was somewhat less. In view of carbamazepine's antikindling effect, this suggests that PTSD symptoms may arise from the effect of trauma in evoking repeated strong emotions, which result in neuronal irritability and inappropriate activation as postulated by Post et al[56] in the pathophysiology of certain mood disorders and borderline personality disorders. Antikindling agents such as valproic acid (Depakene) and clonazepam appear useful as alternatives to lithium and carbamazepine.

Other medications that have been helpful with some PTSD patients include the antihypertensive drugs, clonidine and propranolol, both of which inhibit noradrenergic activity though by different mechanisms.[57] While benzodiazepines would seem useful in anxiety symptoms of PTSD, they have not been systematically studied, probably because of their high abuse potential in this population. Preliminary reports of lithium therapy by Davidson et al[54] reveal encouraging results in diminishing explosiveness, irritability, mood swings, and impulsive behavior, as well as in reducing nightmares and improving sleep. Carbamazepine, valproic acid, and clonazepam appear similarly useful in these symptoms.

At this time, careful assessment and treatment of concurrent conditions and clinical trials with a variety of medications along with psychosocial interventions are warranted for most chronic PTSD patients.

PTSD can occur following any severe stressor; however, prisoners of war represent a special case in which the stressors tend to be chronic as well as severe. They merit special consideration for study and proposed interventions since the entire group suffers similar status and deprivation stressors.

PTSD AMONG PRISONERS OF WAR

Prisoners of war (POWs) frequently develop symptoms of chronic PTSD (see Chapter 17, The Prisoner of War). POWs do not necessarily develop psychiatric disorders; however, follow-up studies of POWs during World War II, the Korean conflict, and the Vietnam conflict indicate an increased risk of such disorders.[58–60] The risk is greatly influenced by the conditions of captivity. Holocaust victims almost universally suffered from PTSD.[61] Soldiers incarcerated by the Japanese during World War II and by the North Koreans (and brainwashed by the Chinese) during the Korean conflict have had increased rates of depressive, anxiety, and psychosomatic disorders, as well as suicide. Conditions of captivity were often excessively harsh with many deaths from malnutrition, infections, and exposure.

Soldiers who had surrendered to the Japanese were treated with absolute contempt because they had violated the samurai warrior code of *Bushido,* which required the fighting man to die in combat, commit *hara kiri* (suicide by disembowelment), or request execution by the less favored method of decapitation.[62] Undoubtedly, brain syndromes caused by malnutrition exacerbated the chronic posttraumatic stress disorders arising from captivity.

During the Korean conflict, captive Americans were not only exposed to malnutrition, disease, and harsh camp conditions but also to a calculated psychological offensive aimed at breaking them that came to be called *brainwashing*. Crude coercive measures involving Pavlovian conditioning, both aversive and positive, with sleep deprivation, physical and psychological torture, and rewards for "acceptable" behavior (such as denouncing capitalism and American "imperialism," and admitting to using chemical and biological warfare) were used in conjunction with sophisticated social manipulation. Officers were separated from enlisted ranks to destroy the influence of leadership. Cohesion was destroyed by rewarding selected soldiers for informing on their fellows. Rewards of food, clothing, and medication might mean the difference between survival and death during the cold Korean winters. Information was carefully controlled; only adverse news (such as race riots in the United States) was presented to the POWs.

Critics of the POWs, not taking into account this new form of psychological warfare and hearing American soldiers denounce America or confess to fabricated war crimes, accused them of lacking willpower and indicted American child-rearing practices as producing psychological weaklings. Such criticisms were even extended to those who died of malnutrition, exposure, and illness; they were accused of having "give-up-itis," moral strength so weak that they would die rather than try to live in adverse circumstances.[63]

Based on his interviews with 20 randomly selected repatriates at the end of the Korean conflict and the work of colleagues who interviewed 300 men, Schein,[64] a researcher at Walter Reed Army Institute of Research, described what was probably the most extensive attempt to destroy unit cohesion and realign social viewpoints ever perpetrated against U.S. prisoners of war. The men were segregated according to race and ethnicity. Military rank was disregarded and the Chinese captors randomly selected small unit leaders. Informers were actively solicited and given special treatment, some of it life sustaining, such as adequate food while others were starving. Such favors were sometimes given noncollaborating soldiers to destroy confidence in them. POWs soon felt that they could not trust anyone. Signed confessions of germ warfare or other war crimes by U.S. forces were solicited and shown to POWs to attack the moral position of the United States. No group association was allowed other than Chinese-orchestrated self-criticism or propaganda lectures. Mail was censored so that only bad news was transmitted. Similarly, all news was from communist sources—press, radio, magazines, and movies. Race riots and criminal acts in the United States were highly publicized.

The postcaptivity evaluations revealed that the communists had little success in changing beliefs and attitudes; however, in producing collaboration they had been much more successful with about 10% to 15% of the men chronically collaborating in giving pro-communist lectures, broadcasting propaganda, giving false confessions, informing on fellow POWs, and so forth. Some attempted to obstruct the communists and they were generally transferred elsewhere. A few developed severe apathy, quit eating, and died. The most common response was neither collaboration nor obstruction of the communists but what the men called "playing it cool"; that is, physical and emotional withdrawal from the whole environment, developing an attitude of watching and waiting rather than hoping and planning.

Schein concluded, "Ultimately that which sustains humans is their personality integration born out of secure and stable group identifications."[64(p30)] Long-term follow-up has revealed that while many POWs improved, symptoms were often life-long.[65–67]

Following the Korean conflict, there was a great deal of media attention focused on the behavior of Korean-era POWs and measures that might be taken for the physical and psychological survival of the POW. In 1955, President Eisenhower issued the Code of Conduct[68] (Figure 16-1) that reaffirmed the basic tenets of resisting the enemy as much as possible and attempting to escape when feasible. It was and is believed that these guidelines actually pro-

THE CODE OF CONDUCT

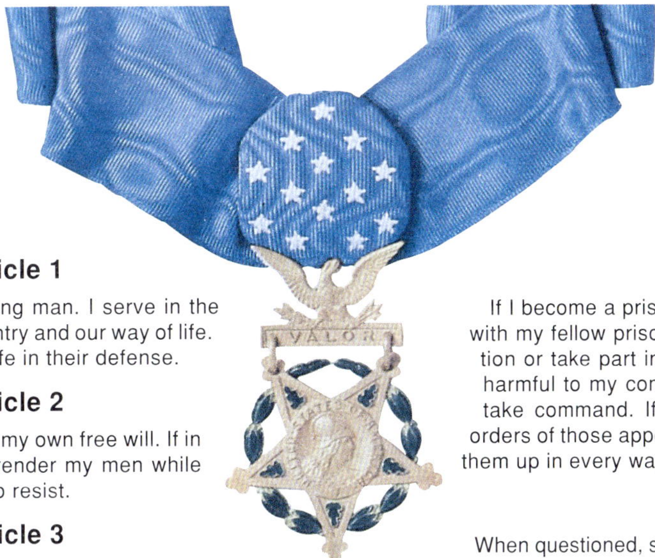

Article 1

I am an American fighting man. I serve in the forces which guard my country and our way of life. I am prepared to give my life in their defense.

Article 2

I will never surrender of my own free will. If in command, I will never surrender my men while they still have the means to resist.

Article 3

If I am captured, I will continue to resist by all means available. I will make every effort to escape and aid others to escape. I will accept neither parole nor special favors from the enemy.

Article 4

If I become a prisoner of war, I will keep faith with my fellow prisoners. I will give no information or take part in any action which might be harmful to my comrades. If I am senior, I will take command. If not, I will obey the lawful orders of those appointed over me and will back them up in every way.

Article 5

When questioned, should I become a prisoner of war, I am required to give name, rank, service number, and date of birth. I will evade answering further questions to the utmost of my ability. I will make no oral or written statements disloyal to my country and its allies or harmful to their cause.

Article 6

I will never forget that I am an American fighting man, responsible for my actions, and dedicated to the principles which made my country free. I will trust in my God and in the United States of America.

Fig 16-1. Code of Conduct for Members of the Armed Forces of the United States. After the Korean conflict, it was realized that coercive "brainwashing" could cause even the most patriotic soldier to be induced to make statements denouncing his country. The code was originally issued by Executive Order 10631 on 17 August 1955 by President Dwight D. Eisenhower and was amended by Executive Order 12017 on 3 November 1977 by President Jimmy Carter. Each soldier is given a copy. Data source: Department of the Army, *Code of Conduct/Survival, Evasion, Resistance, and Escape (SERE) Training*. Washington, DC: DA, 10 December 1985. Army Regulation 350-30.

tect the soldier from undue guilt associated with giving in under a less stringent code. More recently, forced "confessions" and denunciations of America are ignored because they are obtained by coercion.

Most of the American POWs of the Vietnam conflict were aviation officers shot down over North Vietnam. They had succeeded in the rigorous selection and training process for aviation pilots. Not surprisingly, these highly intelligent men invented ingenious methods of resisting the enemy, communicating among themselves even though usually placed in solitary confinement, and strengthening their mental defenses. They often practiced regular physical exercise, meditation, and "mental exercises" such as remembering books, mentally building a home, and writing journals though deprived of writing materials. Follow-up studies conducted after their release revealed that they were healthier than matched controls in all physiological systems other than dental and mental health. They tended to suffer more psychological problems than the controls but the differences were slight.

The relatively small number of POWs who had been captured in South Vietnam consisted primarily of ground troops whose experiences were similar to those captured by the Japanese and North Koreans. Their postcaptivity adjustment resembled that of the World War II and Korean conflict POWs (ie, increased morbidity).

An understanding of and techniques for handling captivity stress have been developed[69–72] based on the experiences of POWs from World War II, the Korean and Vietnam conflicts as well as other groups

(USS *Pueblo* crew members captured by North Korea and the U.S. Embassy personnel taken hostage in Iran). These can be considered in three phases: (1) precaptivity training; (2) captivity adaptation; and (3) postcaptivity recovery.

Precaptivity Training

Precaptivity training is needed for anyone likely to become captive, including military personnel, embassy staff, and others. This should involve learning the expected responses to phases of captivity and methods of adapting optimally to them, and realistic role-playing for purposes of familiarization and desensitization. Generally such training will have survival value. While 30% of American prisoners of the Japanese and North Koreans died in captivity, only 15% of American POWs in North Vietnam died. Although demographic differences (higher education, older, and mostly officers in the Vietnam POW population) and a less hostile climate were predominantly responsible for fewer deaths, soldiers who became POWs in Vietnam had been given captivity training.[71]

Captivity Adaptation

Captivity adaptation generally occurs in certain stages, which have been described by Rahe and Genender[72] as follows:

Stage 1: Startle/Panic—First Seconds to Minutes

Captivity typically occurs as an abrupt transition from normal daily activities to a situation of forceful, often brutal subjugation, a situation that cannot be assimilated quickly. Captors are excitable and have an increased likelihood of killing the captives at this point, producing paralyzing fear, stunned dissociation, or panic flights in captives. Feelings of defenselessness and confusion usually follow actual capture. Successful coping involves rapidly controlling these emotions. This may be facilitated by conscious attempts to count the captors, to memorize their features, and to focus on details of the situation.

Stage 2: Disbelief—First Minutes to Hours

Denial in the form of thinking, "This can't be happening" or "I'm dreaming," may occur. Captives often believe that they will be rescued quickly and are disappointed when this does not occur. Captors engage in various dehumanizing activities such as stripping clothing and personal items, binding, blindfolding, beating, and photographing prisoners for propaganda purposes. Similarly, "confessions" may be extorted by torture for propaganda value. Captives usually cope best by turning their attention inward—thinking of loved ones, home, and freedom—because psychological dissociation from the painful situation is adaptive in this setting.

Stage 3: Hypervigilance—First Hours to Days

The emergence of increased alertness to environmental cues can be useful—attempting to keep track of time, mileage, turns of the vehicle; however, guards are usually highly attentive to possible escape attempts at this time. Generally some form of interrogation will begin with emphasis on intelligence gathering. Hypervigilance can be useful in helping the captive withhold desired intelligence, in orienting to a 24-hour cycle, in assessing the captors, and in possibly eliciting the sympathy of guards who may assist the captive in obtaining reading and writing materials and other basic amenities.

Stage 4: Resistance/Compliance—First Days to Weeks

As the captors attempt to coerce the captives into cooperating, the resistance/compliance stage begins. Interrogations change from intelligence gathering to exploitation with coercive demands for "confessions" of "crimes" or enforced public appearances, often in degrading conditions. Given sufficient physical and psychological torture, virtually anyone can be forced to cooperate with his captors. The degree of cooperation depends on the severity of torture inflicted and the captive's commitment to resist.

The techniques used by captors derive from those used by the Czarist Russian and Stalinist secret police and the state police of Nazi Germany, with refinements added by the Communist Chinese and North Koreans. They include intimidating arrest; imprisonments of indeterminate length; physical, social, and nutritional deprivation; disturbances of body rhythms; physical and sensory isolation; stressful (often brutal) interrogations; unpredictable responses from guards and inquisitors; prolonged fear of death; and attempts to "reeducate" the captive. Settings are usually cramped, filthy, pest-ridden, uncomfortably cold or hot, with poor lighting and ventilation. Communication with fellow captives, or even guards, is prohibited.

Coping in these circumstances involves attempts to keep physically fit, to give the captors just enough information (preferably hard to validate and requiring lengthy time) to prevent severe torture, and attempts to communicate with fellow captives. Religious faith, prayer, meditation, and thoughts of loved ones also play an important role in coping.

Stage 5: Depression—First Weeks to Months

As the extent of his losses (freedom, family, friends, fortune, and possibly future) becomes apparent, the captive may become depressed. The captive may show the classical signs and symptoms of depression, including anorexia, retarded speech and movements, insomnia, fatigue, guilt, self-condemnation, and suicidal thoughts or attempts. Coping is greatly aided by a strong support group, hence the need to establish communication. The captive can use his own intelligence to fight boredom, composing stories and poems, mentally constructing buildings, solving mathematical problems, etc. Captor behavior at this time is primarily custodial.

Stage 6: Gradual Acceptance—First Months to Years

The captive realizes that his captivity may be prolonged and that he must make more productive use of his time if he is to survive. Custodial behavior by captors is usually maintained although "reeducation" efforts may continue. Coping behavior by captives involves living from day to day, taking each day as it comes, and attempting to maintain physical and mental stamina. Group support, if available, is extremely sustaining. Best is group creative work such as crafts, sports, and possibly escape planning.

Postcaptivity Recovery

Rahe and Genender[72] have described six stages of recovery from captivity as follows:

Stage 1. Brief Euphoria—First Seconds to Minutes

The period of elevated spirits of a released captive is usually short-lived. The captive is often mistrustful that the return from captivity may be another false hope. Celebrations may fall flat.

Stage 2: Hyperarousal—First Minutes to Hours

In contrast to the understimulation of the later stages of captivity, the released captive is overwhelmed by stimuli and mentally slowed, causing a "punch-drunk" appearance. Often sleep-deprived on their transition to freedom, the former captives may be confused and exhausted.

Postcaptivity management optimally includes a period of from several days to a week of "decompression." The ex-captive needs protection from the very intrusive media and even from relatives, because he may make remarks that he will later regret. For example, persons still influenced by the "Stockholm Syndrome" (identification with the captors) upon release have made statements favoring the aims of their captors and detrimental to the national interests of their country.

During this decompression time, thorough physical examination and correction of medical problems (eg, infections, infestations, dental care) can be accomplished. Rest and restoration of physiological deficits (sleep, food, fluids) are important just as with combat stress cases. In addition to physical restoration, the principles of proximity and immediacy indicate rapid return to the precaptivity milieu after decompression and positive expectancy. Psychiatric examination must be carefully conducted to avoid an expectation of mental illness, which can lead to a chronic "compensation neurosis." A positive expectation that the ex-captive will soon return to work is important. The psychiatric examination should be both diagnostic and therapeutic, allowing ventilation while providing reassurance.

Stage 3: Compliance/Resistance—First Hours to Days

Captives initially on release are likely to comply with most requests, having been conditioned to do so by their captors. As they regain feelings of individual power and capability, captives will begin to resist activities that appear to have little relevance to their own needs, for example, appointments, psychological testing, and intelligence debriefing. Treatment plans should take into account this emerging independence by allowing free time, the wearing of clothing other than hospital pajamas, time for group meetings with fellow captives, etc. Group cohesion can be fostered by having ex-captives eat together and engage in group "rap sessions." As with Marshall's[73] technique of debriefing troops after a battle, the reconstruction of events and correction of misperceptions can be highly therapeutic. Finally, follow-up reunions may be helpful.

Stage 4: Denial—First Days to Weeks

After an initial candidness about their problems adjusting to freedom, captives are likely to enter a phase of denying that their captivity has produced significant emotional or physical problems. While these statements should not be challenged directly, they should not be taken at face value. Arrangements for ongoing follow-up evaluations and treatment should be made, often through liaison with family members.

Stage 5: Restitution—First Weeks to Months

Attempts at restitution may take a variety of forms, such as gross obesity from overeating, problems with emotional control, and isolation to avoid overstimulation. Employers may attempt restitution by granting long vacations from work when, in actuality, return to a work routine generally helps the ex-captive reestablish feelings of self-worth. The family may attempt restitution by providing all the love and attention they could not show during the captivity. Captives may have difficulty interpreting nonverbal behaviors and the affective content of language. Families should be told to expect disconcerting responses, including crude table manners, and bathroom and sleeping habits acquired in captivity. They should also be told to expect and even encourage the ex-captive to recount his captivity experience because it seems to serve a therapeutic abreactive purpose.

Stage 6: Gradual Readjustment—First Months to Years

Follow-up studies of American POWs from Korea and from World War II Japanese prisons, in both circumstances experiences being extremely severe, revealed increased rates of infectious, cardiovascular, degenerative, and psychiatric disorders and accidental deaths compared to control subjects over the next 25 to 30 years.[72] Depending on the severity of circumstances and the individual's coping skills, some psychological scarring and premature physical disability is likely for the duration of the ex-POW's life. Ongoing follow-up for significantly traumatized individuals may prevent or attenuate disability, but some degree of post-traumatic stress symptoms is inevitable.

SUMMARY AND CONCLUSION

Post-traumatic stress disorder has come to epitomize the blaming and legalistic tendency in modern American society. It is given currency to explain the most outrageous behavior from Vietnam veterans' trafficking in cocaine and narcotics and robbing banks to a sexually promiscuous woman's attributing her behavior to trauma on a San Francisco cable car. Despite these unlikely extensions of the PTSD concept, a core of solid data exists suggesting psychic trauma as underlying much of nonbiologically generated mental illness. Such apparently disparate conditions as multiple personality disorders, panic disorders, and psychogenic depressions may result from early physical and sexual abuse. Psychic trauma occurring in older persons may lead to the development of a constellation of symptoms and behaviors that are termed PTSD. It is often unclear as to who is most responsible for these symptoms, the traumatized person or the original stressor. Attorneys make a living persuading juries and judges one way or the other.

The traumatized person's best hope is to accept responsibility for his symptoms and to develop coping methods to neutralize them. This should be the aim of psychiatric treatment.

REFERENCES

1. Solomon Z. Delayed PTSD among Israeli veterans of the Lebanon war. Biological aspects of non-psychotic disorders. Abstract 51. *Scientific Proceedings, World Federation of Biological Psychiatry*; Jerusalem, Israel: WFBP; April 1989.

2. American Psychiatric Association. *Diagnostic and Statistical Manual of Mental Disorders.* 4th ed. (DSM-IV). Washington, DC: APA; 1994.

3. Charcot JM. Discussed in: Laughlin HP. *The Neuroses.* Baltimore, Md: Butterfield Press; 1967: 847.

4. Oppenheim H. Discussed in: Robitscher J. Mental suffering and traumatic neurosis. In: Leedy JJ, ed. *Compensation in Psychiatric Disability and Rehabilitation.* Springfield, Ill: Charles C Thomas; 1971: 233.

5. Breuer J, Freud S, aus. In: Strachey J, Freud A, eds; Strachey J, trans-ed. *Studies on Hysteria.* New York: Basic Books; 1957.

6. Freud S. Beyond the pleasure principle (1920). In: Strachey J, ed. *Beyond the Pleasure Principle, Group Psychology and Other Works (1920–1922).* Vol 18. *Standard Edition of the Complete Psychological Works of Sigmund Freud.* London, England: Hogarth Press; 1955: 3–64.

7. Freud S. The war neuroses (1919). In: Strachey J, ed. *An Infantile Neurosis and Other Works (1917-1919).* Vol 17. *Standard Edition of the Complete Psychological Works of Sigmund Freud.* London, England: Hogarth Press; 1955: 205–215.

8. American Psychiatric Association. *Diagnostic and Statistical Manual of Mental Disorders.* (DSM-I). Washington, DC: APA; 1952.

9. *Manual of the International Statistical Classification of Diseases, Injuries and Causes of Death.* 9th ed. Originally adopted 1948. Volume 1, Tabular List with Inclusions. Geneva, Switzerland: World Health Organization. American Version: Washington, DC: National Office of Vital Statistics.

10. American Psychiatric Association. *Diagnostic and Statistical Manual of Mental Disorders.* 2nd ed. (DSM-II). Washington, DC: APA; 1968.

11. American Psychiatric Association. *Diagnostic and Statistical Manual of Mental Disorders.* 3rd ed. (DSM-III). Washington, DC: APA; 1980: 250.

12. American Psychiatric Association. *Diagnostic and Statistical Manual of Mental Disorders.* 3rd ed. Revised. (DSM III-R). Washington, DC: APA; 1987.

13. US Army Medical Department. *Nomenclature and Method of Recording Diagnoses.* Washington, DC: War Department Technical Bulletin; 19 October 1945. TB Med 203.

14. Grob GN. Origins of DSM I: A study in appearance and reality. *Am J Psychiatry.* 1991;148(4):421–431.

15. Jones FD. Experiences of a division psychiatrist in Vietnam. *Milit Med.* 1967;132:1003–1008.

16. Jones FD, Johnson AW. Medical and psychiatric treatment policy and practice in Vietnam. *J Soc Issues.* 1975;31(4):49–56.

17. Ellenberger HF. *The Discovery of the Unconscious: The History and Evolution of Dynamic Psychiatry.* New York: Basic Books; 1970: 53–69.

18. Swedo SE. Rituals and releasers. In: Rapoport JL, ed. *Obsessive Compulsive Disorder in Children and Adolescents.* Washington, DC: APA; 1989: 269–288.

19. Kardiner A. The traumatic neuroses of war. In: *Psychosomatic Medicine Monographs.* New York: Paul Harber; 1941: 11–117.

20. Gillespie RD. *Psychological effects of war on citizen and soldier.* New York: WW Norton; 1942.

21. Dobbs D, Wilson WP. Observations on the persistence of war neurosis. *Dis Nerv Syst.* 1960;21:686–691.

22. Kolb LC. The post-traumatic stress disorders of combat: A subgroup with a conditioned emotional response. *Milit Med.* 1984;149:237–243.

23. Kolb LC. Neuropsychological hypothesis explaining posttraumatic stress disorders. *Am J Psychiatry.* 1987; 144:989–995.

24. Van der Kolk B, Greenberg M, Boyd H, Krystal J. Inescapable shock, neurotransmitters, and addiction to trauma: Toward a psychobiology of post-traumatic stress. *Biol Psychiatry.* 1985;20:314–325.

25. Cannon WB. *Bodily Changes in Pain, Hunger, Fear and Rage.* 2nd ed. New York: Appleton; 1929.

26. Krystal JH. Animal models for post-traumatic stress disorder. In: Giller EL, ed. *Biological Assessment and Treatment of Post-traumatic Stress Disorder.* Washington, DC: APA; 1990.

27. Seligman MEP, Maier SF. Failure to escape traumatic shock. *J Exp Psychol (Gen).* 1967;74:1–9.

28. Ross RJ, Ball WA, Sullivan KA, Caroff SN. Sleep disturbance as the hallmark of posttraumatic stress disorder. *Am J Psychiatry.* 1989;146(6):697–707.

29. Van der Kolk BA, Van der Hart O. Pierre Janet and the breakdown of adaptation in psychological trauma. *Am J Psychiatry.* 1989;146(12):1531–1540.

30. Silsby HD, Jones FD. The etiologies of Vietnam post-traumatic stress syndrome. *Milit Med.* 1985;150(1):6–7.

31. Belenky GL. Combat reaction spectrum disorder. Presented at the American Psychiatric Association Annual Meeting; May 1985; Dallas, Tex.

32. Marlowe DH. Personal Communication, 1988.

33. Goodwin J. The etiology of combat-related post-traumatic stress disorders. In: Williams T, ed. *Post-traumatic Stress Disorders of the Vietnam Veteran.* Cincinnati, Ohio: Disabled American Veterans; 1980; 1–23.

34. Morganthau T, Shabad S, Lord M, Young J, Lubenow G. The troubled Vietnam vet. *Newsweek.* 30 March 1981: 24–29.

35. Wilson JP. *Forgotten Warrior Project.* Cincinnati, Ohio: Disabled American Veterans; 1979.

36. Stretch R. PTSD among Vietnam and Vietnam-era veterans. In: Figley CR, ed. *Trauma and its Wake: The Study and Treatment of Post-traumatic Stress Disorder.* New York: Brunner/Mazel; 1986: 156–192.

37. Belenky GL. Varieties of reaction and adaptation to combat experience. *Bull Menninger Clin.* 1987;51(1):64–79.

38. Noy S. Personal Communication, 1985.

39. Ullmann LP, Krasner L. *A Psychological Approach to Abnormal Behavior.* Englewood Cliffs, NJ: Prentice-Hall; 1969.

40. Miller NS. Liability and efficacy from long-term use of benzodiazepines: Documentation and interpretation. *Psychiatr Ann.* 1995;25(3):166–173.

41. Sifneos PE. Affect, emotional conflict and deficit: An overview. *Psychother Psychosom.* 1991;56(3):116–122.

42. Brill NQ, Beebe GW. *A Follow-up Study of War Neuroses.* Washington, DC: US GPO; 1955: 329–333.

43. Glass AJ. Lessons learned. In: Glass AJ, ed. *Overseas Theaters.* Vol 2. In: *Neuropsychiatry in World War II.* Washington, DC: Office of The Surgeon General, US Army; 1973: 989–1027.

44. Stretch R. Incidence and etiology of post-traumatic stress disorder among active duty Army personnel. *J Appl Soc Psychol.* 1986;16:464–481.

45. Horowitz M. *Stress Response Syndromes.* Northvale, NJ: Jason Aronson; 1976.

46. Solomon SD, Gerrity ET, Muff AM. Efficacy of treatments for posttraumatic stress disorder: An empirical review. *JAMA.* 1992;268(5):633–638.

47. Glasser W. *Reality Therapy: A New Approach to Psychiatry.* New York: Harper & Row; 1965.

48. Benson H. *The Relaxation Response.* New York: Wm Morrow; 1975.

49. Sargant WW, Slater E, eds. *An Introduction to Physical Methods of Treatment in Psychiatry.* New York: Science House; 1972: 149.

50. Hogben GL, Cornfield RB. Treatment of traumatic war neurosis with phenelzine. *Arch Gen Psychiatry.* 1981; 38:440–445.

51. Van der Kolk BA. The drug treatment of post-traumatic stress disorder. *J Affective Disord.* 1987;13:203–213.

52. Kosten TR, Frank JB, Dan E, Giller EL. Treating posttraumatic stress disorder with phenelzine or imipramine. In: Giller EL, ed. *Biological Assessment and Treatment of Posttraumatic Stress Disorder.* Washington, DC: APA; 1990: 1–26.

53. Thomson J, Dan E, Rosenheck R, Giller EL. Medication clinic within a Vietnam veteran readjustment counseling center. In: Giller EL, ed. *Biological Assessment and Treatment of Posttraumatic Stress Disorder.* Washington, DC: APA; 1990: 173–183.

54. Davidson JT, Kudler HS, Smith RD. Assessment and pharmacotherapy of posttraumatic stress disorder. In: Giller EL, ed. *Biological Assessment and Treatment of Posttraumatic Stress Disorder.* Washington, DC: APA; 1990: 203–221.

55. Lipper SL, Davidson JRT, Grady TA, et al. Preliminary study of carbamazepine in posttraumatic stress disorder. *Psychosomatics.* 1986;27:849–854.

56. Post RM, Ballenger JC, Uhde TW, et al. Efficacy of carbamazepine in manic-depressive illness: Implications for underlying mechanisms. In: Post RM, Ballenger JC, eds. *Neurobiology of Mood Disorders.* Baltimore, Md: Williams & Wilkins; 1984.

57. Kolb LC, Burris BC, Griffiths S. Propranolol and clonidine in the treatment of post traumatic stress disorders of war. In: Van der Kolk B, ed. *Post Traumatic Stress Disorders: Psychological and Biological Sequelae.* Washington, DC: APA; 1984: 24–42.

58. Beebe GW. Follow-up studies of World War II and Korean War prisoners, II: Morbidity, disability and maladjustments. *Am J Epidemiol.* 1975;101(5):400–422.

59. Ursano RJ, Boydstun JA, Wheatley RD. Psychiatric illness in US Air Force Vietnam prisoners of war: A 5-year follow-up. *Am J Psychiatry.* 1981;138:310–314.

60. Nefzger MD. Follow-up studies of World War II and Korean War prisoners. Part 1: Study plan and mortality findings. *Am J Epidemiol.* 1970;91:123–138.

61. Eitinger L. Pathology of the concentration camp syndrome: Preliminary report. *Arch Gen Psychiatry.* 1961;5:371–379.

62. Nardini JE. Survival factors in American prisoners of war of the Japanese. *Am J Psychiatry.* 1952;109:241–248.

63. Mayer WE. Why did many G.I. captives cave in? *US News and World Report.* 24 February 1956: 56–72.

64. Schein EH. Reaction patterns to severe, chronic stress in American prisoners of war of the Chinese. *J Soc Issues.* 1957;13:21–30.

65. Cohen BM, Cooper MA. A follow-up study of World War II prisoners of war. Veterans Administration Monograph, Washington, DC: US GPO; 1954: 1–70.

66. Sutber BP, Winstead DK, Goist KC, et al. Psychopathology subtypes and symptom correlates among former prisoners of war. *J Psychopathol Behav Assessments.* 1986;8:89–101.

67. Van Kammen WB, Christiansen C, von Kammen DP, Reynolds CF. Sleep and the prisoner-of-war experience—40 years later. In: Giller EL, ed. *Biological Assessment and Treatment of Posttraumatic Stress Disorder*. Washington, DC: APA; 1990: 159–172.

68. Department of the Army, *Code of Conduct/Survival, Evasion, Resistance, and Escape (SERE) Training*. Washington, DC: DA, 10 December 1985. Army Regulation 350-30.

69. Howard NS, Jones FD. The Iranian hostages: Trying to minimize the damage. Presented at the American Psychiatric Association Annual Meeting; May 1984; Los Angeles, Calif.

70. Jones FD, Harris P, Fong YH. Behavioral responses in adaptation to hostage situations. Presented at Third International Conference on Psychological Stress and Adjustment in Time of War and Peace; 3-6 January 1983; Tel-Aviv, Israel.

71. Studies and Analysis Service. *Office of Planning and Program Evaluation: Study of Former Prisoners of War*. Washington, DC: US GPO; 1980.

72. Rahe RH, Genender E. Adaptation to and recovery from captivity stress. *Milit Med*. 1983;148(7):577–585.

73. Marshall SLA. *Pork Chop Hill*. New York: Wm Morrow; 1956: xiv.

Chapter 17

THE PRISONER OF WAR

ROBERT J. URSANO, M.D.[*] AND JAMES R. RUNDELL, M.D.[†]

*Colonel (ret), United States Air Force, Medical Corps, Flight Surgeon; Professor and Chairman, Department of Psychiatry, Uniformed Services University of the Health Sciences, Bethesda, Maryland

†Major, United States Air Force, Medical Corps; Chief, Consultant Liaison of Psychiatry, 89th Medical Group/SGHA, Andrews AFB, Maryland; former Consultant for Psychiatry, Office of the Surgeon General; Associate Professor, Department of Psychiatry, Uniformed Services University of the Health Sciences, Bethesda, Maryland

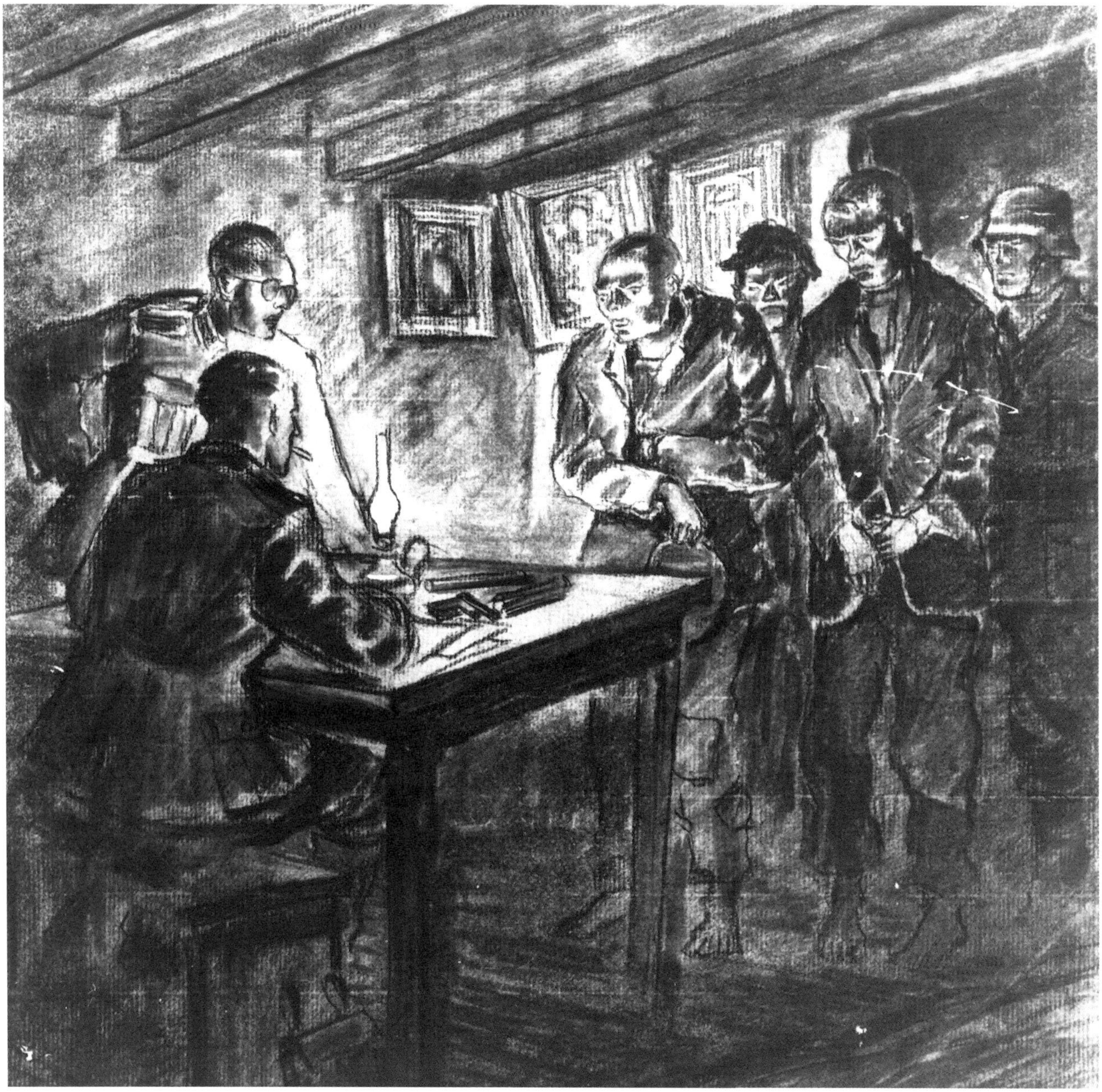

Artist Unknown *Prisoner Interrogation* circa 1943

This sketch is part of an extensive collection of captured German art from World War II in the possession of the U.S. Army Center of Military History. It graphically depicts the questioning of barefoot prisoners of war in what appears to be an underground bunker.

Art: Courtesy of US Army Center of Military History, Washington, DC.

INTRODUCTION

That trauma can be accompanied or followed by psychiatric sequelae is well-established.[1–4] The degree of severity of a traumatic event is positively associated with potential for psychopathology.[3,5–9] This is not a one-to-one association, however. Social supports, cultural variables, and personality also play roles. The prisoner of war (POW) experience can be one of the most traumatic situations in human experience. The study of coping during captivity, as well as psychological health and pathology following repatriation, has implications for psychiatric planning for future wars and for treatment of other stressor-related psychiatric illnesses. In this chapter, the literature on the psychiatric effects of the POW experience, coping behaviors, psychiatric symptoms during imprisonment, psychiatric sequelae after repatriation, etiologic factors producing postrepatriation psychopathology, treatment of the psychiatrically ill former POW, and the effects of imprisonment on the family will be reviewed.

THE PRISON EXPERIENCE

Nature of Captivity

There is no one POW experience. For example, the average duration of POW imprisonment during the Vietnam conflict was substantially longer than during World War II and the Korean conflict. Many POWs were held captive in Vietnam for 6 to 7 years. In addition, the severity of conditions was greater in World War II Pacific Theater POW camps than in European Theater prisons.[10–16] In contrast, the POW experience in the Persian Gulf War was generally no more than 30 days with some, but not all, POWs experiencing torture and others fearing death from bombings by the Allies. It is important to remember that repatriated POWs are a subset of those who are lost, captured, and imprisoned. They are the survivors. Nothing is known about the group that never returned. The nature of captivity plays an important role in determining psychiatric responses both during imprisonment and following repatriation. The types of stressors to which POWs are exposed are dependent on the cultural and socioeconomic status of the captors, the geography, the climate, endemic diseases, the circumstances of capture (aircrew ejection, large group surrender, etc.), the political climate, and the degree of resistance offered by the POW.[17] The degree of stress caused by these experiences depends on the physical conditions, the psychological experience, degree of maltreatment, interpersonal issues, and the individual and cultural appraisal of events.[18] The role of culture itself as a stressor is frequently overlooked.[18] Exposure to a country with limited resources, different rules of interpersonal and group relations, and different day-to-day personal and work habits can be stressful regardless of any intent to deprive or demean a captured soldier.

In order to describe and quantify the stress factors of the Vietnam-era POW experience, Ursano and colleagues reviewed debriefing reports and medical questionnaires completed by repatriated Vietnam-conflict POWs immediately after release.[5] One section of the medical questionnaire included questions on the methods used by the North Vietnamese to control the prisoner's behavior. Each question was answered on a four-point scale that ranged from "never" to "very often." Debriefing reports were coded for frequency and type of maltreatment. Using a factor analytic technique, seven stress factors were identified: (1) psychological maltreatment, (2) physical torture and maltreatment, (3) solitary confinement, (4) interrogation, (5) threats and denials of privileges, (6) high resister status, and (7) duration of maltreatment.

The acute and chronic stresses of captivity must be differentiated. At times, the difference has been referred to as stress (acute) and strain (chronic). Basic animal studies highlight this distinction. Young hamsters separated from their mothers (acute stress) will initially display hyperarousal and make a "separation call." This is eventually followed (chronic stress) by withdrawal and absence of a separation call.[19] Cassem and Hackett have reported a similar pattern of psychological response in humans following the specific stressor of myocardial infarction.[20] An initial period of anxiety and autonomic hyperactivity is followed by withdrawal and neurasthenia.

Readily reversible hyperarousal is a common initial reaction in combat.[21] In contrast, a consistent observation in men exposed to chronic combat is neurasthenia, withdrawal, defeatism, and isolation. A neurasthenic appearance in POWs after prolonged captivity was described[22] by Greenson in World War II POWs[23] and by Strassman in Korean conflict POWs.[24] Both noted an apathy syndrome that was felt to be adaptive in the POW environment. Withdrawal and detachment increased the chances of survival. In this way, energy was conserved and the POW was less likely to stand out, challenge the captors, and elicit threats and torture.

Looking at Minnesota Multiphasic Personality Inventory (MMPI) measures, Ursano et al[25] found that withdrawal and detachment were related to successful coping only in the high but submaximal stress Vietnam-conflict POW group (those captured after 1969). In the maximum stress group, withdrawal and apathy were also present but they were not predictive of successful coping. In this maximum POW stress group, denial, repression, and suspiciousness were associated with better coping. This suggests that cognitive coping strategies may be important in maximal stress settings after withdrawal from the environment has been attempted. With the passage of time, withdrawal and neurasthenia may be less helpful and other strategies such as fantasizing and pondering family concerns more useful.[26]

The stages of the POW captivity experience are as follows: capture, imprisonment, confinement, repatriation, and reintegration. Each stage has unique stressors.[27,28] For instance, at the time of capture, POWs must gain quick emotional control, deal with fears of death, and attend to the tasks necessary for survival. Expectations of rescue fade quickly after removal from the capture site; usually the prisoner is bound and/or blindfolded. A sense of disbelief may result from the rapid sequence of events and the radical change in roles from combatant to captive.

The phase of imprisonment includes the initial "breaking-in" and transport to the final confinement site. The POW is forced to adapt to a lower plane of existence and becomes aware of losing his usual supports and prestige. Feelings of longing for freedom, wishes for sympathy, dissociation, and fantasizing about home or retaliation are common in this phase. This is also the period of hyper-vigilance, alertness, orienting to sur roundings, and attending to detail. The last two can form the basis of a reassuring sense of familiarity over time.

The third phase of the POW experience, confinement, is characterized by exploitative interrogations, confessions, isolation, boredom, demoralization about the uncertainty of the situation, and the need to make decisions regarding resistance and compliance. The hypervigilant state is replaced by apathy, dysphoria, and gradual movement toward accommodation to the situation. During this long phase, POWs often engage in self-developed physical fitness programs, group communication, resistance, humor, creativity through projects and fantasies (learning a language, collaboration, fantasizing about the future, planning escape or sabotage), and also helping other POWs.

The period of repatriation and the subsequent life-long process of reintegration have unique stressors and adaptational strategies as well. They are discussed later in the chapter.

Adaptation and Coping

The stressors of the POW environment are many; often they are terrifying and inhuman, and always they are filled with the unexpected[29,30] as is shown in Exhibit 17-1. Biological stressors can be extreme and vary with both the geographic location and the demeanor of the captors. Psychological stress, including social isolation, is variable. Physiologic stress and emotional duress were both significantly higher in POWs held captive in the Pacific Theater during World War II than in POWs held in the European Theater. Maltreatment is directly related to the extent to which an enemy country sees the POW as politically valuable. In Vietnam, after 1969, conditions improved and torture and maltreatment of the POWs decreased. This change corresponded with the recognition by North Vietnam that the POWs could be an important political tool.

Survival during the POW experience is most related to the degree of injury at the time of capture and the availability of food, shelter, and medical care. For example, 4% of Canadian POWs in World War II died in European prison camps and 27% in the much worse Pacific prisons.[31] The conditions of captivity are strongly influenced by the nature of the combat prior to capture, the economic conditions of the enemy, and whether the POW is seen as politically valuable. Though not all POW experiences are comparable and a single POW experience varies with time, it appears that personality flexibility positively influences survival potential and adaptability. Rigidity is less adaptive. It is not clear whether coping behaviors during captivity affect postrepatriation psychopathology. Ursano[25] found no relationship between postrepatriation psycho-

EXHIBIT 17-1

STRESSES OF CAPTIVITY

Physical
- Crowding
- Diarrhea
- Epidemic diseases
- Exhaustion
- Forced labor
- Infectious organisms
- Injuries
- Medical experimentation
- Nutritional deprivation
- Sleeplessness
- Torture
- Weather extremes
- Wounds

Psychological
- Boredom
- Close long-term affiliation
- Confinement
- Danger
- Family separation
- Fear/terror
- Guilt
- Humiliation
- Isolation
- Threats
- Unpredictability

pathology and resistance stance, "marginal coping" during captivity, or feeling benefited from the POW experience after return.

Exhibit 17-2 summarizes POW coping behaviors.[14,21,22,28–39] Nardini's[10] experience with many of the 12,000 surviving World War II Pacific Theater prisoners of war of the Japanese led him to conclude that there were several attributes that allowed these 12,000 men to survive (there were another 18,000 who did not survive). These included: strong motivation for life, good general intelligence, good constitution, emotional insensitivity or well-controlled and balanced sensitivity, preserved sense of humor, strong sense of obligation to others, controlled fantasy life, courage, successful resistance, opportunism, military experience, and luck.

The POW's personality also affects adaptation and coping. In the crew of the USS *Pueblo*, held by North Korea in 1968, immaturity, passive-dependency, and obsessive-compulsiveness were associated with poor adjustment.[1] Ford and Spaulding[40] examined crew members of the Pueblo just after their release. Men who did well during captivity often had personalities described as "healthy" or "schizoid." They used a wide variety of ego defenses, particularly faith, reality testing, denial, rationalization, and humor. Men who handled the stress poorly were frequently diagnosed as being passive-dependent and were more limited in the number of ego defenses they used.

Schizoid behavior and introversion have been reported to be more adaptive than obsessive-compulsive, passive-dependent, or immature behaviors.[1,31] Passive-dependency has been singled out as a particularly maladaptive response.[1,31,41] Induction of dependency is advantageous to camp leaders in imposing their will.[41] The psychological state of the POW during captivity has been described as dependency, debility, and dread (DDD).[42] Identification of adaptive personality characteristics requires further study. It is clear that personality resiliency and the ability to tolerate passivity is positively related to optimal adaptation.[43-45]

Jones[38] reviewed six books written by former POWs who had been held in North Vietnamese prison camps. He identified coping strategies that sustained the POWs during imprisonment, all having in common that each man had a standard of behavior he set for himself. Ideals that were commonly reported as sustaining were: (*a*) loyalty to country (remembering their heritage, focusing on their patriotic duty to resist), (*b*) idealizing their family (hoping to return with a feeling of having been worthy of them), and (*c*) alliance with fellow prisoners (communications, mutual support, cooperative resistance).

Maintaining military bearing[32] is reported to be an important adaptive behavior. During the Vietnam conflict, identification with military ideals unified POWs in spirit and in their determination. The chain of command formalized and solidified the prisoner society in the camps. The need for internal security became more important as the need for communication privacy grew within the POW system. The Military Code of Conduct, which was modified after the Vietnam conflict, provided guidelines for the prisoners of war.

Probably the single most important adaptive behavior in all POW situations is communication. During the Vietnam conflict, a tap code was devel-

EXHIBIT 17-2

PRISONER OF WAR COPING MECHANISMS

Emphasizing the Greater Good
- Caring for another
- Feeling closer to God
- Focusing on the good
- Loyalty to country/family/POW group
- Motivation for life
- Survival for some purpose

Defenses
- Denial
- Humor
- Intellectualization
- Obsessional thinking
- Rationalization

Relationship to Captors
- Collaboration
- Cultivating relationships with captors
- Resistance
- Study guards' habits and use the knowledge to gain favor
- Withdrawal

Social
- Buddy system
- Chain of command
- Code of conduct
- Communication
- Group activities
- Group affiliation
- Military experience
- Peer pressure
- Withdrawal

Conscious Efforts
- Acceptance of fate
- Communication
- Control of panic
- Discipline
- Flexibility
- Maintaining self-respect
- Maintaining military social structure
- Physical fitness
- Realistic expectations
- Repetitive behaviors
- Rituals
- Self-development activities
- "Talking to family"
- Well-controlled sensitivity
- Will to live

Psychological/Fantasy
- Apathy
- Dissociation
- Fantasies of retaliation
- Fatalism
- Hope
- Idealized expectations of post-release life
- Introversion
- Passive-dependence
- Personality flexibility
- Psychological regression

oped using a 5 X 5 arrangement of the alphabet (the letter k was not used). The row and column of a letter could then be communicated. Ingenious mechanisms were used to spread messages. Coughing, sweeping, and tapping were all important means of using the code. Additionally, the ability to express one's rage in hidden forms—the now historic picture of the Pueblo crew demonstrating a common American gesture of contempt—can provide release from pent-up rage and hostility. There is a fine line, however, between appropriate resistance and provocative resistance (eg, resistance that unnecessarily increases torture and maltreatment). Such poor-coping high resisters often feel they must never comply even to trivial requests. They can bring torture on themselves and their comrades.

Social Isolation

Social isolation and solitude, usually with darkness and silence, are prominent aspects of the POW camp experience. These experiences can greatly contribute to the traumatic stress of captivity.[3] Psychological aspects of isolated living in the Antarctic and other contained environments can shed some light on the POW's social isolation, although there are important differences. The most important difference is that the Antarctic experience is voluntary and the POW experience is not.

Participant observers in expeditions to the Antarctic report that social issues are more important than environmental ones in maintaining the well being of the crew. For example, in one study, the individual's adjustment to the group, the "sameness" of the environment, and the absence of social supports were each more significant than coldness, danger, and other environmental hardships in determining psychological adjustment.[46] The number of sexual remarks made by Antarctic crew members correlated with marital status.[47] The order of frequency of sexual remarks were most frequent in those who were separated, followed by newly married, bachelors, and happily married (high to low).

Singer[39] reviewed journalistic accounts written by former Vietnam-era POWs who had spent a great deal of time in solitary confinement. Several mental phenomena were prominent: (*a*) propensity to review one's life with remorse and guilt, (*b*) recall of the past in vivid detail, (*c*) recall of unused academic or intellectual training, (*d*) extraordinarily vivid dreams with prolonged recall upon awakening, (*e*) intense, vivid, long-enduring fantasies (sometimes lasting days), and (*f*) a splitting of attention and awareness.

The firmer a POW's resistance stance, the more time is spent in isolation. In Vietnam, the greater the POW's duration of isolation, the greater the risk of resulting psychopathology.[33,48] Cause and effect relationships, however, are unclear. Resistant, higher ranking, and older POWs spend more time in solitary confinement and are tortured more often because of their leadership and resistance activities. However, it may also be true that individuals whose personality allows them to survive prolonged solitary confinement are more likely to maintain persistent resistance.

The relationship of social isolation to postrepatriation psychiatric morbidity has been considered by several authors. However, it is difficult to separate out the unique contributions of any one stressor to the development of psychopathology. High social isolation correlates with greater captivity stress in general. Ursano[5] and Hunter[6] both report greater rates of psychopathology among those POWs who spent the greatest time in solitary confinement. Hunter examined 100 former Vietnam conflict POWs and concluded that no definitive statement could be made as to any specific psychiatric disorders resulting from social isolation. However, it was found that former POWs from Vietnam who experienced prolonged periods of isolation had significantly more guilt, ambivalence, suggestibility, superego development, and need for achievement than other former POWs.[49–52]

Psychiatric Symptoms During Captivity

Many psychiatric signs, symptoms, and defense mechanisms have been reported by POWs retro-

EXHIBIT 17-3

PSYCHIATRIC SIGNS AND SYMPTOMS RETROSPECTIVELY REPORTED BY PRISONERS OF WAR

Anxiety
Appetite loss
Boredom
Confusion
Decreased communication
Defeatism
Dependency
Disorganized self-concept
Dissociation
Dysphoric mood
Fear
Guilt
Hyperarousal
Hypersomnia
Hypervigilance
Hypoarousal
Hyporesponsiveness
Hyposomnia
Identification with aggressor
Neurasthenia
Out-of-body experiences
Panic
Regressive behavior
Resignation
Startle response
Suicidal ideation
Weight loss

spectively during debriefings. The distinction between an adaptive coping response and a psychiatric symptom may not be clear. Some POWs experience psychiatric symptoms that may lessen their survival chances, increase their suffering, or lay the groundwork for postrepatriation psychopathology. Symptoms such as anxiety, boredom, and dysphoria are common (Exhibit 17-3).[1,2,22,27,28,31,37]

The prevalence of psychiatric diagnoses in POWs during imprisonment is unknown. Some prisoners do appear to meet criteria for major depression. Anxiety disorders are common. Anticipatory or conditioned anxiety may evolve into panic attacks or an exaggerated startle response. Slightly more than one half of the crew of the Pueblo admitted to significant anxiety or depression during captivity.[1] Psychotic withdrawal has also been reported.[53] Organic mental syndromes are of substantial concern. These may be the result of head trauma during aircrew ejection or torture, food and water deprivation, or untreated physical illnesses such as infections.

RESISTANCE

In Vietnam- and Korean-conflict POWs, high resistance was seen more often among those who were older, held captive longer, experienced longer periods of solitary confinement, and received harsher treatment by captors.[33,48] The high resister may also provoke more mistreatment. For example, in Vietnam, POWs who resisted the Oriental custom of bowing were severely punished. In general, these individuals had difficulty adjusting to the need to be passive and compliant. Their rigidity sometimes made life more dangerous for their fellow prisoners as well.

In 1957 Schein[54] examined 759 POWs shortly after repatriation from Korean prison camps. He compared men who (*a*) collaborated, (*b*) actively resisted, and (*c*) took a neutral course. Both resisters and collaborators had significantly longer internments, had been in service longer, were older, and more intelligent. Additionally they showed more psychopathic deviance (Pd scale of the MMPI). Resisters and collaborators, however, did not differ significantly from one another. No differences among the groups were found in rank, civilian occupation, religion, location of home community, or number of parents present in the home.

Singer[55] studied collaboration and resistance after the Korean conflict using projective psychological testing. She reported the counter-intuitive finding that resisters and collaborators were more alike than different. Both showed less capacity to remain uninvolved with the environment. She suggested that what distinguished resisters and collaborators was not individual variables but rather which group they chose to attach to.

Ursano et al[25] identified high resisters in the maximum stress group of Vietnam U.S. Air Force POWs. The high resisters were older, more senior in rank, pilots, and had spent more days as a prisoner. Using MMPI data, the high resisters showed greater energy, were more outgoing and extroverted, and showed less repression, constraint, and denial. In addition, the high resisters were more likely to experience conflict with authority, be more independent, and less socially conforming. In general, therefore, the high resister tended to be independent, energetic, less likely to bind his energy through cognitive mechanisms, and less attached to the group. These findings are in agreement with those from the Korean conflict.[55,56]

In a study of Vietnam era POWs, Hunter and Phelan,[9] found that only one of several personality traits, need for achievement, correlated with resistance posture. Ursano et al[25] examined high resisters who were successful and those who were unsuccessful based on peer ratings ("marginal copers"). They showed that the unsuccessful high resister in Vietnam was similar to the successful high resister demographically but had a greater need to dominate. The unsuccessful high resister was more like the "marginal coper" group. These findings highlight the utility of separating high resisters into successful and unsuccessful groups as identified by their peers. Future studies should distinguish the "good" high resister and the "poor" high resister who might be compelled to resist and put others at risk.

During the Korean conflict, the concept of "brainwashing" received a great deal of attention with prisoners of the Chinese communists. At the time, the common opinion was that the communists were adept at, and scientific about, inducing collaboration. Some individuals, even after release from Chinese prisons, continued to repeat false confessions, insist on their guilt, praise the justice and leniency they had received, and expound communist doctrine.[57] During the Vietnam conflict, no repatriated POWs could clearly be identified as collaborators in the same sense as the Korean conflict with the exception of one U.S. Marine who voluntarily remained in Vietnam for several years after the war ended.

The term, "brainwashing," has a mystical, magical quality to it. Even when the concept was popular, there was a call for replacing the term with a more elaborate model of interrogation and indoctrination.[58] Many of the "brainwashing" reports of the era are so emotionally charged they are worthless in expanding scientific knowledge about collaboration.[54] Emotionally laden reports appeared on both ends of the opinion spectrum, some maintaining that no one could resist Chinese brainwashing techniques and some saying that individuals who collaborated with the enemy to any degree were cowards. Extensive study by Segal and others[33] showed there was no magical "brainwashing." The term, "coercive persuasion," was subsequently adopted and is more descriptively correct. Productive studies of collaboration and resistance as psychological and interpersonal processes developed from this debate.

Collaboration (and resistance) is a continuum of behaviors, not an all-or-none phenomenon. POWs collaborate in varying degrees. Most commit trivial acts such as signing peace petitions. A small number may engage in more persistent behaviors such as writing, signing, and soliciting signatures for peace petitions, delivering anti-American lectures to fellow prisoners, or aiding in indoctrination programs.[56] Those POWs who collaborate with the enemy do so in part to eliminate the threat of mistreatment and to receive the benefits of preferential treatment.[33]

The concept of collaboration has limited utility except in extreme cases. In Vietnam, all POWs were "broken." For most, this was a profoundly guilt-inducing experience. As a result of the recognition of every individual's breaking point, new strategies to resist interrogation were based on repetitive fall-back positions and giving minor nonsignificant information when resistance was no longer possible. Part of the importance of the communication network and of the military organization in the POW camp was its ability to provide relief from guilt through knowledge that others had broken. In addition, communication fostered the development of guidelines on resistance stance.

The captor's goals are important in determining how POWs are treated. Disrupting the POWs' organizations and their military command through the isolation of prisoner leaders and commanders decreases the POWs' sense of unity and ability to buffer stress and develop coping strategies. Inducing dependency, debility, and dread (DDD)[42] in the individual POW further produces hyporesponsiveness, disruption of time-spanning processes, and disorganization of the self-concept. These may render the prisoner more susceptible to the captor's influence and demands.

SEQUELAE OF THE POW EXPERIENCE

Medical Illness

The first follow-ups of World War II POWs by Cohen and Cooper[12] found significantly greater mortality in Pacific Theater prisoners primarily due to accidents and tuberculosis. No excess mortality was seen in the European group. Gastrointestinal disorders, psychological problems, ophthalmic changes, cardiac disorders, and the effects of malnutrition and tuberculosis were also noted. Similar increased mortality rates were reported in Australian Pacific Theater POWs.[13] The next study by Nefzger,[14] in the mid-1960s, showed that the early excess mortality was decreasing in the Pacific group. However, Korean conflict POWs still had excess mortality.

In the mid-1960s, Beebe, using both records and questionnaires, assessed medical and psychiatric morbidity in the same World War II and Korean POWs.[11] The U.S. Army veterans taken prisoner in the two World War II theaters of action and in the Korean conflict were compared to each other and to controls on the number of hospital admissions between 1946 and 1965 (1954–1965 for Korean conflict POWs), as well as the number of symptoms, amount of disability, and psychosocial maladjustment in 1966 to 1967. Sequelae of the POW experience were found to be both somatic and psychiatric, and were greatest in Pacific Theater POWs. In European Theater POWs, only psychiatric sequelae were apparent in 1966 to 1967. In the 1970s follow-up, Keehn[15] found no excess mortality.

Although somatic problems were most prevalent in the early years after liberation,[11] they persist even today for Pacific Theater veterans.[59] Tennant found higher rates of duodenal ulcers in former Pacific Theater POWs than in a group of noncombat controls, even at 40 years after World War II.[60] This excess medical morbidity correlates with reported weight loss and nutritional deficiency syndromes during the POW period. Current nonspecific somatic symptoms, such as fatigue, are more common in World War II Pacific Theater POWs and in Korean conflict POWs than in non-POW veterans of the same eras.[11] Throughout these studies, the psychiatric signs and symptoms remained the more persistent postliberation findings for both Pacific and European groups.

The findings of greater psychiatric than medical morbidity and the differences between Pacific and European Theater POWs were also evident when Veterans Administration (VA) disability award trends, hospital admission rates, and responses on the Cornell Medical Health Index were examined.

There has been considerable debate over the potential etiologic significance of organic factors in post-traumatic psychiatric disorders of POWs and concentration camp survivors. The term, "concentration camp syndrome," was used to describe concentration camp survivors who show emotional lability, dysphoria, depression, anxiety, insomnia, nightmares, intellectual deterioration, and/or neurasthenia. Eitenger proposed that while psychosocial factors are important in the etiology of these symptoms, nutritional deficiencies, head trauma, infections, etc. also play an important role in reducing the resiliency of the brain, decreasing the ability to cope flexibly with captivity, and to recover normally.[61] However, he was examining concentration camp survivors who suffered the most extreme deprivation. Most POWs, except some in the Pacific Theater in World War II, did not suffer the extreme levels of deprivation of the concentration camp. There is both considerable agreement[62,63] and disagreement[61,64,65] over the degree to which biological factors should be emphasized. No findings supportive of the "KZ (concentration camp) syndrome" were seen in Vietnam-era POWs.[66] It appears most likely that the "KZ syndrome" symptoms of organic impairment are related to the most extreme malnutrition and physical trauma that were seen in the concentration camps of World War II.

Psychiatric Illness

Psychiatric responses to the POW experience include a number of disorders as well as less well defined personality changes.[44,67,68] In the following section, the psychiatric responses seen in POWs are briefly reviewed.

Post-Traumatic Stress Disorder

The fact that traumatic stress can be followed by psychiatric sequelae is well established.[3,4] The recurrent combination of intrusive and avoidant symptoms present in individuals with the diagnosis of post-traumatic stress disorder (PTSD) is well documented in groups of former POWs from several theaters of war up to 40 years after release.[69–71] In one study, 67% to 85% of surviving former World War II POWs were found to have met criteria for PTSD at some time since repatriation.[69] The sample, however, may have been biased because the subjects were solicited by mail. Their psychiatric status may not be representative of former POWs who did not volunteer or former World War II POWs at large. However, the results suggest that PTSD is common following severe POW experiences. White found that 85% of his group of POWs from Japanese camps had suffered at least moderately severe PTSD.[72] Japanese POW camp survivors have consistently been reported to have PTSD symptoms more frequently than other POW groups and the symptoms have been more severe.[13,73–78] Speed et al[76] found the strongest predictors of PTSD were the proportion of body weight lost and the degree of torture. In perhaps the best designed follow-up, Page[75] found high rates of persistent PTSD almost 50 years postrepatriation, particularly in Pacific Theater POWs, when compared to a control group.

PTSD may be acute, chronic, or delayed.[69,79] Although some studies suggest that the risk of PTSD decreases with time,[69] there is some evidence of a late-onset PTSD[80] that may differ from early-onset PTSD in etiology and course. Late-onset PTSD may be more likely to be related to symbolic functioning and the use of war experiences as a symbol of present ongoing conflicts.[81] For example, one Vietnam-era POW presented 10 years after repatriation with anxiety and obsessional symptoms occurring at a time of family conflicts over the raising of children. The former POW was experiencing increased recall of the conflict and anger he felt at his roommate in prison for doing things that annoyed him. At that time, he could not respond to his roommate's behavior because they needed each other. The recall of this experience was explained by the former POW's present life conflicts. It was these present life conflicts that were being expressed in the recall of the memories of the POW experience. Chapter 16, Chronic Post-Traumatic Stress Disorder, discusses this in greater detail.

Post-traumatic stress disorder shows considerable comorbidity with other post-traumatic psychiatric disorders. Alcohol abuse is diagnosed in 41% to 64% of patients with PTSD; depression is diagnosed in 8% to 72%.[67] The relationship of drug abuse, antisocial personality disorder and other personality disorders to PTSD is not yet clear. Most studies do not control enough variables to make an accurate assessment. Because POWs undergo prolonged physiologic stress, a high frequency of medicopsychiatric illness and psychophysiologic symptoms are also common.

The MMPI has been used both clinically and for research on former POWs. In a 1986 study comparing World War II POWs of the Pacific Theater with those held in Europe, the highest elevations were found in Pacific POWs on scales measuring hysteria (Hs), depression (D), hypochondriasis (Hy), psychasthenia (Pt), and schizophrenia (Sc).[69] Both groups were clearly distinguishable from a non-POW control group. There have been attempts to develop an MMPI subscale for PTSD in POWs. This scale has been used in Vietnam conflict and World War II veterans. In one study it could not distinguish Japanese from European POW veterans, although PTSD was diagnosed clinically more often in POWs from the Pacific Theater.[73]

Adjustment Disorder

There is a continuum of response to stress. While major psychiatric illness is frequently studied, minor psychopathology, normal responses to stress, and movement toward psychological health are not well studied.[81] Adjustment disorders should be more closely examined as a paradigm for responses to stress. Identification of stressor-related minor psychopathology may reveal a potential focus for psychotherapy. Just as with major psychiatric diagnoses, the frequency of occurrence of adjustment disorder following the POW experience is positively correlated with the duration and severity of captivity.[82]

In a 1981 study of repatriated U.S. Air Force Vietnam conflict POWs, Ursano et al found that adjustment disorders and marital/occupational problems occurred in 17.2% to 18.2% of the sample at repatriation and in 9.2% to 15.8% at 5-year follow-up.[53] These were the most common psychiatric diagnoses. Hall and Malone closely followed six former POWs and their families for 3 years following return from North Vietnam and found that most experienced cognitive, social, work, emotional, and family difficulties for the first 2 years.[83] These problems, in general, eventually resolved and no major psychiatric illnesses occurred in any of these men.

Depression

Paykel's review of the literature in 1978 revealed that the presence of traumatic events increases subsequent lifetime risk for depression 2-fold and for suicide 6-fold.[84] Although some studies suggest that the prevalence of depression may decline after the first years following a traumatic event,[85,86] the prevalence of major depression in World War II Pacific Theater POWs remains higher than in a non-POW control group even 40 years after release.[87,59] Studies of MMPIs in repatriated POWs reveal elevated depression scales.[88] Page et al,[59] using a large national sample of World War II POWs (Europe and Pacific), Korean-era POWs and non-POW comparison groups, found elevated depressive symptomatology on the CES(D) (Center for Epidemiological Studies [Depression]) scale decades after repatriation. POWs who were younger, less well-educated, and who had received harsher treatment were more likely to report depression.[75]

Depression also frequently accompanies PTSD.[67] A history of concurrent or past depression is seen in 8% to 72% of PTSD patients.[89–93] Many PTSD patients respond to antidepressant medications. It is important to differentiate major depression in the former POW from: (*a*) PTSD, (*b*) adjustment disorder with depressed mood, (*c*) subaffective clinical depression (RDC [Research Diagnostic Criteria] "minor depression"),[94] (*d*) organic mood disorder secondary to nutritional, toxic, or traumatic factors, and (*e*) the neurasthenic syndrome commonly reported during and after traumatic events.

Psychoactive Substance Use Disorders

Alcohol misuse appears to be more common in former POWs than demographically related groups.[11,12,14,15] Studies that control for demographic, socioeconomic, and precaptivity psychiatric history, however, are few. There are morbidity data and other evidence that alcohol abuse is problematic in many former POWs, and should be carefully considered during medical and psychiatric examinations. Kluznik et al reported that 40 years after World War II, a postwar diagnosis of alcoholism was present in 50 of 188 POWs from the Pacific Theater who volunteered for medical and psychiatric examination.[69] Of that group, 67% also had a history of PTSD; therefore, the alcoholism may have been primary or secondary. Alcohol use can be a form of self-medication[95–99] and may suppress nightmares, diminish autonomic hyperactivity, and foster more pleasant nontraumatic fantasies.[97] Alcohol excess frequently accompanies PTSD (41%–80%).[70,87,89–92]

There are few studies of postrepatriation drug abuse in POWs. Potential confounding variables that must be addressed in any such study include demographic data, socioeconomic status, precaptivity substance use, precaptivity prevalence of psychiatric disorders, concurrent psychiatric illness, and presence or absence of captivity-related pain syndromes. Drug abuse following trauma may also represent self-medication of another psychiatric disorder such as depression,[100] an independent phenomenon, or continuation of a preexisting psychoactive substance use disorder. Concurrent drug abuse has been reported in 16% to 50% of veterans with PTSD.[89–92]

Anxiety Disorders

Before DSM-III and the diagnostic category, posttraumatic stress disorder, the most frequent diagnoses given to psychiatrically ill former POWs were anxiety reaction, anxiety state, and anxiety neurosis.[11] Anxiety disorders other than PTSD remain frequent in former World War II POWs (143 of 188 in one study).[31,69,101] Generalized anxiety disorder was most frequently reported (103 of 188) in this group. There was a large degree of overlap with PTSD. In some studies, up to 95% of patients with PTSD meet criteria for at least one other DSM-III-R anxiety disorder.[52,74] Panic attacks and panic disorder are frequent in persons exposed to trauma. Up to half of patients with PTSD also have panic attacks.[102]

Somatoform Disorders

Somatoform disorders, psychophysiologic disorders, and psychiatric disorders due to physical illness associated with POW treatment have all been reported. In one study, 8 of 188 former World War II POWs met criteria for somatization disorder (Briquet's Syndrome), though the severity was usually mild.[69] Interestingly, psychophysiologic disorders present prior to the POW experience do not always recur postrepatriation.[34] Fictitious disorder has been reported in individuals claiming to be POWs. Three men who claimed they were former POWs in Vietnam and reported symptoms of PTSD were found to have never been POWs.[103] For this reason, verifying military history is an important part of the assessment process.

Other Psychiatric Disorders

Adult antisocial behavior, obsessive-compulsive disorder, intermittent explosive disorder, bipolar disorder, schizotypal features, and other psychotic disorders have been reported after trauma.[69,89–92] However, it is unlikely that these disorders are causally related to the POW experience. None of the reports on these disorders adequately control for pre-trauma variables such as psychiatric predisposition, socio-demographic data, or psychoactive substance use patterns.

Personality Change

Personality changes resulting from the POW experience need not be pathological. Many former POWs report that they benefited from captivity,[104] redirecting their goals and priorities and moving toward psychological health.[34,105,106] Particular MMPI profiles have been related to particular POW stressors.[107] In the same manner as the development of psychopathology during and after captivity, nonpathologic personality change appears to be dependent on the nature and severity of the experience at least as much as preexisting personality. As mentioned before, in World War II and Korean conflict POWs a profound apathy syndrome was noticed.[23,24] In contrast, Vietnam-era POWs studied by Ursano[34] showed movement toward character rigidity, decreased interpersonal relatedness, heightened drive to achieve, and the experience of time pressure. Such changes are neither pathological nor beneficial in and of themselves. Sutker et al[107–109] studying Korean conflict POWs found suspiciousness, apprehension, confusion, isolation, detachment, and hostility. Eberly et al[110] found persistent elevated negative affect in World War II POWs 40 years postcaptivity that he interpreted as an adaptational change to accommodate the captivity.

Ursano[34] and Bettelheim[41] have discussed possible reasons for the different personality shifts based on intrapsychic and adaptational shifts. These two types of changes (apathy and rigidity/energy/interpersonal distance) may serve similar adaptive functions, but which type of change develops may depend on the circumstances of imprisonment, such as the amount of physical torture, chronicity (Vietnam-era POWs experienced longer imprisonments than Korean-era POWs), level of deprivation, opportunity for active and passive expressions of aggression, and the types of threats experienced by the POW. These variables depend on the type of war, socioeconomic conditions of the enemy, political climate, and culture of the captors.

From the intrapsychic perspective, conflict within the ego and superego can be seen as the result of heightened aggressive drives bound up during the captivity situation. Such drives are then discharged through the demanding punitive elements of the superego and/or the ambitious, hard-driving pursuit of goals and ideals embodied in the ego ideal. The apathy syndrome seen in Korean conflict POWs may be partially explained as the result of the punitive superego's victory in this intra-superego conflict. In contrast, heightened aggressive drives can also be discharged in the service of the ego-ideal. In this case, determination, character rigidity, and interpersonal distance may be the result.

PREDICTORS OF PSYCHIATRIC DISTRESS

Severity of Captivity

The severity of captivity is a result of both the duration of imprisonment and the degree of maltreatment and deprivation. The length of captivity alone is not a good measure of captivity severity. World War II Pacific Theater POWs were exposed to significantly greater physical, environmental, and psychological stress than were European Theater POWs. Only 40% of 30,000 POWs held by the Japanese survived the war.[10] Disease and malnutrition were common.[11,14] Mortality, owing largely to tuberculosis, was also higher just after repatriation in the Pacific Theater group.[14] Accidents and liver cirrhosis remained significantly more common for many years. Beebe found a higher number of medical and psychiatric symptoms, disability, and maladjustments in Pacific POWs than in European Theater POWs.[11] The former group continues to have higher hospital admission and illness rates. Higher rates of liver cirrhosis suggest a higher frequency of several hepatic diseases and alcoholism in the Pacific group.[14,16] Page[75] has found continued high rates of psychiatric and medical morbidity in the Pacific group into the 1980s.

In Vietnam, POWs captured prior to 1969 had both longer captivity and substantially more deprivation, torture, and maltreatment.[5,6] Wheatley et al[7] and Ursano et al[53] demonstrated a greater degree of psychiatric readjustment problems in repatriated U.S. Air Force POWs captured before 1969 than in those captured after 1969. Pre-1969 captives had a higher frequency of psychiatric diagnoses and abnormal MMPI scales. The overall MMPI profiles of pre-1969 captives also deviated farther from normal than those captured post-1969 on the initial MMPI. Pre-1969 captives showed increased repression, a higher level of denial, greater suspicion, and more distrust. The post-1969 captives' second MMPI profile 5 years later was lower and looked more like aircrew norms. In contrast, the profile of pre-1969 captives had remained essentially unchanged.

Similar findings were reported by Benson et al,[8] in U.S. Navy and U.S. Army Vietnam era POWs. He divided POWs into four groups: (1) officers captured prior to 1969, (2) enlisted personnel captured prior to 1969, (3) officers captured after 1969, and (4) enlisted personnel captured after 1969. These groups were observed for differences in immediate and delayed post-traumatic psychopathology. Enlisted personnel exhibited significantly more postrepatriation psychopathology than commissioned personnel. Significant improvement was noted between the first and the fifth year follow-up only in officers captured after 1969. These results indicate that after controlling for officer-enlisted status, greater captivity stress, as measured by the duration and intensity of captivity, was associated with more negative psychiatric outcome. Vietnam conflict POWs who were exposed to more prolonged isolation had higher rates of psychiatric disorder than did those who experienced more limited solitary confinement.[111] This further indicates the importance of the severity of the captivity experience as a major predictor of psychiatric disturbance.

Predisposition

Determining the role of precaptivity psychopathology and the contribution of genetic, developmental, and interpersonal factors is a difficult process.[112] When examining a patient psychiatrically, the data are retrospective and subject to the effects of being filtered over time. The most valuable sources of information to address this issue are written sources prior to the trauma, such as medical records and evaluations.

In addition to individual developmental factors and the role played by recall of traumatic childhood events, certainly genetic predisposition to psychiatric illness helps determine the phenotypic presentation of an individual following trauma. Life events can precipitate major depressive episodes in susceptible individuals.[111,113] A person who is genetically predisposed to mood disorders is certainly at higher risk for depression after having been a POW than a person not genetically predisposed to mood disorders. To address the more interesting question of trauma as a cause of psychiatric illness, this information must be controlled.

Ursano[34,44] examined six repatriated Vietnam conflict POWs who had been coincidentally evaluated psychiatrically before their captivity. Using the precaptivity psychiatric data, he found that preexisting pathology or identifiable predispositions to psychiatric illness were neither necessary nor sufficient for the development of psychiatric illness after repatriation. Further data on the question of predisposition is provided by studies of captured Vietnam era U.S. Air Force fliers. Fliers are selected for their health and are screened for psychiatric illness. Pre-1969 captives were demographically comparable to the post-1969 group and, in fact, might have been expected to show less illness because they were slightly older and more mature. In fact, they had more psychiatric illness. Because this correlates with the greater degree of stress experienced by this group, these data further support the role of stress over predisposition in the development of psychopathology after severe trauma. Together, these data support the view that psychiatric illness may develop after the POW experience without preexisting illness or identifiable predispositions. Most post-traumatic stress disorder theories have underestimated the role of adult personality growth and resiliency and overestimated the role of preexisting personality in determining the outcome of the POW experience.[7,45]

Social Supports

The importance of social interactions, social supports, group activities, and social isolation during captivity has been discussed. Social factors may be as important as environmental ones in determining coping ability during imprisonment and after return.[57] Recovery from captivity includes the repatriation experience which requires adapting to changes in life directions, career, friendships, and sometimes marital status. These stressors are in addition to the need to psychologically integrate the POW experience into one's life story. Most researchers believe that the more external support available to a former POW, the more likely a positive adjustment will occur.

Davidson studied nonclinical groups of Holocaust survivors in Israel and England in order to evaluate the importance of social support systems in protecting concentration camp survivors from psychiatric morbidity and in facilitating recovery.[114] The subjects of the study were 15 men and 15 women who had been in a concentration camp for 1 to 2 years and had lost virtually all their family members. From interviews of these individuals, he drew two conclusions: (1) supportive bonds have a mitigating and protective influence in the aftermath of the traumatic situation, preserving personality functioning, and (2) the definition of psychic trauma should include social trauma.

Both captivity and reunion with the family are stressful for the POW. Lack of reintegration into the family and society appears to result in higher rates of psychopathology.[6,115] The POW/MIA spouse must first adapt to the absence and unknown status of the active duty member and then adjust to the return. For many POW couples, the readjustment is a difficult transition of reestablishing complementary and supportive roles in family authority and nurturance structures.

READJUSTMENT

Repatriation and Reintegration

As mentioned earlier, most former POWs readjust without clinically significant psychopathology. Some actually use the experience to move toward greater psychological health. Sledge et al[104] identified a distinct group of Vietnam POWs who felt they had benefited from the experience. Those individuals who experienced the greatest stress during captivity were most likely to believe they gained psychologically from the experience. Thus, the subjective sense of having benefited from the experience of being a POW correlated positively with the harshness of the experience.

The stages of repatriation and reintegration are not synonymous with "recovery" in the sense of resolution of psychiatric signs and symptoms. The repatriated POW emerges from what is likely to be a prolonged period of emotional blunting, monotony, apathy, withdrawal, and deprivation, into a rapidly paced series of medical evaluations, family reunions, and public relations activities. The brief period of euphoria upon release is quickly replaced by a period of overstimulation. There may be an attempt to make up for things denied during captivity by activities such as overeating. Initially, released POWs are frequently compliant with the requests of the military and their physicians. But over several days to weeks, they usually begin to take a more active and independent stance.[27,28] There is a tendency for the repatriated POW to minimize potential psychological and psychosocial problems caused by his captivity.

In addition, most repatriated POWs, including those from the Persian Gulf War, have had little experience dealing with the media. The media are a substantial stressor that can have lifelong effects if a later, "Wish-I-had-never-said," statement is broadcast around the world. It is very important to both shield the POW and his family from early intrusive media coverage and to offer training in the management of media requests. This was routinely done for the POWs of the Persian Gulf War. Reminding POWs and their families that it is perfectly acceptable for them to say, "No," can be a most important intervention.

After the tumultuous postrelease period, gradual readjustment and reintegration may continue throughout life. Reintegration occurs gradually and the process is subject to reorganization with changing life circumstances.

Organizers in Adult Personality Development

Personality does not stop developing at the end of childhood or even adolescence.[116] The fact that most neurophysiological and neuroanatomic development is finished before adulthood may provide some protection from radical departures in adult personality, but it is clear from animal studies that changes do occur in neurophysiology and even neuroanatomy during adulthood.[19]

Renee Spitz discussed "organizers" of psychological development—important experiences that structure feelings, thoughts, and behaviors of the present and thus influence future development and psychology.[117] The oedipal phase and childhood traumatic events are two examples. These organizing events are evident in psychotherapy when the therapist and patient identify organizing principles of past experience that are used to guide present behavior. It is useful to conceptualize adult traumas, such as being a POW, as a potential independent organizer of adult personality development.[34] The experience may induce psychopathology or personality growth, or it may resonate with themes already present from earlier organizing events or periods. Later, the symbolic recall of the POW events is the result of a current event activating this "organizer." The recall serves as a symbolic vehicle to express the current conflicts and anxieties.

Recovery

Some data support the idea that recovery is faster when POW trauma is less severe. Wheatley and Ursano[7] found that post-1969 POW returnees experienced more complete and rapid return toward normal and toward expected baseline than did POWs who were captured before 1969. The study of recovery as a process is one of the areas of much needed research. Concentration camp survivors have relatively few instances of complete recovery.[118] They continue to experience less stable working lives, more frequent job changes, more frequent domicile changes, longer sick leaves, and more frequent and long-lasting hospitalization periods than controls.[6] World War II Pacific Theater POWs continue to have more medical and psychiatric morbidity and slower rates of clinical recovery than European Theater POWs.[73] In 188 former World War II POWs examined in 1986, 29% were considered to have fully recovered, 39% still reported mild psychiatric symptoms, and 8% had no recovery or had deteriorated, as seen in Table 17-1.[69] Recently, Page[59] has documented the persistence of high rates of PTSD and depression in World War II Pacific Theater POWs almost 50 years after their captivity.

Supportive social bonds appear to mitigate and protect the ex-POW from long-term psychiatric dysfunction.[114] There may be disillusionment with dreams, hopes, and fantasies about what postcaptivity life would be like.[119] A supportive family and social environment can help blunt that disappointment. Lack of social supports (eg, divorce, loss of idealized lifestyle, death of family or friends) can significantly increase the risk for psychopathology in the postrepatriation period.

At the end of the Persian Gulf War, the first U.S. female prisoner of war returned home. The unique aspects of recovery for women POWs will be of increased concern in future conflicts.

TABLE 17-1

LIFETIME PSYCHIATRIC DIAGNOSES AND ILLNESS COURSES OF 188 FORMER WORLD WAR II PRISONERS OF WAR

	Never Had Disorder	Virtually Complete Recovery	Mild Chronic Condition	Moderate Chronic Condition	Marked Chronic Condition
Post-traumatic stress disorder	63	36	49	30	10
Generalized anxiety disorder	85	11	36	36	20
Alcoholism	138	37	9	2	2
Major depression	143	15	9	14	7
Minor depression with anxiety	165	6	5	10	2
Intermittent depressive disorder	182	0	0	2	4
Panic disorder	173	2	5	7	1
Schizophrenia	187	0	0	0	1
Schizoaffective disorder, mania	187	0	0	1	0
Schizoaffective disorder, depression	186	0	0	2	0
Mania	187	1	0	0	0
Hypomania	184	4	0	0	0
Bipolar I disorder	186	0	1	0	1
Bipolar II disorder	186	0	2	0	0
Cyclothymia	182	1	2	2	1
Labile personality	182	0	3	3	0
Briquet's disorder	180	0	5	2	1
Antisocial personality	181	1	5	1	0
Obsessive-compulsive disorder	183	1	1	3	0
Phobia	168	1	9	1	0
Schizotypal features	177	0	5	4	2
Other psychosis	185	3	0	0	0
Other nonpsychosis	178	1	7	2	0
No psychiatric disorder on examination	49				
Never had a psychiatric disorder	22				

Adapted with permission from Kluznik JC, Speed N, VanValkenburg C, Magraw R. Forty-year follow-up of United States prisoners of war. *Am J Psychiatry*. 1986;143:1444.

TREATMENT OF POSTREPATRIATION ILLNESS

Medical Disorders

Diagnosis and treatment of medical disorders from POW captivity is always the first order of business. These disorders can cause psychiatric symptoms that may mimic psychiatric disorders and have significant morbidity and mortality. Repatriated U.S. Marine POWs from Vietnam (N=26) had an average of 12 medical diagnoses at the time of their return, representing 155 separate diagnostic entities.[120] The 77 U.S. Army repatriated Vietnam-era POWs accumulated 1,149 diagnoses and 386 separate diagnostic entities.[121] The most frequent medical diagnoses made in follow-up medical evaluations of repatriated U.S. Air Force POWs from Vietnam were orthopedic, cardiac, and neurologic.[122]

World War II and Korean conflict POWs had higher mortality rates following release than nonprisoner control groups, owing largely to tuberculosis and effects of physical trauma.[14,15] This excess mortality began to rapidly decline during the first decade following release. However, a current trend toward excess deaths due to liver cirrhosis is emerging, another line of evidence suggesting alcohol misuse remains a problem.[14,15] The confounding factors of malnutrition and parasite infection limit the interpretability of these data. Eitenger compared Norwegian concentration camp survivors and the general population and found significant excess: overall mortality, unstable occupations, job changes, frequency of hospitalizations, sick periods, sick leaves, and the duration of hospitalizations in the concentration camp group.[123]

Nutritional deficiency and physical trauma during captivity increase the risk for postrepatriation medical and psychiatric sequelae.[6,14,15,60,120,124,125] Eitenger maintained that the development of what appeared to be a neurotic outcome, the KZ Syndrome, is actually the result of the extreme organic stressors in the concentration camps.[61]

Because POWs can have lifelong medical morbidity, frequent attention to physical and medical status is important. Yearly physical examinations and monitoring for long-term effects of vitamin deficiencies and malnutrition are important parts of psychiatric follow-up.

Psychiatric Disorders

Debriefing after initial release from captivity[126,127] is now standard treatment. In addition, providing time to learn about how the world has changed and time to become reacquainted with family in a protected environment is important. Briefings to learn how to handle the media are also very important. Group meetings will facilitate discussions and abreaction as well as sharing information about the normal recovery process. This reentry process must be well planned and usually takes one to two weeks or more if possible. Often politics and the POWs' desire to get home shorten this desirable protected stage of recovery. Educating the POW, his or her family, and national leaders may be necessary.

When psychiatric illness exists following captivity, it must be treated. Adjustment disorders are important to diagnose because their evaluation often reveals one or more foci for brief psychotherapy. Treatment is directed toward preventing the development of more severe chronic psychopathology, decreasing the vulnerability to future psychiatric illness, and providing symptomatic relief.

Many forms of psychotherapy have been used in the treatment of post-traumatic stress disorder: supportive, brief focal, behavioral, cognitive, cognitive-behavioral, and long-term insight oriented. The choice of therapy depends on the patient's ability to make use of the treatment as a problem-solving method. Psychodynamic treatments may be of particular import in chronic and late onset PTSD. Five of 12 Cambodian concentration camp survivors who completed a PTSD treatment program combining heterocyclic antidepressants and supportive psychotherapy no longer met criteria for the disorder[128] and symptoms improved in three others. Intrusive symptoms improved more than avoidant symptoms. There have also been numerous reports of spontaneous PTSD symptom resolution 1 to 2 years after repatriation.[69,83]

Some post-traumatic stress disorder symptoms may respond to antidepressant medications. Although no well-controlled studies exist, several case reports and descriptive studies suggest that monoamine oxidase inhibitors, heterocyclic-antidepressants, and a triazolo benzodiazepine (Alprazolam) are effective in ameliorating PTSD symptoms in some patients.[95,97,128–133] The high degree of overlap between PTSD and depression, coupled with the response of some PTSD patients to antidepressant medications, suggests that when there is a positive response to antidepressant medication, it may be because a depressive component is being treated. Many patients, however, say that specific PTSD symptoms such as nightmares, autonomic hyperactivity, and avoidance behaviors improve with drug treatment. In any case, it is important to look for depression. (See Chapter 16 for a further discussion of the pharmacotherapy of PTSD.)

The treatment of depression after trauma must take into account the nature of the symptoms (psychological vs neurovegetative), the presence of a past or family history of depression, the meaning of the traumatic event to the patient, the psychosocial situation at the time of the depression, and the psychological significance of the precipitants of the depressive episode. The particular treatment(s) selected will depend on the biologic vulnerability to depression, severity of neurovegetative symptoms and signs, suitability for psychotherapy, and presence of other psychiatric disorders.

Because alcohol and perhaps other psychoactive substances are often misused following traumatic events, examiners must look closely for behavioral, physiologic, and laboratory evidence of psychoactive substance misuse. Serum glutamic-oxalocetic transaminase (SGOT), serum glutamic-pyruvic transaminase (SGPT), uric acid, triglyceride level, mean corpuscular volume (MCV), hematocrit, and serum gamma-glutamyltranferase (GGT) are valuable in the assessment of current alcohol use. Substance misuse following trauma may be a primary disorder, or as self-medication for the symptoms of other psychiatric disorders.[67,134]

Postrepatriation psychiatric illness may be delayed or episodic.[64] PTSD can be acute, recurrent, chronic, or delayed; alcohol and drug abuse can have similar patterns; depression can be a single episode, recurrent, episodic, or chronic. When recovery appears to have occurred after return home, it may or may not be a permanent condition. Whether recurrent or delayed illnesses are related to symbolic retraumatizations is unknown, but should be considered when evaluating a former POW for treatment.

FAMILY ISSUES

The effect of imprisonment and release on family members and the family system itself can be profound and enduring or minor and transient. One study of POW wives indicated that during the period of captivity, psychological and psychophysiological symptoms were common.[135] Psychological issues included desertion, ambiguity of role, repressed anger, sexuality, censure, and social isolation. Separation anxiety, role distortion, and sleep disorders were common in the children. Male children were significantly more affected than female children.

McCubbin et al interviewed families of 215 U.S. Army, U.S. Navy, and U.S. Marine Corps POWs approximately 1 year prior to the POWs' release.[136] Normal patterns of coping with husband/father absence were disrupted by the unprecedented and indeterminate length of captivity. The social acceptance, stability, and sense of continuity that are taken for granted in the intact family were lacking or severely taxed in the POW family.

Parental preoccupation and overprotectiveness are potential reasons for the occasional presence of higher degrees of overt psychopathology in children of persons exposed to trauma than in the original victim.[137,138] In a study of the offspring of psychiatrically hospitalized concentration camp survivors, 70% had psychopathology severe enough to require hospitalization between the ages of 17 and 22, and 90% prior to the age of 25.[138] A clinical sample of mid-teenage children of concentration camp survivors had more behavioral disturbances and less adequate coping behavior than a clinical control group.[139] A study comparing current effects of long-term father absence during and after the Vietnam conflict due to long-term absence (MIA–missing in action) and temporary absence (POW) revealed significant differences in the children. Both nervous symptoms and community relations were more impaired in the former group.[140]

All of these studies suffer major methodological flaws but should serve as reminders of the potential impact of major life events as they are mediated through parents to children. Adolescents may be particularly sensitive to family tension. Their distress is often visible and can be disruptive in both the family and community.

POW families that present for treatment are frequently in crisis. The resumption of precaptivity roles may be difficult for a mother who has successfully exercised both parental roles for several years, when father has additional individual psychiatric symptoms and/or medical problems, and the children have become accustomed to having their mother to themselves. Treatment focuses on preserving family unity, enhancing the family system, and encouraging individual member development.[141,142]

SUMMARY AND CONCLUSION

The POW has suffered the most severe stressors of war. Repatriated POWs are a select group of survivors who have been able to adapt to captivity and maintain morale, hope, and health for months to years. The ability to communicate with other POWs during captivity is the most important coping strategy. The creative ways in which communication has been established and the content of what is communicated are the basis of many of the POW coping strategies.

Repatriation itself is a stressful event. The POW is faced with the outside world's view of his behavior and situation. He may face a changed world and certainly has much information to catch up on. Some events cannot be "caught up": the birth of a child, the death of a parent, a wife who decided to seek a divorce, or the operational experience necessary to remain current in a profession. These are real losses to which the returning POW must accommodate. Most former POWs adjust well. For some, the experience serves as a personality-organizing focus that results in movement toward emotional growth and maturity, others show no psychological change, while still others develop psychopathology. When psychiatric illness occurs following repatriation, the severity of the trauma and the status of social supports play a large role. Most psychopathology decreases with time, though recurrent, episodic, delayed, and chronic presentations of most of the reported post-traumatic psychiatric disorders are reported.

The stresses on the families of the POW are manifold, both during captivity and after repatriation. The family and the military community are critical elements in the recovery and readaptation of the POW.

Post-traumatic stress disorder, depression, psychoactive substance abuse, somatopsychic disorders, and psychiatric disorders due to captivity-induced medical problems are all seen in returned POWs. The coexistence of two or more of these is the rule. Which is primary or secondary is usually less important than identifying and treating each. Individual psychotherapy (short- and long-term), family therapy, pharmacotherapy, and medical treatment for other diseases and injuries that may have resulted from captivity are all important parts of the medical treatment and follow-up of the former prisoner of war.

REFERENCES

1. Spaulding RC, Ford CV. The Pueblo incident: Psychological reactions to the stresses of imprisonment and repatriation. In: Moos RH, ed. *Human Adaptation: Coping With Life Crises*. Lexington, Mass: DC Heath; 1976: 308–321.

2. Dimsdale JE. The coping behavior of Nazi concentration camp survivors. In: Dimsdale JE, ed. *Survivors, Victims, and Perpetrators*. New York: Hemisphere; 1980: 163–174.

3. Green BL, Wilson JP, Lindy JD. Conceptualizing posttraumatic stress disorder: A psychosocial framework. In: Figley CR, ed. *Trauma and its Wake: Study and Treatment of Post-Traumatic Stress Disorder*. New York: Brunner/Mazel; 1985: 53–72.

4. Simenauer E. Late psychic sequelae of man-made disasters. *Int J Psychoanal*. 1968;49:306–309.

5. Ursano RJ, Wheatley RD, Carlson EH, Rahe AJ. The prisoner of war: Stress, illness, and resiliency. *Psychiatric Annals*. 1987;17:532–535.

6. Hunter EJ. The Vietnam POW veteran: Immediate and long-term effects of captivity. In: Figley CR, ed. *Stress Disorders Among Vietnam Veterans*. New York: Brunner/Mazel; 1978: 188–208.

7. Wheatley RD, Ursano RJ. Serial personality evaluations of repatriated U.S. Air Force Southeast Asia POWs. *Clin Med*. 1982;53:251–257.

8. Benson JW, Bizzell DL, O'Connel PF. Immediate and delayed psychopathology in former prisoners of war. Naval Aerospace Medical Institute. Unpublished manuscript; 1979.

9. Hunter EJ, Phelan JD. Resistance, captor treatment, and personality of the Vietnam prisoner of war. Naval POW Center. Unpublished manuscript; 1978.

10. Nardini JE. Survival factors in American prisoners of war of the Japanese. *Am J Psychiatry*. 1952;92:241–248.

11. Beebe GW. Follow-up studies of World War II and Korean War prisoners II: Morbidity, disability, and maladjustments. *Am J Epidemiol*. 1975;101:400–422.

12. Cohen BM, Cooper MZ. *A Follow-up Study of World War II Prisoners of War*. Washington, DC: US Government Printing Office; 1954. Veterans Administration Medical Monograph.

13. Dent OF, Richardson B, Wilson S, Goulston KJ, Murdoch CW. Postwar mortality among Australian World War II prisoners of the Japanese. *Med J Aust*. 1989;150:378–382.

14. Nefzger MD. Follow-up studies of World War II and Korean War prisoners. *Am J Epidemiol.* 1959;91:123–138.

15. Keehn RJ. Follow-up studies of World War II and Korean Conflict prisoners: III. Mortality to January 1, 1976. *Am J Epidemiol.* 1980;111:194–211.

16. Klonoff H, McDougall G, Clark C, et al. The neuropsychological, psychiatric, and physical effects of prolonged and severe stress: 30 years later. *J Nerv Ment Dis.* 1976;163:246–253.

17. Ursano RJ, Rundell JR. The prisoner of war. *Milit Med.* 1990;155:176–180.

18. Biderman AD. Life and death in extreme captivity situations. In: Appley MH, Trumbull R, eds. *Psychological Stress: Issues in Research.* New York: Appleton-Century-Crofts; 1967: 242–277.

19. Maclean PD. Culminating developments in the evolution of the limbic system. In: Doane BK, Livingston KE, eds. *The Limbic System—Functional Organization and Clinical Disorders.* New York: Raven; 1986: 172–189.

20. Cassem NH, Hackett TP. The setting of intensive care. In: Hackett TP, Cassem NH, eds. *Massachusetts General Hospital Handbook of General Hospital Psychiatry,* 3rd ed. Littleton, Mass: PSG; 1987: 373–400.

21. Rahe RH. Acute versus chronic psychological reactions to combat. *Milit Med.* 1988;153:365–372.

22. Eitinger L. Pathology of the concentration camp syndrome: Preliminary report. *Arch Gen Psychiatry.* 1961;5:371–379.

23. Greenson RR. The psychology of apathy. *Psychoanal Q.* 1949;18:290–302.

24. Strassman AD, Thaler MB, Schein EH. A prisoner of war syndrome: Apathy as a reaction to severe stress. *Am J Psychiatry.* 1956;112:998–1003.

25. Ursano RJ, Wheatley R, Sledge W, et al. Coping and recovery styles in the Vietnam era prisoner of war. *J Nerv Ment Dis.* 1986;174:707–714.

26. Deaton JE. *Coping Strategies of Vietnam POWs in Solitary Confinement.* San Diego, Calif: San Diego State University; 1975. Masters thesis

27. Rahe RH, Genender E. Adaptation to and recovery from captivity stress. *Milit Med.* 1983;148:577–585.

28. Newman FH. The prisoner of war mentality: Its effect after repatriation. *Br Med J.* 1944;1:8–10.

29. Richlin M. Positive and negative residuals of prolonged stress. In: Hunter EJ, ed. *Prolonged Separation: The Prisoner of War and His Family.* San Diego, Calif: Center for Prisoner of War Studies, Naval Health Research Center; 1977: 678–680.

30. Chodoff P. The German concentration camp as a psychological stress. In: Moos RH, ed. *Human Adaptation: Coping with Life Crises.* Lexington, Mass: DC Heath; 1976: 337–349.

31. Weisaeth L. Full documentation of appalling suffering of Canadian ex-POWs. *WVF International Socio-Medical Information Center Newsletter.* 1989;1(1).

32. Coker GT. Prisoners of war. *U.S. Naval Institute Proceedings.* 1974;100:41–48.

33. Segal J. Factors Related to the Collaboration and Resistance Behavior of U.S. Army POWs in Korea. Department of the Army Technical Report 33; 1956.

34. Ursano RJ. The Vietnam War era prisoner of war: Precaptivity personality and the development of psychiatric illness. *Am J Psychiatry.* 1981;138:315–318.

35. Gaither R. *With God in a POW Camp.* Nashville, Tenn: Broadman; 1973.

36. Deaton JE, Berg SW, Richlin M, Litrownik AJ. Coping activities in solitary confinement of US Navy POWs in Vietnam. *J Appl Soc Psychol*. 1977;7:239–257.

37. Rahe RH. Coping with Captivity. Proceedings of Veterans Administration Meeting on POW Affairs; 1984.

38. Jones DR. What the repatriated prisoners of war wrote about themselves. *Aviat Space Environ Med*. 1980;51:615–617.

39. Singer MT. Discussion comments on "The Consequences of War Imprisonment Symposium." In: Levy RA, ed. *Proceedings of the Twenty-Sixth Annual Conference of Air Force Behavioral Scientists*. Brooks AFB, Tex: USAF School of Aerospace Medical Division (AFSC); 1979: 66–79.

40. Ford CV, Spaulding RC. The Pueblo incident: A comparison of factors related to coping with extreme stress. *Arch Gen Psychiatry*. 1973;29:340–343.

41. Bettelheim B. Individuals and mass behavior in extreme situations. In: Maccoby EE, Newcomb TM, Hartley EL, eds. *Readings in Social Psychology*. New York: Henry Holt; 1958: 417–452.

42. Farber IK, Harlow HF. Brainwashing, conditioning, and DDD (debility, dependency, and dread). *Sociometry*. 1957;20:272–285.

43. Ursano RJ. Vietnam era prisoners of war: Studies of U.S. Air Force prisoners of war. In: Sonnenberg SM, Bland AS, Talbott JA, eds. *The Trauma of War: Stress and Recovery in Vietnam Veterans*. Washington, DC: APA; 1985: 339–358.

44. Ursano RJ. An analysis of precaptivity data. In: *Proceedings of the Fifth Joint Medical Meeting Concerning POW/MIA Matters*. Brooks AFB, Tex: Clinical Sciences Division, USAF School of Aerospace Medicine; 1978: 60–66.

45. Singer MT. Vietnam prisoners of war, stress, and personality resiliency. *Am J Psychiatry*. 1981;138:345–346.

46. Mullin CS. Some psychological aspects of isolated Antarctic living. *Am J Psychiatry*. 1960;117:323–325.

47. Palmai G. Psychological observations on an isolated group in Antarctica. *Br J Psychiatry*. 1963;109:364–370.

48. Hunter EJ, Phelan JD, Mowery EC. Resistance posture and the Vietnam prisoner of war. *J Polit Milit Sociol*. 1976;4:295–308.

49. Hunter EJ. The prisoner of war: Coping with the stress of isolation. In: Moos RH, ed. *Human Adaptation: Coping with Life Crises*. Lexington Mass: DC Heath & Co; 1976: 322–332.

50. Hunter EJ. The psychological effects of being a prisoner of war: Vietnam veterans and their families. In: Wilson J, Harel Z, Kahana B, eds. *Human Adaptation to Extreme Stress: From the Holocaust to Vietnam*. New York: Plenum; 1987: 295–308.

51. Hausman W, Rioch D. Military psychiatry—A prototype of social and preventive psychiatry in the United States. *Arch Gen Psychiatry*. 1967;16:727–739.

52. Hunter EJ. *Isolation as a Feature of the POW Experience: A Comparison of Men with Prolonged and Limited Solitary Confinement*. San Diego, Calif: Center for Prisoner of War Studies, Naval Health Research Center; 1975.

53. Ursano RJ, Boydstun JA, Wheatley RD. Psychiatric illness in US Air Force Vietnam prisoners of war: A five-year follow-up. *Am J Psychiatry*. 1981;138:310–314.

54. Schein EH. The Chinese indoctrination program for prisoners of war: A study of attempted "brainwashing." *Psychiatry*. 1956;19:149–172.

55. Singer MT, Schein E. Projective test responses of prisoners of war following repatriation. *Psychiatry*. 1958;21:375–385.

56. Schein EH, Hill WF, Williams HL, Lubin A. Distinguishing characteristics of collaborators and resisters among American prisoners of war. *J Abnorm Soc Psychol* [now *J Abnorm Psychol*]. 1957;55:197–201.

57. Lifton RJ. Thought reform of Western civilians in Chinese communist prisons. *Psychiatry*. 1956;19:173–195.

58. United States Congressional/Senate Committee on Government Operations. *Communist Interrogation, Indoctrination, and Exploitation of American Military and Civilian Prisoners*. Washington, DC: GPO; 1957.

59. Page WF, Engdahl BE, Eberly RE. Prevalence and correlates of depressive symptoms among former prisoners of war. *J Nerv Ment Dis*. 1991;179:670–677.

60. Tennant CC, Goulston KJ, Dent OF. The psychological effects of being a prisoner of war: Forty years after release. *Am J Psychiatry*. 1986;143:618–621.

61. Eitinger L. The concentration camp syndrome: An organic brain syndrome? *Integr Psychiatry*. 1985;3:115–126.

62. Genefke IK. Commentary on # 44. *Integr Psychiatry*. 1985;3:124.

63. Roden RG. Commentary on # 44. *Integr Psychiatry*. 1985;3:125–126.

64. Ewalt JR. Commentary on # 44. *Integr Psychiatry*. 1985;3:119–120.

65. Niederland WG. Commentary on # 44. *Integr Psychiatry*. 1985;3:123.

66. Wheatley R. Intellectual, neuropsychological, and visuomotor assessments of repatriated Air Force SEA POWs. Scientific Proceedings of the Aerospace Medical Association Annual Meeting, San Antonio, Texas; 1981.

67. Rundell JR, Ursano RJ, Holloway HC, Silberman EK. Psychiatric responses to trauma. *Hosp Community Psychiatry*. 1989;40:68–74.

68. Sutker PB, Winstead DK, Goist KC, Malow R, Allain AN Jr. Psychopathology subtypes and symptom correlates among former prisoners of war. *J Psychopathol Behav Assessments*. 1986;8:89–101.

69. Kluznik JC, Speed N, VanValkenburg C, Magraw R. Forty-year follow-up of United States prisoners of war. *Am J Psychiatry*. 1986;143:1443–1446.

70. Laufer RS, Brett E, Gallops MS. Symptom patterns associated with posttraumatic stress disorder among Vietnam veterans exposed to war trauma. *Am J Psychiatry*. 1985;142:1304–1311.

71. Atkinson RM, Sparr LF, Sheff AG, et al. Diagnosis of posttraumatic stress disorder in Vietnam veterans: Preliminary findings. *Am J Psychiatry*. 1984;141:694–696.

72. White NS. Posttraumatic stress disorder (letter to the editor). *Hosp Community Psychiatry*. 1983;34:1061–1062.

73. Eberly R, Engdahl B. Prevalence of somatic and psychiatric disorders among former prisoners of war. *Hosp Community Psychiatry*. 1991;42:807–813.

74. Query WT, Megran J, McDonald G. Applying posttraumatic stress disorder MMPI subscale to World War II POW veterans. *J Clin Psychol*. 1986;42:315–317.

75. Page W. *The Health of Former Prisoners of War*. Washington, DC: National Academy Press; 1992.

76. Speed N, Engdahl BE, Schwartz J, et al. Posttraumatic stress disorder as a consequence of the prisoner of war experience. *J Nerv Ment Dis*. 1989;177:147–153.

77. Goldstein G, van Kammen W, Shelly C, et al. Survivors of imprisonment in the Pacific theater during World War II. *Am J Psychiatry*. 1987;144:1210–1213.

78. Sutker PB, Allain AN Jr, Winstead DK. Psychopathology and psychiatric diagnoses in WW II Pacific theater survivors of POW confinement and combat trauma. *Am J Psychiatry*. 1969;125:59–78.

79. American Psychiatric Association. *Diagnostic and Statistical Manual of Mental Disorders*, 3rd ed. Revised. (DSM III-R). Washington, DC: APA; 1987.

80. Ursano RJ. Posttraumatic stress disorder: The stressor criterion. *J Nerv Ment Dis*. 1987;175:273–275.

81. Holloway HC, Ursano RJ. The Vietnam veteran: Memory, social context, and metaphor. *Psychiatry*. 1984;47:103–108.

82. Berg SW, Richlin M. Injuries and illnesses of Vietnam War POWs IV: Comparison of captivity effects in North and South Vietnam. *Milit Med*. 1977;142:757–761.

83. Hall RCW, Malone PT. Psychiatric effects of prolonged Asian captivity: A two-year follow-up. *Am J Psychiatry*. 1976;133:786–790.

84. Paykel E. Contribution of life events to causation of psychiatric illness. *Psychol Med*. 1978;8:245–254.

85. Helzer JE, Robins LN, Wish E, Hesselbrock M. Depression in Vietnam veterans and civilian controls. *Am J Psychiatry*. 1979;136:526–529.

86. Green BL, Grace MC, Lindy JD, et al. Levels of functional impairment following a civilian disaster: The Beverly Hills Supper Club fire. *J Consult Clin Psychol*. 1983;51:573–580.

87. Breslau N, Davis GC. Chronic stress and major depression. *Arch Gen Psychiatry*. 1986;43:309–314.

88. Klonoff H, Clark C, Horgan J, et al. The MMPI profile of prisoners of war. *J Clin Psychol*. 1976;32:623–627.

89. Behar D. Confirmation of concurrent illnesses in posttraumatic stress disorder. *Am J Psychiatry*. 1984;141:1310–1311.

90. Davidson J, Swartz M, Storck M, et al. A diagnostic and family study of posttraumatic stress disorder. *Am J Psychiatry*. 1985;142:90–93.

91. Escobar JI, Randolph ET, Puente G, et al. Posttraumatic stress disorder in Hispanic Vietnam veterans—clinical phenomenology and sociocultural characteristics. *J Nerv Ment Dis*. 1983;171:585–596.

92. Sierles FS, Chen JJ, McFarland RE, Taylor MA. Posttraumatic stress disorder and concurrent psychiatric illness: A preliminary report. *Am J Psychiatry*. 1983;140:1177–1179.

93. Engdahl BE, Speed N, Eberly RE, Schartz J. Comorbidity of psychiatric disorders and personality profiles of American World War II prisoners of war. *J Nerv Ment. Dis*. 1991;179:181–187.

94. Spitzer RL, Endicott J, Robins E. *Research Diagnostic Criteria for a Selected Group of Functional Disorders*, 3rd ed. New York: Biometrics Research Division, New York State Psychiatric Institute; 1977.

95. Birkheimer LJ, Devane CL, Muniz CE. Posttraumatic stress disorder: Characteristics and pharmacological response in the veteran population. *Compr Psychiatry*. 1985;26:304–310.

96. LaCoursiere RB, Godfrey KE, Ruby LM. Traumatic neurosis in the etiology of alcoholism: Vietnam combat and other trauma. *Am J Psychiatry*. 1980;137:966–968.

97. Van der Kolk BA. Psychopharmacological issues in posttraumatic stress disorder. *Hosp Community Psychiatry*. 1983;34:683–692.

98. Nace EP, O'Brien CP, Mintz J, et al. Adjustment among Vietnam veteran drug users two years post-service. In: Figley CR, ed. *Stress Disorders Among Vietnam Veterans*. New York: Brunner/Mazel; 1978: 71–128.

99. Helzer JE, Robins LN, Davis DH. Depressive disorders in Vietnam returnees. *J Nerv Ment Dis*. 1976;163:177–185.

100. Nace EP, Meyers AL, O'Brien CP, et al. Depression in veterans two years after Vietnam. *Am J Psychiatry*. 1977;134:167–170.

101. Engdahl BE, Page WF, Miller TW. Age, education, maltreatment, and social support as predictors of chronic depression in former prisoners of war. *Soc Psychiatry Psychiatr Epidemiol*. 1991;26:63–67.

102. Horowitz MJ, Wilner N, Kaltreider N, Alvarez W. Signs and symptoms of posttraumatic stress disorder. *Arch Gen Psychiatry*. 1980;37:85–92.

103. Sparr L, Pankratz LD. Factitious posttraumatic stress disorder. *Am J Psychiatry*. 1983;140:1016–1019.

104. Sledge WH, Boydstun JA, Rabe AJ. Self-concept changes related to war captivity. *Arch Gen Psychiatry*. 1980;37:430–443.

105. Van Putten T, Yager J. Posttraumatic stress disorder: Emerging from the rhetoric. *Arch Gen Psychiatry*. 1984;41:411–413.

106. Yager T, Laufer R, Gallops M. Some problems associated with war experience in men of the Vietnam generation. *Arch Gen Psychiatry*. 1984;41:327–333.

107. Sutker PB, Allain AN Jr. MMPI profiles of veterans of WW II and Korea: Comparisons of former POWs and combat survivors. *Psychol Rep*. 1991;68(1):279–284.

108. Sutker PB, Winstead DK, Galina ZH, Allain AN Jr. Assessment of long-term psychosocial sequelae among POW survivors of the Korean conflict. *J Pers Assess*. 1990;54(1&2):170–180.

109. Sutker PB, Winstead DK, Galina ZH, Allain AN Jr. Cognitive deficits and psychopathology among former prisoners of war and combat veterans of the Korean conflict. *Am J Psychiatry*. 1991;148:67–72.

110. Eberly RE, Harkness AR, Engdahl BE. An adaptational view of trauma response as illustrated by the prisoner of war experience. *J Traumatic Stress*. 1991;4:363–380.

111. Lloyd C. Life events and depressive disorder reviewed I: Events as predisposing factors. *Arch Gen Psychiatry*. 1980;37:529–535.

112. Van der Kolk BA. *Post-traumatic Stress Disorder: Psychological and Biological Sequelae*. Washington, DC: APA; 1984.

113. Lloyd C. Life events and depressive disorder reviewed II: Events as precipitating factors. *Arch Gen Psychiatry*. 1980;37:541–548.

114. Davidson S. Massive psychic traumatization and social support. *J Psychosom Res*. 1979;23:395–402.

115. Hunter EJ. The prisoner of war and his family. In: Hunter EJ, ed. *Prolonged Separation: The Prisoner of War and His Family*. San Diego, Calif: Center for Prisoner of War Studies, Naval Health Research Center; 1977: 1–179.

116. Colarusso CA, Nemiroff RA. Clinical applications of adult developmental theory. *Am J Psychiatry*. 1987;144:1263–1270.

117. Spitz R. *The First Year of Life—Normal and Deviant Object Relations*. New York: International University Press; 1965.

118. Penk W, Robinowitz R. Post-traumatic stress disorders (PTSD) among Vietnam veterans: Introduction. *J Clin Psychol*. 1987;43:3–5.

119. Eitinger L. Concentration camp survivors in the postwar world. *Am J Orthopsychiatry*. 1962;32:367–375.

120. Berg SW, Richlin M. Injuries and illnesses of Vietnam War POWs III. Marine Corps POWs. *Milit Med*. 1977;142:678–680.

121. Berg SW. Injuries and illnesses of Vietnam War POWs II. Army POWs. *Milit Med*. 1977;142:598–677.

122. Wetzler HP. Status of Air Force prisoners of war five years post-repatriation. *USAF Med Serv Digest*. 1979;30:26–41.

123. Eitinger L. A follow-up study of the Norwegian concentration camp survivor's mortality and morbidity. *Isr Ann Psychiatry Relat Disciplines* [now *Isr J Psychiatry Relat Sci*]. 1973;11:199–209.

124. Adena MA. The health of Australian veterans. *Med J Aust*. 1989;150:356–357.

125. Dent OF, Tennant CC, Goulston KJ. Precursors of depression in World War II veterans 40 years after the war. *J Nerv Ment Dis*. 1987;175:486–490.

126. Turnbull G. Debriefing British POW's after the Gulf War and released hostages from Lebanon. *WVF International Socio-Medical Information Center Newsletter*. 1992;4:4–16.

127. Weisaeth L. Torture of a Norwegian ship's crew: The torture, stress reactions, and psychiatric after effects. *Acta Psychiatr Scand*. 1989;80(Suppl 355):63–72.

128. Boehnlein JK, Kinzie JD, Ben R, Fleck J. One-year follow-up study of posttraumatic stress disorder among survivors of Cambodian concentration camps. *Am J Psychiatry*. 1985;142:956–959.

129. Hogben GL, Cornfield RB. Treatment of traumatic war neurosis with phenelzine. *Arch Gen Psychiatry*. 1981;38:440–445.

130. Shen WW, Park S. The use of monoamine oxidase inhibitors in the treatment of traumatic war neurosis: Case report. *Milit Med*. 1983;148:430–431.

131. Walker JI. Chemotherapy of traumatic war stress. *Milit Med*. 1982;147:1029–1033.

132. Davidson JRT, Kudler HS, Saunders WB, Erickson L, et al. Predicting response to amitriptyline in posttraumatic stress disorder. *Am J Psychiatry*. 1993;150:1024–1029.

133. Davidson JRT. Pharmacotherapy of posttraumatic stress disorder. *Br J Psychiatry*. 1992;160:309–314.

134. Helzer JE. The impact of combat on later alcohol use by Vietnam veterans. *J Psychoactive Drugs*. 1984;16:183–191.

135. Hall RCW, Simmons WC. The POW wife: A psychiatric appraisal. *Arch Gen Psychiatry*. 1973;29:690–694.

136. McCubbin HI, Hunter EJ, Dahl BB. Residuals of war: Families of prisoners of war and servicemen missing in action. *J Soc Issues*. 1975;31:95–109.

137. Hunter EJ. Long-term effects of parental wartime captivity on children: Children of POW and MIA servicemen. *J Contemp Psychol*. 1988;18:312–328.

138. Menninger K. The academic lecture: Hope. *Am J Psychiatry*. 1959;94:481–491.

139. Axelrod S, Schnipper OL, Rau JH. Hospitalized offspring of Holocaust survivors. *Bull Menninger Clinic*. 1980;44:1–14.

140. Dahl BB, McCubbin HI, Ross KL. Second generational effects of war-induced separations: Comparing the adjustment of children in reunited and non-reunited families. *Milit Med*. 1977;141:146–151.

141. McCubbin HI, Cauble AE, Patterson JM, eds. *Family Stress, Coping, and Social Support*. Springfield, Ill: Charles C Thomas; 1982.

142. McCubbin HI, Patterson JM. Family adaptation to crises. In: McCubbin HI, Cauble AE, Patterson JM, eds. *Family Stress, Coping, and Social Support*. Springfield Ill: Charles C Thomas; 1982: 147–173.

Chapter 18

FOLLOW-UP STUDIES OF VETERANS

ROBERT H. STRETCH, Ph.D.*

*Major, Medical Service Corps, U.S. Army Reserve; Grants Associate, Office of Extramural Research, National Institutes of Health, Bethesda, Maryland; Research Assistant Professor of Psychiatry, Uniformed Services University of the Health Sciences, Bethesda, Maryland

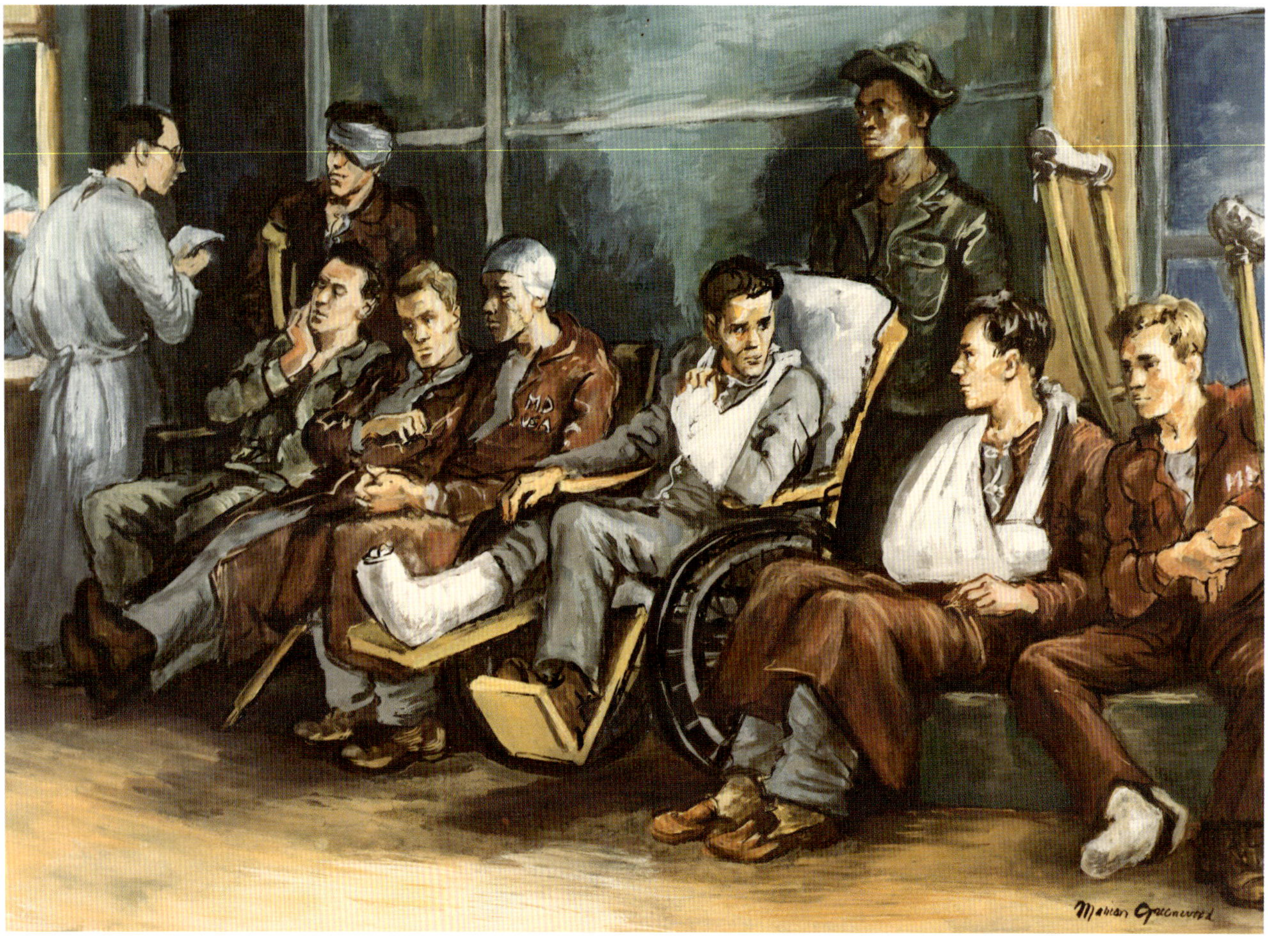

Marion Greenwood *The Dental Front* 1945

Marion Greenwood created a series of watercolors depicting the work of the U.S. Army Medical Department at the England General Hospital in Atlantic City, New Jersey during World War II. This watercolor portrays wounded soldiers waiting for their next medical procedure, in this case a visit with the dentist. Many of these seriously-wounded soldiers will be separated from the service for medical reasons and will receive their follow-up care through Veterans Administration hospitals.

Art: Courtesy of US Army Center of Military History, Washington, DC.

INTRODUCTION

The role of "soldier" has been glorified throughout the ages as a noble and honorable calling. The age of modern warfare, beginning with World War I, has been no exception. Soldiers such as Alvin York and Audie Murphy have been immortalized for their heroic deeds on the battlefield. The late actor, John Wayne, became the idol of millions for his combat soldier portrayals in countless movies. These romanticized depictions of wars and the men who fought in them tend to make one forget that war is a brutal and dehumanizing experience for many men.

Soldiers are often simply common men driven by geopolitical forces beyond their control into the role of combatant and, as such, typify the strengths and weaknesses inherent in all men. The vast majority of soldiers are not career military men. After wars' end, soldiers once again become civilians and return to their families to try to pick up where they left off. It is this process of readjustment that has more often than not been ignored by society. It is the soldier who is prized and valued, not the ex-soldier. The purpose of this chapter is to document the scientific attempts to follow up on veterans since the end of World War I to gain insight into the readjustment process and the successes and failures of veterans who were affected to different degrees by their war experiences.

WORLD WAR I STUDIES

Follow-up studies of veterans in the modern age of warfare began with the work of Salmon and Fenton[1] on the psychological adjustment of veterans of World War 1. In 1919, and again in 1924, Salmon and Fenton studied the postwar adjustment of a sample of veterans who had been hospitalized for war neuroses at Base Hospital No. 117 in France. Base Hospital No. 117 was the third-echelon facility which received those stress casualties who had not been returned to duty immediately by the division psychiatrist or after 3 to 5 days at the field hospital in the division rear. They had either failed to recover in 3 weeks at one of the three neurological hospitals or had been evacuated to the nonpsychiatric hospitals in the rear and therefore had been transferred to Base Hospital No. 117. They were the most severe cases.

The 1919–1920 Study

Preparation for the study was begun shortly after the armistice was signed. The purpose of the study was to determine the condition of a typical group of diagnosed war neurosis cases after their return to the civilian community in the United States. Questionnaire data were used to determine how well or poorly these men were getting along in terms of ability to work and contribute to society. The data do not provide for adequate clinical conclusions for a medical diagnosis of neurosis during follow-up, but do provide insight into problems and difficulties in attempts at readaptation. Data were collected from 758 veterans out of the 2,590 veterans who had been hospitalized at Base Hospital No. 117 in France.

Subjects were classified according to social status and ability to work and be self-supporting. These classifications were normal, neurotic, fatigued, disabled, and psychotic. The "normal" group consisted of men who went back to work to support themselves and their families and readjusted easily to civilian life. Many of these men noted tendencies to become angry or easily excited, nervous, restless, forgetful, and suffered from slight headaches or dizziness. For the most part these men were in good health, self-supporting, and happy.

The "neurotic" group consisted of those men who had only partially adjusted to their way of life prior to entering the military. They continued to suffer from one or more nervous difficulties and were either under a physician's care or had consulted one about their problems. They were able to return to work but were often unhappy because of their neurotic problems. These men tended to exhibit some of the same symptoms shown in France: tremors and tics, speech defects, weakness, insomnia, jumpiness, inability to concentrate, and memory disorders. These men also reported a great many minor injuries and serious accidents resulting from their nervous condition. Many men in this group were no longer able to function in their former jobs in machine shops or factories, but found working outdoors as salesmen, farmers, laborers, etc. less difficult.

The "fatigued" group consisted of men who could not work regularly without suffering and being bedridden. These men experienced fatigue, severe headaches, lack of ambition, depression, and were only able to work about one half of the time. The "disabled" group consisted of those men who were rehospitalized for psychoneurosis or reported a "nervous breakdown" or some incapacitating disease such as tuberculosis. The last group, the "psychotics," consisted of men who suffered from conditions such as dementia praecox, psychopathic personality, and epilepsy.

The current adjustment of these men according to the preceding classifications was then compared to the military classifications used by the U.S. Army in France to estimate the man's future military usefulness at the time of his discharge from Base Hospital No. 117. These men had been classified in one of four categories, as follows:

- Class A: Officers and enlisted men fit for combat service.
- Class B: Officers and enlisted men temporarily unfit for combat service but physically fit for other duty and restorable to Class A status within 6 months.
- Class C: Officers and enlisted men permanently unfit for combat service but capable of other supply-oriented service.
- Class D: Officers and enlisted men unfit for any duty within the American Expeditionary Forces.

This classification system took into account factors such as health, strength, and endurance which would be of significance in both U.S. Army and civilian life. The authors reasoned that if the classifications were adequately made, then some positive correlation should exist between these classifications and the men's later (1919–1920) conditions. The percentages of veterans in each group in the follow-up sample were very similar to the percentages of all cases at the hospital assigned to each group. These percentages for follow-up vs all cases were as follows:

Category	Follow-up Cases	All Cases
Class A	24.8%	19.6%
Class B	36.6%	39.2%
Class C	29.3%	31.8%
Class D	7.5%	6.6%

An additional 1.8% of the follow-up group and 2.9% of the total group had been transferred to another hospital unclassified.

In the 1919 to 1920 time frame, the veterans' groups were adjusting as follows:

- Class A: 68.1% were adjusting adequately (45.2% were normal, 22.9% were neurotic).
- Class B: 64.8% were adjusting adequately (41.8% were normal, 23% were neurotic).
- Class C: 55.4% were adjusting adequately (33.3% were normal, 22.1% were neurotic).
- Class D: 40.3% were adjusting adequately (21% were normal, 19.3% were neurotic).

The next stage in the study consisted of an inquiry into the question of mental disease diagnosis at discharge and its relation to functioning levels for the 1919 to 1920 period. For this comparison subjects were divided into two groups. Working veterans were those in the normal and neurotic categories. Disabled veterans were those in the fatigued, disabled, and psychotic categories. An examination of the percentages of various mental diagnoses associated with the working veterans revealed that the typical war neuroses at that time, primarily concussion, gas, and anxiety types, ranked very high in terms of successful readaptation (75% of veterans diagnosed as having anxiety neurosis, 73.4% of veterans with gas neurosis, and 67.8% of veterans with concussion neurosis at discharge were among the working veterans in 1919–1920). The less successfully readapted veterans were those whose diagnoses were of the more pronounced constitutional types such as hypochondriasis, neurasthenia, psychasthenia, and hysteria. Thus, veterans whose diagnosis reflected a recent onset of symptoms in response to war-related trauma exhibited a greater degree of readjustment than those veterans whose diagnoses reflected a certain constitutional susceptibility.

Additional observations revealed a slight tendency for younger men to do better in their readjustment than the older men, as well as a tendency for those of "good stock" and make-up to readapt themselves better to civilian life than those from "poor stock" and make-up. It was also found that men whose occupations required somewhat more intelligence for performance were better able to readapt than men whose occupations demanded less intelligence.

The 1924–1925 Study

A second follow-up of veterans from Base Hospital No. 117 was conducted in the period 1924 to 1925. Data were obtained from 763 subjects. Hospital estimates of potential military value at time of discharge were again compared to current functioning. As before, the veterans' current functioning was determined relative to their original classification grade as follows:

- Class A: 83% were functioning adequately (40.7% normal, 42.3% neurotic)
- Class B: 85.9% were functioning adequately (39.1% normal, 46.8% neurotic)
- Class C: 73.9% were functioning adequately (30% normal, 43.9% neurotic)
- Class D: 72.7% were functioning adequately (40.9% normal, 31.8% neurotic)

Thus, these hospital estimates of future U.S. Army potential again were predictive of future civilian readjustment.

A follow-up comparison of the relationship of specific mental diagnoses to current functioning again revealed that veterans with typical war neuroses of that time (gas syndrome, exhaustion, concussion, anxiety) showed greater evidence of recovery than those with more pronounced constitutional types (neurasthenia, psychasthenia, hypochondriasis). More important is the observation that practically every diagnostic group showed an increase in the percentage of veterans who had readapted adequately from the first period (1919–1920) to the second period (1924–1925).

Whereas in the 1919 to 1920 follow-up younger veterans seemed to be readapting better than older veterans, the 1924 to 1925 follow-up found a tendency for the extreme age groups, both younger and older, to make poorer readaptations than men in the middle age range. The finding in the 1919 to 1920 study of a positive relationship between family history and current functioning was not found in the 1924 to 1925 study. Personal and family histories were not in themselves predictive of future civilian readjustment.

Occupational data from the 1924 to 1925 study revealed that former war neurotics who had difficulty working at manufacturing trades in urban areas were able to readapt fairly successfully in agricultural work. Overall, the 5 years between follow-up studies showed evidence of a great deal of improvement among veterans of Base Hospital No. 117. The percentage of veterans who were able to function adequately increased from 60.9% to 80.8%. The fatigued veterans, who were able to work only about one half the time, decreased from 17.3% to 9.8% while the disabled and psychotic groups, who were not able to work, decreased from 21.7% to 9.4%. Salmon and Fenton[1] speculated that the most important factor underlying this marked improvement was the focus of various governmental and social agencies on the problems of soldiers that led to their becoming an asset rather than a burden upon society.

WORLD WAR II STUDIES

The conclusion of World War II saw a continued interest in the postwar psychological adjustment of servicemen. The most comprehensive follow-up study to emerge from the World War II literature is that of Brill and Beebe.[2] This study was generated as a result of the establishment by the National Research Council of a Committee on Veterans Medical Problems whose task was to develop a program of medical follow-up studies based on the medical experience of the Armed Forces and the Veterans Administration.

The study was conducted using subjects drawn from representative samples of 8,000 U.S. Army (including U.S. Air Force) and 2,216 U.S. Navy and Marine Corps veterans who had been diagnosed as suffering from a psychoneurosis during service (both combat and noncombat) in World War II. Psychoneurosis included the following types of disorders: hysteria; anxiety state; hypochondriasis; neurasthenia; neurocirculatory asthenia; obsessive–compulsive; psychasthenia; phobias; reactive depression; psychoneurosis; and others, unqualified, unspecified, including combat exhaustion.

From these U.S. Army and U.S. Navy rosters a "clinical" sample of 955 veterans with psychoneurosis was selected to receive a 4-hour examination by one of 225 psychiatrists nationwide who had agreed to participate in the project. A second "record" sample of 520 U.S. Army and U.S. Navy cases of psychoneurosis was selected to be studied on the basis of military records.

A control group of 397 U.S. Army enlisted men was chosen at random such that the number among them who saw service during each month in 1944 was proportional to the number of psychiatric admissions during each month of that year. Data for controls consisted of information on their military and medical histories during service. A second control group was added in 1951 in response to the Korean mobilization. This group consisted of 502 new recruits who were given psychiatric examinations as they were received in large training divisions immediately after induction.

The first objective of the study was to determine the characteristics of the clinical and record samples and the ways they differed from the general military population both before and during military service in relation to the chance of breakdown in service. The second objective was to determine the etiology of combat breakdown, its progression during service, and its effects on subsequent military performance. The third major goal was to learn what happened to these men after they left the service and to describe their follow-up psychiatric status approximately 5 years after breakdown. Of particular importance to this review are the results of this third goal. For data regarding the first two objectives the reader is referred to Brill and Beebe.[2]

Mortality

A mortality check on the 1,475 U.S. Army and U.S. Navy veterans in the clinical and record samples was made in 1953. A total of 36 deaths were discovered in comparison to an expected 31 deaths among same age males in the general population. An examination of cause of death revealed a relatively high suicide rate for subjects in the study (six suicides compared to only two expected).

Symptom Prevalence

During the examination, only 8.7% of examined cases and an estimated 10.1% of the entire clinical sample reported experiencing no psychiatric symptoms. The most common symptoms reported by the subjects were anxiety (45.3%); depression (29.6%); nightmares (22.1%); insomnia (31.9%); headache (42.8%); irritability (48.6%); difficulty in concentration (20.1%); restlessness (45.4%); and psychogenic somatic complaints of the gastrointestinal (41.7%), cardiovascular (21.9%), and musculoskeletal systems (34.8%). In addition, 9.5% of subjects reported alcoholism, 10.1% reported hysteria, and 9.8% reported phobias.

The examiners traced these psychiatric symptoms and psychogenic somatic complaints back to their origin to determine which were evident before service, which first appeared during service, and which appeared after discharge. Rather than examining the origin of each symptom, a summary was made for each subject and a significant number (19%) presented different complaints originating both before and during service. All symptoms originated before service for 24% of subjects and during service for 43% of subjects. Only 4% of subjects had all symptoms develop after discharge.

When asked to assess their own health, the subjects indicated that, when compared to entry into the service, they were currently in better health than they had been at time of separation. At time of separation, 81% regarded their health as poorer than at entry into service, 45% described their health as "much worse," and only 19% felt their health was the same or better. During the follow-up 5 years later, 71% described their health as poorer than at entry, 31% felt "much worse," and 29% reported their health as the same or better. Although their health had tended to improve, the vast majority of the subjects still did not regard themselves as being well at follow-up.

Occupational Adjustment

Examiners assessed occupational adjustment by focusing on the veteran's ability to handle his job, avoidance of interpersonal difficulties, attitudes toward his work (including security, pay, working conditions), and employer satisfaction with the veteran. Satisfactory occupational adjustment was exhibited by 67% of the subjects, while 7% had a questionable adjustment, and 26% had an impaired adjustment. At the time of examination, 76% of the subjects were employed full-time, 9% part-time, and 15% were unemployed. Illness was a factor in preventing full-time employment for 14% of the sample.

Economic Adjustment

A veteran was considered to have a satisfactory economic adjustment if he could support his family, and if any dissatisfaction with his income was within normal limits or neurotic in origin. Using these criteria, 74% of the subjects had made a satisfactory adjustment, 5% were questionable, and 21% were impaired.

Marital Adjustment

Only 15% of the subjects were still single at follow-up in comparison to 46% at separation and 62%

at entry into the service. Examiners reported finding less satisfactory adjustment in this area than in most others. Only 60% of married subjects were regarded as having satisfactory adjustment, 22% were questionable, and 18% were impaired.

Family Adjustment

Assessment of family adjustment was made on the basis of the subject's attitudes and behavior toward either his own wife and children, if any, or with his parental family. A veteran was considered to be impaired if he ran away from home before the end of adolescence, quarreled often with parents or siblings, refused to cooperate within the family in a normal fashion (contributing to its support), or was too dependent upon his family, unable to make independent decisions or to engage in normal activities outside the family. On this basis, 67% of veterans were adjusting satisfactorily, 21% were questionable, and 12% were impaired.

Community and General Social Adjustment

This area of adjustment refers to the boundaries of socially acceptable behavior and mores. Only 56% of the subjects were deemed to have adjusted satisfactorily, 25% were questionable, and 19% were impaired.

Psychiatric Disability

A veteran was considered psychiatrically disabled if his psychiatric symptomatology caused him to either lose time from work or prevented him from carrying out his role as a student or father. The degree of impairment or disability also involved how the veteran's adjustment in other areas such as family and community adjustment was affected. Disability in one or more minor areas of activity without work disruption was usually labeled as mild disability, while a moderate degree of disability usually affected work time or efficiency appreciably.

The results revealed that less than 30% of the veterans in the follow-up study were more than slightly disabled due to psychiatric symptoms, and only 8.1% were more than moderately disabled. Thus, while there was a great deal of psychiatric symptomatology present in these veterans, this symptomatology did not translate into disability.

In looking at changes in psychiatric conditions since discharge from the service, it was found that most veterans who were not psychiatrically disabled at discharge either remained the same or improved. Of those veterans who were disabled at discharge, 60% appeared to have improved, 24% remained the same, and 14% became worse.

Treatment Issues

At follow-up it was determined that 36% of the veterans in the study had sought some type of psychiatric or other treatment for relief of symptoms. When asked whether they felt the need for further psychiatric treatment, 56% of the veterans reported that they did not. Of the 40% who did express a need for further treatment (4% expressed no opinion), less than a third felt their need was great.

The basic conclusions of this large-scale follow-up study of World War II veterans are similar to those reported by Salmon and Fenton[1] on World War I veterans. Both studies revealed a marked tendency for significant improvement among psychiatrically troubled veterans 5 years since discharge from the service. Not only have their conditions improved, but their ability to function as contributing members rather than as burdens to society has also improved. This is not to imply that they have not been significantly affected by their war-related service. It merely means that for the majority of impaired veterans, their negative experiences have not served to prevent them from coping in a satisfactory fashion.

Ripley and Wolf[3] conducted a follow-up of 100 veterans who had been hospitalized with schizophrenia or schizophrenic-like reactions while participating in combat campaigns in New Guinea and the Philippines from 1943 to 1945. Follow-up data over a period of 5 to 8 years after hospitalization were gathered from records, questionnaires, and personal interviews. Many of these veterans had functioned in the military for long periods prior to their breakdown despite the presence of a high degree of psychopathologic symptomatology.

Upon evacuation to the United States, marked symptomatic improvement was noticed in one fifth of the patients. More than one third of the patients had been discharged after 2 months of hospitalization, and only four had not been released after more than a year. In comparing the prewar and postwar adjustment of these veterans, it was found that their general health, ability to function at work, family relationships, and social adaptation were all poorer.

Evidence was found for a gradual trend toward decreased disability, although several common symptoms persisted: vague somatic complaints, irritability, headaches, seclusiveness, insomnia, difficulty in concentration, dejection, excessive fantasy, suspiciousness, anxiety, restlessness, hallucinations, and resentment toward authority. Eleven patients had had further hospitalizations. Over one fifth of the veterans were severely disabled by these symptoms after 5 or more years. The most important factors in promoting a good readjustment were a warm, tolerant, helpful attitude on the part of a wife or other family member, satisfactory work situation, and success in school and social contacts.

Additional evidence concerning the long-term effects of war neuroses can be found in the report of a 5-year follow-up study by Futterman and Pumpian-Mindlin.[4] This study of 200 combat veterans seeking treatment at the Veterans Administration Mental Hygiene Clinic in Los Angeles provided evidence of fresh cases of traumatic war neuroses that had not previously sought treatment since the war. Common symptomatology among these veterans included: intense anxiety, recurrent combat-related dreams, startle reactions, depression, guilt, and a tendency to sudden, violent behavior. Secondary symptoms included a tendency to avoid people, fear of criticism, difficulty in making decisions, and various sleep disturbances.

Similar findings were reported by Archibald, Long, Miller, and Tuddenham[5] in their 15-year follow-up report on gross stress reactions resulting from combat during World War II. Questionnaire data were obtained from 57 combat veterans and 48 noncombat control subjects. The data indicated that the combat veterans were bothered by problems of tension, irritability, depression, diffuse anxiety symptoms, headaches, startle reactions, dizziness, blackouts, avoidance of activities similar to combat experience, internalization of feelings, insomnia, and nightmares. Eighty-two percent of the combat veterans reported that their psychological symptoms had interfered with their abilities to provide for their families.

Ponteva[6] conducted a follow-up study of Finnish soldiers who had been treated for psychiatric reasons during the war with Russia (1941–1944). Approximately 15,700 soldiers had been hospitalized for psychiatric causes. Subjects for the follow-up study were selected at random from these hospitalized veterans using records maintained at the War Casualties Archives. A control group was also picked at random from pneumonia patients because of the lack of correlation between pneumonia and psychiatric disorders.

Data were obtained from 373 patients and 372 controls. It was found that at the time of follow-up (1971) approximately 43% of the psychiatric patients and 23% of the controls were either partially or entirely unable to work. The two most important causes of disability for the patients were cardiovascular diseases and mental diseases. Ponteva concluded that the adaptation of wartime psychiatric patients to civil life after the war was very good in the subgroups of veterans suffering from neurotic and reactive disorders. The more severely disturbed veterans, however, were not as successful in their readjustment.

Long-term reactions to modern warfare are by no means limited to American or European veterans. Meguro[7] conducted a 20-year follow-up study of war neurosis cases discharged from the former Konodai Army Hospital in Japan between 1941 and 1945. Questionnaires and interviews were used to collect data from 104 Japanese veterans selected at random from the total population of 2,205 war neurosis patients. Results revealed that, of those who had developed war neuroses and were unable to adapt to military life, more than 56% were now considered medically healthy and socially adapted. Approximately 68% of the veterans reported that their war neurosis symptoms had, in the medical sense, been cured. Meguro noted, however, that about one sixth of this group was still jobless and single in their middle age and could not be considered socially adapted. Among those veterans who were found "cured" of their former principal symptoms, the data indicated that the whole group still tended to be more neurotic than a normal group.

KOREAN CONFLICT STUDIES

Little research has been conducted on the follow-up status of Korean conflict veterans. Archibald and Tuddenham[8] investigated the long-term effects of combat stress on veterans of the Korean conflict as part of a further follow-up on an earlier study of World War II veterans.[5] All subjects were seen as outpatients at the Oakland, California Veterans Administration (VA) mental hygiene clinic. Included in the study were 15 Korean conflict veterans showing evidence of combat fatigue and 17 Korean conflict noncombatants with various psychiatric diagnoses representative of the clinic population.

Archibald and Tuddenham were interested in assessing the existence of a poststress syndrome of restlessness, irritability, tension, headaches, sleep disturbance, overreactive startle reflex, feelings of isolation and distrust, sense of inadequacy, and restriction of social contacts and activities. Questionnaire data revealed that the combat-fatigued veterans showed a significantly higher incidence than the noncombat veterans of sweaty hands, dizziness, depression, irritability, combat dreams, restlessness, and difficulty in concentration and in memory. At time of sampling the combat-fatigued veterans had a higher incidence of every one of the symptoms than they did during combat.

On a rating of changes in health status, fewer combat-fatigued veterans reported improvement and more reported deterioration than did the noncombat veterans. Significant differences were also found between the combat fatigued veterans and noncombat veterans in response to noises of airplanes, sudden loud noises such as firecrackers, combat portrayals on television or in movies, and going through a highway tunnel. These results among Korean conflict veterans confirm the findings for similar groups of World War II veterans.

Thienes-Hontos, Watson, and Kucala[9] assessed the prevalence of stress symptomatology among a sample of 29 Korean veterans and 29 Vietnam veterans who had been hospitalized for psychiatric reasons at the St. Cloud, Minnesota VA medical center between 9 and 36 months after their military separation dates. Hospital files for these veterans were examined to determine the incidence of the following stress-related symptoms: recurrent dreams and recollections of a traumatic event, intrusive thoughts, constricted affect, feelings of estrangement from others, diminished interest in one or more significant activities, hyperalertness, sleep disturbance, survivor guilt, memory impairment, and trouble concentrating. Results indicated that constricted affect, memory impairment/trouble concentrating, and diminished interests were more commonly reported by Korean rather than Vietnam veterans. Recurrent dreams were more often reported by Vietnam rather than Korean veterans. Overall, nearly identical percentages of Korean (42.2%) and Vietnam (42.3%) veterans reported symptoms that were found to be stress-related.

VIETNAM CONFLICT STUDIES

The period since the end of U.S. involvement in Vietnam has witnessed an unparalleled amount of research interest in the readjustment of its veterans. The impetus for this interest stems largely from the myriad of controversies and mystiques that surround both the conduct of the war and the men who fought in it. Never before in the history of the United States has there been such an unpopular and divisive conflict as expressed by the antiwar demonstrations of the late 1960s. Perhaps more important was the way in which the public outcry against the war carried over to the men who fought in it. The veterans of Vietnam did not return to the victory parades of an adoring nation. Far too often they returned alone and afraid of the very society they had fought to protect. As with the diversity of opinions about the war itself, a dichotomy of opinions existed among researchers interested in the prevalence and severity of apparent stress reactions experienced by returning Vietnam veterans. Figley[10] delineated two diverse perspectives that emerged from the literature in the 1970s: *stress evaporation* and *residual stress*.

The stress evaporation perspective holds that the Vietnam veteran probably did suffer some psychological readjustment problems during and immediately after military service, but any problems disappeared since returning home. Representative studies of this perspective include those by Worthington,[11,12] and Borus.[13-16] These studies found no significant differences between veterans who served in Vietnam and those who did not on a wide range of psychosocial behaviors. These studies did not, however, always include control groups or assess for combat experience.

The residual stress perspective holds that the nature of the Vietnam combat experience is such that it has a significant impact on the veteran, making the transition back to civilian life difficult. Studies representative of this perspective include those by Wilson,[17] Strayer and Ellenhorn,[18] Haley,[19] and Figley and Southerly[20] which have documented significantly more problems of adjustment among Vietnam combat veterans than among noncombat Vietnam-era veterans.

There are two basic conclusions that can be drawn from these studies of the readjustment of Vietnam veterans in the 1970s. If one looks at Vietnam-era veterans as a group, there do not appear to be any significant differences in comparison to nonveterans in most areas of interpersonal and intrapersonal adjustment.[11–16] However, if one controls for either service in Vietnam in general, or combat experience in particular, then there is considerable evidence that suggests that Vietnam combat veterans, when compared to Vietnam-era veterans or nonveterans, exhibit significantly more (*a*) negative general and specific orientations toward violence,[21] (*b*) psychological symptoms,[17,20,22] (*c*) indices of depression,[23] (*d*) political alienation,[4,24,25] and (*e*) adjustment problems.[10,17,18,20]

Research on Vietnam veterans in the 1980s witnessed a shift in emphasis brought about by the inclusion of the category of Post-Traumatic Stress Disorder (PTSD), both Acute and Chronic/Delayed, in the third edition of the American Psychiatric Association's *Diagnostic and Statistical Manual of Mental Disorders* (DSM-III) in 1980.[26]

Briefly, PTSD is characterized by the development of common symptomatology following a psychologically traumatic event that is outside the range of normal human experience. The characteristic symptoms involve reexperiencing the traumatic event through intrusive memories, recurrent dreams, or "flashbacks" caused by environmental or ideational stimuli; numbing of responsiveness to or reduced involvement with the external world as evidenced by diminished interest in activities, feelings of detachment or estrangement, constricted affect; and a variety of autonomic, dysphoric, or cognitive symptoms such as exaggerated startle response, sleep disturbances, survivor guilt, difficulty concentrating, memory impairment, or avoidance of activities that arouse recollection of the traumatic event.

The inclusion of the category of PTSD in DSM-III has resulted in fewer studies whose purpose is to either document or refute the existence of readjustment problems among Vietnam veterans. More studies are attempting to determine how prevalent these problems are in the veteran population as well as their etiologies and appropriate treatment modalities.

One of the most comprehensive studies of the readjustment of Vietnam veterans is the five-volume report by the Center for Policy Research,[27] which examined educational and occupational adjustment, social and psychological problems, long-term stress reactions, and how veterans have dealt with their war experiences. The data for this project consist of in-depth interviews with over 1,400 Vietnam and Vietnam-era veterans from various parts of the country, both urban and rural.

The results of this study reveal that Vietnam veterans have not attained as high a degree of education as their peers and tend to hold jobs that are of lower levels than both Vietnam-era veterans (those who did not serve in Vietnam) and nonveterans. Unemployment is a particularly acute problem among black Vietnam veterans, while a greater proportion of whites have not fully utilized the educational opportunities available to them under the "GI Bill" (the Veterans Readjustment Benefits Act of 1966).

Combat was found to have a significant impact on the social and psychological adjustment of Vietnam veterans. Evidence was found documenting a direct, significant relationship between combat and current drug and alcohol use, arrests, medical problems, and stress-related symptoms. This latter relationship to stress-related symptoms seemed to be concentrated primarily among veterans who served in combat during and after 1968 when public opinion and support for the war became highly negative. Reactions to combat among Vietnam veterans also differed along racial lines. Increased combat exposure among white veterans was characterized by excessive alcohol use while among black veterans drug abuse was found more frequently.

An examination of long-term stress reactions among these Vietnam veterans revealed that differences in family stability and the amount and intensity of combat experiences interacted to affect veterans to different degrees. Supportive relationships with others were found to have a significant effect in reducing the incidence and severity of stress reactions for all veterans, regardless of amount of combat experience. For veterans residing in large cities, interaction with other Vietnam veterans was found to alleviate stress reactions, while veterans in smaller cities and rural areas tended to be helped by the presence of a highly supportive network of close friends.

Additional data reveal that Vietnam veterans have attempted to deal with their war experiences in different ways. Some veterans have tried to simply forget or block out the past; others cling to it tenaciously; while still others have attempted to work through their past experiences by reflection and dialogue with others. It appears, however, that the majority of Vietnam veterans interviewed in this study have not made substantial progress in resolving the conflicts and problems resulting from their war experiences. Many men still tend to avoid emotional conflicts, blame others for their problems, or have fallen victim to self-pity or self-flagellation.

Among the recommendations generated by this study to improve the readjustment of Vietnam veterans are to extend the period of eligibility for "GI Bill" education and training benefits, develop training programs for chronically unemployed veterans, promote the use of fellow veterans as mental health counselors and therapists, and develop more expertise in understanding and treating psychosocial aftereffects of traumatic war experiences.

Recent estimates of the prevalence of stress reactions such as PTSD among the 2.8 million veterans who served in Vietnam range from 500,000[28] to 700,000[29] to as many as 1.5 million.[30,31] These figures indicate that anywhere from 18% to 54% of Vietnam veterans are currently experiencing symptoms of PTSD.

Additional information on the prevalence of PTSD in Vietnam veterans is contained in the summary of preliminary findings from the National Vietnam Veterans Readjustment Study (NVVRS).[32] This study was conducted under contract with the Veterans Administration (now the Department of Veterans Affairs) and mandated by Congressional legislation (Public Law 98-160). The study was designed to be the most rigorous and comprehensive examination to date of the prevalence of PTSD and other psychological problems in the readjustment to civilian life of Vietnam veterans. In-depth interviews averaging 3 to 5 hours were conducted with over 3,000 men and women representing three major groups of interest: Vietnam-theater veterans, Vietnam-era veterans, and nonveterans or civilian counterparts.

Among the many findings of this study are that the majority of Vietnam-theater veterans have successfully readjusted to civilian life and currently experience few symptoms of PTSD or other readjustment problems. Male Vietnam-theater veterans typically do not differ from Vietnam-era veterans on various indices of current life adjustment. Female Vietnam veterans, however, currently experience more readjustment problems than female Vietnam-era veterans matched for age and military occupation.

Employing multiple assessment procedures, the results indicate that 15.2% of all male Vietnam-theater veterans are currently experiencing symptoms of PTSD. Among female Vietnam-theater veterans, the current PTSD prevalence is estimated to be 8.5%. These rates are considerably higher than the rates for either Vietnam-era veterans (males = 2.5%, females = 1.1%) or civilian counterparts (males = 1.2%, females = 0.3%). These figures represent individuals with symptoms that qualify for a clinical diagnosis of PTSD. If one looks at those individuals who have clinically significant stress reaction symptoms that are insufficient to qualify as full PTSD, but still may require professional attention, an additional 11.1% of male and 7.8% of female Vietnam-theater veterans can be classified as currently experiencing "partial PTSD."

Additional analyses indicate that 30.6% of male and 26.9% of female Vietnam-theater veterans have had PTSD at some point in their lives. This means that of all the male and female Vietnam-theater veterans who have ever had PTSD, over one third of these males and over one fourth of these females still have PTSD today. Other findings reveal a strong relationship between PTSD and other postwar readjustment problems. Individuals with PTSD have a greater tendency to exhibit other specific psychiatric disorders and other postwar readjustment problems. This is particularly true among those Vietnam-theater veterans who have high levels of exposure to combat and other war zone stressors.

Significant differences were also found for minority group veterans. The current PTSD prevalence rate for PTSD is estimated to be 27.9% for Hispanic veterans, 20.6% for blacks, and 13.7% for whites. It is believed that the differences between blacks and whites can be explained by differing levels of exposure to war zone stress, but this does not explain the differences between Hispanics and either blacks or whites.

Overall, this study provides evidence that nearly 500,000 of the 3.14 million men and women who served in the Vietnam theater are currently suffering from PTSD and nearly 1,000,000 have had PTSD at some point in their lives.

Over the past several years this author has been conducting an epidemiologic study of the psychosocial adjustment of Vietnam and Vietnam-era veterans.[33–38] These studies represent a programmatic research effort into the assessment of the prevalence and severity of post-traumatic stress disorder as well as the factors involved in its etiology among Vietnam veterans.

The major hypothesis of this research is that the prevalence and severity of PTSD is affected by a combination of different factors that include combat/war zone experience, and social support system legitimization of experiences both during service in Vietnam and upon reentry (primarily the first year back). The importance of combat experience has already been demonstrated in the literature and in this review.

The importance of supportive relationships in reducing the incidence of stress reactions among Vietnam veterans has already been noted by the

Center for Policy Research.[27] It may be that stress reactions such as PTSD involve the failure of social support systems to promote the catharsis or abreaction of stressful combat experiences. Without validation or legitimization of these experiences, Vietnam veterans may be unable to cope successfully.

In addition to its epidemiologic orientation, the studies by Stretch differ from previous reports in that they examine populations of Vietnam veterans that have been largely ignored in the past. More specifically, these studies examine PTSD and factors involved in its development among Vietnam and Vietnam-era veterans still on active duty in the U.S. Army (including a subsample of nurses), U.S. Army Reservists, prior-service civilians, and more recently, Canadians who joined and served in the U.S. military in Vietnam.

The results of these ongoing studies indicate that not all Vietnam veterans are currently experiencing PTSD to the degree determined among the civilian veteran population. A questionnaire, the Vietnam-Era Veterans Adjustment Survey (VEVAS), was sent to all Vietnam and Vietnam-era veterans assigned to a moderate-sized U.S. Army post on the East Coast in the Spring of 1982. Data were gathered on attitudes and opinions about the war, combat experience, past and current psychosocial health problems, and social support experiences both during and after service in Vietnam. Using the DSM-III criteria for assessing PTSD, it was determined that 12 of the 238 Vietnam veterans (5.1%) are currently experiencing symptoms related to PTSD and 25 veterans (10.5%) report symptoms of PTSD that occurred during service in Vietnam.

VEVAS data were also collected from 667 Vietnam veterans assigned to U.S. Army Reserve troop units nationwide in the Spring of 1982. Results indicate that 73 of these randomly selected veterans (10.9%) report current symptoms of PTSD and 84 (12.4%) report having been bothered in Vietnam. Similar data were collected from 361 active duty Vietnam veteran nurses in the Spring of 1983. Again using DSM-III criteria, it was determined that 12 out of 361 Vietnam veteran nurses (3.3%) are currently suffering from PTSD and 33 nurses (9.1%) were bothered by symptoms of PTSD during Vietnam. Additional data were collected from 499 Vietnam veterans with no current military affiliation who were obtained at random from VA medical benefits files. Of these latter veterans, 160 (32.1%) were found to be currently suffering from PTSD and 127 (25.5%) report symptoms of PTSD during their service in Vietnam.

Another group of Vietnam veterans that has been ignored by other researchers until now, consists of the estimated 10,000 to 40,000 Canadians who enlisted in the U.S. military and served in Vietnam.[39] The study of PTSD among these Canadian Vietnam veterans is important for several reasons. One is the nature of their homecoming and subsequent readjustment experiences. While many Americans returned home to face rejection and hostility for their role in the war, Canadians found neither rejection nor recognition. No one knew they had been in Vietnam so they were ignored and isolated from other veterans. Because they served with the U.S. military, they were denied veteran status in Canada and are not eligible for any veterans benefits from the Canadian government. They are also not eligible to join veterans groups such as the Royal Canadian Legion and have been labeled "mercenaries" and "traitors." Among 164 Canadian Vietnam veterans who responded to a modified version of the VEVAS, 90 Canadians (55%) are currently experiencing symptoms of PTSD. A total of 83 veterans (51%) report experiencing symptoms of PTSD during their Vietnam service.

Table 18.1 presents the PTSD prevalence rates for these five different groups of Vietnam veterans. "Acute" PTSD refers to those veterans who reported experiencing PTSD during Vietnam service, but do not report symptoms at the present time. These rates range from a low of 6.6% for Reserve veterans to a high of 10.4% among Canadian Vietnam veterans. "Delayed" PTSD refers to veterans who did not report PTSD symptoms during Vietnam, but are currently bothered by PTSD. The delayed PTSD rates range from 1.4% among U.S. Army nurses to 14.8% among prior-service civilian veterans. "Chronic" PTSD is represented by those veterans who were bothered by symptoms of PTSD during their Vietnam service, and are still bothered by PTSD at the present time. Chronic PTSD rates vary from 1.9% for U.S. Army nurses to 40.2% for Canadian veterans. These mutually exclusive categories may be combined to yield an "Overall" PTSD rate representing the percentage of veterans who have experienced symptoms of PTSD at any time during or after service in Vietnam. As can be seen, the overall prevalence of PTSD ranges from 10.5% among U.S. Army Nurse Corps Vietnam veterans to 65.2% among Canadian Vietnam veterans.

The results of these studies suggest that factors other than combat affect the attenuation of PTSD. Social support, particularly during the first year back from Vietnam, was found to be just as predictive of current PTSD symptomatology as combat

TABLE 18-1

PREVALENCE OF POST-TRAUMATIC STRESS SYNDROME (PTSD) AMONG VIETNAM VETERANS

Prevalence Rates	Army Nurses N=361 (%)	Army Troops N=238 (%)	Army Reserve N=677 (%)	Civilians N=499 (%)	Canadians N=164 (%)
Current PTSD	3.3	5.1	11.2	32.1	54.9
Vietnam PTSD	9.1	10.5	12.4	25.5	50.6
Acute PTSD	7.2	7.1	6.6	8.2	10.4
Delayed PTSD	1.4	1.7	5.5	14.8	14.6
Chronic PTSD	1.9	3.4	5.8	17.2	40.2
Overall PTSD	10.5	12.2	17.9	40.2	65.2

Adapted with permission from Stretch R. Effects of service in Vietnam on Canadian Forces military personnel. *Armed Forces Society*. 1990;16:582.

experience. The data suggest that initially PTSD does result from traumatic combat/war zone experiences, but the veteran's ability to either successfully cope with or succumb to this disorder depends upon social support. Veterans in the studies who had received positive social support from friends and relatives reported fewer symptoms of PTSD than did veterans who reported encountering negative or hostile reactions from others upon return from Vietnam.

Active duty veterans had high levels of social support and low levels of PTSD. The significantly greater percentage of U.S. Army Reserve Vietnam veterans reporting symptoms of PTSD is likely to be the result of their having been exposed to more negative or hostile societal reactions to their service in Vietnam than their active duty counterparts. Vietnam veterans who remained on active duty were able to interact with fellow veterans in an affirming military culture on a daily basis. Being full-time members of the civilian community and only "part-time soldiers" provided reservists with fewer opportunities to work through their Vietnam experiences in a supportive nonjudgmental atmosphere. The Vietnam veteran subjects obtained from the VA severed their ties with the military early on and likely received less social support for their service than their active duty or reserve counterparts. They also have much greater rates of PTSD than these other groups.

The Canadian Vietnam veterans have the most serious PTSD prevalence rates of any group studied. This is surprising in that they cannot be accused of faking symptoms in order to gain compensation because their lack of legal status as "veterans" has made them ineligible for compensation. Based on data from questionnaires and corroborating evidence from veterans' letters and informal interviews, it is likely that this higher prevalence of PTSD is due to three reasons: (1) lack of social support and recognition from Canadian society and the government of Canada, (2) isolation from other Vietnam veterans in Canada, and (3) lack of availability of any medical or psychological readjustment counseling services in Canada.

The data also suggest that further research is needed to clarify what is meant by "combat experience." Few would disagree that combat is traumatic, but what exactly is it that is traumatic? This author's research also focused on nurses who served in Vietnam. Nurses are not normally considered to have experienced "combat." While they certainly differ from infantry troops in that they do not carry weapons or actively engage in firefights with enemy soldiers, they do share many common experiences. Nurses stationed in hospitals and field units in Vietnam were not always in safe, secure locations and were often subjected to enemy shelling.

More importantly, nurses were often exposed to the horrors and carnage of war on a daily basis. One does not have to fire a weapon or kill someone to become traumatized by war. Constant exposure to maimed, dying, and dead soldiers is certainly in itself traumatic. This was confirmed by Futterman and Pumpian-Mindlin[4] who reported that traumatic war neuroses were more common among certain groups of noncombatants such as medical first-aid men who were exposed to the violent effects and results of combat, but had not been active participants in combat.

The data demonstrate that duty in Vietnam by nurses was just as traumatic as combat duty for the other active duty and reserve Vietnam veterans. VEVAS data on PTSD symptoms exhibited during Vietnam duty reveal no significant differences among the number of nurses (9.1%), other active duty veterans (10.5%), and Reservists (12%) experiencing PTSD at that time.

SUMMARY AND CONCLUSION

This review of follow-up studies on the readjustment of veterans has demonstrated that while weaponry and tactics may change from war to war, the impact of war on its participants remains largely unchanged. Medical and psychiatric nomenclature of reactions to war experiences also change, but the reactions themselves are remarkably similar. Veterans of World War I suffered from "shell shock," World War II and Korean veterans suffered from "war neuroses," and Vietnam veterans suffer from "post-traumatic stress disorder."

These past studies demonstrate that the majority of veterans are able to make a satisfactory adjustment to civilian life. This does not mean that they emerged from war unscathed. It is unrealistic to expect someone to not be affected by the inhumanity and brutality of war. It is also unrealistic to assume that veterans cannot put these experiences into their proper perspective by acknowledging their impact and then using that perspective to continue on with their lives. Supportive relationships with others appears to be the key to successful readjustment for these veterans.

In many ways veterans of previous war eras may have had a better opportunity for successful readjustment than Vietnam veterans. Vietnam veterans did not return from their war en masse on transport ships which often took weeks to arrive in the States. They returned on jetliners as individuals denied the therapeutic opportunity to work through their war experiences with their fellow veterans. They also returned to a society that did not greet them as conquering heroes or even acknowledge the sacrifices they made.

For these reasons and others it appears that Vietnam veterans have been less successful than veterans of previous war eras in readjusting to civilian life. As society begins to realize that the veterans who served in Vietnam were not necessarily responsible for the mistakes made there, then many more Vietnam veterans will be able to put the past behind them and look to the future more confidently.

REFERENCES

1. Salmon TW, Fenton N, eds. In the American Expeditionary Forces [Section 2]. *Neuropsychiatry*. Vol 10. In: *The Medical Department of the United States Army in the World War*. Washington, DC: Office of The Surgeon General, US Army; 1929.

2. Brill NQ, Beebe GW. *A Follow-up Study of War Neuroses*. Washington, DC: US Government Printing Office; 1955.

3. Ripley HS, Wolf S. Long-term study of combat area schizophrenic reactions. *Am J Psychiatry*. 1951;108:409–416.

4. Futterman S, Pumpian-Mindlin E. Traumatic war neuroses five years later. *Am J Psychiatry*. 1951;108:401–408.

5. Archibald HC, Long DM, Miller C, Tuddenham RD. Gross stress reactions in combat: A 15-year follow-up. *Am J Psychiatry*. 1962;119:317–322.

6. Ponteva M. After-effects of mental disorders of war. Presented at VI World Congress of Psychiatry; August 28–September 3, 1977; Honolulu, Hawaii.

7. Meguro K. War neurosis: A 20-year follow-up study. *Seishinigaku*. 1967;8:999–1007 and 9:39–42.

8. Archibald HC, Tuddenham RD. Persistent stress reaction after combat. A 20-year follow-up. *Arch Gen Psychiatry*. 1965;12:475–481.

9. Thienes-Hontos P, Watson CG, Kucala T. Stress-disorder symptoms in Vietnam and Korean war veterans. *J Consult Clin Psychol*. 1982;50:558–561.

10. Figley CR. Symptoms of delayed combat stress among a college sample of Vietnam veterans. *Milit Med.* 1978;143:107–110.

11. Worthington ER. The Vietnam-era veteran, anomie and adjustment. *Milit Med.* 1976;141:169–170.

12. Worthington ER. Demographic and pre-service variables as predictors of post-military service adjustment. In: Figley CR, ed. *Stress Disorders Among Vietnam Veterans.* New York: Brunner/Mazel; 1978: 173–187.

13. Borus JF. Re-entry I. *Arch Gen Psychiatry.* 1973;28:501–506.

14. Borus JF. Re-entry II: "Making it" back in the States. *Am J Psychiatry.* 1973;130:850–854.

15. Borus JF. Re-entry III: Facilitating healthy readjustment in Vietnam veterans. *Psychiatry.* 1973;36:428–429.

16. Borus JF. Incidence of maladjustment in Vietnam returnees. *Arch Gen Psychiatry.* 1974;30:554–557.

17. Wilson JP. *Identity, Ideology, and Crisis: The Vietnam Veteran in Transition: Part II.* (Report to Disabled American Veterans Association). Cleveland: Cleveland State University, Forgotten Warrior Project; 1978.

18. Strayer R, Ellenhorn L. A study exploring adjustment patterns and attitudes. *J Soc Issues.* 1975;31:81–94.

19. Haley, S. Treatment implications of post-combat stress response syndromes for mental health professionals. In: Figley CR, ed. *Stress Disorders Among Vietnam Veterans.* New York: Brunner/Mazel; 1978: 254–257.

20. Figley CR, Southerly WT. Psychosocial adjustment of recently returned veterans. In: Figley CR, Leventman S, eds. *Strangers at Home: Vietnam Veterans Since the War.* New York: Praeger; 1980: 167–180.

21. Brady D, Rappoport L. Violence and Vietnam: A comparison between attitudes of civilians and veterans. *Hum Relat.* 1974;26:735–752.

22. DeFazio VJ, Rustin S, Diamond A. Symptom development in Vietnam era veterans. *J Orthopsychiatry.* 1975;45:158–163.

23. Helzer JE, Robins LN, Wish E, Hesselbrock M. Depression in Vietnam veterans and civilian controls. *Am J Psychiatry.* 1979;136:526–529.

24. Pollock, JC, White D, Gold F. When soldiers return: Combat and political alienation among white Vietnam veterans. In: Schwartz D, Schwartz S, eds. *New Directions in Political Socialization.* New York: Free Press; 1975: 317–333.

25. Wikler NJ. Vietnam and the veterans consciousness. Paper presented at the annual meeting of the Pacific Sociological Association, San Jose, California. March 1974.

26. American Psychiatric Association. *Diagnostic and Statistical Manual of Mental Disorders DSM-III,* 3rd ed. Washington, DC: APA; 1980.

27. *Legacies of Vietnam: Comparative Adjustment of Veterans and Their Peers.* New York: Center for Policy Research; 1981.

28. Disabled American Veterans Association. Forgotten warriors: America's Vietnam era veterans. *DAV.* 1980;Jan.

29. Walker JI, Cavenar JO. Vietnam veterans: Their problems continue. *J Nerv Ment Disease.*1980;170:174–180.

30. Harris L, and Associates. *Myths and Realities: A Study of Attitudes Toward Vietnam Era Veterans.* Submitted by the Veterans Administration to the Committee on Veterans Affairs, U.S. Senate, Senate Committee Print No. 29. Washington, DC: US Government Printing Office; 1980.

31. Schindler FE. Treatment by systematic desensitization of a recurring nightmare of a real life trauma. *J Behav Ther Exp Psychiatry.* 1980;2:53–54.

32. Kulka RA, Schlenger WE, Fairbank JA, et al. *Executive Summary: Contractual Report of Findings from the National Vietnam Veterans Readjustment Study.* Research Triangle Park, NC: Research Triangle Institute; 1988.

33. Stretch R. Post-traumatic stress disorder among US Army Reserve Vietnam and Vietnam-era veterans. *J Consult Clin Psychol.* 1985;53:935–936.

34. Stretch R. Incidence and etiology of post-traumatic stress disorder among active duty Army personnel. *J Appl Soc Psychol.* 1986;16:464–481.

35. Stretch R. PTSD among Vietnam and Vietnam-era veterans. In: Figley CR, ed. *Trauma and Its Wake: The Study and Treatment of Post-Traumatic Stress Disorder.* New York: Brunner/Mazel; 1986: 156–192.

36. Stretch R. Post-traumatic stress disorder and the Canadian Vietnam veteran. *J Traumatic Stress.* 1990;3:239–254.

37. Stretch R. Psychosocial readjustment of Canadian Vietnam veterans. *J Consult Clin Psychol.* 1991;59:188–189.

38. Stretch R, Vail J, Maloney J. Post-traumatic stress disorder among Army Nurse Corps Vietnam veterans. *J Consult Clin Psychol.* 1985;53:704–708.

39. McAndrew B. Viet Nam vets in Canada still feel isolated. *Toronto Star.* 6 July 1986; A9.

Chapter 19

SUMMATION

FRANKLIN D. JONES, M.D., F.A.P.A.* AND GREGORY L. BELENKY, M.D.†

*Colonel (ret), Medical Corps, U.S. Army; Clinical Professor, Uniformed Services University of the Health Sciences, Bethesda, Maryland; Past President and Secretary and currently Honorary President, Military Section of the World Psychiatric Association; formerly Psychiatry and Neurology Consultant, Office of The Surgeon General, U.S. Army

†Colonel, Medical Corps, U.S. Army; Associate Professor, Department of Psychiatry, Uniformed Services University of the Health Sciences, Bethesda, Maryland; Director, Division of Neuropsychiatry, Walter Reed Army Institute of Research, Washington, D.C.; Secretary, Military Section, World Psychiatric Association

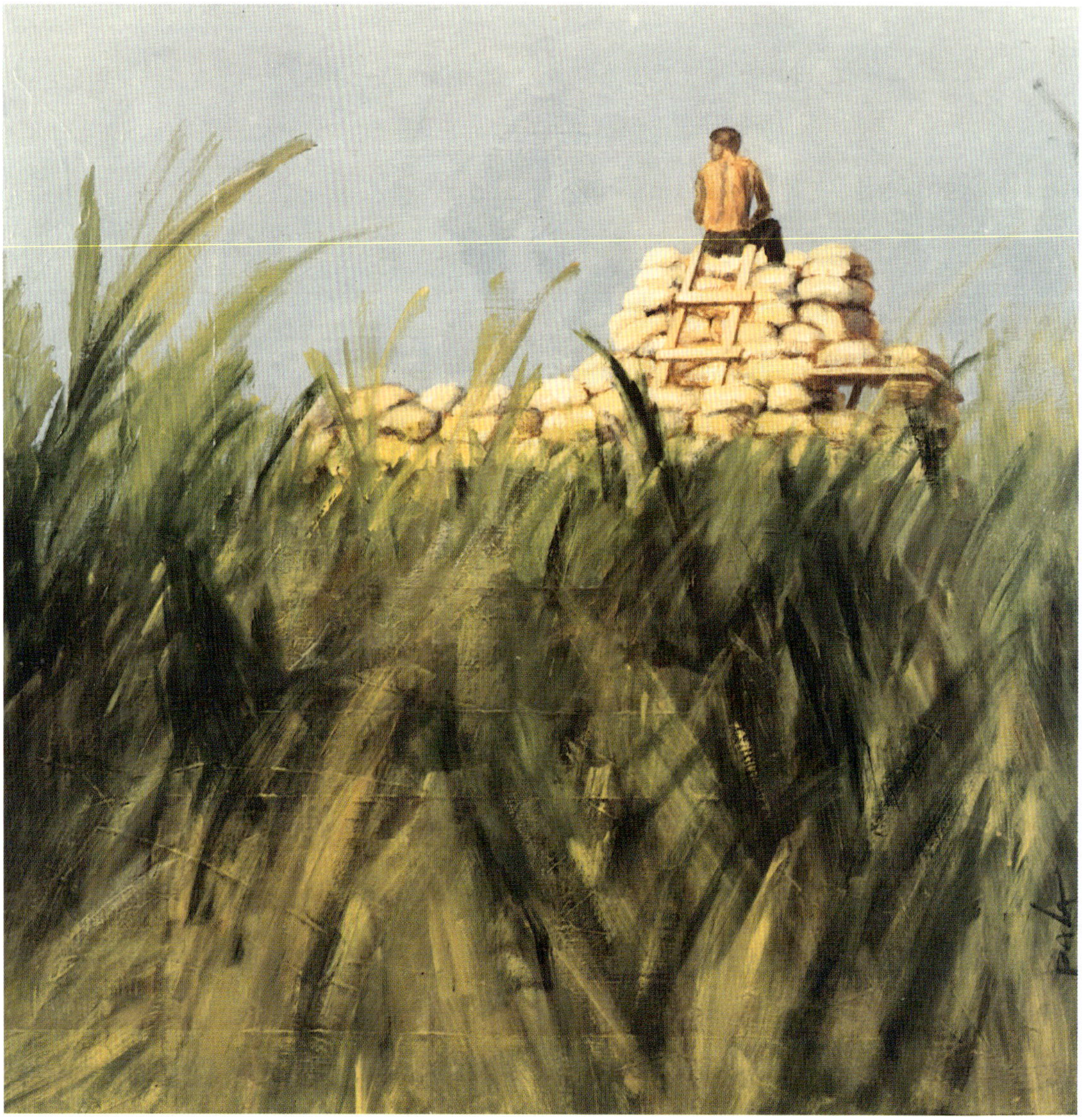

Michael Pala *Sentinel* 1968

Michael Pala was a member of Combat Artist Team #6 in Vietnam during February and March of 1968. His serene painting depicts the individual soldier, on sentry duty, alone with his thoughts. It is the goal of combat psychiatry to provide that soldier with every possible psychological defense against the horrors of the battlefield, and should those defenses fail, to provide him with the timely, caring treatment necessary for his recovery.

Art: Courtesy of US Army Center of Military History, Washington, DC.

LESSONS OF WAR

Role of the Military

The study of civilization is the study of war, preparation for war, and recovery from war. While a few fortunate nations have been spared from the direct ravages of war for a few centuries, most countries have almost continuously been in one of war's stages. Theories of war have considered individual leaders' ambitions, instinctual behaviors, economic forces, religious forces, and cultural forces[1,2] in attempts to understand and control what has largely become not only human but also economic waste. Although in the distant past, wars may have served the winnowing purpose of evolution, most thinkers believe that the few things solved by war are better solved by peace. Furthermore, with the development of atomic weaponry, the existence of humankind itself is threatened. Prevention of war, therefore, is the paramount role of modern military forces.

The authors take the position that the foreseeable future includes the potential for conflict, that preparation for war is paradoxically more likely to result in peace, and that the medical role in this endeavor is critical to its success. For the mental health disciplines, this role encompasses identification and elimination of unfit personnel, improvement of marginal personnel to standards of acceptability, prevention of psychiatric casualties, and treatment of casualties when prevention fails. All of these efforts must be guided by past experience and sound principles of human behavior. Failures have occurred in all of these categories.

Selection of Personnel

Many studies reviewed by Arthur[3] reveal that mass psychiatric screening of personnel for induction into the military beyond minimal testing for normal intelligence, absence of psychotic disorders, and absence of significant criminal behavior is markedly inefficient. Following World War I, which had resulted in large numbers of psychiatric casualties, an attempt was made at the beginning of World War II to reject draft registrants who might break down in combat.

The identification and elimination of allegedly mentally unfit personnel threatened the war effort early in the United States' entry into World War II. Guided by the theory that soldiers who had exhibited any prior symptoms of anxiety would be prone to breakdown, medical personnel were at one point eliminating almost as many soldiers as were being recruited.[4,5] By contrast, the less stringent screening of soldiers in World War I resulted in adequate soldiers for the fight. Furthermore, review of casualty breakdown in World War II[6] revealed that breakdown was largely related to unit and battle conditions rather than predisposition, while studies of casualties from World War II[7] and the Arab-Israeli wars[8] revealed that soldiers who had broken down in combat, when properly treated, were at no greater risk of another breakdown than their cohorts who had not broken down.

Menninger[9] reviewed World War I and World War II statistics and showed that the liberal selection policy of World War I resulted in the rejection of about 2% of soldiers at induction for neuropsychiatric reasons and about 2% breakdown of the total, while the more stringent policy of World War II resulted in the rejection of 11% of inductees but a higher rate of breakdown of 12% of the total.[9]

Although about 1,600,000 registrants were classified as unfit for induction during World War II because of mental disease or educational deficiency (a disqualification rate about 7.6 times as high as in World War I), separation rates for psychiatric disorders in World War II were 2.4 times as high as in World War I.[6] Not only was screening ineffective in preventing breakdown, but also the liberal separation policy for those presenting with neurotic symptoms threatened the war effort.[6] For instance, in September 1943 almost as many soldiers were being eliminated from the U.S. Army as accessed; most of those separated were for psychoneurosis (35.6/1,000/y).[6(p740)]

Studies attempting to find predisposition to psychiatric breakdown in combat have revealed more similarities between psychiatric casualties and their fellow soldiers than differences. For example, in a comparison of the combat records of 100 men who suffered psychiatric breakdowns requiring evacuation to a U.S. Army hospital in the continental United States and an equivalent group of 100 surgical casualties, Pratt[10] found no significant difference in numbers of awards for bravery. Glass remarked, "Out of these experiences came an awareness that social and situational determinants of behavior were more important than the assets and liabilities of individuals involved in coping with wartime stress and strain."[7(p1024)]

Improvement of marginal personnel to meet standards has been successful in at least two conflicts. During the Vietnam conflict, Secretary of Defense McNamara ordered the recruitment of soldiers with minor unfitting conditions (most were slow learners or soldiers with personality disorders) who were to be given special training and to serve in combat (Project 100,000). While a higher percentage of these soldiers had to repeat basic training and had general discharges for unfitness, the great majority served in a satisfactory fashion. The program was successful enough that the number of drafted lower-functioning soldiers exceeded the original 100,000 planned: 320,000 were inducted. While many low-aptitude veterans did well in the military, their postmilitary civilian adjustment was not as good as that of a comparable nonveteran civilian comparison group, being disproportionately unemployed, unmarried, underpaid, and undereducated.[11]

Israel has developed special programs to train soldiers who otherwise could not serve. Most of these men are from families displaced from Arabic countries. They are often illiterate and don't speak Hebrew. Also they are often poorly motivated. The program utilizes women drill sergeants to inspire the soldiers' best efforts. The training includes also a basic education in Hebrew literacy and Israeli cultural values. These soldiers have acquitted themselves well in Israel's ongoing conflicts with Arab neighbors. An important aspect of soldier support is the family. It is known that family stress can adversely affect a soldier and lead to combat breakdown.

Training of Personnel

Training of personnel involves several important dimensions: technical proficiency, personality characteristics, strength and endurance, group cohesiveness, and stress inoculation. There is considerable overlap in all of these areas; for example, technical proficiency, which may require strength and endurance, leads to the personality characteristic of self-confidence, which, along with technical proficiency, produces a sense of mastery and value to the group, promoting group cohesion. All of these characteristics are positively associated with the ability to withstand combat stress.

Much of military training addresses all of these dimensions. Shared vigorous training not only increases strength and endurance and builds self-confidence, but also increases group affiliation and cohesion.[12] Aware of the importance of cohesion, the military has kept personnel together in cohort units from basic training to deployment. In addition, efforts have been made to keep commanders with the same unit for longer periods of time to enhance not only horizontal (peers) but also vertical (hierarchical) cohesion.

An important aspect of combat training is the need for realism. Troops new to combat are known to be more vulnerable to combat stress reactions than experienced troops. Realistic training with live ammunition and actual danger is believed to act as an "inoculation" against battlefield stress. Unfortunately such training inevitably results in an irreducible small number of casualties. Technical proficiency is increasingly being accomplished with computer simulations. With technological innovations involving "virtual reality," perhaps the desired realism in combat simulations is on the horizon. Or could training with no element of real fear and physical discomfort lead to a false sense of confidence which shatters in the face of imminent life threat? Some combination of "live" and "virtual" reality may be needed.

Rediscovery and Extensive Application of Principles

The United States became involved in World War II (1939–1945) 2 years after its outbreak. Over 20 years had passed since the end of World War I, and at the onset of American involvement in World War II, military medical personnel were unprepared to carry out the program of forward psychiatry that had been devised by World War I psychiatrists.[9] No psychiatrists were assigned to combat divisions and no provisions for special psychiatric treatment units at the field army level or communications zone had been made.[6] American planners had believed that potential psychiatric casualties could be screened out prior to induction.

World War I style forward treatment was relearned during two battles of the Tunisian Campaign in March and April 1943.[13] Captain Fred Hanson avoided evacuation and returned more than 70% of 494 neuropsychiatric patients to combat after 48 hours of treatment, which basically consisted of resting the soldier and indicating to him that he would soon rejoin his unit.[13] General Omar Bradley issued a directive that established a holding period of 7 days for psychiatric patients and further prescribed the term "exhaustion" as the initial diagnosis for all combat psychiatric cases. The World War I principles had been rediscovered!

Discovery of Mediating Principles

In addition to rediscovering the principles of treatment applied so effectively in World War I, and the ineffectiveness of large-scale screening, World War II psychiatrists learned about the epidemiology of combat stress casualties (direct relationship to intensity of combat, modified by physical and morale factors) and the importance of unit cohesion both in preventing breakdown and in enhancing combat effectiveness.

Another finding during World War II was the chronology of breakdown in combat. It had long been recognized that "new" and "old" men in combat units were more prone to breakdown. "New" or inexperienced troops were more likely to become stress casualties and have usually accounted for over three fourths of stress casualties; however, with increasing exposure to combat after 1 or 2 combat months, an increasing rate of casualty generation also occurs.

From studies of cumulative stress such as these as well as observations of the efficacy of a "point system" (so many points of credit toward rotation from combat per unit of time in combat or so many combat missions of aircrews) used during World War II, the value of periodic rest from combat and of rotation came to be understood and applied in the Korean and Vietnam conflicts with fixed combat tours. The final and perhaps most important lesson of World War II was the importance of group cohesion not only in preventing breakdown, but also in producing effectiveness in combat.[7]

Prevention of Psychiatric Casualties

Prevention of psychiatric casualties must address the factors known to be important in soldier efficiency and breakdown. These can be grouped into biological, interpersonal, and intrapsychic factors. In terms of biological factors, commanders must enforce salt and water discipline to avoid dehydration and sleep discipline to prevent exhaustion and to counter time-zone dislocation. During the U.S. invasion of Grenada, dehydration and accidents accounted for a majority of U.S. casualties.[14]

Interpersonal factors may be the most critical in terms of preventing psychiatric casualties. Soldiers living and working together in conditions of shared danger and hardship will foster unit cohesion. During the 1973 surprise attack by Arab forces, the Israelis had to be quickly mobilized. This resulted in some tank crews going into battle with teammates who were strangers. Such crews, who obviously lacked cohesion, had far higher psychiatric casualty rates than those in which soldiers had trained together, sometimes for years. The leader must partake of these dangers and hardships, display concern for his soldiers, and demonstrate expertise in battle. In a survey of Israeli soldier factors in morale, the commander's battle competence was the most highly rated attribute.[15]

When combat is imminent, the commander should brief the small unit on what is to be expected. This briefing should be realistic but not pessimistic. After combat, the commander should lead the small group in a debriefing in which each combatant has an opportunity to describe the action. This group debriefing allows correction of misinterpretations, recognition of individual performance, and consolidation of lessons learned. It also strengthens cohesive bonds.

Another important aspect of prevention is arranging for rest from battle, preferably on a unit basis. During World War II, aircrews were relieved of duty after a fixed number of combat flights, roughly the number at which on a statistical basis there was a better than 50% chance of survival. During the Korean conflict the combat tour was 9 months while the support troops served 13 months. During the Vietnam conflict the tour for all was 12 months with 4 to 6 days of "R and R" (rest and recreation) approximately midway through the tour. Unfortunately, rest from the combat zone and completion of the tour were on an individual rather than unit basis, degrading cohesion.

Impediments to Cohesion

Among the alleged impediments to unit cohesion are race, gender, ethnicity, and sexual preference. The military has adopted policies to overcome all of these issues except the last. All units have been racially integrated since the Korean conflict. Women have entered all military roles other than ground combat and submarine warfare. Educational programs such as Black History, Hispanic History, Native American History, and Asian-Pacific History weeks are overcoming ethnic stereotypes. Homosexuality remains controversial, being viewed as detrimental to morale and discipline. Change in this area may occur through judicial or legislative action; however, President Clinton has indicated his desire to end discrimination against homosexuals in the military.[16] Because there is no law against homosexuality in the military, this could be accomplished by executive order; however, the Uniform Code of Military Justice describes sodomy, homosexual or heterosexual, as a felony. Changing this would require an act of Congress.

There is speculation that the ability to bond in small groups for relatively brief periods of time for hunting or fighting is to an extent gender specific. This might explain the observation that women have never been a significant element in front line combat forces in hundreds of societies for which there are records. The female child-bearing role, leading ultimately to social role differentiation of males and females, however, does not allow the determination of whether there are any biologically determined differences between males and females in group bonding. Although averages of physical differences between males and females such as upper body strength (greater in males) and rate of secretion of medullary adrenal hormones (more rapid in males) may be significant, individuals often excel in feats of skill and strength regardless of sex.

Future wars may require the military to select individuals for roles based on innate and learned differences rather than sexual stereotypes. Such selections may place women in leadership positions that involve skills in communication and vigilance tasks as well as direct combat roles. As an example, tanks with a lower profile on the horizon are more difficult to sight and hit. The former Soviets reportedly selected short men for tank crews in order to fit them into a lower tank profile. Perhaps short women will some day fill such roles. With the expected reduction of the combat age demographic pool, the United States will be under even greater pressure to utilize women in combat roles. In the assignment of combat pilots General H. Norman Schwartzkopf, commander of coalition forces in the Persian Gulf War, has indicated that women should have been assigned combat roles.[17]

Personal Factors in Combat Stress

The soldier brings with him many, sometimes conflicting, intrapsychic beliefs and attitudes that must be modified by skillful training to produce the most effective soldier. The late adolescent soldier has been a preferred recruit in the past because of malleability and certain inherent attitudes. The malleability applies to the normal lack of career definition and identity of most late adolescents. Furthermore, these older adolescents usually have a sense of invulnerability which Masserman[18] has termed one of the Ur-defenses (or delusions) of humans. The first author has argued in Chapter 1, Psychiatric Lessons of War, that it is the loss of such defenses that produces breakdown on an individual basis. Shaw[19] has pointed out that the treatment of the combat psychiatric casualty near the front with replenishment of physiological deficits and expectation of return to one's unit shores up these failing defenses.

Stress Inoculation

Another aspect of prevention is exposure to realistic combat training. It is well-known that so called "green troops" not previously in combat become stress casualties in disproportionately high numbers. This was recognized by U.S. Civil War commanders who sought to "blood" their men in combat to improve their fighting efficiency.[20] It was argued that this "blooding" increased feelings of comradeship and desire for revenge against the enemy. Some forms of severe stress do not inoculate but increase vulnerability to subsequent stress as seen in a study[21] of elderly holocaust survivors who were exposed to missile strike threats during the Persian Gulf War. This would be in consonance with the observation that repeated severe trauma leads to breakdown as seen in the "old sergeant syndrome."[22] As mentioned earlier, the advent of computer simulations exposing combatants to virtual reality (VR) training may be the most realistic training short of combat.

Another potent effect deriving from our current understanding of the theory of behavior therapy involves the process of habituation.[23] Exposure to a situation producing severe anxiety results in reduction of anxiety when no aversive stimulation occurs. This may account for the observation that combat veterans are less likely to be overwhelmed by anxiety. Paradoxically, however, repeated exposure to combat may eventually result in breakdown, presumably due to the erosion of feelings of invulnerability (loss of Ur-defenses) occasioned by the deaths of comrades. Thus an aspect of prevention is the removal of soldiers from combat periodically to prevent breakdown. A fixed tour of 12 months in the Vietnam conflict and a week of "R and R" (rest and recreation) about one half of the way through the year's tour may have resulted in combat stress casualties that were among the lowest of any conflict (11/1,000/y).[24] This rate was about the same as that for soldiers not in combat stationed in Korea at the same time (13/1,000/y).[24]

TREATMENT OF PSYCHIATRIC CASUALTIES

The deceptively simple measures employed since World War I and embodied in Artiss'[4] proximity, immediacy, and expectancy ("PIE") conceptualization, broadened into D. Jones' "BICEPS" acronym (brevity, immediacy, centrality, expectancy, proximity, simplicity as discussed in Chapter 8, U.S. Air Force Combat Psychiatry) remain the mainstay of traditional treatment of psychiatric casualties. Chapter 2, Traditional Warfare Combat Stress Casualties, has shown that the therapeutic basis of these measures is expectancy. A casualty treated briefly and immediately has less opportunity to dwell on the potential for death and maiming. Such treatment involving simple measures of replenishment of nutrition and sleep, taking place in a safe area near the battle area (and near the soldier's own unit), produces a powerful and explicit expectancy that after a period of rest the soldier will return to his own unit for which the cohesive bonds have not been attenuated. Centrality carries the additional principle that prior to evacuation out of the combat zone psychiatric casualties are collected at a centralized location at which skilled mental health professionals are expected to return a significant portion of such casualties back to combat zone duty.

Technological advances have jeopardized the applicability of these principles in modern warfare. Sophisticated intelligence gathering (sometimes by satellites), highly mobile forces, and continuous fighting even at support levels in the battlefield may not allow for a safe forward treating area or the return of a soldier to his own unit. In such circumstances, new principles of intervention involving prevention, "buddy aid," and possible use of medications may be required.

In summary, World War II taught combat psychiatrists that psychiatric casualties are an inevitable consequence of life-threatening hostilities; that they cannot be efficiently screened out ahead of time; that their numbers depend on individual, unit, and combat environmental factors; and that appropriate interventions can return the majority to combat duty.

Low-Intensity vs Traditional Combat Stress

The authors have used terms such as low-, mid-, and high-intensity combat somewhat differently from many military writers. For example, high-intensity combat is restricted to nuclear and chemical/biological warfare by some writers. The authors feel that conventional warfare is of high intensity when it involves continuous or near continuous fighting with numerous pulses of battle in a 24-hour period. Similarly, the authors feel that battle is of low intensity when battles are brief and infrequent, allowing for recuperation between battles. Thus, terrorist attacks would be of low intensity even though resulting in large numbers of killed and wounded as occurred in the bombing of a U.S. Marine Corps barracks in Beirut in 1985.[25]

Just as in the initial battles of World War II, provisions had not been made for psychiatric casualties in the early months of the Korean conflict (1950–1953). As a result they were evacuated from the combat zone. Because only 5 years had elapsed, the lessons of World War II were still well known and the principles learned during that war were applied appropriately after the initial period of confusion, due to the efforts of Colonel Albert J. Glass, the Neuropsychiatry Consultant and a World War II veteran.[26] Psychiatric casualties accounted for only about 5% of medical out-of-country evacuations, and some of these (treated in Japan) were returned to the combat zone. To prevent the "old sergeant syndrome," a rotation system was in effect—9 months in combat or 13 months in support units. Attempts were made to rest individuals ("R and R" or rest and recreation) and, if tactically possible, whole units.

In the Korean conflict many soldiers also presented with frostbite, a usually preventable disorder. These physical disorders were often actually masked psychiatric casualties. It is important to identify and avoid evacuation of hidden psychiatric casualties. Such casualties may be as transparent as one with a helmet headache or as subtle as development of malaria from failure to take chemo-prophylaxis or development of frostbite or immersion foot from failure to maintain foot hygiene.

Low-Intensity Combat Stress Casualties

An unrecognized portent of psychiatric problems of future wars was the psychiatric problems of rear-area support troops. As the Korean conflict progressed, U.S. support troops increased in number until they greatly outnumbered combat troops. These support troops were seldom in life-endangering situations. Their psychological stresses were related more to separation from home and friends, social and sometimes physical deprivations, and boredom. Paradoxically, support troops who may have avoided the stress of combat, according to a military historian[27] and a combat veteran,[28] were deprived of the enhancement of self-esteem provided by such exposure. To an extent the situation resembled that of the nostalgic soldiers of prior centuries. In these circumstances the soldier sought relief in alcohol abuse and, in coastal areas, in drug abuse, and sexual stimulation. These often resulted in disciplinary infractions. Except for attempts to prevent venereal diseases, these problems were scarcely noticed at the time, a lesson not learned.

The Korean conflict confirmed that the appropriate use of the principles of combat psychiatry could result in the return to battle of up to 90% of combat psychiatric casualties; however, there was a failure to recognize the types of casualties that can occur among rear-echelon soldiers. These "garrison casualties" later became the predominant psychiatric casualties of the Vietnam conflict.[29,30] Vietnam and the Arab-Israeli wars revealed limitations to the traditional principles of combat psychiatry.

The epidemiology of psychiatric casualties among troops in battle emphasizes those that resulted from battlefield stress (eg, anxiety, fatigue, hysterical syndromes). However, casualties resulting from less dramatic causes had been recognized since World War I. These less dramatic casualties, more common in rear-echelon or garrison settings, presented with problems of alcohol and drug abuse, disciplinary infractions, venereal diseases, personality disorders, and "self-inflicted" medical disorders (for example, malaria from failure to use prophylaxis). Not until the Vietnam conflict were these casualties recognized as potentially serious causes of ineffectiveness.

It is not surprising then that various authors have called such casualties "garrison casualties"[29,31] and "nostalgic casualties."[32] Nostalgic casualties occur in soldiers separated from their home environment with attendant loss of social reinforcement. Rosen[33] has pointed out that one need not be a soldier for this to occur and that displaced persons and other groups often suffer from this "forgotten" psychological disorder. Situations such as the fighting of an unpopular war of indefinite duration are likely to increase these casualties, particularly in the absence of strong cohesive forces, which usually develop from shared hardship and danger.[12] In combat situations, cohesion needs little encouragement to flourish. Low-intensity warfare, often characterized by long periods of idleness without the shared experience of cohesion-building danger, should produce more nostalgic casualties. This situation probably also accounts for the higher incidence of such casualties among support than among combat troops.[34]

PSYCHIATRIC SYNDROMES

Combat fatigue was designed as a nonspecific label carrying an implication that the soldier is normal and will recover with rest. It subsumes a great variety of behaviors that in modern nomenclatures might be given such labels as adjustment disorders, somatoform disorders (conversion reaction), dissociative disorders, or post-traumatic stress disorder (PTSD). Because conversion disorders and PTSD have presented in most wars and their mismanagement can be devastating, they deserve special consideration. Similarly, psychological reactions to maiming injuries and central nervous system (CNS) injuries were considered separately.

Post-Traumatic Stress Disorders

Chronic PTSD has come to be recognized as a common sequel of severe stress whether experienced in combat, disasters, prisoner of war or hostage status, torture, or sexual and physical assault. Perhaps because of the potential for "secondary gain" or inadvertent positive reinforcement of the invalid or sickness role, militaries have been ambivalent about expending medical resources for such casualties. For example, following World War I German psychiatrists gave generous treatment and pensions to psychiatric casualties and were rewarded by seeing their numbers grow. After World War II, however, and based on World War I experience, German psychiatrists did not grant pensions for nonpsychotic conditions; their numbers then were few.[35] Despite the potential for abuse of the PTSD diagnosis, those calculating the gains and losses from combat must include these casualties in their deliberations. Figures from World War I and World War II reveal that about one fourth of those seeking chronic care in Veterans Administration hospitals would fall into this group although they were usually given various neurotic diagnoses.

To the heterogeneous syndromes of substance abuse, indiscipline, and sexual problems found in low-intensity wars that have been labeled disorders of frustration and loneliness or "nostalgic casualties" should be added chronic and delayed post-traumatic stress disorders (chronic and delayed PTSD). PTSD is usually and appropriately thought of in the context of acute overwhelming stress; however, the frequent morale problems of low-intensity, ambiguous wars may carry over into the postwar lives of the former combatants. The current discontents of these war veterans may find expression in the reappearance or new appearance of symptoms associated with combat: anxiety and fears, autonomic hyperactivity, reliving of psychologically traumatic events, and a variety of other malaises. Such symptoms often follow service in wars of high intensity as well, particularly when the outcome was unsatisfactory or there is psychological or financial gain from such symptoms.

Prevention and Treatment of Low-Intensity Combat Stress Disorders

Although successful treatments for low-intensity combat stress casualties were developed as early as the Napoleonic Wars, circumstances can prevent the application of remedies. For example, during the Vietnam conflict the 1-year rotation policy, ostensibly for the purpose of preventing psychiatric casualties due to cumulative stress, the policy of rotating commanders out of combat units after 6 (and later only 3) months in order to give more officers combat experience, and the policy of individual replacement of losses rather than unit replacements all interacted to impair unit cohesion, which might have prevented some of the nostalgic casualties.

Vietnam revealed the limits of World War II type psychiatric treatment policy in a low-intensity, prolonged, unpopular conflict. Such conflicts, if they cannot be avoided, must be approached with primary prevention as the focus. Career soldiers with strong unit cohesion will not endanger themselves, their fellows, or their careers by abusing alcohol or drugs.

While prevention through development of unit cohesion and morale is as important for disorders of loneliness and frustration as for combat stress casualties, likewise treatment follows principles of disallowing evacuation from the combat zone, and measures to strengthen unit cohesion. A preventive measure among support troops would involve allowing them to function in combat roles. Unlike the handling of combat stress treatment failures through medical evacuation, disorders of loneliness and frustration may be handled through administrative and disciplinary measures.

Sexually transmitted diseases (venereal diseases or VD) have been a major cause of lost soldier strength in wars of the twentieth century. While modern medicine has markedly reduced the time lost and complications of venereal diseases, it has not reduced the infection rates. Although unlikely to have immediate effects on combat efficiency, the HIV virus poses severe problems in long-term prevention. Many of the world social tensions and ongoing wars are occurring in Africa, where the HIV infection is reaching epidemic proportions. Unlike in the United States, where the populations at risk are mainly homosexuals and intravenous drug abusers and their consorts, the spread of HIV in Africa is primarily through heterosexual intercourse.

In South America, another politically troubled area with narcoterrorism, or communist insurgencies, or both, in several countries, acquired immunodeficiency syndrome (AIDS) is emerging as a difficult public health problem. Because urban areas in these third-world countries are being hit hardest by AIDS, there is concern that the professional and leadership classes of African, and to a lesser extent South American, countries could experience severe setbacks in goals of industrialization and democratic reforms. Internal unrest in Latin America frequently has led to U.S. military deployment beginning before 1900.

The main lessons from the U.S. experience in managing substance abuse in Vietnam are that treatment should be in country to prevent an evacuation syndrome and that the factors that prevent breakdown in general—cohesion, effective leadership, and good morale—may protect soldiers from substance abuse. Avoidance of idleness and medical supervision of brothels may further minimize nostalgic casualties.

The appropriate treatment of acute combat stress casualties will decrease the later development of chronic post-traumatic stress disorders. Other measures to prevent chronic PTSD include the previously mentioned combat stress debriefing (see Chapter 11, Debriefing Following Combat), which has been adapted to civilian critical incident stress debriefing. In treating the maimed or disfigured, or patients with physical losses (amputees, blinded, paralyzed), prevention of chronic PTSD is assisted by avoiding an invalid role and emphasizing what the person can do rather than cannot do.

FUTURE COMBAT

Future wars may differ drastically from previous wars. Although the former Soviet nation states are mostly considered allies or at least neutral to the North Atlantic Treaty Organization (NATO) allies and NATO has overwhelming military superiority, conflicts with nations that have advanced military technology are possible. This was demonstrated in the Persian Gulf War in which Iraq launched missiles resulting in military and civilian casualties and posed the potential risk of mass casualties.

Future wars that pose the risk of use of weapons of mass destruction will require dispersion and mobility of allied forces. Furthermore, a technologically advanced enemy may possess sensors capable of detecting aggregations of materials and personnel. This scenario would severely challenge the traditional applications of the principles of combat psychiatry. Prevention and far-forward consultation and intervention must be given maximal emphasis in the future.

Combat psychiatric treatment requires a relatively safe setting near the battle area in which mental health personnel can render simple supportive treatment followed by return of the casualty to his own unit. The ability to target aggregations of personnel and equipment will mean that treatment settings must be mobile or be left far from the battlefield. The dispersion and mobility of tactical units will make it very difficult to return casualties to their own units.

Despite strenuous efforts of prevention including strengthening unit cohesion, avoiding physiological deficits, and optimizing personality variables, psychiatric casualties will occur. Treatment of these casualties requires development of new principles of management. Combatants will need to recognize combat stress reactions in themselves and their comrades and take remedial action. This may be as simple as arranging for nutritional and sleep replenishment. It may include reassurance from a squad leader, commander, or medical aidman. It is possible that a rapid-acting, nonsedating, nonaddictive antianxiety drug may be developed to treat soldiers on the battlefield.

Currently buspirone (BuSpar), an azapirone, with partial serotonin agonist actions, is a nonsedating, nonaddicting anxiolytic; however, it has an approximately 10-day latency prior to its therapeutic effects. Furthermore, buspirone's activating effects may not be desirable and may interfere with sleep. It may prove useful in returning refractory cases to duty. The recent development of a benzodiazepine antagonist, flumazenil (Romazicon), that can rapidly reverse benzodiazepine hypnotics, may allow the use of such hypnotics on or near the battlefield. The notion that medicated soldiers would lack compassion and would release inappropriate aggression[36] has little basis in fact or theory.

If a combat stress casualty is evacuated and cannot be returned to his own unit, it may be possible to incorporate him into a newly created unit of such casualties under suitably trained senior leaders. This may be necessary anyway if units are markedly degraded in mass casualty actions. Creating such units would be a formidable but accomplishable task utilizing known techniques to create cohesion and morale; however, it would probably require several weeks of intensive work with mental health professionals.

Areas of Current Study and Suggestions for Future Research

While the military has learned much about sustaining the combat member and treating those who break down, there are many areas that need clarification. Issues include not only ideal socialization of the soldier but training targeted to individual strengths and weaknesses, a full understanding of the biology at the molecular level of combat sustenance, and breakdown and ideal treatment of the ineffective combatant. Research in these areas is ongoing.

Prevention of Combat Stress Casualties: Sustaining the Soldier in Combat

Anything that improves soldier effectiveness decreases combat stress casualties and conversely anything that degrades soldier effectiveness increases combat stress casualties. Thus, the net of prevention of combat stress casualties can be cast broadly to include almost all improvements in doctrine, command, control, communications, and intelligence (C^3I), training; logistics; rations; and equipment.

In the biobehavioral area, improvements in the means of sustaining the soldier physiologically and psychologically all contribute to increased combat effectiveness and decreased combat stress casualties. Social psychological research into ways of enhancing unit morale, leadership, and cohesion could better sustain the soldier by improving his unit. Similarly, research into better ways of sustaining the soldier physiologically in terms of nutrition, hydration, rest, and recuperation could improve soldier performance and thus enhance the unit. Neurobiological investigations into brain changes accompanying acute combat stress reactions and in particular those associated with the development of PTSD would be of great value in suggesting new means of prevention and treatment.

A productive area of current research in the realm of physiological sustainment is in sleep, sleep deprivation, and continuous operations. It is representative of a number of areas in which advances in biomedicine are finding application in sustaining soldiers in combat. Sleep deprivation is a frequent associated finding in cases of acute combat stress reaction. Sleep deprivation-induced decrements in performance frequently contribute to the occurrence of incidents of friendly fire. In the work on sleep, sleep deprivation, and continuous operations, experimentation and modeling are being combined to advance the understanding of the effect of sleep deprivation on performance.

Recent laboratory work has shown that caffeine is effective in sustaining performance in continuous operations and has led to the recommendation that caffeine-containing bars or tablets be added to the meal-ready-to-eat (MRE). Recent modeling of company-sized unit performance has shown that although soldiers can fight while averaging 4 hours of sleep each night, their performance degrades rapidly. For indefinite sustainability of performance without degradation over time, soldiers need 8 hours of sleep each night. This suggests that while some sleep deprivation may be inevitable in continuous combat operations, depriving soldiers of sleep should be as a result of the exigencies of the combat situation, and not a result of deliberate policy.

Work is underway to identify the physiological changes in the brain that accompany the performance degradation in sleep deprivation. These studies involve positron emission tomography (PET), fast magnetic resonance imaging (fMRI), and other physiological as well as behavioral measures. Initial findings show that the performance degradation in sleep deprivation is associated with a decrease in global brain energy metabolism. These studies of basic mechanisms will lead to the development of novel, safe, and effective pharmaceuticals to sustain soldier performance during continuous operations.

Work is also underway to develop safe and effective sleep-inducing drugs to promote brief, recuperative sleep during continuous operations. As sleep's recuperative value depends both upon duration and continuity, the hope is to find a nonaddictive, nonperformance-impairing, sleep-inducing drug that will initiate and sustain unfragmented sleep in the nonsleep conducive conditions of continuous combat operations. Work is currently underway, as suggested earlier in this chapter, to study the effectiveness of triazolam (a benzodiazepine) for initiating and maintaining sleep in combination with flumazenil (a benzodiazepine antagonist) for rapidly restoring alertness upon awakening.

As part of a broad effort to develop unobtrusive, robust, field-deployable biomedical telemetry to monitor soldier status during combat operations, work is underway on the application of artificial neural networks to the discrimination of alert from drowsy electroencephalograms, to provide an online, real-time assessment of soldier alertness for feedback to the soldier and for relay up the chain of command. These systems would be an integral part of the soldier computer, which in turn will be standard equipment for the soldier in the 21st century. Information about each soldier's status would be fed back to the soldier and shared with his comrades and his chain of command through a radiofrequency, local area network (RF-LAN).

Treatment of Acute Combat Stress and Prevention of PTSD

As is clear from previous chapters, the treatment of acute combat stress casualties and the prevention of PTSD are often one and the same thing. Anecdotal accounts from World War I to the present and the few formal studies that have been conducted clearly indicate that successful brief, forward treatment of an acute combat stress casualty reduces the risk of that casualty's subsequently developing PTSD. However, soldiers develop PTSD without having an antecedent history of an acute combat stress reaction. Because traumatic events are unavoidable in combat operations, are there means of preventing the later development of PTSD in soldiers who continue to perform well during the actual events and hence do not come for immediate treatment? Here, anecdotally, the routine application of after-action debriefings and event reconstructions after every major battle, engagement, or otherwise traumatic event, appears to be useful. Carefully controlled studies of the value of after-action debriefings and event reconstructions following traumatic events in the prevention of later PTSD would confirm the value of this technique.

A further, heretofore almost untouched, area for research is the utility of psychotropic medications in the treatment of acute combat stress reactions and in the prevention of PTSD. Anecdotally, benzodiazepines appear to delay recovery of acute combat stress reactions and to foster evolution of the stress reaction into PTSD. Benzodiazepines may be the pharmacological equivalent of evacuation to the rear in terms of their deleterious effects. Whether antidepressant drugs, especially the new selective serotonergic, noradrenergic, and dopaminergic reuptake inhibitors, could play a useful role in the treatment of acute combat stress reactions remains to be investigated. Whether these agents alone, or in combination with after-action debriefing and event reconstruction, could be of use in the prevention of PTSD is an open question as well and one well worth investigating.

CONCLUSION

This review of warfare reveals certain recurring themes concerning soldiers who persevere in combat vs those who break down in combat. Both groups are often quite similar as individuals (and may even be the same individuals); however, their social situations are markedly different. The social situations consist of a matrix of factors that determine whether the soldier excels or breaks down.

Thus, in adapting to combat, as in all survival-relevant activities, humans respond holistically. Their physical, intrapsychic, and social states form this matrix of factors that influences their responses to environmental danger. In combat, deep urgings for individual survival often conflict with socially conditioned expectations, requirements, and desires for "soldierly conduct," that have been embodied in ideals such as patriotism, discipline, loyalty to comrades, and identification with the leader.

To prevent combat breakdown the presence of mission-oriented small group cohesion is essential. Cohesion is fostered by good leadership and by having soldiers train, live, and experience stress together. Further preventive measures include adequate rest, sleep, and nutrition so that chronic or acute fatigue does not develop. Rest from battle should ideally occur through small group rotation so that group support is continuous. Commanders should be open and honest with their subordinates to build trust and vertical cohesion and to enhance the soldier's understanding of the importance of his contribution to the unit mission and the national interest. The soldier must believe that the entire society supports him in suffering privations and sacrifices.

Factors that foster psychiatric breakdown are the negatives of the preventive factors: poor leadership, cohesion, and training; inadequate social support; and the buildup of fatigue. Factors that emphasize perceptions of individual or collective vulnerability increase the probability of psychiatric breakdown. This accounts for the strong relationship between intensity of combat (as measured by wounded and killed in action) and numbers of stress casualties. It also accounts for the observation that death of a comrade was the most common precipitant of breakdown during World War II. A feeling of helplessness in controlling one's fate also exacerbates stress and weakens resistance. This is seen in the increased stress casualties that occur in circumstances of indirect fire such as artillery or bombing barrages, or gas attacks compared with the direct fire situation (even though the wounded and killed rate may be the same or higher than under indirect fire).

After a soldier has become a psychiatric casualty, it is important to restore as many positive factors as possible: rest, sleep, and nutrition. Bonds to the unit are kept intact with expectation of return to the unit, hence the importance of treating as far forward and as quickly as possible. Treatment must be kept simple to emphasize the normality of the soldier's experience rather than give an imputation of mental illness. In garrison or rear-echelon settings, prevention is even more important because the disorders that occur (alcohol and drug abuse, character disorders, and sexual problems) are even more difficult to treat than combat stress disorders. In rear-echelon settings, attention should be paid to discipline, morale-enhancing activities, and recognition of the critical role played by support troops. Communication between support troops and those they support should be encouraged. Temporary assignment to combat units should be available. Infractions should be dealt with through forward rather than rearward evacuation to minimize secondary gain from misbehavior.

Prevention of combat stress casualties is primarily a command responsibility but the medical person, through consultation with command and avoidance of medical "evacuation syndromes," plays a critical role in this endeavor. The psychiatric lessons of war can profitably be applied to military communities during peacetime as well as to civilian communities.

REFERENCES

1. Freud S. *Civilization and its Discontents 1930*. New York: WW Norton; 1962.

2. Lorenz K. *On Aggression*. New York: Bantam; 1966: 228–265.

3. Arthur RJ. Success is predictable. *Milit Med*. 1971;136(6):539–545.

4. Artiss KL. Human behavior under stress: From combat to social psychiatry. *Milit Med*. 1963;128(10):1011–1015.

5. Ginsberg E, Anderson JK, Ginsberg SW, Herma JL. *The Ineffective Soldier: Patterns of Performance*. New York: Columbia University Press; 1959: 11.

6. Glass AJ. Lessons learned. In: Glass AJ, Bernucci R, eds. *Zone of Interior*. Vol 1. In: *Neuropsychiatry in World War II*. Washington, DC: Office of The Surgeon General, US Army; 1966: 735–759.

7. Glass AJ. Lessons learned. In: Glass AJ, ed. *Overseas Theaters*. Vol 2. In: *Neuropsychiatry in World War II*. Washington, DC: Office of The Surgeon General, US Army; 1973: 989–1027.

8. Belenky GL, Tyner CF, Sodetz FJ. *Israeli Battle Shock Casualties: 1973 and 1982*. Report WRAIR NP-83-4. Washington, DC: Walter Reed Army Institute of Research; Defense Technical Information Center Document ADA133359; 1983.

9. Menninger WC. *Psychiatry in a Troubled World*. New York: McMillan; 1948: 10–12.

10. Pratt D. Combat record of psychoneurotic patients. *Bull US Army Med Dept*. 1947;7:809–811.

11. McAllister B. 1990. Disadvantaged veterans gain little in military, study finds. *The Washington Post*, 24 February 1990, pp. A1, A10.

12. Belenky GL, Kaufman LW. Cohesion and rigorous training: Observations of the Air Assault School. *Milit Rev*. 1983;63:24–34.

13. Drayer CS, Glass AJ. Introduction. In Glass AJ, ed. *Overseas Theatres*. Vol 2. In *Neuropsychiatry in World War II*. Washington, DC: Medical Department, US Army, Office of The Surgeon General and Center of Military History; 1973: 1–23.

14. Rumbaugh J. Personal Communication, 1985.

15. Gal R. Unit morale: From a theoretical puzzle to an empirical illustration—an Israeli example. *J Appl Soc Psychol*. 1986;16(6):549–564.

16. Gillman B. 1992. Clinton says he'll "consult" on allowing gays in military. *The Washington Post*. 13 November 1992: A1, A11.

17. Schwartzkopf HN. 1992. During interview by Diane Rehm on Public Broadcasting Service, 1 October 1992.

18. Masserman JH. Faith and delusion in psychotherapy: The Ur-defenses of man. *Am J Psychiatry*. 1953;110:324–333.

19. Shaw JA. Psychodynamic considerations in the adaptation to combat. In: Belenky GL, ed. *Contemporary Studies in Combat Psychiatry*. New York: Greenwood; 1987: 117–132.

20. Calhoun JT. Nostalgia as a disease of field service. *Med Surg Rept*. 1864;11:130–132.

21. Solomon Z, Prager E. Elderly Israeli holocaust survivors during the Persian Gulf War: A study of psychological distress. *Am J Psychiatry*. 1992;149(12):1707–1710.

22. Sobel R. Anxiety-depressive reactions after prolonged combat experience: The "old sergeant syndrome." Supplement on Combat Psychiatry. *Bull US Army Med Dept.* 1949;9:137–146.

23. Marks IN. Behavioral psychotherapy. *Am J Psychiatry.* 1976;133(3):260.

24. Tiffany W, Allerton W. Army psychiatry in the mid-60's. *Am J Psychiatry.* 1967;123:810–819.

25. Jenkins BM. *The Lessons of Beirut: Testimony Before the Long Commission.* Santa Monica, Calif: Rand Corporation; 1984.

26. Glass AJ. Psychiatry in the Korean campaign (installment 1). *US Armed Forces Med J.* 1953;4:1387–1401.

27. Kirkland FR. Personal Communication, July 1991.

28. Glass AJ. Personal Communication, January 1982.

29. Jones FD, Johnson AW. Medical and psychiatric treatment policy and practice in Vietnam. *J Soc Issues.* 1975;31(4):49–65.

30. Renner JA. The changing patterns of psychiatric problems in Vietnam. *Comprehensive Psychiatry.* 1973;14(2):169–180.

31. Jones FD. Combat stress: Tripartite model. *Int Rev Army Navy Air Force Med Serv.* 1982;55:247–254.

32. Jones FD. Psychiatric lessons of low-intensity wars. *Ann Med Milit Fenn* [Finland]. 1985;60(4):128–134.

33. Rosen G. Nostalgia: A "forgotten" psychological disorder. *Psychol Med.* 1975;5:340–354.

34. Jones FD. Reactions to stress: Combat vs combat-support psychiatric casualties. Presented at 6th World Congress of Psychiatry; August 28–September 3, 1977; Honolulu, Hawaii.

35. Kalinowsky LB. War and post-war neuroses in Germany. *Med Bull US Army, Europe.* 1980; 7(3):23–29.

36. Gabriel RA. *No More Heroes: Madness and Psychiatry in War.* New York: Hill and Wang; 1987.

ACKNOWLEDGEMENTS

A book of this nature is indebted to numerous students of and contributors to the study of man's adaptation to war. Lieutenant General Charles Pixley, then the Surgeon General of the U.S. Army, assigned the author and first editor (FDJ) to Walter Reed Army Institute of Research (WRAIR) in 1981, and his successors, Lieutenant General Bernhard Mittemeyer, Lieutenant General Quinn Becker, Lieutenant General Frank Ledford, and Lieutenant General Alcide LaNoue continued the assignments, making the undertaking and development of the project possible. Brigadier General (then Colonel) Russ Zajtchuk approached the editors in 1989 to request modification of the manuscript to enable the project to become part of the Textbook of Military Medicine series. Donald Jenkins, Ph.D., of the Borden Institute, guided the early efforts. His successor, Colonel Ronald Bellamy, M.D., saw the project to its completion.

The members of the Combat Stress Work Group (1981–1983) in the Department of Military Psychiatry at WRAIR provided an atmosphere of inquiry and intellectual ferment. This group included many distinguished foreign visitors (Colonel Pinchas Harris, Lieutenant Colonel Shabtai Noi, and Colonel Reuven Gal, Ph.D., Israel; Lieutenant Colonel Stanislav Nikic, M.D., Yugoslavia; Colonel Carlos Collazo, M.D., Argentina; Brigadier General Olukayode Adelaja, M.D. and Major Bgenga Okulate, M.D., Nigeria; General Louis Crocq, M.D., France; Lieutenant Colonel Yeng Hoi Fong, M.D., Chief Medical Officer, Singapore Armed Forces; and others). Also contributing were former WRAIR members (the late Colonel Albert Julius Glass, M.D.; the late David McK. Rioch, M.D.; Edwin Weinstein, M.D.; Colonel Frederick Tyner, M.D.; Colonel Frederick Manning, Ph.D.; and Colonel Norman H. Camp, M.D.), and current members of WRAIR (Colonel Gregory Belenky, M.D.; Fred Hegge, Ph.D.; and many others). Special thanks are given for the contributions of the late William Datel, Ph.D., of WRAIR. Many of the ideas presented are distilled from their knowledge and experience.

We are particularly indebted to David Marlowe, Ph.D., Chief, Department of Military Psychiatry, WRAIR, for providing support through the many years of this project. He shared with us numerous educational experiences, not the least of which were his own spirited exegeses of complex material, and also reviewed some of the productions. In a similar vein, Colonel Frederick Manning, Ph.D.; Lieutenant Colonel (Ret) Faris Kirkland, Ph.D.; and Colonel Larry Ingraham, Ph.D. applied their considerable analytical skills to the material.

We were fortunate to have the assistance of Colonel Robert Gifford, Ph.D., and Major Elias Nimmer, Ph.D., who provided us with superb administrative support necessary to keep the project viable. We also owe thanks to the many individuals who reviewed drafts, suggested resource materials, and, in general, gave us the support necessary to complete this project: Colonel David Armitage, M.D.; Colonel (Ret) Kenneth Artiss, M.D.; Colonel (Ret) Mike Bain, M.D.; Colonel (Ret) Stewart Baker, M.D.; Doug Bey, M.D.; Colonel James Collins, M.D.; Colonel (Ret) Manuel Febo, M.D.; Don Ferguson, Ph.D.; Colonel Richard Fragala, M.D.; Lieutenant Colonel (Ret) Terry Fullerton, Ph.D.; Colonel (Ret) Harry Holloway, M.D.; Colonel (Ret) Steve Hursh, Ph.D.; Colonel (Ret) Craig Llewellyn, M.D.; Colonel (Ret) Matt Parrish, M.D.; Colonel Norman Ream, M.D.; Major E. Cameron Ritchie, M.D.; the late Major General James Rumbaugh, M.D.; and Captain (Ret) Robert Strange, M.D. We also wish to thank Mrs. Ann Robinson for her clerical assistance, Mr. Rich Howard for his assistance in locating library materials, and Mr. Verne Schwartz of the U.S. Army Center for Military History for his assistance with locating the artwork featured in this volume. And finally, thanks to those who provided graphics support for the project: Charles Hoover, Joe Fritz, and Helen Sing.

Despite the debt owed to these colleagues, the authors and editors are solely responsible for any erroneous interpretation or misuse of data. We hope that the fruit of these labors is a document that is both lucid and fluent.

—The Specialty Editors

ACRONYMS AND ABBREVIATIONS

A

AA: Alcoholics Anonymous
AA: anterograde amnesia
AAD: after-action debriefing
AAR: after-action review
AEF: American Expeditionary Forces
AIDS: acquired immunodeficiency syndrome
AMA: American Medical Association
AMEDD: Army Medical Department
AMTRAC: amphibious transport craft
APC: armored personnel carrier
ARCENT: U.S. Army Central Command
ARMA: Adaptability Rating for Military Aviation
ATH: air transportable hospital
ATLS: advanced trauma life support
AWACS: Airborne Warning and Control System
AWOL: absent without leave

B

BAS: battalion aid station
BBB: blood-brain barrier
BDZ: benzodiazepine
BFB: basal forebrain
BFC: battle fatigue center
BI & W: battle injury and wounding
BICEPS: brevity, immediacy, centrality, expectancy, proximity, simplicity
BUMED: Bureau of Medicine and Surgery
BZ: 3-quinuclidinyl benzilate

C

66C: psychiatric nurse
66C7T: clinical nurse specialist
C^3I: command, control, communications, and intelligence
CA: Cocaine Anonymous
CACO: casualty assistance calls officer
CATF: Commander, Amphibious Task Force
CCI: civilian critical incidents
CED: critical event debriefing
CES(D): Center for Epidemiological Studies (Depression)
CHI: closed head injury
CIA: Central Intelligence Agency
CIB: Combat Infantryman Badge
CINCLANTFLT: Commander in chief, U.S. Atlantic Fleet
CINCPACFLT: Commander in Chief, U.S. Pacific Fleet
CISD: critical incident stress debriefing
CLF: Commander, Land Forces
CMC: Commandant of the Marine Corps
CMHS: Community Mental Health Services
CMTC: Combat Maneuver Training Center
CNO: Chief of Naval Operations
CNS: central nervous system
CO: commanding officer
COHORT: cohesion, operational readiness, training
COMMZ: communications zone
CONUS: continental United States
CQ: charge-of-quarters
CSC: combat stress control
CSCP: combat stress control preventive
CSH: combat support hospital
CSR: combat stress reaction
CSS: combat service support
CSU: combat stress unit
CT: computed tomography

D

D: depression scale on the Minnesota Multiphasic Personality Inventory
DA: Department of the Army
DAI: diffuse axonal injury
DBMS: Director of Base Medical Services
DDD: dependency, debility, and dread
DEPMEDS: deployable medical systems
DEROS: date of expected return from overseas station
DNBI: disease/nonbattle injury
DON: Department of the Navy
DPICM: dual purpose improved conventional munition
DPTSD: delayed post-traumatic stress disorder
DSM-I: Diagnostic and Statistical Manual, 1st ed
DSM-II: Diagnostic and Statistical Manual, 2nd ed
DSM-III: Diagnostic and Statistical Manual, 3rd ed
DSM-III-R: Diagnostic and Statistical Manual, 3rd ed rev
DSM-IV: Diagnostic and Statistical Manual, 4th ed

E

1-E: first echelon
2-E: second echelon
3-E: third echelon
4-E: fourth echelon
ECT: electroconvulsive therapy
EDRF: endothelium-derived relaxing factor
EEG: electroencephalogram
EMP: electromagnetic pulse
EOD: explosive ordnance disposal
EOTD: end-of-tour debriefing
ETO: European Theater of Operations

F

91F: psychiatric specialist
FAC: forward air controllers
FBI: Federal Bureau of Investigation
FDC: fire direction center
FEMA: Federal Emergency Management Agency
fMRI: fast magnetic resonance imaging
FSSG: Force Service Support Group

G

91G: behavioral science specialist
G-1: Assistant Chief of Staff (Personnel)
G-4: Assistant Chief of Staff (Logistics)
Ga: Tabun
GABA: γ-aminobutyric acid
Gb: Sarin
Gd: Soman

GGT: gamma-glutamyltranferase
GOAT: Galveston Orientation and Amnesia Test
GP: general purpose

H

HERD: Historical Event Reconstruction Debriefing
HIP: high-induction profile
HIV: human immunodeficiency virus
HMMWV: high mobility multipurpose wheeled vehicle
HQ: headquarters
Hs: hysteria scale on the Minnesota Multiphasic Personality Inventory
Hy: hypochondriasis scale on the Minnesota Multiphasic Personality Inventory

I

ICBM: intercontinental ballistic missile
ICD-9: Manual of International Statistical Classification of Diseases, Injuries, and Causes of Death
IDF: Israeli Defence Forces
IFV: infantry fighting vehicle
IQ: intelligence quotient
IRR: Individual Ready Reserve
IV: intravenous

J

JRTC: Joint Readiness Training Center
JTF: Joint Task Force

K

KIA: killed in action
KO: mobile psychiatric detachment
KZ: concentration camp syndrome

L

91L: occupational therapy specialist
LCC: Amphibious Command Ships [landing ships, command, communication]
LHA: landing ship, helicopter, assault
LKA: Amphibious Cargo Ships [landing ships, cargo, amphibious]
LPH: landing ship, platform, helicopter
LRRP: long-range reconnaissance patrol
LSD: Dock Landing Ships [landing ships, dock]
LST: Tank Landing Ships [landing ships, tank]

M

I MEF: I Marine Expeditionary Force
II MEF: II Marine Expeditionary Force
III MEF: III Marine Expeditionary Force
MAO: monoamine oxidase
MAOI: monoamine oxidase inhibitors
MARFORLANT: U.S. Marine Corps Forces Atlantic
MARFORPAC: U.S. Marine Corps Forces Pacific
MASF: mobile aeromedical staging facility
MASH: Mobile Army Surgical Hospital
MCV: mean corpuscular volume
MEB: Marine Expeditionary Brigade
MEB: medical evaluation board
MEDCAP: medical civic action program
MEDDAC: Medical Department activity
MEDIC: computer-based patient management system for isolated environments
MEF: Marine Expeditionary Force
MEU: Marine Expeditionary Unit
MF2K: Medical Force 2000
MH/CSC: mental health/combat stress control
MHCS: Mental Hygiene Consultation Service
MIA: missing in action
MILES: multiple integrated laser engagement system
MLRS: multiple launch rocket system
MMART: Mobile Medical Augmentation Readiness Teams
MMPI: Minnesota Multiphasic Personality Inventory
MOOTW: military operations other than war
MOPP: mission-oriented protective posture
MOS: military occupational specialty
MP: military police
MRE: meal-ready-to-eat
MRI: magnetic resonance imaging
MTO: Mediterranean Theater of Operations

N

NA: Narcotics Anonymous
NATO: North Atlantic Treaty Organization
NBC: nuclear, biological, and chemical
NCO: noncommissioned officer
NCOIC: noncommissioned officer in charge
NFT: neurofibrillary tangles
NP: neuropsychiatry
NSAID: nonsteroidal antiinflammatory drug
NTC: National Training Center
NUMI: Naval Undersea Medical Institute
NVVRS: National Vietnam Veterans Readjustment Study
NYD (nervous): not yet diagnosed (nervous)

O

O & M: orientation and mobilization
OD: right eye
OJC: Operation Just Cause
OM: psychiatric detachment team
OOTW: operation other than war
OT: occupational therapist

P

PA: physician assistant
PCRTS: primary casualty receiving treatment ships
Pd: psychopathic deviance scale on the Minnesota Multiphasic Personality Inventory
PDF: Panamanian Defense Force
PET: positron emission tomography
PFC: private first class
PHI: penetrating head injury
PIE: proximity, immediacy, and expectancy
PIES: proximity, immediacy, expectancy, simplicity
POMCUS: pre-positioned overseas material configured unit sets
POW: prisoner of war
PROFIS: Professional Officer Filler Sytem
PSYOPS: psychological operations
PT : physical training
Pt: psychasthenia scale on the Minnesota Multiphasic Personality Inventory
PTA: post-traumatic amnesia
PTSD: post-traumatic stress disorder
PX: post exchange

R

R and R: rest and recreation
RA: retrograde amnesia
RAF: Royal Air Force
RDC: Research Diagnostic Criteria
REM: rapid eye movement
REMF: rear-echelon mother f—er
RF-LAN: radio-frequency, local area network
RIMA: reversible inhibitor of monoamine oxidase-A
RTDTD: return to duty to die

S

1SG: first sergeant
SAC: Strategic Air Command
SAP: Specialty Advisor for Psychiatry
Sc: schizophrenia scale on the Minnesota Multiphasic Personality Inventory
SCI: spinal cord injury
SCRTS: secondary casualty receiving treatment ships
SEALS: SEa Air Land commandoS
SECNAV: Secretary of the Navy
SFC: sergeant first class
SGOT: serum glutamic-oxalocetic transaminase
SGPT: serum glutamic-pyruvic transaminase
SIW: self-inflicted wounds
SOD: superoxide dismutase
SOF: special operations forces
SOP: standing operating procedure
SP4: specialist 4th class
SPRINT: special psychiatric rapid intervention team
SSC: Surgical Support Companies
SSRI: selective serotonin reuptake inhibitors

T

T&R: training and rehabilitation
TAB: TMB-4 [an oxime], atropine, and benactyzine
TBI: traumatic brain injury
TBS: total body surface
TCA: tricyclic antidepressant
TEMPER: tent, extendable, modular, personnel
TENS: transcutaneous electrical nerve stimulation
TGA: transient global amnesia
TO&E: Table of Organization and Equipment
TOC: tactical operations center
TSOP: tactical standing operating procedure

U

UCMJ: Uniform Code of Military Justice
USAFE: U.S. Air Force, Europe
USARV: U.S. Army Vietnam

V

VA: Veterans Administration (since 1985, Department of Veterans Affairs)
VC: Viet Cong
VD: venereal disease
VEVAS: Vietnam-Era Veterans Adjustment Survey
VR: virtual reality

W

WIA: wounded in action
WRAIR: Walter Reed Army Institute of Research
WSO: weapons systems operator

INDEX

A

E

F

G

H

I

J

K

L

M

N

O

P

R

T

U